# Injectable Drugs Guide

# *Injectable Drugs Guide* on MedicinesComplete

As well as being available as a print version the *Injectable Drugs Guide* is also available to access on-line via MedicinesComplete. Updates will be placed on the electronic version periodically in between new editions of the printed version being released.

MedicinesComplete provides immediate access to up-to-date drug information sourced from an extensive range of the world's most trusted resources. Intuitive, flexible and cost-effective, MedicinesComplete is the definitive solution empowering informed, safe and fast decisions. Contact sales@medicinescomplete.com for further information, trials and details of our subscription based pricing.

# Injectable Drugs Guide

## Alistair Gray
BSc(Hons) MRPharmS DipClinPharm
Clinical Services Lead Pharmacist
East Lancashire Hospitals NHS Trust, UK

## Jane Wright
BSc(Hons) MRPharmS DipClinPharm
Lead Pharmacist
Lancashire Care NHS Foundation Trust, UK

## Vincent Goodey
BSc(Hons) MRPharmS MSc
Deputy Director of Pharmacy
East Lancashire Hospitals NHS Trust, UK

## Lynn Bruce
BSc MRPharmS DipClinPharm
Pharmacy Team Leader
Medical Assessment Unit, Royal Blackburn Hospital
East Lancashire Hospitals NHS Trust, UK

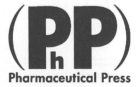

London • Chicago  **Pharmaceutical Press**

**Published by Pharmaceutical Press**

1 Lambeth High Street, London SE1 7JN, UK
1559 St Paul Avenue, Gurnee, IL 60031, USA

© Royal Pharmaceutical Society of Great Britain 2011

(**PhP**) is a trade mark of Pharmaceutical Press

Pharmaceutical Press is the publishing division of the Royal Pharmaceutical Society

First published 2011

Typeset by Thomson Digital, Noida, India
Printed in Great Britain by TJ International, Padstow, Cornwall

ISBN 978 0 85369 787 9

A catalogue record for this book is available from the British Library.

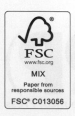

FSC
www.fsc.org
MIX
Paper from
responsible sources
FSC® C013056

# Contents

# Preface

The *Injectable Drugs Guide* provides a user-friendly, single point of reference for health-care professionals in the prescribing, preparation, administration and monitoring of injectable medicines.

The idea for such a book grew out from some of the entries in our sister book *Clinical Pharmacy Pocket Companion*, which, as well as covering many clinical topics such as electrolyte disturbances and perioperative management of medicines, also deals with a number of medicines requiring therapeutic monitoring. It became apparent that the benefits of such an approach could be rolled out to a greater number of medicines. At around the same time the UK National Patient Safety Agency issued a patient safety alert entitled 'Promoting safer use of injectable medicines' (NPSA/2007/20). This requires organisations to risk assess individual parenteral drugs and put procedures in place to allow them to be handled more safely.

The *Injectable Drugs Guide* is a handbook supporting the risk assessment process (each drug has a risk rating). It also provides a holistic approach to injectable medicines to meet the needs of the many disciplines involved in the clinical use of injectables and also those providing advice about injectable drug use.

The book comprises primarily individual drug monographs. There are a number of appendices giving further guidance on specific aspects of injectable therapy and additional clinical information (the full list of these is found on the Contents page).

In the main, cancer chemotherapy agents are not covered in the monographs. This is because there are tight controls around the use of these agents in clinical practice. Their handling in clinical settings is highly protocol driven and locality specific; use by inexperienced individuals is inappropriate.

Alistair Gray
Jane Wright
Vince Goodey
Lynn Bruce
November 2010

Each monograph is presented in a format that sequences the information as needed by healthcare professionals from *contemplation* of treatment, through preparation and administration, to the monitoring that may be required during and after therapy. Monographs are generally presented in the following order:

**Drug name and form(s)** of the preparation(s)

**Background information** about each medicine including,
* Type of drug
* What it is used to treat (licensed and unlicensed indications and routes)
* Additional miscellany of interest to the user
* If appropriate, how doses of the drug are usually expressed

**Pre-treatment checks** including,
* Contraindications and cautions to be considered prior to use
* Any measures and/or tests that should be undertaken before commencing therapy. In some cases these tests are mandatory; in others they are dependent on the circumstances in which the drug is being used. These are listed alphabetically.
* Pregnancy and breast-feeding information has not been included except in a few special cases (standard reference sources or the advice of a Medicines Information department should be sought if this information is needed).

**Dose** including indication-specific information and any adjustments required in renal or hepatic impairment. Unless otherwise stated, doses are for adults (child and neonatal doses have not been included).

**Routes of administration**
* A series of headings outline the route(s) by which a particular drug may be given; the specifics of preparation and administration are provided for each route. In some cases the individual heading indicates the circumstances in which a particular route is appropriate.
* For drugs given by infusion, most monographs specify the quantity of infusion fluid to use. However, some monographs use the phrase 'dilute in a suitable volume of compatible infusion fluid'. In this case the prescriber should choose a volume and fluid that is appropriate to the patient's needs and clinical condition (compatibility data are given further down the monograph in the Technical Information table).

**Technical information** includes details of:

* **Incompatibilities** with fluids, other drugs by Y-site administration and also some-times with materials
* **Compatibilities** with infusion fluids and also drugs where co-administration and concentrations are likely to be used in practice. Drugs for which compatibility is concentration-specific are *not* included in this list. More detailed sources such as Trissel[1] should be used to clarify these.
* **pH**, particularly for drugs which are given intravenously
* **Sodium content** is stated if it is ≥1 mmol per likely dose; information about other significant electrolytes is given where appropriate
* **Osmolarity** for the most significantly hyperosmolar products
* **Excipients** where allergy is a possibility or where these could have significant side-effects in certain individuals
* **Storage conditions** advised for long-term and in-use storage plus, in some cases details on the significance of any change in appearance
* **Displacement value** for dry powder products
* **Special handling and management of spillage** information if appropriate
* **Stability after preparation information.** This is *not* provided so that infusions can be prepared significantly prior to use in a clinical area, but rather to indicate how long a preparation is stable if it is not possible to administer it immediately. Stability information is also provided for reconstituted multidose vials.

**Monitoring** includes the measures required to ensure the medicine is used safely throughout therapy, the clinical outcome and other parameters that need consideration, e.g. certain adverse effects. The frequency of monitoring of each parameter is stated and the rationale for monitoring. In some cases the frequency is precise, e.g. 'daily', in others the frequency is not clearly defined in the literature and an individual clinician will need to decide what is reasonable. In these cases the term 'periodically' has been used.

**Additional information** includes

**Common and serious undesirable effects including:**

* **Immediate adverse reactions** or those that may occur shortly after administration
* **Injection- or infusion-related** adverse events, either due to rapid administration or those which are injection-site related
* **Other adverse reactions**

**Pharmacokinetics** in the main provides an indication of the elimination half-life of the drug, which can be useful in determining duration of effect. Some monographs provide information on other pharmacokinetic or pharmacodynamic parameters where these might be helpful.

**Significant interactions** drugs are grouped together under subheadings to give an indication of likely effect of the interaction. These lists are not comprehensive and more detailed sources such as *Stockley's Drug Interactions*[2] should be used if required.

**Action in case of overdose** gives guidance on managing *therapeutic* overdose of the drug and in most cases lists general supportive measures required. For the management of significant overdose an on-line source such as Toxbase[3] should always be consulted.

**Counselling** points are intended to provide a prompt for healthcare professionals as they speak to patients about their therapy.

**Risk rating.** Each medicine has been risk-assessed, considering the worst case scenario, to provide an overall risk rating based on the NPSA tool for risk assessment of individual injectable medicine products prepared in clinical areas.[4] The assessment is displayed pictorially with icons and as a risk score. See Appendix 11 for more information on the risk rating used.

**References.** In general the main reference source used to assemble the information has been the manufacturer's product literature (in the UK this is the Summary of Product Characteristics or SPC) and MedicinesComplete (see below). In the main, SPCs mentioned can be accessed on-line at http://www.medicines.org.uk/EMC/. To save space references have not been included if information has been sourced from MedicinesComplete, although the SPCs used have been stated for clarity. Any other reference source used is stated in the normal way using the Vancouver system of referencing.

## References

1. Trissel L, ed. *Handbook on Injectable Drugs*, 14th edn. Bethesda, MD: American Society of Health-System Pharmacists, 2007 (accessible via MedicinesComplete).
2. Baxter K, ed. *Stockley's Drug Interactions 9* (accessible via MedicinesComplete).
3. Toxbase accessible at http://www.toxbase.org.
4. National Patient Safety Agency. *Promoting safer use of injectable medicines* (NPSA/2007/20) (accessible at www.npsa.nhs.uk/health/alerts).

# Feedback

Feedback on any aspect of the book would be welcome via the e-mail address pharmpresseditorial@rpharms.com.

# About the authors

**Lynn Bruce** studied pharmacy at Aston University. The first 20 years of her working life were based in secondary care variously as MI pharmacist, clinical pharmacy lead, clinical economist and latterly in various management positions. She migrated across the divide to primary care in 1997 becoming PCG and then PCT prescribing advisor. Hospital clinical pharmacy beckoned her back to secondary care in 2002: she is now Pharmacy Team Leader on the Medical Assessment Unit at the Royal Blackburn Hospital.

Lynn is married and, when she's not writing pharmacy books, loves studying wildlife and travelling and is addicted to puzzles of all types.

**Vince Goodey** graduated in 1985 from the London School of Pharmacy, and has since worked primarily in the hospital sector in clinical and managerial roles. As a postgraduate Vince studied at the University of Manchester to attain an MSc in Pharmacy Practice in 1996.

Although hailing originally from Essex, Vince is currently Deputy Director of Pharmacy at East Lancashire Hospitals NHS Trust.

**Alistair Gray** is from Sunderland. He studied pharmacy at Sunderland Polytechnic, graduating in 1988 with first-class honours, and then completed his pre-registration year with Boots in Newcastle-upon-Tyne. He continued working for Boots in a variety of pharmacy and store management positions in the North West of England. In 2002 he changed disciplines and became Community Services pharmacist at Queens Park Hospital in Blackburn. He completed a Diploma in Clinical & Health Services Pharmacy at the University of Manchester in 2008 and subsequently became Clinical Services Lead Pharmacist for East Lancashire Hospitals NHS Trust in 2009 based at the now re-named Royal Blackburn Hospital.

Alistair is married with two children and loves spending time with his family. He follows Formula One motor racing closely, enjoys reading, eating out, going to the movies, playing guitar and songwriting.

**Jane Wright**, after working for 18 years in the Civil Service, attended the University of Manchester to study pharmacy. Jane graduated in 1994 and did her pre-registration year at the Royal Preston Hospital. For the next ten years Jane worked in Blackburn hospitals in a variety of clinical roles, her last being Clinical Services Manager with responsibility for education and training. In 1999 she obtained a Diploma in Clinical & Health Services Pharmacy at the University of Manchester. She moved to Lancashire Care NHS Foundation Trust in April 2005 where she is currently employed as Lead Pharmacist for East Lancashire.

Jane is married and in her spare time enjoys playing with Molly and Polly (two very lively dogs).

# Contributors

**Catherine Strong** MRPharmS DipClinPharm, Lead Clinical Pharmacist (acute medicine) based at Fairfield General Hospital (The Pennine Acute Hospitals NHS Trust), Bury, UK.

**Katy Hand** BSc(Hons) MRPharmS MSc in Clinical Pharmacy, Critical Care Pharmacist, Southampton General Hospital, Southampton, UK.

**Kevin Johnson** MRPharmS DipClinPharm, Medical Admissions Unit Pharmacist, Royal Blackburn Hospital, Blackburn, UK.

**Joanna Wallett** MRPharmS DipClinPharm, Senior Clinical Pharmacist, East Lancashire Hospitals NHS Trust, Royal Blackburn Hospital, Blackburn, UK.

# Acknowledgements

All the authors would like to thank Cat, Katie, Joanna and Kevin (our contributors) for all their time, expertise and patience.

The advice and assistance provided by Sue Keeling and the pharmacy department of the Imperial College Healthcare NHS Trust and the pharmacy departments of Epsom and St Helier University Hospitals NHS Trust in producing the guidelines in the appendices is gratefully acknowledged.

The advice and assistance provided by the National Extravasation Information Service in producing Appendix 6 is gratefully acknowledged. Thanks also to Bruce Burnett who put the original draft of Appendix 6 and Appendix 7 together for the *Clinical Pharmacy Pocket Companion*.

We would like to acknowledge our respective employers: East Lancashire Hospitals NHS Trust and Lancashire Care NHS Foundation Trust.

Alistair thanks Rachel, Amelia and Imogen for all their support throughout the creation of this publication. It took just a little bit longer than expected!

Jane thanks Steve for his tolerance, and apologies to Molly and Polly for all the missed walkies opportunities.

Lynn thanks John for scraping her off the ceiling during moments of stress.

Vince thanks Joanne and Josh for their support and Marm for all her well-intentioned but aberrant key padding.

Finally we would like to thank everyone at the Pharmaceutical Press who has had a hand in this publication, particularly Christina De Bono, Louise McIndoe, Rebecca Perry and Linda Paulus.

# Abbreviations

| | |
|---|---|
| ↑ | increased, raised or hyper- (as in ↑K = hyperkalaemia) |
| ↓ | decreased or hypo- (as in ↓K = hypokalaemia) |
| ABGs | arterial blood gases |
| ABW | actual bodyweight |
| ACE | angiotensin-converting enzyme |
| ACS | acute coronary syndromes |
| ACT | activated clotting time |
| ACTH | adrenocorticotrophic hormone, corticotrophin |
| ADH | anti-diuretic hormone; vasopressin |
| ADR | adverse drug reaction |
| AF | atrial fibrillation |
| AIDS | acquired immune deficiency syndrome |
| Alk Phos | alkaline phosphatase |
| ALT | alanine transaminase (alanine aminotransferase) |
| AML | acute myeloid leukaemia |
| ANC | absolute neutrophil count |
| ANTT | aseptic non-touch technique |
| APTT | activated partial thromboplastin time |
| ARDS | adult respiratory distress syndrome |
| AST | aspartate transaminase (aspartate aminotransferase) |
| AUC | area under the curve |
| AV | atrioventricular |
| AZT | azidothymidine (zidovudine) |
| BAL | British anti-Lewisite (dimercaprol) |
| BCG | Bacillus Calmette–Guérin |
| BMD | bone mineral density |
| BP | blood pressure |
| bpm | beats per minute |
| Ca | calcium |
| CABG | coronary artery bypass graft |
| CAPD | continuous ambulatory peritoneal dialysis |
| L-carnitine | levocarnitine |
| CCPD | continuous cyclic peritoneal dialysis |
| CHM | Commission on Human Medicines |
| CHMP | Committee for Medicinal Products for Human Use |
| CIVAS | Centralised Intravenous Additive Service |
| CK | creatine kinase, creatine phosphokinase, CPK |
| CKD | chronic kidney disease |

| | |
|---|---|
| Cl | chloride |
| CMV | cytomegalovirus |
| CNS | central nervous system |
| $CO_2$ | carbon dioxide |
| COPD | chronic obstructive pulmonary disease |
| CPR | cardiopulmonary resuscitation |
| Cr | creatinine |
| CrCl | creatinine clearance |
| CRP | C-reactive protein |
| CSF | cerebrospinal fluid |
| CSII | continuous subcutaneous insulin infusion |
| CSM | Committee on Safety of Medicines |
| cSSTI | complicated skin and soft-tissue infections |
| CTZ | chemoreceptor trigger zone |
| CVA | cerebrovascular accident |
| CVP | central venous pressure |
| DAFNE | dose adjustment for normal eating |
| DAS | disease activity score |
| DIC | disseminated intravascular coagulation |
| DKA | diabetic ketoacidosis |
| DMARDs | disease-modifying anti-rheumatic drugs |
| DVT | deep vein thrombosis |
| ECG | electrocardiogram |
| ECT | electroconvulsive therapy |
| EFAD | essential fatty acid deficiency |
| eGFR | estimated glomerular filtration rate |
| EMD | electromechanical dissociation |
| EPSE | extrapyramidal side-effects (e.g. muscle shakes and tremor) |
| ESR | erythrocyte sedimentation rate |
| FBC | full blood count |
| FU | fluorouracil |
| G6PD | glucose-6-phosphate dehydrogenase |
| GCS | Glasgow Coma Scale |
| G-CSF | granulocyte colony-stimulating factor |
| GFR | glomerular filtration rate |
| GGT | gamma-glutamyl transpeptidase |
| GH | growth hormone |
| GI | gastrointestinal |
| Gluc | glucose |
| GORD | gastro-oesophageal reflux disease |
| GP | glycoprotein |
| GVHD | graft-versus-host disease |
| HACA | human anti-chimeric antibody |
| Hartmann's | Sodium lactate intravenous infusion, compound |
| Hb | haemoglobin |
| HbA1c | glycosylated (glycated) haemoglobin |
| HBV | hepatitis B virus |
| HCG | human chorionic gonadotrophin |
| $HCO_3$ | bicarbonate |
| HDL | high-density lipoprotein |
| HHS | hyperosmolar hyperglycaemic state (formerly HONS or HONK) |
| HIPAA | heparin-induced platelet activation assay |

| | |
|---|---|
| HIT | heparin-induced thrombocytopenia |
| HIV | human immunodeficiency virus |
| HRT | hormone replacement therapy |
| HSCT | haematopoietic stem cell transplantation |
| HSV | herpes simplex virus |
| IBW | ideal bodyweight (see Appendix 10 for calculation) |
| IgE | immunoglobulin E |
| IGF | insulin-like growth factor |
| IgG | immunoglobulin G |
| IHD | ischaemic heart disease |
| IM | intramuscular |
| INR | international normalised ratio |
| IV | intravenous |
| JVP | jugular venous pressure |
| K | potassium |
| KCl | potassium chloride |
| KGF | human keratinocyte growth factor |
| LDL | low-density lipoprotein |
| LFTs | liver function tests |
| LHRH | luteinising hormone releasing hormone |
| LMWH | low-molecular-weight heparin |
| LRTI | lower respiratory tract infection |
| LVEF | left-ventricular ejection fraction |
| LVF | left ventricular failure |
| MAOI | monoamine oxidase inhibitor |
| MCV | mean cell volume |
| Mg | magnesium |
| MHRA | Medicines and Healthcare products Regulatory Agency |
| MI | myocardial infarction |
| MIC | minimum inhibitory concentration |
| min | minute |
| mmHg | millimetres of mercury (used in blood pressure readings) |
| MRSA | methicillin-resistant *Staphylococcus aureus* |
| Na | sodium |
| NaCl | sodium chloride |
| NBM | nil by mouth |
| NG | nasogastric |
| NICE | National Institute for Health and Clinical Excellence |
| NIHSS | NIH Stroke Scale |
| NMS | neuroleptic malignant syndrome e.g. hyperthermia, muscle rigidity & altered consciousness |
| NPIS | National Poisons Information Service (tel: 0844 892 0111) |
| NPSA | National Patient Safety Agency |
| NQMI | non-Q wave myocardial infarction |
| NRTI | nucleoside reverse transcriptase inhibitor |
| NSAID | non-steroidal anti-inflammatory drug |
| NSTEMI | non ST-segment elevation myocardial infarction |
| NYHA | New York Heart Association |
| $O_2$ | oxygen |
| OHSS | ovarian hyperstimulation syndrome |
| PA | tissue plasminogen activator |
| PBPC | peripheral blood progenitor cell |

| | |
|---|---|
| PCA | patient-controlled analgesia |
| PCI | percutaneous coronary intervention |
| PCV | packed cell volume |
| PE | pulmonary embolism |
| PE | phenytoin sodium equivalents *(only in the Fosphenytoin monograph)* |
| PEA | pulseless electrical activity |
| PICC | peripherally inserted central intravenous catheter |
| PML | progressive multifocal leucoencephalopathy |
| PN | parenteral nutrition |
| $PO_4$ | phosphate |
| PONV | postoperative nausea and vomiting |
| PPH | primary pulmonary hypertension |
| PPI | proton pump inhibitor |
| PRCA | pure red cell aplasia |
| PSA | prostate-specific antigen |
| PT | prothrombin time |
| PTH | parathyroid hormone |
| PVC | poly(vinyl chloride) |
| r-DNA | recombinant DNS |
| RIE | right-sided infective endocarditis |
| Ringer's | Ringer's solution for injection |
| SA | sinoatrial |
| SBECD | sulfobutylether beta cyclodextrin sodium |
| SC | subcutaneous |
| SIADH | syndrome of inappropriate ADH secretion |
| SLE | systemic lupus erythematosus |
| SPC | summary of product characteristics |
| STEMI | ST-segment elevation myocardial infarction |
| SVT | supraventricular tachycardia |
| $T_3$ | tri-iodothyronine; liothyronine |
| $T_4$ | tetra-iodothyronine; levothyroxine |
| TFTs | thyroid function tests |
| TIA | transient ischaemic attack |
| TIH | tumour-induced hypercalcaemia |
| TIVAD | totally implantable venous access device |
| TNF | tumour necrosis factor |
| TPN | total parenteral nutrition |
| TRH | thyrotrophin-releasing hormone |
| TSH | thyroid-stimulating hormone, thyrotrophin |
| U | urea |
| UA | unstable angina |
| U&Es | urea and electrolytes |
| UFH | unfractionated heparin |
| ULN | upper limit of normal |
| VEP | visual evoked potentials |
| VT | ventricular tachycardia |
| VTE | venous thromboembolism |
| WCC | white cell count |
| WFI | water for injections |
| WPW | Wolff–Parkinson–White syndrome |

# Abciximab

**2 mg/mL solution in 5-mL vials**

- Abciximab is a platelet aggregation inhibitor of the glycoprotein (GP IIb/IIIa) receptor inhibitor class.
- It is used to prevent ischaemic cardiac complications in patients undergoing PCI and for short-term prevention of MI in patients with unstable angina not responding to conventional treatment and who are scheduled for PCI.

## Pre-treatment checks

- Avoid in active internal bleeding; major surgery, intracranial or intraspinal surgery or trauma within the past 2 months; stroke within the past 2 years; intracranial neoplasm, arteriovenous malformation or aneurysm, severe ↑BP, haemorrhagic diathesis, thrombocytopenia, vasculitis, hypertensive retinopathy; breast feeding.
- Caution with concomitant use of drugs that ↑ risk of bleeding, in elderly patients; in hepatic and renal impairment; and in pregnancy.
- The number of vascular punctures and IM injections should be minimised during the treatment.
- IV access should be obtained only at compressible sites of the body.
- All vascular puncture sites should be documented and monitored closely (caution if there is puncture of non-compressible vessels within 24 hours).
- The use of urinary catheters, nasotracheal intubation and nasogastric tubes should be critically considered before commencing therapy.

*Biochemical and other tests*

| | |
|---|---|
| ACT | FBC (including platelets, Hb and haematocrit) |
| APTT | LFTs |
| Blood pressure and pulse | Prothrombin time |
| Bodyweight | Renal function: U, Cr, CrCl (or eGFR) |
| ECG | |

## Dose

Abciximab is used in combination with aspirin and heparin.

**Standard dose:** initially 0.25 microgram/kg by IV injection over 1 minute, followed immediately by IV infusion at a rate of 0.125 microgram/kg/minute (maximum 10 micrograms/minute).

**For prevention of ischaemic complications:** start 10–60 minutes before PCI and continue infusion for 12 hours.

**For unstable angina:** start up to 24 hours before possible PCI and continue infusion for 12 hours after intervention.

**Concomitant aspirin therapy:** at least 300 mg daily.

**Concomitant therapy with unfractionated heparin**

- *Before and during PCI:* see product literature for details.
- *Unstable angina:* heparin is given by IV infusion throughout the abciximab infusion to maintain APTT at 60–85 seconds.

**Dose in renal impairment:** use with caution in severe impairment: ↑risk of bleeding.

**Dose in hepatic impairment:** avoid in severe impairment: ↑risk of bleeding.

## Intravenous injection

*Preparation and administration*

1. Do not shake the vial.
2. Withdraw the required dose.
3. The solution should be clear and colourless. Inspect visually for particulate matter or discoloration before administration and discard if present.
4. Give by IV injection over 1 minute through a non-pyrogenic low-protein-binding 0.2-, 0.22- or 5.0-micron filter.

## Continuous intravenous infusion

*Preparation and administration*

> *Filter *either* at the preparation *or* at the administration stage.

1. Do not shake the vial.
2. Withdraw the required dose and add to a suitable volume of NaCl 0.9% or Gluc 5% through a non-pyrogenic low-protein-binding 0.2-, 0.22- or 5-micron filter*. Mix well.
3. The solution should be clear and colourless. Inspect visually for particulate matter or discoloration before administration and discard if present.
4. Give at the calculated rate via a volumetric infusion device through an in-line non-pyrogenic low-protein-binding 0.2- or 0.22-micron filter* (if not filtered at the preparation stage).

## Technical information

| | |
|---|---|
| Incompatible with | No information |
| Compatible with | **Flush**: NaCl 0.9%<br>**Solutions**: NaCl 0.9%, Gluc 5%<br>**Y-site**: Adenosine, atropine sulfate, bivalirudin, fentanyl, metoprolol, midazolam |
| pH | 7.2 |
| Sodium content | Negligible |
| Storage | Store at 2-8°C in original packaging. Do not freeze. Do not shake. |
| Stability after preparation | From a microbiological point of view, should be used immediately; however, prepared infusions may be stored at 2-8°C and infused (at room temperature) within 24 hours. |

## Monitoring

| Measure | Frequency | Rationale |
|---|---|---|
| ACT | Every 30 minutes and a minimum of 2 minutes after each *heparin* bolus | • If the ACT is <200 seconds, additional heparin boluses of 20 units/kg may be given until an ACT ≥200 seconds is achieved.<br>• If higher doses of heparin are considered clinically necessary (despite a greater bleeding risk), the heparin can be carefully titrated using weight-adjusted boluses to a target ACT not exceeding 300 seconds. |

*(continued)*

## Monitoring (continued)

| Measure | Frequency | Rationale |
|---------|-----------|-----------|
| Platelets | 2-4 hours after the initial dose and at 24 hours | • Thrombocytopenia may occur. If platelets drop to:<br>• 60 000 cells/mm³ (60 × 10⁹/L), heparin and aspirin should be stopped.<br>• <50 000 cells/mm³ (50 × 10⁹/L), transfusion of platelets should be considered.<br>• <20 000 cells/mm³ (20 × 10⁹/L), platelets should be transfused. |
| Hb and haematocrit | 12 and 24 hours after bolus dose | • To check for any adverse events or bleeding. |
| ECG | Shortly after catheterisation and 24 hours after bolus dose | |
| Vital signs (including BP and pulse) | Hourly for the first 4 hours, and then at 6, 12, 18, and 24 hours after bolus dose | |

## Additional information

| | |
|---|---|
| Common and serious undesirable effects | *Immediate:* Anaphylaxis and other hypersensitivity reactions have rarely been reported.<br>*Common:* Thrombocytopenia, ↓pulse, nausea, vomiting, chest pain, pyrexia, puncture site pain, back pain, headache, bleeding, ↓BP. |
| Pharmacokinetics | Initial elimination half-life is 10 minutes, followed by a second phase of about 30 minutes. |
| Significant interactions | • The following may ↑abciximab levels or effect (or ↑side-effects):<br>thrombolytics, coumarin anticoagulants, antiplatelet drugs. |
| Action in case of overdose | *Symptoms to watch for:* Allergy, thrombocytopenia or uncontrolled bleeding.<br>*Antidote:* No specific antidote. Stop administration and give supportive therapy as appropriate, including platelet transfusion if necessary. |
| Counselling | Administration may result in the formation of human anti-chimeric antibody (HACA), which could potentially cause allergic or hypersensitivity reactions (including anaphylaxis), thrombocytopenia, or diminished benefit upon re-administration. |

| Risk rating: **RED** | Score = 6<br>High-risk product: Risk-reduction strategies are required to minimise these risks. |
|---|---|

This assessment is based on the full range of preparation and administration options described in the monograph. These may not all be applicable in some clinical situations.

## Bibliography

SPC Reopro 2 mg/mL solution for injection or infusion (accessed 30 March 2010).

# Acetylcysteine

**200 mg/mL solution in 10-mL ampoules (20% solution)**

- Acetylcysteine is used for the prevention of hepatotoxicity in the treatment of paracetamol (acetaminophen) overdosage.
- It protects the liver if infused within 24 hours of paracetamol ingestion. It is most effective if given within 8 hours of ingestion, after which effectiveness declines sharply.
- If more than 24 hours have elapsed since ingestion, advice should be sought from the National Poisons Information Service (NPIS) or from a liver unit on the management of serious liver damage.
- Acetylcysteine can be nebulised (unlicensed) for use as a mucolytic.

## Pre-treatment checks

- Administer with caution to any patient with asthma or a history of bronchospasm or peptic ulcer disease (↑risk of GI haemorrhage). However, do not delay necessary treatment in these patients.
- Previous anaphylactoid reaction to acetylcysteine is *not* an absolute contraindication for a further treatment course: NPIS advice is to pretreat with an antihistamine, e.g. chlorphenamine 10 mg IV.
- In pregnancy, appropriate maternal treatment is important for the wellbeing of both the mother and the fetus. If the blood levels of paracetamol indicate that acetylcysteine is required, it should be given.

*Biochemical and other tests (not all are necessary in an emergency situation)*

Bodyweight
INR
LFTs

The plasma paracetamol concentration in relation to time after overdose is used to determine whether a patient is at risk of hepatotoxicity and should therefore receive acetylcysteine.

As there is a risk of increased acetylcysteine side-effects, it is unwise to institute treatment before paracetamol levels are known unless more than 8 hours have elapsed since ingestion or levels are likely to be delayed.

NB: Blood samples taken <4 hours after a paracetamol overdose give unreliable estimates of the serum paracetamol concentration.

Refer to the poisoning treatment graph (Figure A1) at the end of the monograph:

- Otherwise healthy patients whose plasma paracetamol concentrations fall on or above the 'Normal treatment line' should receive acetylcysteine. If there is doubt about the timing of the overdose, consideration should be given to treatment with acetylcysteine.
- Sufferers from chronic alcoholism and patients taking enzyme-inducing drugs, e.g. phenytoin, phenobarbital, primidone, carbamazepine, rifampicin and St John's wort, are susceptible to paracetamol-induced hepatotoxicity at lower plasma paracetamol concentrations and should be treated if plasma paracetamol concentrations fall on or above the 'High-risk treatment line'.
- The 'High-risk treatment line' should also be used to guide treatment in patients with malnutrition, e.g. patients with anorexia or AIDS, as they are likely to have depleted glutathione reserves.
- In patients who have taken staggered overdoses, blood levels are meaningless in relation to the treatment graph, and these patients should be considered for treatment with acetylcysteine.

## Dose

> It is essential to consult a poisons information service, e.g. Toxbase at www.toxbase.org (password or registration required) for full details of the management of paracetamol toxicity.

**Treatment for paracetamol poisoning by IV infusion** (refer to Table A1 below):
**Bag 1:** 150 mg/kg bodyweight given in 200 mL of infusion fluid over 15 minutes
**Bag 2:** 50 mg/kg bodyweight in 500 mL infusion fluid over the next 4 hours
**Bag 3:** 100 mg/kg bodyweight in 1 L infusion fluid over the next 16 hours

**Treatment for paracetamol poisoning by the oral route (unlicensed):** in the USA, acetylcysteine is licensed for oral use in paracetamol overdose. An initial dose of 140 mg/kg as a 5% solution is followed by 70 mg/kg every 4 hours for an additional 17 doses.

**As a mucolytic via nebuliser (unlicensed):** the adult dose is 3–5 mL acetylcysteine 20% injection, nebulised 3–4 times daily using air (use of concentrated oxygen causes degradation).
Acetylcysteine may cause bronchospasm. This can be avoided either by giving a lower dose – diluting 1 mL acetylcysteine 20% in 5 mL NaCl 0.9% and giving 3–4 mL – or pre-administering a nebulised bronchodilator.

## Intravenous infusion

*Preparation and administration*

1. Withdraw the required dose and add to the appropriate volume of infusion fluid. Mix well.
2. The solution should be clear and colourless. Inspect visually for particulate matter or discoloration before administration.
3. Give by IV infusion over the time period stated above.

## Oral administration (unlicensed)

*Preparation and administration*

1. Withdraw the required dose.
2. Dilute the injection to 4 times its volume with diet soft drink and give to the patient to drink; if given via a nasogastric tube, water may be used as the diluent.

## Nebulisation (unlicensed)

*Preparation and administration*

1. Withdraw the required dose and dilute with NaCl 0.9% if required (see dose above).
2. Give via a nebuliser using air (not oxygen).

## Technical information

| | |
|---|---|
| Incompatible with | Equipment made of rubber and some metals, e.g. iron, copper and nickel. Otherwise no information. |
| Compatible with | Equipment made of plastic, glass and stainless steel. **Flush**: NaCl 0.9% **Solutions**: Gluc 5% (preferred), NaCl 0.9% (both including added KCl) **Y-site**: No information |
| pH | 6–7.5 |
| Sodium content | 12.8 mmol/10 mL |

*(continued)*

## Technical information (*continued*)

| | |
|---|---|
| Storage | Store below 25°C. A change in colour to light purple is not thought to indicate significant impairment of safety or efficacy. |
| Stability after preparation | From a microbiological point of view, prepared infusions should be used immediately; however, solutions are known to be stable at room temperature for up to 24 hours. |

## Monitoring

| Measure | Frequency | Rationale |
|---|---|---|
| Liver function and INR | To determine completion of antidote | • ↑Transaminases (ALT or AST) and ↑INR indicate hepatotoxicity. Acetylcysteine can also cause a marginally elevated INR. <br> • An INR of ≤1.3 with normal transaminases does not warrant further treatment. If all measures are raised, then 'bag 3' should be repeated over 16 hours. |
| ECG | If indicated | • ECG changes have been reported in patients with paracetamol poisoning, irrespective of the treatment given. |
| Renal function and serum K | | • ↓K has been reported in patients with paracetamol poisoning, irrespective of the treatment given. <br> • Renal failure is a recognised complication of paracetamol overdose. |
| Serum bicarbonate | | • Metabolic acidosis can be a complication of paracetamol overdose. |

## Additional information

| | |
|---|---|
| Common and serious undesirable effects | *Immediate:* Anaphylactoid or hypersensitivity-like reactions have been reported in 0.3-3% of patients, in patients with hepatic cirrhosis, and in patients with low or absent paracetamol concentrations. <br> • Symptoms include nausea/vomiting, injection-site reactions, flushing, itching, rashes/urticaria, angioedema, bronchospasm/respiratory distress, ↓BP and, rarely, ↑pulse or ↑BP. These have usually occurred 15-60 minutes after the start of infusion. Symptoms have often been relieved by stopping the infusion, but occasionally an antihistamine or corticosteroid may be necessary. <br> • Once the reaction has settled, the infusion can normally be restarted at 50 mg/kg over 4 hours. Further reactions are almost unknown. <br> *Infusion-related:* Too rapid administration: Higher incidence of hypersensitivity reactions. |
| Pharmacokinetics | Elimination half-life of 2-6 hours reported after IV dosing, with 20-30% of the administered dose being recovered unchanged in the urine. |
| Significant interactions | No known interactions. |
| Action in case of overdose | *Symptoms to watch for:* effects similar to the anaphylactoid reactions noted above, but they may be more severe. <br> There is a theoretical risk of hepatic encephalopathy. |

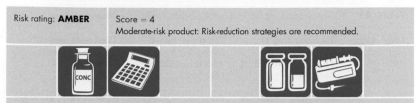

Risk rating: **AMBER** | Score = 4
Moderate-risk product: Risk-reduction strategies are recommended.

This assessment is based on the full range of preparation and administration options described in the monograph. These may not all be applicable in some clinical situations.

## Bibliography

SPC Parvolex (accessed 17 August 2008).
Toxbase at www.toxbase.org (accessed 18 August 2008).

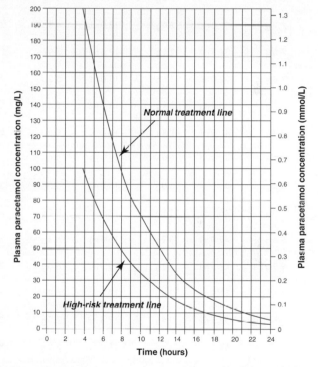

**Figure A1** Patients whose plasma paracetamol concentrations are above the normal treatment line should be treated with acetylcysteine by IV infusion (or, if acetylcysteine cannot be used, with methionine by mouth, provided the overdose has been taken within 10-12 hours and the patient is not vomiting).

Patients on enzyme-inducing drugs (e.g. carbamazepine, phenobarbital, phenytoin, primidone, rifampicin, alcohol and St John's wort) or who are malnourished (e.g. in anorexia, in alcoholism, or those who are HIV positive) should be treated if their plasma paracetamol concentration is above the high-risk treatment line.

The prognostic accuracy after 15 hours is uncertain, but a plasma paracetamol concentration above the relevant treatment line should be regarded as carrying a serious risk of liver damage.

(Graph reproduced courtesy of Professor Philip Routledge, Therapeutics and Toxicology Centre, Cardiff and taken from BNF 60 (September 2010).)

**Table A1**  Acetylcysteine dosing table for paracetamol overdose

| Bodyweight (kg) | 1st dose 'Bag 1' 150 mg/kg over 15 minutes in 200 mL Gluc 5% | | 2nd dose 'Bag 2' 50 mg/kg over 4 hours in 500 mL Gluc 5% | | 3rd dose 'Bag 3' 100 mg/kg over 16 hours in 1 L Gluc 5% | |
|---|---|---|---|---|---|---|
| | Parvolex (dose) | Parvolex (volume) | Parvolex (dose) | Parvolex (volume) | Parvolex (dose) | Parvolex (volume) |
| 40 | 6.0 g | 30.0 mL | 2.0 g | 10.0 mL | 4.0 g | 20 mL |
| 42 | 6.3 g | 31.5 mL | 2.1 g | 10.5 mL | 4.2 g | 21 mL |
| 44 | 6.6 g | 33.0 mL | 2.2 g | 11.0 mL | 4.4 g | 22 mL |
| 46 | 6.9 g | 34.5 mL | 2.3 g | 11.5 mL | 4.6 g | 23 mL |
| 48 | 7.2 g | 36.0 mL | 2.4 g | 12.0 mL | 4.8 g | 24 mL |
| 50 | 7.5 g | 37.5 mL | 2.5 g | 12.5 mL | 5.0 g | 25 mL |
| 52 | 7.8 g | 39.0 mL | 2.6 g | 13.0 mL | 5.2 g | 26 mL |
| 54 | 8.1 g | 40.5 mL | 2.7 g | 13.5 mL | 5.4 g | 27 mL |
| 56 | 8.4 g | 42.0 mL | 2.8 g | 14.0 mL | 5.6 g | 28 mL |
| 58 | 8.7 g | 43.5 mL | 2.9 g | 14.5 mL | 5.8 g | 29 mL |
| 60 | 9.0 g | 45.0 mL | 3.0 g | 15.0 mL | 6.0 g | 30 mL |
| 62 | 9.3 g | 46.5 mL | 3.1 g | 15.5 mL | 6.2 g | 31 mL |
| 64 | 9.6 g | 48.0 mL | 3.2 g | 16.0 mL | 6.4 g | 32 mL |
| 66 | 9.9 g | 49.5 mL | 3.3 g | 16.5 mL | 6.6 g | 33 mL |
| 68 | 10.2 g | 51.0 mL | 3.4 g | 17.0 mL | 6.8 g | 34 mL |
| 70 | 10.5 g | 52.5 mL | 3.5 g | 17.5 mL | 7.0 g | 35 mL |
| 72 | 10.8 g | 54.0 mL | 3.6 g | 18.0 mL | 7.2 g | 36 mL |
| 74 | 11.1 g | 55.5 mL | 3.7 g | 18.5 mL | 7.4 g | 37 mL |
| 76 | 11.4 g | 57.0 mL | 3.8 g | 19.0 mL | 7.6 g | 38 mL |
| 78 | 11.7 g | 58.5 mL | 3.9 g | 19.5 mL | 7.8 g | 39 mL |
| 80 | 12.0 g | 60.0 mL | 4.0 g | 20.0 mL | 8.0 g | 40 mL |

*(continued)*

**Table A1**   Acetylcysteine dosing table for paracetamol overdose *(continued)*

| Bodyweight (kg) | 1st dose 'Bag 1' 150 mg/kg over 15 minutes in 200 mL Gluc 5% | | 2nd dose 'Bag 2' 50 mg/kg over 4 hours in 500 mL Gluc 5% | | 3rd dose 'Bag 3' 100 mg/kg over 16 hours in 1 L Gluc 5% | |
|---|---|---|---|---|---|---|
| | Parvolex (dose) | Parvolex (volume) | Parvolex (dose) | Parvolex (volume) | Parvolex (dose) | Parvolex (volume) |
| 82 | 12.3 g | 61.5 mL | 4.1 g | 20.5 mL | 8.2 g | 41 mL |
| 84 | 12.6 g | 63.0 mL | 4.2 g | 21.0 mL | 8.4 g | 42 mL |
| 86 | 12.9 g | 64.5 mL | 4.3 g | 21.5 mL | 8.6 g | 43 mL |
| 88 | 13.2 g | 66.0 mL | 4.4 g | 22.0 mL | 8.8 g | 44 mL |
| 90 | 13.5 g | 67.5 mL | 4.5 g | 22.5 mL | 9.0 g | 45 mL |
| 92 | 13.8 g | 69.0 mL | 4.6 g | 23.0 mL | 9.2 g | 46 mL |
| 94 | 14.1 g | 70.5 mL | 4.7 g | 23.5 mL | 9.4 g | 47 mL |
| 96 | 14.4 g | 72.0 mL | 4.8 g | 24.0 mL | 9.6 g | 48 mL |
| 98 | 14.7 g | 73.5 mL | 4.9 g | 24.5 mL | 9.8 g | 49 mL |
| 100 | 15.0 g | 75.0 mL | 5.0 g | 25.0 mL | 10.0 g | 50 mL |
| 102 | 15.3 g | 76.5 mL | 5.1 g | 25.5 mL | 10.2 g | 51 mL |
| 104 | 15.6 g | 78.0 mL | 5.2 g | 26.0 mL | 10.4 g | 52 mL |
| 106 | 15.9 g | 79.5 mL | 5.3 g | 26.5 mL | 10.6 g | 53 mL |
| 108 | 16.2 g | 81.0 mL | 5.4 g | 27.0 mL | 10.8 g | 54 mL |
| 110 | 16.5 g | 82.5 mL | 5.5 g | 27.5 mL | 11.0 g | 55 mL |
| >110 | If weight is >110 kg, dose as for 110 kg | | | | | |

# Aciclovir (acyclovir)

**25 mg/mL solution in 10-mL, 20-mL and 40-mL vials; 250-mg and 500-mg dry powder vials**

* Aciclovir sodium is a synthetic purine nucleoside analogue structurally related to guanine.
* It is used mainly for the treatment of viral infections due to herpes simplex virus (types 1 and 2) and varicella-zoster virus (herpes zoster and chickenpox).
* Doses are expressed in terms of the base: Aciclovir 1 g $\cong$ 1.1 g aciclovir sodium.

## Pre-treatment checks

* Check that the patient is not hypersensitive to aciclovir or valaciclovir; caution in patients with neurological abnormalities or substantial hypoxia.
* Hydration status (patient **must** be adequately hydrated).

*Biochemical and other tests*

Bodyweight
FBC

LFTs
Renal function: U, Cr, CrCl (or eGFR)

## Dose

> To avoid excessive dosing, doses should be calculated on the basis of ideal bodyweight (IBW) in obese patients. See Appendix 10.

**Treatment of herpes simplex in immunocompromised patients, severe initial genital herpes, and varicella-zoster:** 5 mg/kg by IV infusion every 8 hours, usually for 5 days.
**Treatment of varicella-zoster in immunocompromised patients and simplex encephalitis:** 10 mg/kg by IV infusion every 8 hours (usually for at least 10 days in encephalitis).
**Prophylaxis of herpes simplex in immunocompromised patients:** 5 mg/kg by IV infusion every 8 hours.
**Dose in renal impairment:** adjusted according to creatinine clearance:

* CrCl >25–50 mL/minute: 5–10 mg/kg every 12 hours.
* CrCl 10–25 mL/minute: 5–10 mg/kg every 24 hours.
* CrCl <10 mL/minute: 2.5–5 mg/kg every 24 hours.

## Intermittent intravenous infusion

*Preparation and administration*

> See Special handling below.

1. If using dry powder vials, reconstitute each 250-mg vial with 10 mL WFI (use 20 mL for each 500-mg vial). Shake gently to dissolve to give a solution containing 25 mg/mL.
2. Withdraw the required dose and add to a suitable volume of compatible infusion fluid (usually NaCl 0.9%). The final concentration must be no more than 5 mg/mL (i.e. add doses ≤500 mg to 100 mL; add doses >500 mg to 250 mL).
3. The solution should be clear, light yellow and slightly opalescent. Inspect visually for particulate matter or discoloration before administration and discard if present.
4. Give by IV infusion over a minimum of 1 hour.

## Intermittent intravenous infusion via a syringe pump

*Preparation and administration*

See Special handling in the table below.

1. If using dry powder vials, reconstitute each 250-mg vial with 10 mL WFI or NaCl 0.9% (use 20 mL for each 500-mg vial). Shake gently to dissolve to give a solution containing 25 mg/mL.
2. Withdraw the required dose into a syringe pump without further dilution.
3. The solution should be clear, light yellow and slightly opalescent. Inspect visually for particulate matter or discoloration before administration and discard if present.
4. Give by IV infusion over a minimum of 1 hour. Periodically inspect for turbidity or crystallisation; discard if present.

## Technical information

| | |
|---|---|
| Incompatible with | WFI containing parabens or benzyl alcohol. Aztreonam, cisatracurium, dobutamine, dopamine, foscarnet, levofloxacin, meropenem, morphine sulfate, ondansetron, pantoprazole, pethidine, piperacillin with tazobactam, tramadol. |
| Compatible with | **Flush**: NaCl 0.9% <br> **Solutions**: NaCl 0.9%, Gluc 5%, Gluc-NaCl, Hartmann's (including added KCl) <br> **Y-site**: Amikacin, ampicillin, benzylpenicillin, cefotaxime, ceftazidime, ceftriaxone, cefuroxime, chloramphenicol sodium succinate, clindamycin, co-trimoxazole, dexamethasone, erythromycin, fluconazole, gentamicin, granisetron, hydrocortisone sodium succinate, imipenem with cilastatin, magnesium sulfate, methylprednisolone sodium succinate, metoclopramide, metronidazole, propofol, ranitidine, remifentanil, tobramycin, vancomycin |
| pH | 11 |
| Sodium content | About 1.1 mmol/250-mg vial. |
| Storage | Store below 25°C in original packaging. Do not refrigerate (may precipitate). |
| Special handling | Avoid contact with eyes and unprotected skin. |
| Stability after reconstitution | From a microbiological point of view, should be used immediately; however, prepared infusions may be stored at 25°C and infused within 12 hours. Check for signs of precipitation. |

## Monitoring

| Measure | Frequency | Rationale |
|---|---|---|
| U&Es, serum creatinine | After initiation, then periodically | • Urea and creatinine levels may transiently rise. If serious, they are usually reversed by rapid rehydration, dose reduction or withdrawal. |
| LFTs | Periodically | • Reversible increases in liver-related enzymes may occur. |
| FBC | | • Anaemia, thrombocytopenia and leucopenia have been reported (rarely). |

(continued)

## Monitoring (continued)

| Measure | Frequency | Rationale |
|---------|-----------|-----------|
| Signs and symptoms of encephalopathy | On presentation | • Typical symptoms include lethargy, obtundation, tremors, confusion, hallucinations, agitation, seizures and coma. They are usually reversible. |

## Additional information

| | |
|---|---|
| Common and serious undesirable effects | *Infusion-related:* Local: Inflammation or phlebitis at infusion site. *Other:* Headache, nausea, vomiting, diarrhoea, rash, pruritus, urticaria. |
| Pharmacokinetics | Elimination half-life is 3.8 hours in normal adults (19.5 hours if CrCl <15 mL/minute). |
| Significant interactions | No significant interactions. |
| Action in case of overdose | *Symptoms to watch for:* Aciclovir crystals may precipitate in renal tubules, causing renal tubular damage, if the maximum solubility of free aciclovir is exceeded. Maximum urine concentration occurs within the first few hours of infusion; therefore, ensure adequate urine flow during that period (with good hydration). Other nephrotoxic drugs, pre-existing renal disease and dehydration increase the risk of further renal impairment. *Antidote:* No known antidote, but haemodialysis can remove aciclovir from the circulation. |

| Risk rating: **AMBER** | Score = 3 Moderate-risk product: Risk-reduction strategies are recommended. |
|---|---|

 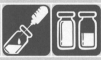

This assessment is based on the full range of preparation and administration options described in the monograph. These may not all be applicable in some clinical situations.

## Bibliography

SPC Aciclovir 250 mg powder for solution for infusion, Wockhardt UK Ltd (accessed 23 February 2010).

SPC Aciclovir 25 mg/mL sterile concentrate, Hospira UK Ltd (accessed 23 February 2010).

SPC Zovirax IV 250mg, 500 mg (accessed 23 February 2010).

# Adalimumab

**40 mg solution in pre-filled pen or syringe**

Adalimumab should be used under specialist supervision only.

- Adalimumab is a cytokine modulator.
- Adalimumab is licensed for use in the treatment of disease states where raised TNF levels are seen: active rheumatoid arthritis, ankylosing spondylitis, psoriatic arthritis, plaque psoriasis and Crohn's disease.
- Adalimumab has been assessed by NICE and in the UK should be used in accordance with the appropriate guidance.

## Pre-treatment checks

- Screen for tuberculosis (TB): do not give in active TB or other severe infections.
- Do not use in moderate to severe heart failure.
- Caution in hepatitis B virus: reactivation of hepatitis B has occurred in patients who are carriers.
- Caution should be exercised with demyelinating CNS disorders, as there is a risk of exacerbating symptoms.

*Biochemical and other tests*

| | |
|---|---|
| ESR and CRP | Tender joint count, swollen joint count (if being |
| FBC | used for psoriatic or rheumatoid arthritis) |
| LFTs | U&Es |
| Skin assessment (if being used for psoriasis) | |

## Dose

**Rheumatoid arthritis:** 40 mg by SC injection every 2 weeks in combination with methotrexate. If methotrexate is inappropriate or not tolerated, adalimumab dose may be increased to 40 mg every week.

**Psoriatic arthritis and ankylosing spondylitis:** 40 mg every 2 weeks.

**Crohn's disease:** initially 80 mg by SC injection, then 40 mg 2 weeks after initial dose. Accelerated regimen: initially 40 mg by SC injection for four doses over 1–2 days, then 80 mg 2 weeks after initial dose; maintenance, 40 mg every 2 weeks, increased if necessary to 40 mg every week. To induce remission, adalimumab is usually given in combination with a corticosteroid, but it may be given as monotherapy if a corticosteroid is inappropriate or not tolerated.

**Psoriasis:** 80 mg by SC injection initially, then 40 mg every 2 weeks commencing 1 week after initial dose.

This drug has not been studied in patients with renal or hepatic impairment; therefore no dose recommendations can be made.

## Subcutaneous injection

*Preparation and administration*

1. The solution should be clear and colourless. Inspect visually for particulate matter or discoloration before administration and discard if present.
2. Give by SC injection into the thigh or abdomen. Avoid areas that are reddened, bruised or hard. If using the abdomen, give at least 5 cm from the umbilicus. Rotate injection sites for subsequent injections, ensuring they are at least 3 cm from a previous site.

## Technical information

| | |
|---|---|
| Incompatible with | Not relevant |
| Compatible with | Not relevant |
| pH | Not relevant |
| Sodium content | Negligible |
| Storage | Store at 2-8°C in original packaging. Do not freeze. |

## Monitoring

| Measure | Frequency | Rationale |
|---|---|---|
| Clinical improvement | Periodically | • Discontinue treatment if there is no clinical response after 12 weeks for all licensed indications except psoriasis, where the treatment may continue for 16 weeks. |
| Infections | During and after treatment | • Serious infections, including tuberculosis, may occur. Adalimumab may take up to 5 months to be eliminated from the body; therefore monitoring should be continued during this period. |
| Injection sites | Post injection | • In controlled trials 15% of patients developed injection site reactions such as erythema, itching, haemorrhage, pain or swelling. |
| FBC, LFTs, U&Es, ESR and CRP | 3 months after initiation and then every 6 months or in accordance with local policy | • Can affect liver function.<br>• May cause ↓haemoglobin.<br>• The other measures are used to assess therapeutic benefit or disease progression. |

## Additional information

| | |
|---|---|
| Common and serious undesirable effects | *Injection/infusion-related:* Local: injection-site reactions, i.e. erythema, itching, pain, swelling.<br>*Other:* Cough, headache, diarrhoea, abdominal pain, stomatitis, mouth ulcer, nausea, rash, pruritus, musculoskeletal pain, respiratory infections, fever, fatigue, ↑Alk Phos, ↑pulse. |
| Pharmacokinetics | Mean terminal half-life is about 2 weeks; it may take up to 5 months for adalimumab to be eliminated from the body. |
| Significant interactions | • The following may ↑adalimumab levels or effect (or ↑side-effects): abatacept (↑risk of infections), anakinra (↑risk of infections), live vaccines (avoid combination). |
| Action in case of overdose | No dose-limiting toxicity was observed during clinical trials. |

*(continued)*

## Additional information (continued)

| Counselling | Report signs or symptoms of infection, especially tuberculosis infection during or after treatment with adalimumab, e.g. persistent cough, wasting/weight loss, low-grade fever.<br>Patients should be given a special alert card.<br>Patients may receive concurrent vaccinations, except for live vaccines. |
| --- | --- |

| Risk rating: **GREEN** | Score = 1<br>Lower-risk product: Risk-reduction strategies should be considered. |
| --- | --- |

This assessment is based on the full range of preparation and administration options described in the monograph. These may not all be applicable in some clinical situations.

## Bibliography

SPC Humira (accessed 21 October 2008).

# Adenosine

### 3 mg/mL solution in 2-mL and 10-mL vials

* Adenosine is an endogenous nucleoside that is present in all cells of the body and is involved in many biological processes. It acts as an antiarrhythmic by stimulating adenosine A1-receptors and slowing conduction through the AV node.
* It is used to restore sinus rhythm in the treatment of paroxysmal SVT, including that associated with the Wolff–Parkinson–White syndrome. It is also used for the differential diagnosis of SVTs and in myocardial imaging.

## Pre-treatment checks

* Contraindicated in patients with second- or third-degree AV block (except in patients with a functioning artificial pacemaker); sick sinus syndrome (except in patients with a functioning artificial pacemaker); asthma.
* Caution in atrial fibrillation or flutter with accessory pathway (conduction down anomalous pathway may increase).
* Caution in heart transplant, prolonged QT interval or obstructive pulmonary disease.

*Biochemical and other tests*

Bodyweight in certain indications

## Dose

### Reversion to sinus rhythm in paroxysmal SVT:

* *Initial dose:* 6 mg by rapid IV injection (3 mg in patients with heart transplant as very sensitive to effects of adenosine). If it is essential to co-administer with dipyridamole, the initial dose should be reduced to 0.5–1 mg.

- *Second dose:* 12 mg by rapid IV injection, if the first dose is not effective within 1–2 minutes (6 mg in patients with heart transplant).
- *Third dose:* 12 mg by rapid IV injection if the second dose is not effective within 1–2 minutes.

**Aid to diagnosis of broad or narrow complex SVT:** the above ascending dosage schedule is given until sufficient diagnostic information has been obtained.

**In conjunction with radionuclide myocardial perfusion imaging:** 140 micrograms/kg/minute by IV infusion for 6 minutes (see Table A2). The radionuclide is injected after 3 minutes of infusion.

## Intravenous injection

*Preparation and administration*

For administration via a central or large peripheral vein only.

1. Withdraw the required dose.
2. The solution should be clear and colourless. Inspect visually for particulate matter or discoloration before administration and discard if present.
3. Give by rapid IV injection over 2 seconds into a central or large peripheral vein at a site as close to the cannulation site as possible.
4. Follow by a rapid flush of 20 mL NaCl 0.9%.
5. Discard any unused solution immediately.

**Table A2**  Dose of adenosine 3 mg/mL for myocardial perfusion scanning in mL/minute

| Bodyweight (kg) | Infusion rate (mL/minute) | Bodyweight (kg) | Infusion rate (mL/minute) |
|---|---|---|---|
| 45-49 | 2.1 | 75-79 | 3.5 |
| 50-54 | 2.3 | 80-84 | 3.8 |
| 55-59 | 2.6 | 85-89 | 4.0 |
| 60-64 | 2.8 | 90-94 | 4.2 |
| 65-69 | 3.0 | 95-99 | 4.4 |
| 70-74 | 3.3 | 100-104 | 4.7 |

## Intravenous infusion via a syringe pump (myocardial perfusion imaging)

*Preparation and administration*

For administration via a large peripheral vein only

1. Withdraw the required injection volume into a suitable syringe.
2. The solution should be clear and colourless. Inspect visually for particulate matter or discoloration prior to administration and discard if present.
3. Give by IV infusion over 6 minutes into a large peripheral vein at the rate specified above. Separate venous infusion sites for adenosine and radionuclide administration are recommended to avoid an adenosine bolus effect.

## Technical information

| | |
|---|---|
| Incompatible with | No information |
| Compatible with | **Flush**: NaCl 0.9%<br>**Solutions**: NaCl 0.9%, Gluc 5%, Hartmann's<br>**Y-site**: Abciximab |
| pH | 4.5-7.5 |
| Sodium content | Negligible |
| Storage | Store below 30°C but do not refrigerate (risk of crystal formation).<br>Discard unused injection solution immediately. |

## Monitoring

| Measure | Frequency | Rationale |
|---|---|---|
| ECG | During administration | • Possibility of transient cardiac arrhythmias arising during conversion of the SVT to normal sinus rhythm.<br>• Increments should not be given if high-level AV block develops at any particular dose. |
| Heart rate and blood pressure | Every minute during IV administration | • To avoid an adenosine bolus effect BP should be measured in the arm opposite to the infusion.<br>• May rarely produce significant ↓BP and reflex ↑pulse. |

## Additional information

| | |
|---|---|
| Common and serious undesirable effects | *Immediate:* Include transient facial flush, chest pain, dyspnoea, bronchospasm, choking sensation, nausea, light-headedness; severe ↓pulse reported (requiring temporary pacing); ECG may show transient rhythm disturbances. |
| Pharmacokinetics | Elimination half-life is <10 seconds. |
| Significant interactions | • Dipyridamole may ↑adenosine effect (or ↑side-effects): initial dose should be reduced to 0.5-1 mg.<br>• The following may ↓adenosine effect: aminophylline, theophylline and other xanthines such as caffeine are known potent inhibitors of adenosine. |
| Action in case of overdose | No cases of overdosage have been reported. |
| Counselling | Advise of the potential for the above undesirable effects and advise avoidance of methylxanthines, e.g. coffee, tea. |

| Risk rating: **AMBER** | Score = 4<br>Moderate-risk product: Risk-reduction strategies are recommended. |
|---|---|

This assessment is based on the full range of preparation and administration options described in the monograph. These may not all be applicable in some clinical situations.

## Bibliography

SPC Adenocor (accessed 25 February 2010).
SPC Adenoscan (accessed 25 February 2010).

# Adrenaline (epinephrine)

**1 mg/mL (1 in 1000) solution in ampoules and pre-filled syringes**
**1 mg/mL (1 in 1000) solution in 0.15-mL and 0.3-mL auto-injector**
**0.1 mg/mL (1 in 10000) solution in 3-mL and 10-mL pre-filled syringes**

* Adrenaline is an endogenous substance that is produced in the adrenal medulla and has direct-acting sympathomimetic activity.
* It is used in the emergency treatment of acute allergy, anaphylactic shock and for cardiac resuscitation.
* The IM route is preferred in shock and allergy because absorption from this route is more reliable than from SC injection.
* The IV route is used for advanced cardiac life support and where there is doubt regarding circulatory adequacy and absorption from IM dosing. The IV route is also used in critical care for low cardiac output states.

## Pre-treatment checks

* Contraindications are relative as the drug is used in life-threatening emergencies.
* Outside of emergency situations, the following contraindications should be considered: hyperthyroidism, hypertension, ischaemic heart disease, arrhythmias, diabetes mellitus and closed-angle glaucoma.
* Do not inject into fingers, toes, ears, nose or genitalia owing to the risk of ischaemic tissue necrosis.

*Biochemical and other tests (not all are necessary in an emergency situation)*

None practical in emergency scenarios

## Dose

Selection of the correct strength of adrenaline injection is crucial.

**Acute anaphylaxis in adults by IM route:** 500 micrograms (0.5 mL of the 1 in 1000 injection) by IM injection. The dose may be repeated if necessary at 5- to 15-minute intervals. Alternatively, 300 micrograms (0.3 mL of the 1 in 1000 injection) may be given using an auto-injector in patients with history or at risk of anaphylaxis.
**Acute anaphylaxis in adults by IV route (use with extreme care only if the IM route is clearly ineffective):** 50 micrograms (0.5 mL of the 1 in 10000 injection) over 2–3 minutes. Repeat according to response. Consider infusion if multiple doses are required.
**Advanced cardiac life support:** refer to local resuscitation guidelines for use in CPR via IV or intraosseous routes.
**Intraosseous route:** doses are the same as those used IV.
**Endotracheal route (only if circulatory access cannot be obtained):** 2–3 mg diluted to 20–30 mL with NaCl 0.9% via *endotracheal tube*, repeated as necessary. Intracardiac injection is no longer recommended.

**Low cardiac output states:** 0.01–0.3 microgram/kg/minute by IV infusion. Adjust dose according to clinical response: heart rate, BP, cardiac output, presence of ectopic beats and urine output.

## Intramuscular injection

*Preparation and administration*

> Selection of the correct strength of adrenaline injection is crucial.

1. Withdraw the required dose or, if using an auto-injector device, follow the manufacturer's instructions for preparation of the dose.
2. Give by IM injection into the mid-point of the anterolateral aspect of the thigh through clothing if necessary (avoid injecting into the buttock because of the risk of tissue necrosis).

## Intravenous injection in acute anaphylaxis (only if the IM route is ineffective)

*Preparation and administration*

> For administration via a central line if possible. If a peripheral vein is used, flush with NaCl 0.9% immediately after injection.
> Selection of the correct strength of adrenaline injection is crucial.

1. Withdraw the required dose. Dilute to 5 mL with NaCl 0.9% to facilitate slow administration.
2. The solution should be clear and colourless. Inspect visually for particulate matter or discoloration prior to administration and discard if present.
3. Give by IV injection over 2–3 minutes into a central vein if possible (if a peripheral vein is used, flush immediately afterwards with 20 mL NaCl 0.9%).

## Continuous intravenous infusion via syringe pump

*Preparation of a 80 microgram/mL solution (various regimens may be used)*

> For administration via a central line.
> Selection of the correct strength of adrenaline injection is crucial.

1. Withdraw 4 mg and make up to 50 mL in a syringe pump with a compatible infusion solution.
2. Cap the syringe and mix well to give a solution containing 80 micrograms/mL.
3. The solution should be clear and colourless. Inspect visually for particulate matter or discoloration prior to administration and discard if present.

*Administration*

Give by IV infusion into a central vein using a syringe pump.

| Technical information | |
|---|---|
| Incompatible with | Sodium bicarbonate.<br>Aminophylline, ampicillin, pantoprazole, micafungin. |
| Compatible with | **Flush**: NaCl 0.9%<br>**Solutions**: NaCl 0.9%, Gluc 5%, Gluc-NaCl, Hartmann's, Ringer's (including added KCl)<br>**Y-site**: Amikacin, atracurium, calcium chloride, calcium gluconate, cisatracurium, clonidine, dobutamine, dopamine, fentanyl, furosemide, glyceryl trinitrate, hydrocortisone sodium succinate, labetalol, midazolam, milrinone, noradrenaline, propofol, ranitidine, remifentanil, tigecycline, tirofiban, vecuronium, verapamil |

*(continued)*

## Technical information (*continued*)

| | |
|---|---|
| pH | 2.2-5 |
| Sodium content | Negligible |
| Excipients | Contains sulfites (may cause hypersensitivity reactions). |
| Storage | Store below 25°C in original packaging.<br>Discoloured solutions or solutions containing a precipitate should not be used. |
| Stability after preparation | From a microbiological point of view should be used immediately; however, prepared infusions may be stored at 2-8°C and infused (at room temperature) within 24 hours. |

## Monitoring

| Measure | Frequency | Rationale |
|---|---|---|
| Respiratory function and airway patency | Continuously | • Response to therapy - anaphylaxis. |
| Blood pressure | | • ↑BP desired response to therapy. |
| Heart rate/ECG | | • ↑Pulse desired response to therapy.<br>• Arrhythmias may occur. |
| Cardiac and urine output | Hourly | • Response to therapy. |
| Blood glucose | 12 hourly | • Hyperglycaemia may occur. |

## Additional information

| | |
|---|---|
| Common and serious undesirable effects | *Injection/infusion-related:* Local: Tissue necrosis at injection site.<br>*Other:* Hyperglycaemia, ↓K, palpitations, ↑pulse, arrhythmias, ↑BP, cold extremities, tremor, anxiety, headache, cerebral haemorrhage, dyspnoea, angle-closure glaucoma, nausea |
| Pharmacokinetics | Serum half-life 2-3 minutes. After SC or IM injection effects may be delayed due to vasoconstriction. |
| Significant interactions | • The following may ↑adrenaline levels or effect (or ↑side-effects): dopexamine, MAOIs (risk of hypertensive crisis), moclobemide (risk of hypertensive crisis), rasagiline (avoid combination).<br>• Beta-blockers may ↓adrenaline levels or effect.<br>• Adrenaline may ↑levels or effect of the following drugs (or ↑side-effects): anaesthetics, general-volatile (↑risk of arrhythmias); antidepressants-tricyclic (risk of arrhythmias and ↑BP); beta-blockers (risk of severe ↑BP and ↓pulse); tolazoline (avoid combination). |
| Action in case of overdose | *Symptoms to watch for:* Effects are short lived and typically require supportive measures only. Stop administration and give supportive therapy as appropriate. |
| Counselling | Correct technique for use of auto-injector. |

| Risk rating: **GREEN** | Score = 1<br>Lower-risk product: Risk-reduction strategies should be considered. |
|---|---|

This assessment does not cover IV infusion technique.

## Bibliography

SPC Adrenaline (Epinephrine) Injection BP 1 in 1000, Hameln Pharmaceuticals Ltd (accessed 30 April 2009).

SPC Epinephrine (Adrenaline) Injection 1:10000, International Medication Systems (UK) Ltd (accessed 30 April 2009).

SPC EpiPen Jr. Auto-Injector 0.15 mg (accessed 30 April 2009).

# Alfacalcidol (1α-hydroxycholecalciferol)

**1 microgram/0.5 mL and 2 micrograms/mL solution in ampoules**

* The term vitamin D is used for a range of closely related sterol compounds including alfacalcidol, calcitriol, colecalciferol and ergocalciferol. Vitamin D compounds possess the property of preventing or curing rickets.
* Alfacalcidol injection is indicated in the treatment of renal osteodystrophy; hyperparathyroidism (with bone disease); hypoparathyroidism; nutritional and malabsorptive rickets and osteomalacia; pseudo-deficiency (vitamin D-dependent) rickets and osteomalacia; hypophosphataemic vitamin D-resistant rickets and osteomalacia

## Pre-treatment checks

* Do not give to patients with hypercalcaemia, including hypercalcaemia of malignancy.
* In patients with renal bone disease, relatively high initial plasma Ca levels may indicate autonomous hyperparathyroidism, which is often unresponsive to alfacalcidol.

*Biochemical and other tests*

Electrolytes: serum Ca, $PO_4$
Liver function: Alk Phos
Renal function: U, Cr, CrCl (or eGFR)

## Dose

**Initial adult dose**: 1 microgram/day. Adjust dose according to biochemical response taking care to avoid ↑Ca. Maintenance doses are generally in the range of 250 nanograms to 1 microgram/day.
**Initial dosage in elderly patients:** 500 nanograms/day.

**Patients undergoing haemodialysis:** the initial dosage for adults is 1 microgram/dialysis. The maximum recommended dose is 6 micrograms/dialysis and not more than 12 micrograms/ week. The injection is given into the return line from the haemodialysis machine at the end of each dialysis.

## Intravenous injection

*Preparation and administration*

1. Withdraw the required dose.
2. Give by IV injection over approximately 30 seconds.

## Technical information

| | |
|---|---|
| Incompatible with | No information |
| Compatible with | No information |
| pH | No information |
| Sodium content | Negligible |
| Excipients | Contains ethanol (may interact with metronidazole, possible religious objections). Contains propylene glycol (adverse effects seen in ↓renal function, may interact with disulfiram and metronidazole). |
| Storage | Store at 2-8°C in original packaging. |

## Monitoring

| Measure | Frequency | Rationale |
|---|---|---|
| Serum Ca and PO$_4$ | Initially weekly until dose and plasma Ca and PO$_4$ are stable, then monthly; also whenever nausea or vomiting occurs. | • ↑Ca and ↑PO$_4$ can occur during treatment with pharmacological doses of compounds having vitamin D activity.<br>• Plasma PO$_4$ concentrations should be controlled to reduce the risk of ectopic calcification. |
| Alk Phos | Monthly | • A fall in serum Alk Phos level often precedes the appearance of ↑Ca. |
| Renal function | Periodically | • Increased risk of ↑Ca in renal impairment. |
| Ophthalmological examination | | • To check for ectopic calcification. |
| Signs/symptoms of toxicity | | • Typically these are: persistent constipation or diarrhoea, constant headache, loss of appetite, mental changes. |

## Additional information

| | |
|---|---|
| Common and serious undesirable effects | ↑Ca (persistent constipation or diarrhoea, constant headache, vertigo, loss of appetite, polyuria, thirst, sweating), rash. Rarely nephrocalcinosis, pruritus, urticaria. |
| Pharmacokinetics | Formation of 1,25 dihydroxycholecalciferol occurs within 1 hour after IV injection and peak concentrations are reached in 2-5 hours. Elimination half-life of the formed 1,25 dihydroxycholecalciferol is 14-30 hours. |
| Significant interactions | Injectable preparation contains ethanol and propylene glycol: may interact with disulfiram and metronidazole. |
| Action in case of overdose | *Symptoms to watch for:* ↑Ca. Stop treatment until plasma Ca levels return to normal (about 1 week). Restart treatment at half the previous dose if appropriate. |
| Counselling | Advise to report symptoms of ↑Ca: persistent constipation or diarrhoea, constant headache, vertigo, loss of appetite, polyuria, thirst, sweating. Advise of the need for further blood tests. |

| | |
|---|---|
| Risk rating: **GREEN** | Score = 1 <br> Lower-risk product: Risk-reduction strategies should be considered. |

This assessment is based on the full range of preparation and administration options described in the monograph. These may not all be applicable in some clinical situations.

## Bibliography

SPC One-Alpha injection (accessed 25 January 2009).

# Alteplase (recombinant tissue-type plasminogen activator, rt-PA, TPA)

**10-mg, 20-mg and 50-mg dry powder vials with solvent (WFI)**

- Alteplase is a form of endogenous tissue plasminogen activator produced by recombinant DNA technology. It has thrombolytic activity.
- It is licensed for the dissolution of clots in MI, acute massive PE with haemodynamic instability and acute ischaemic stroke.
- It has also been used (unlicensed) to dissolve clots in a variety of other circumstances.
- Each 1 mg of alteplase provides 580 000 units of human recombinant tissue plasminogen activator activity.

## Pre-treatment checks

* Contraindicated in recent haemorrhage, trauma, or surgery (including dental extraction); coagulation defects; bleeding diatheses; aortic dissection; aneurysm; coma; history of cerebrovascular disease, especially recent events or with any residual disability; recent symptoms of possible peptic ulceration; heavy vaginal bleeding; severe ↑BP; active pulmonary disease with cavitation; acute pancreatitis; pericarditis; bacterial endocarditis; severe liver disease; and oesophageal varices.
* Caution in acute stroke; monitor for intracranial haemorrhage; monitor BP (antihypertensive recommended if systolic >180 mmHg or diastolic >105 mmHg).
* Use with caution if there is a risk of bleeding including that from venepuncture or invasive procedures.
* Caution in external chest compression, pregnancy, elderly (contraindicated if >80 years), ↑BP, conditions in which thrombolysis might give rise to embolic complications such as enlarged left atrium with atrial fibrillation (risk of dissolution of clot and subsequent embolisation), and recent or concurrent use of drugs that ↑risk of bleeding.
* Administration of aspirin or IV heparin should be avoided in the first 24 hours after treatment but if heparin is required for other indications the dose should not exceed 10 000 units per day SC.

**Additional contraindications in acute myocardial infarction/acute pulmonary embolism:** known history of ischaemic stroke or TIA in the preceding 6 months, except current acute ischaemic stroke within 3 hours.

**Additional contraindications in acute ischaemic stroke:** convulsion accompanying stroke, severe stroke, history of stroke in patients with diabetes, stroke in last 3 months, hypoglycaemia, hyperglycaemia.

*Biochemical and other tests (not all are necessary in an emergency situation)*

Blood glucose – do not give if <2.8 or >22 mmol/L.

Blood pressure and pulse – do not give if systolic BP >185 or diastolic BP >110 mmHg, or if aggressive management (IV pharmacotherapy) is necessary to reduce BP to these limits.

Bodyweight (in certain indications).

FBC – do not give if platelets <100 000/mm$^3$.

LFTs – do not give in severe disease.

## Dose

**Myocardial infarction within 6 hours of symptom onset (patients ≥65 kg):** 15 mg by IV injection, then 50 mg by IV infusion over 30 minutes, then 35 mg by IV infusion over 60 minutes (total dose 100 mg over 90 minutes).

**Myocardial infarction within 6 hours of symptom onset (patients <65 kg):** 15 mg by IV injection, then 0.75 mg/kg by IV infusion over 30 minutes, then 0.5 mg/kg by IV infusion over 60 minutes (maximum total dose 100 mg over 90 minutes).

**Myocardial infarction between 6 and 12 hours of symptom onset (patients ≥65 kg):** 10 mg by IV injection, then 50 mg by IV infusion over 60 minutes, then 40 mg by IV infusion over 2 hours (total dose 100 mg over 3 hours).

**Myocardial infarction between 6 and 12 hours of symptom onset (patients <65 kg):** as above up to a total dose of 1.5 mg/kg over 3 hours.

**Pulmonary embolism (patients ≥65 kg):** 10 mg by IV injection followed by 90 mg by IV infusion over 2 hours.

**Pulmonary embolism (patients <65 kg):** as above up to a total dose of 1.5 mg/kg (maximum total dose 100 mg).

**Acute ischaemic stroke within 3 hours of symptom onset:** calculate the total dose, i.e. 900 micrograms/kg (maximum total dose 90 mg). Give 10% of the total dose by IV injection and the remainder by IV infusion over 60 minutes.

**Central venous catheter occlusion (unlicensed):** a 1 mg/mL solution has been used instilled into the catheter. A typical dose is 2 mg, repeated after 2 hours if necessary (maximum total dose 4 mg).

**Intracardiac thrombosis of prosthetic heart valves (unlicensed):** 100 mg has been given by IV infusion over 2 hours.

**Peripheral arterial thromboembolism (unlicensed):** doses of 0.2–1 mg/hour by intra-arterial infusion have been commonly used.

**Removal of distal clots during a surgical procedure (unlicensed):** alteplase has been given intra-arterially as three doses of 5 mg at 10-minute intervals.

## Intravenous injection

*Preparation and administration*

Alteplase is incompatible with Gluc solutions.

1. Calculate the volume of solvent (WFI) to produce a solution containing 1 or 2 mg/mL.
2. Using a syringe and wide-bore needle or the manufacturer's transfer device (only for 1 mg/mL solutions), direct the stream of WFI directly into the lyophilised cake.
3. Gently swirl the vial (do not shake) to dissolve the drug. Allow to stand if necessary to dissipate bubbles.
4. Withdraw the required dose.
5. The solution should be clear and colourless to pale yellow. Inspect visually for particulate matter or discoloration prior to administration and discard if present.
6. Give by IV injection over 1–2 minutes.

## Intravenous infusion

*Preparation and administration*

Alteplase is incompatible with Gluc solutions.

1. Calculate the volume of solvent (WFI) to produce a solution containing 1 mg/mL.
2. Using a syringe and wide-bore needle or the manufacturer's transfer device (if available), direct the stream of WFI directly into the lyophilised cake.
3. Gently swirl the vial (do not shake) to dissolve the drug. Allow to stand if necessary to dissipate bubbles.
4. Withdraw the required dose (bearing in mind that infusion solutions are only stable for up to 8 hours at room temperature).
5. The solution may be infused at the 1 mg/mL concentration as prepared.
6. Alternatively dilute to 5 times the volume with NaCl 0.9% to give a solution containing 0.2 mg/mL.
7. The solution should be clear and colourless to pale yellow. Inspect visually for particulate matter or discoloration prior to administration and discard if present.
8. Give by IV infusion via a volumetric infusion device at a rate appropriate to the indication. Prepare a fresh infusion solution every 8 hours if required.

| Technical information | |
|---|---|
| Incompatible with | Alteplase is incompatible with Gluc solutions.<br>Bivalirudin, dobutamine, dopamine, glyceryl trinitrate, heparin sodium. |
| Compatible with | **Flush**: NaCl 0.9%<br>**Solutions**: NaCl 0.9%<br>**Y-site**: Lidocaine, metoprolol |
| pH | 6.8–7.8 |

*(continued)*

## Technical information (continued)

| | |
|---|---|
| Sodium content | Negligible |
| Storage | Store below 25°C in original packaging. Protect from light. |
| Displacement value | Negligible |
| Stability after preparation | From a microbiological point of view, should be used immediately; however: Reconstituted vials and prepared infusions may be stored at 2-8°C and given (at room temperature) within 24 hours. Prepared infusions are stable at room temperature for up to 8 hours. |

## Monitoring

| Measure | Frequency | Rationale |
|---|---|---|
| **In treatment of myocardial infarction** | | |
| Heart rate | Continuously | • ↓Pulse may result from reperfusion. |
| ECG | | • Arrhythmias may result from reperfusion. |
| Blood pressure | | • ↓BP may occur. Raise legs and slow or stop infusion temporarily. |
| **In treatment of ischaemic stroke** | | |
| Blood pressure and neurological observations | Continuously | STOP infusion if: <br> • Marked ↓BP. <br> • Neurological deterioration, i.e. <br>   – Conscious level (2 points GCS eye/motor score) <br>   – NIHSS >4 points. <br> • ↑BP >185/110 mmHg if sustained or associated with neurological deterioration. |

## Additional information

| | |
|---|---|
| Common and serious undesirable effects | *Immediate:* Anaphylaxis and other hypersensitivity reactions have been reported rarely. <br> *Injection/infusion-related:* Local: Haemorrhage at injection site. <br> *Other:* Bleeding, ↓BP, ↑or ↓pulse, coronary artery reperfusion events, e.g. rhythm disorders, nausea, vomiting, headache, muscle pain, fever. |
| Pharmacokinetics | Elimination half-life is around 40 minutes. |
| Significant interactions | • The following may ↑risk of haemorrhage with alteplase: anticoagulants, heparins, antiplatelet agents, e.g. aspirin, clopidogrel, dipyridamole, GP IIb/IIIa inhibitors. |
| Action in case of overdose | *Symptoms to watch for:* Severe bleeding. <br> *Antidote:* No specific antidote. Stop administration and give supportive therapy as appropriate including fresh frozen plasma, fresh blood and tranexamic acid if necessary. |
| Counselling | Report bleeding events. |

| Risk rating: **AMBER** | Score = 3<br>Moderate-risk product. Risk-reduction strategies are recommended |
|---|---|

This assessment is based on the full range of preparation and administration options described in the monograph. These may not all be applicable in some clinical situations.

## Bibliography

SPC Actilyse (accessed 31 March 2010).

# Amikacin

**100 mg/2 mL, 500 mg/2 mL solution in vials**
* Amikacin sulfate is a semi-synthetic aminoglycoside antibiotic derived from kanamycin A.
* It is used similarly to gentamicin in the treatment of severe Gram-negative and other infections.
* Doses are expressed in terms of the base: Amikacin 1 g $\cong$ 1.3 g amikacin sulfate.

## Pre-treatment checks

* Do not use in myasthenia gravis.
* Use with caution in patients with eighth cranial nerve damage.
* Ensure patient is well hydrated prior to during treatment.

*Biochemical and other tests*

Bodyweight
Renal function: U, Cr, CrCl (or eGFR)

## Dose

**Standard dose**: 7.5 mg/kg every 12 hours, increased to 7.5 mg/kg every 8 hours in severe infections.
**Life-threatening infections and/or those caused by *Pseudomonas*:** up to 500 mg every 8 hours and for no more than 10 days (maximum total treatment dose should not exceed 15 g).
**Dose in renal impairment**: adjusted according to creatinine clearance.[1]
* CrCl > 20–50 mL/minute: 5–6 mg/kg every 12 hours
* CrCl 10–20 mL/minute: 3–4 mg/kg every 12 hours
* CrCl <10 mL/minute: 2 mg/kg every 24–48 hours

## Intramuscular injection (preferred route, unless not feasible or in life-threatening infections)

*Preparation and administration*

1. Withdraw the required dose.
2. Give by deep IM injection into the upper outer quadrant of the buttocks.

## Intravenous injection

*Preparation and administration*

> If used in combination with a penicillin or cephalosporin, administer at a different site. If this is not possible then flush the line thoroughly with a compatible solution between drugs.

1. Withdraw the required dose.
2. The solution should be clear and colourless to pale yellow. Inspect visually for particulate matter or discoloration prior to administration and discard if present.
3. Give by IV injection over 2–3 minutes.

## Intermittent intravenous infusion

*Preparation and administration*

> If used in combination with a penicillin or cephalosporin, administer at a different site. If this is not possible then flush the line thoroughly with a compatible solution between drugs.

1. Withdraw the required dose and add to a suitable volume of compatible infusion fluid (usually 100 mL NaCl 0.9%).
2. The solution should be clear and colourless to pale yellow. Inspect visually for particulate matter or discoloration prior to administration and discard if present.
3. Give by IV infusion over 30 minutes.

## Technical information

| | |
|---|---|
| Incompatible with | Potassium chloride.<br>Aminophylline, amphotericin B, ampicillin, benzylpenicillin, cefotaxime, ceftazidime, ceftriaxone, cefuroxime, gentamicin, heparin sodium, Pabrinex, pantoprazole, phenytoin sodium, propofol, tobramycin. |
| Compatible with | **Flush**: NaCl 0.9%<br>**Solutions**: NaCl 0.9%, Gluc 5%, Hartmann's<br>**Y-site**: Aciclovir, adrenaline (epinephrine), calcium gluconate, chloramphenicol sodium succinate, ciprofloxacin, cisatracurium, clindamycin, dexamethasone, esmolol, fluconazole, furosemide, granisetron, hydrocortisone sodium succinate, labetalol, magnesium sulfate, metronidazole, midazolam, noradrenaline (norepinephrine), ondansetron, phytomenadione (mixed micelles), ranitidine, remifentanil, tigecycline, sodium bicarbonate, vancomycin, verapamil |
| pH | 3.5-5.5 |
| Sodium content | Negligible |
| Excipients | Contains sulfites (may cause hypersensitivity reactions). |
| Storage | Store below 25°C in original packaging. |
| Stability after reconstitution | From a microbiological point of view should be used immediately; however, prepared infusions may be stored at 2-8°C and infused (at room temperature) within 24 hours. |

## Monitoring

| Measure | Frequency | Rationale |
|---|---|---|
| Vestibular and auditory function | Daily | • Ototoxicity is a potential effect of over exposure to amikacin.<br>• Check there is no deterioration of balance or hearing - if there is this may be indicative of toxic levels. |
| Signs of nephrotoxicity | | • If signs of renal irritation occur, e.g. albumin, casts, red or white blood cells in urine: increase hydration and consider dosage reduction.<br>• If azotaemia or a progressive decrease in urine output occurs: stop therapy. |
| Amikacin serum concentration | See right-hand column for details of first measurement. Twice weekly in normal renal function; more frequently if renal function is impaired | • For meaningful interpretation of results the laboratory request form **must** state:<br>the time the previous dose was given<br>the time the blood sample was taken<br>• The first measurements should be made around the third dose.<br>• A trough level is taken just before this dose and should be <10 mg/L.<br>• A peak level is taken 1 hour after the dose has been given and should not exceed 30 mg/L (35 mg/L is stated in USA). |
| Renal function | Periodically | • If CrCl (or eGFR) changes a dose adjustment may be necessary. |

## Additional information

| | |
|---|---|
| Common and serious undesirable effects | Common vestibular and auditory damage, nephrotoxicity. |
| Pharmacokinetics | Elimination half-life is 2-3 hours in normal renal function. |
| Significant interactions | • Amikacin may ↑risk of nephrotoxicity with the following drugs: ciclosporin, platinum compounds, tacrolimus.<br>• Amikacin may ↑levels or effect of the following drugs (or ↑side-effects): diuretics-loop (↑risk of ototoxicity), muscle relaxants non-depolarising, suxamethonium.<br>• Amikacin may ↓levels or effect of the following drugs: neostigmine, pyridostigmine. |
| Action in case of overdose | *Antidote:* None, but haemodialysis may be effective.<br>Stop administration and give supportive therapy as appropriate. |

Risk rating: **AMBER**

Score = 3
Moderate-risk product: Risk-reduction strategies are recommended.

This assessment is based on the full range of preparation and administration options described in the monograph. These may not all be applicable in some clinical situations.

## Reference

1. Ashley C, Currie A, eds. *The Renal Drug Handbook*, 3rd edn. Oxford: Radcliffe Medical Press, 2009.

## Bibliography

SPC Amikacin 250 mg/mL injection, Hospira UK Ltd (accessed 23 February 2009).
SPC Amikin injection 100 mg/2 mL and 500 mg/2 mL (accessed 23 February 2009).

# Aminophylline

**25 mg/mL solution in 10-mL ampoules; 250 mg/mL solution in 2-mL ampoules**

* Aminophylline is a soluble complex of theophylline and rapidly liberates theophylline after injection or infusion. It relaxes bronchial smooth muscle, relieves bronchospasm, and has a stimulant effect on respiration. It also stimulates the myocardium and CNS, ↓peripheral resistance and venous pressure, and causes diuresis.
* Aminophylline IV may be used to treat acute bronchospasm including acute severe asthma and acute exacerbation of COPD.
* Aminophylline has a low therapeutic index, i.e. there is a narrow effective range outside which a dose is toxic or sub-therapeutic. Serum levels should be monitored regularly, particularly during initiation of therapy. The pharmacokinetics of theophylline are affected by several factors including age, smoking, disease, diet, and drug interactions.
* If therapeutic doses of aminophylline and/or theophylline are administered simultaneously by more than one route or in more than one preparation, the hazard of serious toxicity is increased.
* *In the UK* doses are usually expressed in terms of the base:
  Aminophylline 1 mg ≡ 1.09 mg aminophylline hydrate.
* *In the USA* aminophylline is required to be labelled in terms of anhydrous *theophylline* content:
  Aminophylline 600 micrograms ≅ 500 micrograms theophylline.

## Pre-treatment checks

* Do not use in patients hypersensitive to ethylenediamine or those allergic to xanthine derivatives, e.g. theophylline, caffeine.
* Do not use in acute porphyria.
* In patients currently receiving theophylline preparations, the loading dose should be deferred until a serum theophylline concentration can be attained or the clinician must carefully select a dose based on the potential benefits and risks. Knowledge of the time, route of administration and dosage form of the patient's last theophylline dose may inform this decision.
* Caution in patients undergoing influenza immunisation or who have active influenza infection or acute febrile illness – theophylline clearance may be reduced.
* Caution in patients with cardiac failure, COPD, renal or hepatic dysfunction and in chronic alcoholism – theophylline clearance may be reduced.
* Use with caution in patients with peptic ulcer, hyperthyroidism, glaucoma, diabetes mellitus, severe hypoxaemia, ↑BP, compromised cardiac or circulatory function and epilepsy, as these conditions may be exacerbated.
* Smoking status (tobacco or marijuana) should be determined: theophylline clearance may be increased in smokers and in those regularly exposed to tobacco smoke.

*Biochemical and other tests (not all are necessary in an emergency situation)*

*Electrolytes:* serum K

Ideal bodyweight (and therefore patient's height)

LFTs

Plasma theophylline concentration for patients already taking therapy (especially if previous dose within the past 24 hours)

## Dose

*Severe acute asthma or acute exacerbation of COPD*

> A 250 mg/mL injection is available for IM use but this route causes intense local pain and is not recommended.
> To avoid excessive dosing, doses should be calculated on the basis of ideal bodyweight (IBW) in obese patients.

**Loading dose for patients not on oral theophylline/aminophylline:** 250–500 mg ($\cong$5 mg/kg IBW) by slow IV injection over at least 20 minutes with close monitoring. Follow immediately by a maintenance infusion (see below). Loading doses are based on the expectation that 0.5 mg/kg of theophylline will result in a 1 microgram/mL increase in serum theophylline concentration.

**Loading dose for patients already on oral theophylline/aminophylline:**
- Defer treatment until serum theophylline level is available. Adjust loading dose on the basis that each 600 microgram/kg IBW of aminophylline will increase plasma theophylline concentration by 1 mg/L. Follow immediately by a maintenance infusion (see below).
- Alternatively, if there are compelling reasons to proceed omit the loading dose and start the maintenance infusion (see below).

**Maintenance dose by continuous IV infusion:**
- Initial dose:
  - Otherwise healthy non-smoking adults: 500 micrograms/kg IBW/hour
  - Elderly persons, in cor pulmonale, heart failure, or liver disease: 300 micrograms/kg IBW/hour
  - Children 10–16 years of age and young adult smokers: 700–800 micrograms/kg IBW/hour
- Adjust dose according to plasma theophylline concentration – see Monitoring in the table below.

## Intravenous injection via a syringe pump

> This method is used for the *loading* dose only – the infusion rate must be reduced after the initial 20-minute loading infusion.

*Preparation of a 10 mg/mL solution (other strengths may be used according to local policies)*

1. Withdraw 500 mg aminophylline (20 mL of 25 mg/mL solution) into a 50-mL syringe.
2. Make up to a final volume of 50 mL with Gluc 5% or NaCl 0.9%.
3. Cap the syringe and mix well to give a solution containing 10 mg/mL.
4. The solution should be clear and colourless. Inspect visually for particulate matter or discoloration prior to administration and discard if present.

*Administration*

1. Give by IV infusion using a syringe pump for 20 minutes only at the rate specified in the chart below. The rate should never exceed 25 mg/minute (150 mL/hour). If patients experience acute adverse effects while the loading dose is being infused, either stop the infusion for 5–10 minutes or give at a slower rate. Table A3 gives further guidance.
2. Discard any infusion remaining at the end of 20 minutes.

**Fluid restriction:** the maximum concentration that can be given is 25 mg/mL via a central line.

**Table A3** Aminophylline loading dose: rate of infusion using a 10 mg/mL solution

| Ideal bodyweight (kg) | Dose (mg) | Volume of 10 mg/mL containing required dose (mL) | Loading dose infusion rate for 20 minutes only (mL/hour) |
|---|---|---|---|
| 40 | 200 | 20 | 60 |
| 45 | 225 | 22.5 | 67.5 |
| 50 | 250 | 25 | 75 |
| 55 | 275 | 27.5 | 82.5 |
| 60 | 300 | 30 | 90 |
| 65 | 325 | 32.5 | 97.5 |
| 70 | 350 | 35 | 105 |
| 75 | 375 | 37.5 | 112.5 |
| 80 | 400 | 40 | 120 |
| 85 | 425 | 42.5 | 127.5 |
| 90 | 450 | 45 | 135 |

## Continuous intravenous infusion (maintenance infusion)

*Preparation of a 1 mg/mL solution (other strengths may be used according to local policies)*

1. Remove 20 mL from a 500-mL bag of Gluc 5% or NaCl 0.9% and discard.
2. Withdraw 500 mg aminophylline (20 mL of 25 mg/mL solution) and add to the prepared infusion bag.
3. Mix well to give a solution containing 1 mg/mL.
4. The solution should be clear and colourless. Inspect visually for particulate matter or discoloration prior to administration and discard if present.
5. Give by IV infusion via a volumetric infusion device at the required rate (see Table A4).
6. Prepare a fresh infusion bag at least every 24 hours if required.

**Fluid restriction:** the maximum concentration that can be given is 25 g/mL via a central line.

**Table A4** Aminophylline maintenance dose: rate of infusion using a 1 mg/mL solution

| Ideal bodyweight (kg) | 300 micrograms/kg/hour (mL/hour) | 500 micrograms/kg/hour (mL/hour) | 800 micrograms/kg/hour (mL/hour) |
|---|---|---|---|
| 40 | 12 | 20 | 32 |
| 45 | 13.5 | 22.5 | 36 |
| 50 | 15 | 25 | 40 |
| 55 | 16.5 | 27.5 | 44 |
| 60 | 18 | 30 | 48 |
| 65 | 19.5 | 32.5 | 52 |
| 70 | 21 | 35 | 56 |
| 75 | 22.5 | 37.5 | 60 |
| 80 | 24 | 40 | 64 |
| 85 | 25.5 | 42.5 | 68 |
| 90 | 27 | 45 | 72 |

## Technical information

| | |
|---|---|
| Incompatible with | Should not be allowed to come into contact with metals. Amiodarone, ciprofloxacin, cisatracurium, clarithromycin, dobutamine, hydralazine, ondansetron. |
| Compatible with | **Flush**: NaCl 0.9%<br>**Solutions**: NaCl 0.9%, Gluc 5%, Hartmann's (all with added KCl)<br>**Y-site**: Aztreonam, ceftazidime, fluconazole, foscarnet, linezolid, meropenem, micafungin, piperacillin with tazobactam, ranitidine, remifentanil, vecuronium bromide |
| pH | 8.6-10 (precipitation occurs at pH <8) |
| Sodium content | Nil |
| Excipients | Contains ethylenediamine (may cause hypersensitivity reactions). |
| Storage | Store below 25°C in original packaging. Protect from light. Do not freeze. Discard ampoule if contents discoloured. |
| Stability after preparation | Use prepared infusions immediately; change every 24 hours. |

## Monitoring

| Measure | Frequency | Rationale |
|---------|-----------|-----------|
| Plasma theophylline concentration | 30 minutes after loading dose then 4-6 hours after the start of IV infusion until target concentration is achieved. Re-check 24 hours after dose adjustments. | • Target plasma-theophylline concentration for optimum response: 10-20 mg/L (55-110 micromol/L). Toxicity is most likely to occur when plasma concentration exceeds 20 micrograms/mL.<br>• There is marked inter-patient variation in the dosage required to achieve plasma levels of theophylline within the desired therapeutic range.<br>• If theophylline concentrations are<br>  • <9.9 mg/L (<55 micromol/L): increase infusion rate by 25% if symptoms are *not* controlled and current dosage is tolerated.<br>  • 10-14.9 mg/L (55-82 micromol/L): maintain infusion rate if symptoms are controlled and current dosage is tolerated.<br>  • 15-19.9 mg/L (82.5-109 micromol/L): consider 10% decrease in infusion rate to provide greater margin of safety even if current dosage is tolerated.<br>  • 20-24.9 mg/L (110-137 micromol/L): decrease infusion rate by 25% even if no adverse effects are present.<br>  • 25-30 mg/L (137.5-165 micromol/L): stop infusion for 24 hours (in adults); re-check level before resuming. Decrease previous infusion rate by about 25%.<br>  • >30 mg/L (>165 micromol/L): stop infusion and treat overdose as indicated. If therapy is resumed, decrease subsequent infusion rate by about 50% and recheck serum concentration after 24 hours.<br>• If switching to an oral formulation, measure theophylline level at least 5 days after starting oral treatment (trough concentrations of theophylline should be taken just before the next dose). |
| ECG | During loading dose | • Can cause cardiac arrhythmias. |
| Serum K | Daily | • During regular therapy serum K levels must be monitored as ↓K may occur rapidly.<br>• This is particularly important during combination therapy with beta$_2$-agonists, corticosteroids or diuretics, or in the presence of hypoxia. |

## Additional information

| | |
|---|---|
| Common and serious undesirable effects | *Immediate:* Anaphylaxis has been reported rarely.<br>*Injection/infusion-related:*<br>• Too rapid administration: nausea, vomiting, arrhythmias, convulsions.<br>• Local: IM injections are very painful and should not be used.<br><br>*Other:* ↑Pulse, palpitations, nausea and other GI disturbances, headache, CNS stimulation, insomnia, arrhythmias. |
| Pharmacokinetics | Elimination half-life is about 8 hours in non-smoking adults; about 10-12 hours in elderly patients; about 32 hours in liver cirrhosis; about 3-5 hours in smokers. |

(continued)

## Additional information *(continued)*

| | |
|---|---|
| Significant interactions | • The following may ↑theophylline levels or effect (or ↑side-effects): aciclovir, allopurinol, azithromycin, calcium-channel blockers, cimetidine, ciprofloxacin, clarithromycin, disulfiram, doxapram, erythromycin, fluconazole, fluvoxamine, halothane, influenza vaccine, interferon alfa, isoniazid, ketamine, ketoconazole, methotrexate, norfloxacin, oestrogens, pentoxifylline, propafenone, verapamil, zafirlukast.<br>• The following may ↓theophylline levels or effect: barbiturates, carbamazepine, phenytoin, primidone, rifampicin, ritonavir, St John's Wort, sulfinpyrazone, tobacco.<br>• Risk of ↓K with the following: acetazolamide, corticosteroids, diuretics, beta2-sympathomimetics.<br>• Theophylline may ↓levels or effect of the following drugs: adenosine, benzodiazepines, lithium, phenytoin, zafirlukast. |
| Action in case of overdose | *Symptoms to watch for:* ↑Pulse, nausea, vomiting, arrhythmias and seizures (may occur even without preceding symptoms of toxicity and often result in death). Profound ↓K may develop rapidly.<br>*Antidote:* No known antidote. Consider charcoal haemoperfusion if plasma theophylline concentration >80 mg/L (acute) or >60 mg/L (chronic), or if >40 mg/L in elderly patients. Stop administration and give supportive therapy as appropriate. |

| Risk rating: **AMBER** | Score = 5<br>Moderate-risk product: Risk-reduction strategies are recommended. |
|---|---|

This assessment is based on the full range of preparation and administration options described in the monograph. These may not all be applicable in some clinical situations.

## Bibliography

SPC Aminophylline Injection, Hameln Pharmaceuticals Ltd (accessed 3 May 2010).
SPC Aminophylline Injection BP 250 mg/10 mL, Goldshield plc (accessed 3 May 2010).
SPC Aminophylline Injection BP 500 mg/2 mL, Goldshield plc (accessed 3 May 2010).

# Amiodarone hydrochloride

**50 mg/mL solution in 3-mL and 6-mL ampoules; 300 mg/10 mL solution in pre-filled syringes**
• Amiodarone hydrochloride is an antiarrhythmic with mainly class III properties.
• It is used in the control of ventricular and supraventricular arrhythmias, including arrhythmias associated with Wolff–Parkinson–White syndrome.

## Pre-treatment checks

- Do not use in: ↓pulse, sinoatrial block, AV block or other severe conduction disorders (unless the patient has a pacemaker), severe ↓BP, and severe respiratory failure.
- Caution in heart failure.
- Electrolyte disorders should be corrected before starting treatment.

*Biochemical and other tests (not all are necessary in an emergency situation)*

| | |
|---|---|
| Blood pressure and pulse | Electrolytes: serum Na, K, Ca, Mg |
| Bodyweight | LFTs (especially transaminases) |
| Chest X-ray | TFTs |
| ECG | |

## Dose

**Arrhythmias:**

- *Initial infusion:* 5 mg/kg by IV infusion over 20–120 minutes via a central venous catheter. The faster rate is used if rapid control of arrhythmias is required.
- *Subsequent infusion:* the initial dose may be followed by a subsequent infusion of approximately 15 mg/kg (up to a maximum of 1.2 g) over 24 hours. Adjust the rate according to clinical response.

As soon as an adequate response has been obtained oral therapy should be initiated concomitantly at the usual loading dose (e.g. 200 mg three times a day although this may be dependent on the duration of the IV therapy). IV therapy should then be phased out gradually according to clinical response.

**Cardiopulmonary resuscitation:** for ventricular fibrillation or pulseless tachycardia unresponsive to other interventions 150–300 mg or 5 mg/kg by IV injection. This should not be repeated for at least 15 minutes.

## Intravenous infusion

*Preparation and administration*

> Amiodarone is incompatible with NaCl 0.9%.
> Very irritant: repeated or continuous infusions should be given via a central line.

1. Withdraw the required dose and add to a suitable volume of Gluc 5% (use 250 mL for the initial infusion; use up to 500 mL for the subsequent infusion). Solutions containing less than 600 micrograms/mL in Gluc 5% are unstable.
2. The solution should be clear and colourless to pale yellow. Inspect visually for particulate matter or discoloration prior to administration and discard if present.
3. Give by IV infusion via a volumetric infusion device at the rate specified above. Do not use a drop-counting infusion device because amiodarone affects drop size.

## Intravenous injection (cardiopulmonary resuscitation only)

*Preparation and administration*

1. The pre-filled syringe containing 300 mg/10 mL is ready for use. Expel any excess amiodarone. Alternatively withdraw 3–6 mL of 50 mg/mL solution from an ampoule, dilute to 10–20 mL with Gluc 5% and mix well.
2. The solution should be clear and colourless to pale yellow. Inspect visually for particulate matter or discoloration prior to administration and discard if present.
3. Give by IV injection over a minimum of 3 minutes.

## Technical information

| | |
|---|---|
| Incompatible with | Amiodarone is incompatible with NaCl 0.9%. <br> Avoid equipment containing the plasticiser diethylhexyl phthalate (DEHP). <br> Aminophylline, bivalirudin, ceftazidime, digoxin, drotrecogin alfa (activated), furosemide, heparin sodium, imipenem with cilastatin, magnesium sulfate, micafungin, pantoprazole, piperacillin with tazobactam, sodium bicarbonate. |
| Compatible with | **Flush**: Gluc 5% <br> **Solutions**: Gluc 5% (including added KCl) <br> **Y-site**: Amikacin, benzylpenicillin, clindamycin, dobutamine, dopamine, glyceryl trinitrate, lidocaine, noradrenaline, tobramycin, vancomycin |
| pH | 4 |
| Sodium content | Nil |
| Excipients | Contains benzyl alcohol. |
| Storage | Store below 25°C in original packaging. |
| Stability after preparation | From a microbiological point of view should be used immediately; however, prepared infusions may be stored at 2-8°C and infused (at room temperature) within 24 hours. Solutions containing less than 600 micrograms/mL in Gluc 5% are unstable. |

## Monitoring

| Measure | Frequency | Rationale |
|---|---|---|
| ECG during the loading dose for: heart rate, PR, QRS, and QT interval prolongation | Continuously | • Prolongation of the QT interval is indicative of a therapeutic antiarrhythmic effect. <br> • It has been suggested that initial loading doses be continued until significant prolongation of the QT interval (10-15%) is observed; further adjustments in dosage should be based upon maintaining this percentage of QT prolongation. |
| Blood pressure | Continuous during loading dose, periodically thereafter | • ↓BP and in rare instances cardiovascular collapse can occur. |
| TFTs | 6 monthly if on long-term therapy | • Monitoring of $T_4$, $T_3$, and TSH levels is required as changes in thyroid function commonly occur requiring corrective action. <br> • Continue monitoring for several months following its discontinuation (this is particularly important in elderly patients). |
| LFTs and pulmonary function | | • Long-term therapy with oral amiodarone requires periodic monitoring for thyroid, hepatic and pulmonary function. |

## Additional information

| | |
|---|---|
| Common and serious undesirable effects | *Immediate:* Anaphylaxis has very rarely been reported. Also angioedema. *Injection/infusion-related:* <br>• Too rapid administration: ↓BP, hot flushes, sweating, nausea. <br>• Local: discomfort and inflammation if given via a peripheral vein - central line advised. Injection site reactions are common (pain, erythema, oedema, necrosis, thrombophlebitis, phlebitis). Local tissue damage may occur following extravasation. <br><br>*Other:* ↓Pulse. Long-term use: pulmonary toxicity (pneumonitis, fibrosis, pleuritis), changes in thyroid function, corneal micro deposits, photosensitivity |
| Pharmacokinetics | *Elimination half-life:* (single dose) 25 days; (chronic dose) 14-107 days (mean 52 days). |
| Significant interactions | • The following may ↑risk of ventricular arrhythmias with amiodarone (avoid combination): <br>amisulpride, antidepressants-tricyclic, arsenic trioxide, artemether with lumefantrine, atomoxetine, benperidol, chloroquine, co-trimoxazole, disopyramide, droperidol, erythromycin-parenteral, fosamprenavir, haloperidol, hydroxychloroquine, ivabradine, levofloxacin, lithium, mefloquine, mizolastine, moxifloxacin, nelfinavir, pentamidine isetionate, phenothiazines, pimozide, quinine, ritonavir, sertindole, sotalol, sulfamethoxazole, sulpiride, tolterodine, zuclopenthixol. <br>• The following may ↑amiodarone levels or effect (or ↑side-effects): atazanavir, beta-blockers (↑risk of ↓pulse and AV block), diltiazem (↑risk of ↓pulse and AV block), indinavir (avoid combination), verapamil (↑risk of ↓pulse and AV block). <br>• Amiodarone may ↑levels or effect of the following drugs (or ↑side-effects): acenocoumarol (monitor INR), dabigatran (↓dabigatran dose), digoxin (halve digoxin dose), flecainide (halve flecainide dose), phenindione (monitor INR), phenytoin (monitor levels), warfarin (monitor INR), simvastatin (↑risk of myopathy). |
| Action in case of overdose | Besides supportive measures, prolonged surveillance of the patient is required because of the long biological half of amiodarone. <br>Severe ↓pulse; if necessary beta-agonists or glucagon may be given. |
| Counselling | Phototoxicity awareness. <br>Report respiratory symptoms after long-term therapy. <br>Advise of the need for regular blood tests and for an annual ophthalmic examination. |

| | |
|---|---|
| Risk rating: **RED** | Score = 6 <br>High-risk product: Risk-reduction strategies are required to minimise these risks. |

This assessment is based on the full range of preparation and administration options described in the monograph. These may not all be applicable in some clinical situations.

**Bibliography**

SPC Cordarone X intravenous (accessed 11 March 2010).

# Amoxicillin (amoxycillin)

**250-mg, 500-mg, 1-g dry powder vials**

* Amoxicillin sodium is a penicillin.
* It is used for the treatment of infections caused by susceptible Gram-negative bacteria (e.g. *Haemophilus influenzae*, *Escherichia coli*, *Proteus mirabilis*, *Salmonella*) and also for susceptible Gram-positive bacteria (e.g. *Streptococcus pneumoniae*, enterococci, non penicillinase producing staphylococci, *Listeria*).
* Amoxicillin must not be given intrathecally (potentially fatal encephalopathy has been reported).
* Doses are expressed in terms of the base:
  Amoxicillin 1 g ≡ 1.06 g amoxicillin sodium.

## Pre-treatment checks

* Do not give if there is known hypersensitivity to penicillins.
* Caution in erythematous rashes common in glandular fever, cytomegalovirus infection, and acute or chronic lymphocytic leukaemia.
* Maintain adequate hydration with high doses.

*Biochemical and other tests*

FBC
Renal function: U, Cr, CrCl (or eGFR)

## Dose

**Standard dose**: 500 mg by IM or IV injection or IV infusion every 8 hours.

**Severe infections:** 1 g by IV injection or infusion every 6 hours.

**Listerial meningitis** (in combination with another antibiotic): 2 g by IV infusion every 4 hours for 10–14 days.

**Endocarditis** (in combination with another antibiotic if indicated): 2 g by IV infusion every 6 hours, increased to 2 g every 4 hours, e.g. in enterococcal endocarditis or in monotherapy.

**Surgical prophylaxis:** 1 g by IM or IV injection immediately before induction, followed by 500 mg 6 hours later. Check local policies.

**Dose in renal impairment**: adjusted according to creatinine clearance:[1]

* CrCl >20–50 mL/minute: Dose as in normal renal function.
* CrCl 10–20 mL/minute: dose as in normal renal function.
* CrCl <10 mL/minute: 250 mg–1 g every 8 hours (maximum 6 g/day in endocarditis).

## Intravenous injection

*Preparation and administration*

See Special handling below.

If used in combination with an aminoglycoside (e.g. amikacin, gentamicin, tobramycin), preferably administer at a different site. If this is not possible then flush the line thoroughly with a compatible solution between drugs.

1. Reconstitute each 250-mg vial with 5 mL WFI (use 10 mL for each 500-mg vial; use 20 mL for each 1-g vial).
2. Withdraw the required dose.
3. The solution should be clear and a pale straw colour (a transient pink colour or slight opalescence may appear during reconstitution). Inspect visually for particulate matter or discoloration prior to administration and discard if present.
4. Give by IV injection over 3–4 minutes.

## Intermittent intravenous infusion

*Preparation and administration*

> See Special handling below.
> Amoxicillin is incompatible with Gluc 5%, Hartmann's and KCl.
> If used in combination with an aminoglycoside (e.g. amikacin, gentamicin, tobramycin), preferably administer at a different site. If this is not possible then flush the line thoroughly with a compatible solution between drugs.

1. Reconstitute each 250-mg vial with 5 mL WFI (use 10 mL for each 500-mg vial; use 20 mL for each 1-g vial).
2. Withdraw the required dose and add to a suitable volume of NaCl 0.9% (usually 100 mL).
3. The solution should be clear and colourless to pale straw in colour (a transient pink colour or slight opalescence may appear during reconstitution). Inspect visually for particulate matter or discoloration prior to administration and discard if present.
4. Give by IV infusion over 30–60 minutes.

## Intramuscular injection

*Preparation and administration*

> See Special handling below.

1. Add 1.5 mL WFI to a 250-mg vial (use 2.5 mL for a 500-mg vial) and shake vigorously. If pain occurs, 1% lidocaine may be used for reconstitution (see the monograph Lidocaine for cautions and monitoring). Do not use the 1-g vial for IM use (two separate 500-mg injections should be given if a 1-g dose is required).
2. Withdraw the required dose.
3. Give by deep IM injection.

## Technical information

| | |
|---|---|
| Incompatible with | Amoxicillin is incompatible with Gluc 5%, Hartmann's and KCl.<br>Amikacin, ciprofloxacin, gentamicin, midazolam, tobramycin. |
| Compatible with | **Flush**: NaCl 0.9%<br>**Solutions**: NaCl 0.9%<br>**Y-site**: Lorazepam, ofloxacin |
| pH$^2$ | 8-10 |
| Sodium content | 3.3 mmol/1-g vial |
| Storage | Store below 25°C in original packaging. |

*(continued)*

## Technical information (continued)

| | |
|---|---|
| Displacement value | 0.2 mL for every 250 mg |
| Special handling | Avoid skin contact as may cause sensitisation. |
| Stability after preparation | Reconstituted vials should be used immediately.<br>From a microbiological point of view, prepared infusions should be used immediately; however, they may be stored at 2-8°C and infused (at room temperature) within 24 hours. |

## Monitoring

| Measure | Frequency | Rationale |
|---|---|---|
| Renal function | Periodically, especially if for extended duration | • Impaired renal function may occur: consider dose adjustment.<br>• Electrolyte disturbances may occur (high Na content). |
| FBC | | • Transient leucopenia, thrombocytopenia, haemolytic anaemia, neutropenia may occur. |
| Prothrombin time | | • Possible prolongation of bleeding time and defective platelet function (monitor closely if anticoagulated). |
| Signs of supra-infection or superinfection | Throughout treatment | • May result in the overgrowth of non-susceptible organisms: appropriate therapy should be commenced; treatment may need to be interrupted. |
| Development of diarrhoea | Throughout and up to 2 months after treatment | • Development of severe, persistent diarrhoea may be suggestive of *Clostridium difficile*-associated diarrhoea and colitis (pseudomembranous colitis). Discontinue drug and treat. Do not use drugs that inhibit peristalsis. |
| Patency of bladder catheters | Regularly in affected patients | • May precipitate in catheters at high doses. |

## Additional information

| | |
|---|---|
| Common and serious undesirable effects | *Immediate:* Anaphylaxis and other hypersensitivity reactions have been reported.<br>*Other:* Diarrhoea, nausea, urticaria, maculopapular rashes (often appearing > 7 days after commencing treatment), fever, joint pains and angioedema. |
| Pharmacokinetics | Elimination half-life is about 1 hour (7-20 hours in severe renal impairment). |
| Significant interactions | No significant interactions. |
| Action in case of overdose | *Symptoms to watch for:* Large doses have been associated with seizures.<br>*Antidote:* None but haemodialysis may be effective. Stop administration and give supportive therapy as appropriate. |

(continued)

## Additional information (*continued*)

| | |
|---|---|
| Counselling | During administration of high doses of amoxicillin maintain adequate fluid intake and urinary output to reduce the possibility of amoxicillin crystalluria. Women taking the combined contraceptive pill should be should be advised to take additional precautions during and for 7 days after the course. |

| | |
|---|---|
| Risk rating: **GREEN** | Score = 2<br>Lower-risk product: Risk-reduction strategies should be considered. |

This assessment is based on the full range of preparation and administration options described in the monograph. These may not all be applicable in some clinical situations.

### References

1. Ashley C, Currie A, eds. *The Renal Drug Handbook*, 3rd edn. Oxford: Radcliffe Medical Press, 2009.
2. Communication with GSK Medicines Information department.

### Bibliography

SPC Amoxicillin sodium for injection, Wockhardt UK Ltd (accessed 30 March 2010).
SPC Amoxil vials for injection 500 mg and 1 g (accessed 30 March 2010).

# Amphotericin (amphotericin B)

**See specific preparations on the following pages for injectable forms available.**
* Amphotericin is a polyene antifungal.
* It is given by IV infusion in the treatment of severe systemic fungal infections. It is the usual treatment of choice in fungal endocarditis, meningitis, peritonitis, or severe respiratory tract infections. It may be given with flucytosine in severe infections.

Amphotericin is available in four commercial forms and these preparations are **not** interchangeable. They each have specific instructions for reconstitution, test dosing (to check for potential anaphylaxis) and dosing, as stated in the sub-monographs on the following pages. Pre-treatment checks and subsequent monitoring parameters are, however, the same for all.

### Pre-treatment checks

* Do not give if there is known hypersensitivity to amphotericin or any excipients, unless in the opinion of the physician the advantages of using it outweigh the risks of hypersensitivity.
* Assess sodium status and correct any deficiency before commencing therapy to counter potential amphotericin B-induced nephrotoxicity. Some authorities recommend pre-hydrating with 1 L NaCl 0.9%.

*Biochemical and other tests*

Bodyweight

LFTs

Electrolytes: serum Na, K, Mg

Renal function: U, Cr, CrCl (or eGFR)

FBC

## Dose, preparation and administration, technical Information

See the following individual product monographs *for Abelcet, AmBisome, Amphocil* and *Fungizone* which all follow this main monograph.

| Monitoring | | |
|---|---|---|
| **Measure** | **Frequency** | **Rationale** |
| Anaphylactoid reaction | With test dose | • Although anaphylaxis is rare, a test dose followed by 30 minutes of observation is necessary. If a severe allergic reaction occurs no further doses of the preparation should be given. Ensure facilities for cardiopulmonary resuscitation are readily to hand. |
| Renal function | Daily initially, then two to three times weekly | • ↓K is common. Strategies that have been adopted to counter this include giving spironolactone or amiloride (varying doses have been used).<br>• ↓Na may occur but pre-hydrating with 1 L NaCl 0.9% may be sufficient to prevent this.<br>• If clinically significant ↓renal function consideration should be given to dose reduction or discontinuation until renal function improves, taking into account any concomitant therapy with known nephrotoxic drugs. |
| Serum magnesium | | • ↓Mg is common and may require supplementation. |
| LFTs | Weekly | • A clinical decision to discontinue therapy may be needed if abnormal LFTs are observed, i.e. ↑bilirubin, ↑Alk Phos. |
| FBC | | • A normocytic anaemia can occur due to suppression of erythropoietin production. If treatment cannot be stopped, blood transfusions or recombinant erythropoietin have been used. |
| Chills, fever, rigor, nausea and other infusion-related reactions | Observe with each infusion | • Infusion reactions are common. Prophylactic measures should only be advocated when symptoms first arise and then as premedication for subsequent infusions, e.g.<br>  • Pretreating with paracetamol, antihistamines, antiemetics may lessen these reactions, or running the infusion at a slower rate.<br>  • An IV dose of 25 mg hydrocortisone is sometimes given before or during the infusion to ↓febrile reactions.<br>  • Pethidine injection (0.5 mg/kg) has been given in patients likely to develop chills, usually 20 minutes before expected onset of chills. Some centres recommend adding 50 mg pethidine to the infusion bag (*Fungizone* only).<br>  • 500-1000 units of heparin sodium is sometimes added to the infusion bag (*Fungizone* only) to help prevent thrombophlebitis - but not if pethidine is used. |

## Additional information

| | |
|---|---|
| Common and serious undesirable effects | *Immediate:* anaphylactoid reactions.<br>*Infusion-related:* Local: pain and thrombophlebitis at injection site.<br>*Other:*<br>• Common: Headache, ↓K, ↓Mg, ↓Ca, hyperglycaemia, ↓Na, ↑pulse, vasodilatation, flushing, ↓BP, dyspnoea, diarrhoea, abdominal pain, ↑bilirubin, rash, back pain, pyrexia, rigors, chest pain.<br>• Rare: Anorexia, nausea and vomiting, diarrhoea, muscle and joint pain; anaemia; renal toxicity; also cardiovascular toxicity (including arrhythmias, BP changes), blood disorders, neurological disorders (including hearing loss, diplopia, convulsions, peripheral neuropathy, encephalopathy), abnormal liver function (see above). |
| Significant interactions | • The following may ↑side-effects with amphotericin:<br>Corticosteroids may ↓K. Acute pulmonary reactions occasionally occur during or shortly after leucocyte transfusions - try to separate these infusions over time as far as possible and monitor pulmonary function.<br>• Amphotericin may ↑effect/side-effects of the following drugs:<br>May potentiate the toxicity of digoxin due to ↓K (monitor). May enhance the curariform actions of skeletal muscle relaxants due to ↓K. |
| Action in case of overdose | No specific antidote and not haemodialysable. Monitor cardiorespiratory, ECG, ABG, renal, liver function, haematological status and serum electrolytes and give supportive therapy as required. Correct ↓BP by raising the foot of the bed and fluid resuscitation. |

| | |
|---|---|
| Risk rating: **RED** | Score = 8<br>High-risk product: Risk-reduction strategies are required to minimise these risks. |

This assessment is based on the full range of preparation and administration options described in the monograph. These may not all be applicable in some clinical situations.

### Bibliography

SPC Abelcet (accessed 3 April 2009).<br>SPC AmBisome (accessed 3 April 2009).<br>SPCs Amphocil 50 mg and 100 mg (accessed 3 April 2009).<br>SPC Fungizone Intravenous (accessed 3 April 2009).

# Abelcet (amphotericin B-phospholipid complex)

### 5 mg/mL concentrate for infusion in 20-mL vials

Amphotericin is available in four commercial forms and these preparations are **not** interchangeable. They each have specific instructions for reconstitution, test dosing (to check for potential anaphylaxis) and dosing.

Pre-treatment checks and subsequent monitoring parameters are, however, the same for all and are listed in the main Amphotericin monograph.

## Dose

**Severe systemic fungal infections in patients not responding to conventional amphotericin or to other antifungal drugs, or where toxicity or renal impairment precludes conventional amphotericin:** initial test dose of 1 mg over 15 minutes then 5 mg/kg once daily for at least 14 days.

## Intermittent intravenous infusion

*Preparation*

Check that the prescription specifies Abelcet and that the product you are using is Abelcet. Amphotericin is incompatible with NaCl 0.9% and all electrolyte solutions.

1. Allow suspension to reach room temperature then shake gently to ensure there is no yellow sediment at the bottom of the vial.
2. Withdraw the required dose (using 17- to 19-gauge needles) into one or more 20-mL syringes.
3. Replace the needles on the syringes with a 5-micron filter needle provided by the manufacturer (use a fresh needle for each syringe) and transfer to a suitable volume of Gluc 5% to give a solution containing 1 mg/mL (2 mg/mL can be used in children, patients with cardiovascular disease or patients with fluid restriction).
4. The solution should be clear and yellow in colour. Inspect visually for particulate matter or discoloration prior to administration and discard if present.

*Administration*

1. Flush the existing IV line with Gluc 5% (or use a separate line).
2. Initial test dose (prior to first dose only): Give 1 mg over 15 minutes via a volumetric infusion device, stop the infusion and observe patient carefully for signs of allergic reactions for at least 30 minutes; if no adverse effects are seen, give the remainder of the infusion.
3. Give by IV infusion via a volumetric infusion device at a rate of 2.5 mg/kg/hour (an in-line membrane filter of pore size 15 microns or more may be used).
4. Flush line again with Gluc 5% when infusion has finished.

## Abelcet – technical information

| | |
|---|---|
| Incompatible with | Amphotericin is incompatible with NaCl 0.9% and all electrolyte solutions. Amphotericin is incompatible with most drugs; care must be taken to avoid inadvertent contact in infusion lines. |
| Compatible with | **Flush**: Gluc 5%<br>**Solutions**: Gluc 5%<br>**Y-site**: Not recommended |
| pH | 5-7 |
| Sodium content | Approximately 3 mmol/vial |
| Storage | Store at 2-8°C in original packaging. Do not freeze. |
| Stability after preparation | From a microbiological point of view, should be used immediately; however, prepared infusions may be stored at 2-8°C and infused (at room temperature) within 24 hours. Shake vigorously before use. |
| Pharmacokinetics | Elimination half-life is 7 days. |

| Risk rating: **RED** | Score = 8 |
|---|---|
| | High-risk product: Risk-reduction strategies are required to minimise these risks. |

This assessment is based on the full range of preparation and administration options described in the monograph. These may not all be applicable in some clinical situations.

## Bibliography

SPC Abelcet (accessed 30 march 2010).

# AmBisome (liposomal amphotericin B)

**50-mg dry powder vials**

Amphotericin is available in four commercial forms and these preparations are **not** interchangeable. They each have specific instructions for reconstitution, test dosing (to check for potential anaphylaxis) and dosing.

Pre-treatment checks and subsequent monitoring parameters are however the same for all and are listed in the main amphotericin monograph.

## Dose

**Severe systemic or deep mycoses where toxicity (particularly nephrotoxicity) precludes use of conventional amphotericin**: initial test dose 1 mg over 10 minutes then 1 mg/kg daily increased gradually if necessary to 3 mg/kg daily; maximum 5 mg/kg daily (unlicensed dose).

**Suspected or proven infection in febrile neutropenic patients unresponsive to broad-spectrum antibacterials**: initial test dose 1 mg over 10 minutes then 3 mg/kg daily until afebrile for three consecutive days; maximum period of treatment 42 days; maximum 5 mg/kg daily (unlicensed dose).

### Intermittent intravenous infusion

*Preparation*

Check that the prescription specifies AmBisome and that the product you are using is AmBisome. Amphotericin is incompatible with NaCl 0.9% and all electrolyte solutions.

1. Reconstitute each 50-mg vial with 12 mL WFI.
2. Shake the vial vigorously for 30 seconds to completely disperse; the resultant preparation contains 4 mg/mL.
3. Visually inspect for particulate matter and continue shaking if necessary.
4. Withdraw the required dose and add (via the 5-micron filter provided) to a suitable volume of Gluc 5% to give a solution containing 0.2–2 mg/mL.
5. The solution should be clear and yellow in colour. Inspect visually for particulate matter or discoloration prior to administration and discard if present.

*Administration*

1. Flush the existing IV line with Gluc 5% (or use a separate line).
2. Initial test dose (prior to first dose only): Give 1 mg over 10 minutes via a volumetric infusion device; stop infusion for 30 minutes and observe patient carefully for signs of allergic reactions; if no adverse effects are seen give the remainder of the infusion.

3. Give by IV infusion via a volumetric infusion device over 30–60 minutes (an in-line membrane filter of pore size 1 micron or more may be used). Give doses >5 mg/kg over 2 hours.
4. Flush the line again with Gluc 5% when infusion has finished.

## AmBisome – technical information

| | |
|---|---|
| Incompatible with | Amphotericin is incompatible with NaCl 0.9% and all electrolyte solutions. Amphotericin is incompatible with most drugs; care must be taken to avoid inadvertent contact in infusion lines. |
| Compatible with | **Flush**: Gluc 5%<br>**Solutions**: Gluc 5%<br>**Y-site**: Not recommended |
| pH | 5-6 |
| Sodium content | < 0.5 mmol/vial |
| Storage | Store below 25°C in original packaging. Do not freeze. |
| Displacement value | 0.5 mL/vial but this is already accounted for in the initial reconstitution of the vial |
| Stability after preparation | From a microbiological point of view, should be used immediately; however:<br>• Reconstituted vials are single use only but may be stored at 2-8°C for 24 hours.<br>• Prepared infusions may be stored at 2-8°C and infused (at room temperature) within 24 hours. |
| Pharmacokinetics | Elimination half-life: 7-10 hours after first dose; 100-153 hours after several doses. |

| | |
|---|---|
| Risk rating: **RED** | Score – 8<br>High-risk product: Risk-reduction strategies are required to minimise these risks. |

This assessment is based on the full range of preparation and administration options described in the monograph. These may not all be applicable in some clinical situations.

## Bibliography

SPC AmBisome (accessed 30 March 2010).

# Amphocil (amphotericin B-sodium cholesteryl sulfate complex)

### 100-mg and 50-mg dry powder vials

Amphotericin is available in four commercial forms and these preparations are **not** interchangeable. They each have specific instructions for reconstitution, test dosing (to check for potential anaphylaxis) and dosing.

Pre-treatment checks and subsequent monitoring parameters are, however, the same for all and are listed in the main amphotericin monograph.

## Dose

**Severe systemic fungal infections in patients not responding to conventional amphotericin or to other antifungal drugs, or where toxicity or renal impairment precludes conventional amphotericin:** initial test dose 2 mg over 10 minutes then 1 mg/kg daily increased gradually if necessary to 3–4 mg/kg daily. Doses as high as 6 mg/kg daily have been used in some patients.

## Intermittent intravenous infusion

*Preparation*

Check that the prescription specifies Amphocil and that the product you are using is Amphocil. Amphotericin is incompatible with NaCl 0.9% and all electrolyte solutions.

1. Reconstitute each vial by rapidly injecting WFI (10 mL for a 50-mg vial; 20 mL for a 100-mg vial)
2. Shake gently to until the yellow fluid becomes clear (fluid may be opalescent); the resultant solution contains 5 mg/mL.
3. Visually inspect for particulate matter; do not use if any present.
4. Withdraw the required dose from the vial(s) and add to a suitable volume of Gluc 5% to give a solution containing 625 micrograms/mL, i.e. add each 1 mL of prepared solution to 7 mL Gluc 5%.
5. The solution should be clear and yellow in colour. Inspect visually for particulate matter or discoloration prior to administration and discard if present.

*Administration*

1. Flush the existing IV line with Gluc 5% (or use a separate line).
2. Initial test dose (prior to first dose only): Give 3.2 mL (2 mg) of the prepared infusion over 10 minutes via a volumetric infusion device then stop the infusion and observe the patient carefully for signs of allergic reaction for 30 minutes; if no adverse effects are seen give the remainder of the infusion.
3. Give by IV infusion at a rate of 1–2 mg/kg/hour via a volumetric infusion device or slower if not tolerated. Amphocil should not be filtered prior to administration and should not be given using an in-line filter.
4. Flush line again with Gluc 5% when infusion has finished.

### Amphocil – technical information

| | |
|---|---|
| Incompatible with | Amphotericin is incompatible with NaCl 0.9% and all electrolyte solutions. Amphotericin is incompatible with most drugs; care must be taken to avoid inadvertent contact in infusion lines. |
| Compatible with | **Flush**: Gluc 5%<br>**Solutions**: Gluc 5%<br>**Y-site**: Not recommended |
| pH | 6.5-7.5 |
| Sodium content | <0.5 mmol/vial |
| Storage | Store below 30°C in original packaging. |
| Displacement value | Negligible |

(continued)

## Amphocil – technical information (*continued*)

| | |
|---|---|
| Stability after preparation | From a microbiological point of view, should be used immediately; however:<br>• Reconstituted vials are single use only but may be stored at 2-8°C for 24 hours.<br>• Prepared infusions may be stored at 2-8°C and infused (at room temperature) within 24 hours. |
| Pharmacokinetics | Elimination half-life is 28-29 hours. |

| | |
|---|---|
| Risk rating: **RED** | Score = 8<br>High-risk product: Risk-reduction strategies are required to minimise these risks. |

This assessment is based on the full range of preparation and administration options described in the monograph. These may not all be applicable in some clinical situations.

## Bibliography

SPCs Amphocil 50 mg and 100 mg (accessed 30 March 2010).

# Fungizone Intravenous (conventional amphotericin B)

**50-mg (50 000 units) dry powder vials**

Amphotericin is available in four commercial forms and these preparations are **not** interchangeable. They each have specific instructions for reconstitution, test dosing (to check for potential anaphylaxis) and dosing.
Pre-treatment checks and subsequent monitoring parameters are, however, the same for all and are listed in the main amphotericin monograph.

## Dose

**Systemic fungal infections:** initial test dose of 1 mg by IV infusion over 20–30 minutes, then 250 micrograms/kg by IV infusion once daily, gradually increased over 2–4 days, if tolerated, to 1 mg/kg daily. Generally patients are maintained on the highest dose which is not accompanied by unacceptable toxicity. If there is a gap in therapy of more than 7 days, then the dose must be re-titrated up.
**Severe infections:** the daily dose may be increased to a maximum of 1.5 mg/kg either once daily or on alternate days (as the drug is excreted slowly).

### Intermittent intravenous infusion

*Preparation*

Check that the prescription specifies Fungizone and that the product you are using is Fungizone. Amphotericin is incompatible with NaCl 0.9% and all electrolyte solutions.

1. The Gluc 5% infusion fluid to be used must be pH 4.2 or above. Check each container and if pH < 4.2 add 1–2 mL of a sterile buffer solution*.
2. Rapidly add 10 mL WFI to each vial directly into the powder cake using a needle of minimum diameter 20G.
3. Shake immediately until clear to produce a 5 mg/mL colloidal solution.
4. Withdraw the required dose and add to a suitable volume of Gluc 5% (pH already checked) to give a concentration of 10 mg/100 mL or less. If given via a central line, concentrations up to 40 mg/100 mL (unlicensed) have been used.
5. The solution should be clear and yellow in colour. Inspect visually for particulate matter or discoloration prior to administration and discard if present.
6. Begin infusion immediately after dilution and protect the infusion container from light throughout administration. It is not necessary to protect giving sets from light as short-term exposure should not affect stability.

*Buffer solution contains: dibasic sodium phosphate (anhydrous) 1.59 g, monobasic sodium phosphate (anhydrous) 0.96 g, WFI to 100 mL.

*Administration*

1. Flush existing IV line with Gluc 5% (or use a separate line).
2. Initial test dose (prior to first dose only): Give 1 mg by IV infusion via a volumetric infusion device over 20–30 minutes, stop the infusion and observe patient carefully for signs of allergic reactions for at least 30 minutes; if no adverse effects are seen give the remainder of the infusion.
3. Give by IV infusion via a volumetric infusion device over 2–4 hours or longer if not tolerated (an in-line membrane filter of pore size 1 micron or greater may be used).
4. Flush line again with Gluc 5% when the infusion has finished.

## Fungizone Intravenous – technical information

| | |
|---|---|
| Incompatible with | Amphotericin is incompatible with NaCl 0.9% and all electrolyte solutions. Amphotericin is incompatible with most drugs; care must be taken to avoid inadvertent contact in infusion lines. |
| Compatible with | **Flush**: Gluc 5%<br>**Solutions**: Gluc 5%<br>**Y-site**: Not recommended |
| pH | 5.7 |
| Sodium content | <0.5 mmol/vial |
| Storage | Store at 2–8°C in original packaging. |
| Displacement value | Negligible |
| Stability after preparation | From a microbiological point of view, should be used immediately; however:<br>• Reconstituted vials are single use only but may be stored protected from light at 2–8°C for 24 hours.<br>• Use prepared infusions immediately and protect from light. |
| Pharmacokinetics | Elimination half-life is 15 days. |

| Risk rating: **RED** | Score = 8 |
|---|---|
| | High-risk product: Risk-reduction strategies are required to minimise these risks. |

This assessment is based on the full range of preparation and administration options described in the monograph. These may not all be applicable in some clinical situations.

## Bibliography

SPC Fungizone intravenous (accessed 30 March 2010).

# Ampicillin

### 500-mg dry powder vials

- Ampicillin sodium is a penicillin.
- It is used for the treatment of infections including those caused by susceptible Gram-positive organisms. It is sometimes used synergistically with aminoglycoside antibiotics.
- Doses are expressed in terms of ampicillin:
  Ampicillin 1 g $\cong$ 1.06 g ampicillin sodium.

### Pre-treatment checks

- Do not give if there is known hypersensitivity to penicillins.
- Caution in erythematous rashes common in glandular fever, cytomegalovirus infection, and acute or chronic lymphocytic leukaemia.

*Biochemical and other tests*

FBC
LFTs
Renal function: U, Cr, CrCl (or eGFR)

### Dose

If used in combination with an aminoglycoside (e.g. amikacin, gentamicin, tobramycin), preferably administer at a different site. If this is not possible then flush the line thoroughly with a compatible solution between drugs.

**Standard dose**: 500 mg by IM or IV injection or IV infusion every 4–6 hours.
**Listerial meningitis** (in combination with another antibiotic): 2 g by IV infusion every 4 hours for 10–14 days.

**Endocarditis** (in combination with another antibiotic if indicated): 2 g by IV infusion every 6 hours, increased to 2 g every 4 hours, e.g. in enterococcal endocarditis or in monotherapy.

**Dose in renal impairment**: adjusted according to creatinine clearance,[1]

*   CrCl > 20–50 mL/minute: dose as in normal renal function.
*   CrCl 10–20 mL/minute: 250 mg–2 g every 6 hours.
*   CrCl <10 mL/minute: 250 mg–1 g every 6 hours.

## Intravenous injection

*Preparation and administration*

See Special handling in Technical information below.

Ampicillin is incompatible with Hartmann's. It is incompatible with Gluc 5% (but may be injected into drip tubing over 3–4 minutes).

If used in combination with an aminoglycoside (e.g. amikacin, gentamicin, tobramycin), preferably administer at a different site. If this is not possible then flush the line thoroughly with a compatible solution between drugs.

1.  Reconstitute each 500-mg vial with 5 mL WFI.
2.  Withdraw the required dose.
3.  The solution should be clear and colourless. Inspect visually for particulate matter or discoloration prior to administration and discard if present.
4.  Give by IV injection over 3–5 minutes.

## Intermittent intravenous infusion

*Preparation and administration*

See Special handling below.

Ampicillin is incompatible with Gluc 5% and Hartmann's.

If used in combination with an aminoglycoside (e.g. amikacin, gentamicin, tobramycin), preferably administer at a different site. If this is not possible then flush the line thoroughly with a compatible solution between drugs.

1.  Reconstitute each 500-mg vial with 5 mL WFI.
2.  Withdraw the required dose and add to a suitable volume NaCl 0.9% (usually 100 mL).
3.  The solution should be clear and colourless. Inspect visually for particulate matter or discoloration prior to administration and discard if present.
4.  Give by IV infusion over 30–60 minutes.

## Intramuscular injection

*Preparation and administration*

See Special handling below.

1.  Add 1.8 mL WFI to a 500-mg vial and shake vigorously to give a solution containing 250 mg/mL.
2.  Withdraw the required dose.
3.  Give by deep IM injection.

## Technical information

| | |
|---|---|
| Incompatible with | Ampicillin is incompatible with Hartmann's. It is incompatible with Gluc 5% (but may be injected into drip tubing over 3-4 minutes). Sodium bicarbonate. Adrenaline (epinephrine), amikacin, amphotericin, calcium gluconate, cisatracurium, dopamine, erythromycin lactobionate, fluconazole, gentamicin, hydralazine, hydrocortisone sodium succinate, metoclopramide, midazolam, ondansetron, tobramycin, verapamil. |
| Compatible with | **Flush**: NaCl 0.9% <br> **Solutions**: NaCl 0.9% (including added KCl) <br> **Y-site**: Aciclovir, aztreonam, chloramphenicol sodium succinate, clarithromycin, clindamycin, esmolol, flucloxacillin, furosemide, labetalol, magnesium sulfate, metronidazole, pantoprazole, phytomenadione, propofol, remifentanil, vancomycin |
| pH | 8 10 |
| Sodium content | About 1.3 mmol/500-mg vial |
| Storage | Store below 25°C |
| Displacement value | 0.2 mL/500 mg |
| Special handling | Avoid skin contact as may cause sensitisation. |
| Stability after preparation | Reconstituted vials should be used immediately. From a microbiological point of view, prepared infusions should be used immediately; however, they may be stored at 2-8°C and infused (at room temperature) within 24 hours. |

## Monitoring

| Measure | Frequency | Rationale |
|---|---|---|
| Renal function | Periodically, especially if for extended duration | • Impaired renal function may occur: may require a dose adjustment. <br> • Electrolyte disturbances may occur (high Na content). |
| FBC | | • Transient leucopenia, thrombocytopenia, haemolytic anaemia, neutropenia may occur. |
| Prothrombin time | | • Possible prolongation of bleeding time and defective platelet function (monitor closely if anticoagulated). |
| LFTs | | • Moderate ↑AST and ↑ALT have been reported (rarely). |
| Development of diarrhoea | Throughout and up to 2 months after treatment | • Development of severe, persistent diarrhoea may be suggestive of *Clostridium difficile*-associated diarrhoea and colitis (pseudomembranous colitis). Discontinue drug and treat. Do not use drugs that inhibit peristalsis. |

*(continued)*

## Monitoring (continued)

| Measure | Frequency | Rationale |
|---------|-----------|-----------|
| Signs of supra-infection or superinfection | Throughout treatment | • May result in the overgrowth of non-susceptible organisms - appropriate therapy should be commenced; treatment may need to be interrupted. |
| Development of rash | | • A maculopapular rash sometimes occurs (often appearing more than 7 days after commencing treatment), which may or may not be related to a hypersensitivity reaction. In practice clinicians discontinue if this occurs.<br>• It should preferably not be given to patients with infectious mononucleosis since they are especially susceptible to ampicillin-induced skin rashes. |

## Additional information

| | |
|---|---|
| Common and serious undesirable effects | *Immediate:* Anaphylaxis and other hypersensitivity reactions have been reported.<br>*Other:* Diarrhoea, nausea, urticaria, maculopapular rashes (often appearing > 7 days after commencing treatment), fever, joint pains and angioedema. |
| Pharmacokinetics | Elimination half-life is 1-1.9 hours. |
| Significant interactions | No significant interactions. |
| Action in case of overdose | *Symptoms to watch for:* Large doses have been associated with seizures.<br>*Antidote:* None, haemodialysis may be effective. Stop administration and give supportive therapy as appropriate. |
| Counselling | Women taking the combined contraceptive pill should be should be advised to take additional precautions during and for 7 days after the course. |

| Risk rating: **GREEN** | Score = 2<br>Lower-risk product: Risk-reduction strategies should be considered. |
|---|---|

This assessment is based on the full range of preparation and administration options described in the monograph. These may not all be applicable in some clinical situations.

## Reference

1. Ashley C, Currie A, eds. *The Renal Drug Handbook*, 3rd edn. Oxford: Radcliffe Medical Press, 2009.

# Anidulafungin

**100-mg dry powder vials**

- Anidulafungin is a semi-synthetic echinocandin antifungal agent active against *Aspergillus* and *Candida* spp.
- It is used in the treatment of candidaemia, oesophageal candidiasis and other forms of invasive candidiasis.

## Pre-treatment checks

Do not give if there is known hypersensitivity to any echinocandin-class medicines.

*Biochemical and other tests*

Fungal culture (unknown causative organism does not prevent empirical treatment).
LFTs

## Dose

**Treatment of invasive candidiasis in adult non-neutropenic patients**: 200 mg by IV infusion on the first day, then 100 mg by IV infusion daily. The duration of therapy should be based on the patient's clinical response and usually continues for at least 14 days after the last positive culture.

## Intermittent intravenous infusion

*Preparation and administration*

NB: Anidulafungin was previously available as a dry powder vial accompanied by an ethanol-containing solvent. The preparation instructions are different for that product.

1. Reconstitute each vial with 30 mL WFI (this can take up to 5 minutes). The reconstituted solution must be further diluted within 1 hour.
2. Withdraw the entire contents of each vial to be used and add to 100 mL NaCl 0.9% or Gluc 5% (i.e. if giving a 200-mg dose, use two 100-mL bags). Each bag now contains 130 mL.
3. The solution should be clear and colourless. Inspect visually for particulate matter or discoloration prior to administration and discard if present.
4. Give each bag by IV infusion over a minimum of 90 minutes, i.e. give each bag at a maximum rate of 87 mL/hour. If giving a 200-mg dose give the bags one after the other.

## Technical information

| Incompatible with | Sodium bicarbonate. Amphotericin. |
|---|---|
| Compatible with | **Flush**: NaCl 0.9%<br>**Solutions**: NaCl 0.9%, Gluc 5%<br>**Y-site**: No information |
| pH | 3.5-5.5 |
| Sodium content | Negligible |
| Storage | Store at 2-8°C in original packaging. Do not freeze. |
| Displacement value | Negligible |

*(continued)*

## Technical information (continued)

| | |
|---|---|
| Stability after preparation | From a microbiological point of view, should be used immediately; however:<br>• Reconstituted vials may be stored at 2-8°C for 1 hour.<br>• Prepared infusions may be stored at 2-8°C and infused (at room temperature) within 24 hours. |

## Monitoring

| Measure | Frequency | Rationale |
|---|---|---|
| LFTs | Periodically | • ↑ALT, ↑AST, ↑Alk Phos, ↑bilirubin, ↑GGT are seen commonly.<br>• Patients with ↑LFTs should be monitored for evidence of worsening hepatic function and the risk/benefit of continuing therapy considered. |

## Additional information

| | |
|---|---|
| Common and serious undesirable effects | Diarrhoea, nausea, vomiting; flushing; convulsion, headache; coagulopathy, ↓K, ↑serum creatinine; rash, pruritus |
| Pharmacokinetics | Elimination half-life is about 24 hours. |
| Significant interactions | No significant interactions. |
| Action in case of overdose | No specific antidote; use general supportive measures. It is not dialysable. |

| | |
|---|---|
| Risk rating: **AMBER** | Score = 5<br>Moderate-risk product: Risk-reduction strategies are recommended. |

This assessment is based on the full range of preparation and administration options described in the monograph. These may not all be applicable in some clinical situations.

### Bibliography

SPC ECALTA 100 mg powder for concentrate for solution for infusion (accessed 9 March 2010).

# Apomorphine hydrochloride

**10 mg/mL solution in 2-mL and 5-mL ampoules, 3-mL pen injector**
**5 mg/mL solution in 10-mL pre-filled syringe (for infusion only)**

Apomorphine should be used under specialist supervision only.

- Apomorphine is a dopamine agonist.
- It is used in Parkinson disease to treat disabling motor fluctuations (or the 'on–off' phenomenon) where treatment with levodopa (plus peripheral decarboxylase inhibitor) and/or other dopamine agonists has diminished. It may be used for long-term treatment in advanced disease, or as a palliative treatment near the end of life.

## Pre-treatment checks

- Do not give to patients with respiratory depression, dementia, psychotic diseases or hepatic impairment.
- Do not give to patients who have an 'on' response to levodopa that is marred by severe dyskinesia or dystonia.
- Ensure that the patient has been initiated on domperidone (usually 20 mg three times a day) at least 2 days before therapy begins (nausea and vomiting occurs in up to 10% of patients, particularly at initiation). It may be possible to reduce or withdraw domperidone altogether once treatment is established.
- Caution in renal, pulmonary or cardiovascular disease and in patients prone to nausea and vomiting.

*Biochemical and other tests*

Blood pressure

ECG if there are any cardiovascular disorders

FBC – screen for haemolytic anaemia

LFTs

Renal function: U, Cr, CrCl (or eGFR)

## Dose

**Initiation of therapy (in hospital):**

- When the patient has received domperidone 20 mg three times a day for at least 2 days, withhold existing antiparkinsonian medication overnight to provoke an 'off' episode.
- To determine the threshold dose give 1 mg (0.1 mL) by SC injection and observe for 30 minutes for a motor response. If there is no response or an inadequate response, give 2 mg by SC injection and observe for an additional 30 minutes. Continue to increase the dose in an incremental manner, leaving a minimum of 40 minutes between injections until a satisfactory motor response is obtained.

**Maintenance therapy:**

- The previously determined dose (maximum recommended single dose 10 mg) may be given at the first signs of an 'off' episode. Absorption may vary with different injection sites so observe for 60 minutes to assess quality of response.
- The usual daily dose varies according to the patient's response, but is typically in the range of 3–30 mg given as 1–10 injections/day (sometimes as many as 12). The maximum recommended daily dose is 100 mg.

**Continuous infusion:**

- Used for patients who have shown a good 'on' response but whose overall control remains unsatisfactory using intermittent injections or who require more than 10 injections/day.
- Start at 1 mg/hour by SC infusion and increase in increments of not more than 0.5 mg/hour leaving a minimum of 4 hours between increases. Usual rate is 1–4 mg/hour. Additional intermittent injections may be given if required.
- Continuous infusions are normally given during the patient's waking hours. 24-hour infusions are not recommended unless there are severe night time problems.

## Subcutaneous injection (intermittent injection)

*Preparation and administration*

1. Withdraw the required dose from an ampoule, or if using the pen injector set the dose in accordance with the manufacturer's instructions.
2. The solution should be clear and colourless; do not use if the solution has turned green or if particles can be seen.
3. Give by SC injection into the lower abdomen or outer thigh. Rotate sites for subsequent injections.

## Subcutaneous infusion (continuous infusion)

Apomorphine injection must not be given by the IV route.
Do not mix with WFI – this can lead to nodule formation and ulceration.

*Preparation and administration*

1. Withdraw the required dose using ampoules or the 5 mg/mL pre-filled syringe.
2. If using 10 mg/mL ampoules the solution may be diluted with an equal volume of NaCl 0.9% before administration to reduce local SC reactions.
3. The solution should be clear and colourless; do not use if the solution has turned green or if particles can be seen.
4. Give by continuous SC infusion by a mini pump or syringe driver, changing the infusion site every 12 hours.

## Technical information

| | |
|---|---|
| Incompatible with | Do not mix with WFI - this can lead to nodule formation and ulceration. |
| Compatible with | **Flush**: Not relevant<br>**Solutions**: NaCl 0.9%<br>**Y-site**: Not relevant |
| pH | 3-4 |
| Sodium content | Negligible |
| Excipients | Contains sulfites (may cause allergic reactions). |
| Storage | Store below 25°C in original packaging.<br>Discard each pen injector no more than 48 hours from first use. Ampoules and pre-filled syringe are for single use only: discard any unused solution. |
| Stability after preparation | From a microbiological point of view, should be used immediately; however, prepared infusions may be stored at 2-8°C and infused (at room temperature) within 24 hours. |

## Monitoring

| Measure | Frequency | Rationale |
|---|---|---|
| Reduction in rigidity, tremor and gait disturbance | At initiation then periodically | • To ensure clinical improvement. |
| Renal function | | • Use with caution in renal impairment. |
| LFTs | | • Do not give to patients with hepatic impairment. |
| Blood pressure | | • Can cause ↓BP. |
| ECG | | Use with caution in cardiovascular disease, may cause QT prolongation. |

*(continued)*

## Monitoring (continued)

| Measure | Frequency | Rationale |
|---------|-----------|-----------|
| FBC | 6 monthly | • May cause haemolytic anaemia (if this occurs refer to haematologist for advice - may need to stop treatment). |

## Additional information

| | |
|---|---|
| Common and serious undesirable effects | *Injection/infusion-related:* Local: SC nodules, induration, erythema, tenderness, irritation, itching, bruising, pain.<br>*Other:* Nausea, vomiting, sedation (including sudden onset of sleep) and neuropsychiatric disturbances. |
| Pharmacokinetics | Elimination half-life is 30-60 minutes. |
| Significant interactions | No significant interactions are known. |
| Action in case of overdose | There is little experience of overdose by the SC route. Give supportive therapy as appropriate. |
| Counselling | Instruct on how to use the device.<br>Discuss side-effects as stated above. |

Risk rating: **AMBER**    Score = 5
Moderate-risk product: Risk-reduction strategies are recommended.

This assessment is based on the full range of preparation and administration options described in the monograph. These may not all be applicable in some clinical situations.

### Bibliography

SPC APO-go Ampoules (accessed 6 October 2008).
SPC APO-go PFS (accessed 6 October 2008).
SPC APO-go Pen (accessed 6 October 2008).

# Aripiprazole

**7.5 mg/mL solution in 1.3-mL vial**
• Aripiprazole is an atypical antipsychotic.
• It is used IM for the rapid control of agitation and disturbed behaviour in patients with schizophrenia or mania when oral therapy is not appropriate.

## Pre-treatment checks

- Review physical health; aripiprazole should be used with caution in patients with cerebrovascular disease, conditions that would predispose patients to ↓BP (dehydration, hypovolaemia, and treatment with antihypertensive medications) or ↑BP, including accelerated or malignant.
- Caution should be taken if patient is already taking medication which is known to cause QT prolongation or electrolyte imbalance.
- Seizures are rare with aripiprazole but it should be used with care in those with a history of seizures or with conditions that lower the seizure threshold.
- Consider medication already administered for maintenance or acute treatment of schizophrenia or mania.

*Biochemical and other tests (not all are necessary in an emergency situation)*

Blood pressure                                    Pulse
ECG                                               Respiratory rate

## Dose

**Initial dose:** usual dose is 9.75 mg (1.3 mL) by IM injection, although the effective dose range is 5.25–15 mg (0.7–2 mL).

**Further doses:** if required a second injection may be given 2 hours after the first injection but no more than three injections should be given in any 24-hour period. The maximum daily dose is 30 mg by all routes.

Patients should be switched to oral therapy as soon as possible if ongoing treatment is required.

## Intramuscular injection

*Preparation and administration*

1. Withdraw the required dose.
2. Give by IM injection into the deltoid muscle or deep within the gluteus maximus muscle.

## Technical information

| Incompatible with | Not relevant |
|---|---|
| Compatible with | Not relevant |
| pH | Not relevant |
| Sodium content | Negligible |
| Storage | Store below 30°C in original packaging. Use opened vials immediately and discard any unused solution. |

## Monitoring

| Measure | Frequency | Rationale |
|---|---|---|
| Blood pressure | For at least 4 hours after injection | • May cause orthostatic ↓BP. |
| Pulse | | • May cause ↑pulse. |
| Respiratory rate | | • May cause sedation. |
| Level of consciousness | | • May cause sedation; particular care should be taken if IM benzodiazepine also administered. |

## Additional information

| | |
|---|---|
| Common and serious undesirable effects | Somnolence, dizziness, headache, akathisia, nausea, vomiting, ↑pulse, neuroleptic malignant syndrome. |
| Pharmacokinetics | Peak plasma levels are reached between 1-3 hours. Elimination half-life is 75-146 hours. |
| Significant interactions | • The following may ↑aripiprazole levels or effect (or ↑side-effects): anaesthetics-general (↑risk of ↓BP), artemether with lumefantrine (avoid combination), lorazepam (↑risk of ↓BP), ritonavir, sibutramine (avoid combination). <br> • The following may ↑aripiprazole levels (↓aripiprazole dose): atazanavir, fluoxetine, fosamprenavir, indinavir, itraconazole, ketoconazole, lopinavir, nelfinavir, paroxetine, ritonavir, saquinavir. <br> • The following may ↓aripiprazole levels (↑aripiprazole dose): carbamazepine, efavirenz, nelfinavir, nevirapine, phenobarbital, phenytoin, primidone, rifabutin, rifampicin, St. John's Wort. <br> • Aripiprazole may ↓levels or effect of levodopa. <br> • Aripiprazole may ↑risk of ventricular arrhythmias with the following drugs: antiarrhythmics, antidepressants-tricyclic, atomoxetine, methadone. <br> • Aripiprazole ↓convulsive threshold and may ↓effect of the following drugs: barbiturates, carbamazepine, ethosuximide, oxcarbazepine, phenytoin, primidone, valproate. |
| Action in case of overdose | Give supportive therapy as appropriate. |

| | |
|---|---|
| Risk rating: **AMBER** | Score = 2 <br> Moderate-risk product: Risk-reduction strategies are recommended. |

This assessment is based on the full range of preparation and administration options described in the monograph. These may not all be applicable in some clinical situations.

## Bibliography

SPC Abilify (accessed 15 April 2009).

# Ascorbic acid (vitamin C)

**500 mg/5 mL solution ampoule**

• Ascorbic acid and its calcium and sodium salts have vitamin C activity. Vitamin C is a water-soluble vitamin essential for the synthesis of collagen and intercellular material.
• Deficiency leads to the development of scurvy characterised by capillary fragility, bleeding (especially from small blood vessels and the gums), normocytic or macrocytic anaemia, cartilage and

bone lesions, and slow healing of wounds. Deficiency develops when dietary intake is inadequate and may occur in infants and alcoholics. It is rare in adults, but less florid manifestations of vitamin C deficiency are commonly found, particularly in elderly patients.

* Patients taking high-dose ascorbic acid for prolonged periods may become tolerant to it and exhibit symptoms of deficiency when intake is reduced to normal.

## Pre-treatment checks

* Large doses can cause haemolysis in patients with G6PD deficiency.
* Large doses may cause hyperoxaluria and renal oxalate calculi. This is more likely in dehydrated individuals.

## Dose

Ascorbic acid is usually given orally. If oral administration is not feasible or when malabsorption is suspected, utilisation is reportedly better after IM administration.

**For scurvy:** 250 mg (parenteral) once or twice daily should reverse skeletal changes and haemorrhagic disorders within 2–21 days.

**Prevention of scurvy:** 50–200 mg daily (oral or parenteral).

## Intramuscular injection (preferred route if parenteral administration is necessary)

*Preparation and administration*

1. Withdraw the required dose.
2. Inject slowly high into the gluteal muscle, 5 cm below the iliac crest. Rotate injection sites for subsequent injections.

## Intermittent intravenous infusion

*Preparation and administration*

1. Withdraw the required dose and add to 100 mL NaCl 0.9% or Gluc 5%.
2. The solution should be clear and colourless. Inspect visually for particulate matter or discoloration prior to administration and discard if present.
3. Give by IV infusion over 15–30 minutes.

## Subcutaneous injection

*Preparation and administration*

1. Withdraw the required dose.
2. Give by SC injection.

| Technical information | |
|---|---|
| Incompatible with | Aminophylline, benzylpenicillin, chloramphenicol sodium succinate, doxapram, erythromycin lactobionate, hydrocortisone sodium succinate, propofol, sodium bicarbonate. |
| Compatible with | **Flush**: NaCl 0.9%<br>**Solutions**: NaCl 0.9%, Gluc 5%, Gluc-NaCl, Hartmann's, Ringer's<br>**Y-site**: Amikacin, calcium gluconate, metoclopramide, verapamil |
| pH | 5.5–6.5 |

(continued)

## Technical information (continued)

| | |
|---|---|
| Sodium content | Negligible |
| Excipients | Contains sulfites (may cause allergic reactions). |
| Storage | Store below 25°C in original packaging. |
| Stability after preparation | From a microbiological point of view, should be used immediately; however, prepared infusions may be stored at 2-8°C and infused (at room temperature) within 24 hours. |

## Monitoring

| Measure | Frequency | Rationale |
|---|---|---|
| Fluid balance | Regularly during treatment | • Dehydration increases the likelihood of renal oxalate calculi formation. |
| Ability to urinate | Daily | • High-dose ascorbic acid can cause renal oxalate calculi. |

## Additional information

| | |
|---|---|
| Common and serious undesirable effects | Large doses of ascorbic acid have resulted in haemolysis in G6PD deficiency. |
| Pharmacokinetics | Ascorbic acid is widely distributed in the body tissues. Doses in excess of the body's needs are rapidly eliminated unchanged in the urine; this generally occurs with intakes exceeding 100 mg daily. |
| Significant interactions | • Ascorbic acid should not be given for the first month after starting desferrioxamine as it can initially worsen iron toxicity.<br>• Ascorbic acid may interfere with a number of tests based on oxidation-reduction reactions. |
| Action in case of overdose | Stop treatment and give supportive therapy as appropriate. |

| | |
|---|---|
| Risk rating: **GREEN** | Score = 1<br>Lower-risk product: Risk-reduction strategies should be considered. |

This assessment is based on the full range of preparation and administration options described in the monograph. These may not all be applicable in some clinical situations.

## Bibliography

SPC Ascorbic acid 500 mg/5 mL BPC UCB Pharma (accessed 20 October 2008).
SPC Pabrinex Intravenous High Potency Injection, Archimedes Pharma (accessed 20 October 2008).
SPC Desferal Novartis (accessed 20 October 2008).

# Atenolol

**500 micrograms/mL solution in 10-mL ampoules**
* Atenolol is a cardioselective beta-adrenoceptor blocker.
* It is used IV for the early management of suspected acute myocardial infarction within 12 hours of onset of chest pain, and in management of arrhythmias.

## Pre-treatment checks

* Atenolol is likely to worsen pre-existing uncontrolled heart failure, ↓BP, bradyarrhythmias or obstructive airways disease and the risk/benefits should be considered before use.
* Use with extreme caution in asthmatics.
* Dosage requirements may be reduced in patients with impaired renal function.

*Biochemical and other tests*

Blood pressure                          Pulse
Bodyweight (for infusion)               Renal function: U, Cr, CrCl (or eGFR)

## Dose

**Myocardial infarction:** 5 mg (10 mL) by IV injection followed by oral beta-blocker therapy as appropriate.
**Cardiac arrhythmias, by IV injection:** 2.5 mg (5 mL) by IV injection. This dose may be repeated at 5-minute intervals until an adequate response is attained, up to a maximum dosage of 10 mg. The cumulative dose can be repeated every 12 hours until oral beta-blocker therapy is appropriate.
**Cardiac arrhythmias, by IV infusion:** 150 micrograms/kg by intermittent IV infusion.
Required dose of atenolol injection in mL: (150 micrograms/kg) = bodyweight (kg) × 0.3.
This dose can be repeated every 12 hours until oral beta-blocker therapy is appropriate.

## Intravenous injection

*Preparation and administration*

1. Withdraw the required dose.
2. The solution should be clear and colourless. Inspect visually for particulate matter or discoloration prior to administration and discard if present.
3. Give by IV injection at a maximum rate of 1mg/minute (2 mL/minute).

## Intermittent intravenous infusion

*Preparation and administration*

1. Withdraw the required dose.
2. Add to a suitable volume (usually 100 mL) of NaCl 0.9% or Gluc 5%.

3. The solution should be clear and colourless. Inspect visually for particulate matter or discoloration prior to administration and discard if present.
4. Give by IV infusion over 20 minutes.

## Technical information

| | |
|---|---|
| Incompatible with | Amphotericin |
| Compatible with | **Flush**: NaCl 0.9%<br>**Solutions**: NaCl 0.9%, Gluc 5%, Gluc-NaCl<br>**Y-site**: Meropenem, morphine sulfate |
| pH | 5.5-6.5 |
| Sodium content | Negligible |
| Storage | Store below 25°C in original packaging. |
| Stability after preparation | From a microbiological point of view, should be used immediately; however, prepared infusions may be stored at 2-8°C and infused (at room temperature) within 24 hours. |

## Monitoring

| Measure | Frequency | Rationale |
|---|---|---|
| Pulse | Continuously | • Consider withholding therapy if pulse drops to 50-55 bpm or lower.<br>• Excessive ↓pulse can be countered with IV atropine sulfate in doses of 600 micrograms repeated every 3-5 minutes up to a maximum of 2.4 mg. |
| Blood pressure | | • Stop dosing if ↓BP occurs that requires corrective measures. |
| Respiratory function or oxygen saturation in at risk individuals | After initial dosing | • May cause bronchoconstriction in susceptible individuals, e.g. patients with history of bronchospasm or respiratory disease. |

## Additional information

| | |
|---|---|
| Common and serious undesirable effects | • ↓Pulse, ↓BP, cold extremities.<br>• Bronchospasm may occur in patients with asthma or other respiratory disease. |
| Pharmacokinetics | Approximately 6 hours (longer in renal impairment) |
| Significant interactions | • The following may ↑atenolol levels or effect (or ↑side-effects): adrenaline (risk of severe ↑BP and ↓pulse), alpha-blockers (severe ↓BP), amiodarone (risk of ↓pulse and AV block), antiarrhythmics (risk of myocardial depression), clonidine (↑risk of withdrawal ↑BP), diltiazem (risk of ↓pulse and AV block), dobutamine (risk of severe ↑BP and ↓pulse), flecainide (risk of myocardial depression and ↓pulse), moxisylyte (severe ↓BP), nifedipine (severe ↓BP and heart failure), noradrenaline (risk of severe ↑BP and ↓pulse), verapamil (risk of asystole and severe ↓BP). |

(continued)

## Additional information (*continued*)

| | |
|---|---|
| Action in case of overdose | *Symptoms to watch for:* ↓Pulse, ↓BP, acute cardiac insufficiency and bronchospasm.<br>*Antidote:*<br>• Excessive ↓pulse can be countered with IV atropine sulfate (see Monitoring above and the Atropine sulfate monograph).<br>• Glucagon or dobutamine are further options for unresponsive ↓pulse - seek specialist advice.<br>• Bronchospasm can usually be reversed by bronchodilators. |
| Counselling | Patients may experience fatigue and cold extremities during maintenance therapy, and should report wheezing. |

| | |
|---|---|
| Risk rating: **AMBER** | Score = 3<br>Moderate-risk product: Risk-reduction strategies are recommended. |

This assessment is based on the full range of preparation and administration options described in the monograph. These may not all be applicable in some clinical situations.

### Bibliography

SPC Tenormin (accessed 5 January 2009).

# Atosiban

**6.75 mg/0.9 mL solution in vials**
**7.5 mg/mL solution in 5-mL vials**

• Atosiban is a peptide analogue of oxytocin, which acts as an oxytocin receptor antagonist.
• It is used to delay imminent uncomplicated premature labour presenting at 24–33 weeks' gestation.
• Atosiban is given IV as the acetate, but doses are expressed in terms of the base.

## Pre-treatment checks

• Contraindicated in eclampsia and severe pre-eclampsia, intrauterine infection, intrauterine fetal death, antepartum haemorrhage (requiring immediate delivery), placenta praevia, abruptio placenta, intrauterine growth restriction with abnormal fetal heart rate, premature rupture of membranes after 30 weeks' gestation.
• Atosiban is not licensed for use in any conditions of the mother or fetus in which continuation of pregnancy is hazardous, so a full examination of mother and fetus should be carried out to ensure that the presentation is uncomplicated.

*Biochemical and other tests*

Cervical dilatation (1–3 cm, or 0–3 cm for women who have not previously given birth), cervical effacement ($\geq$50%).

Gestational age (from 24 to 33 completed weeks).

LFTs (there is insufficient clinical trial data to support use in hepatic impairment, so caution is advised).

Patient age ($\geq$18 years).

Rate and duration of uterine contractions (minimum 30 seconds duration at a rate of $\geq$4 per 30 minutes).

Renal function: U, Cr, CrCl (or eGFR) (there is insufficient clinical trial data to support use in renal impairment, so caution is advised).

## Dose

Treatment is divided into three stages:

1. An initial dose of 6.75 mg/0.9 mL is given by IV injection over 1 minute.
2. A loading dose of 300 micrograms/minute is given by IV infusion for 3 hours.
3. A further 100 micrograms/minute by IV infusion is given for up to 45 hours. The total duration of treatment should not exceed 48 hours, and the total dose of atosiban should not exceed 330 mg per course of treatment.

## Intravenous injection

*Preparation and administration*

1. Using the 6.75 mg/0.9 mL vial withdraw the required dose.
2. The solution should be clear and colourless. Inspect visually for particulate matter or discoloration prior to administration and discard if present.
3. Give by IV injection over 1 minute.

## Intravenous infusion

*Preparation*

1. Remove 10 mL from a 100-mL bag of NaCl 0.9% or Gluc 5% and discard.
2. Using two 5-mL vials withdraw 75 mg (10 mL) of atosiban and add to the prepared infusion bag. Mix well to give a solution containing atosiban 750 micrograms/mL.
3. The solution should be clear and colourless. Inspect visually for particulate matter or discoloration prior to administration and discard if present.

*Administration*

1. Give by IV infusion using a volumetric infusion device at a rate of 24 mL/hour (18 mg/hour) for the 3-hour loading period.
2. Reduce the rate of infusion to 8 mL/hour (6 mg/hour) for up to 45 hours as required.
3. Prepare replacement infusion bags as necessary to ensure that the infusion can continue to run.

| Technical information | |
|---|---|
| Incompatible with | No information |
| Compatible with | **Flush**: NaCl 0.9%<br>**Solutions**: NaCl 0.9%, Gluc 5%, Hartmann's<br>**Y-site**: No information |
| pH | 4.5 |

*(continued)*

## Technical information (*continued*)

| | |
|---|---|
| Sodium content | Nil |
| Storage | Store at 2-8°C in original packaging.<br>Use opened vials immediately and discard any unused solution. |
| Stability after preparation | From a microbiological point of view, should be used immediately; however, prepared infusions may be stored at 2-8°C and infused (at room temperature) within 24 hours. |

## Monitoring

| Measure | Frequency | Rationale |
|---|---|---|
| Physical evidence of labour | Throughout infusion | • E.g. cervical examination, uterine contractions via external tocodynamometry.<br>• Discontinuation is warranted if cervical dilatation of ≥1 cm occurs during therapy, or if contractions continue for 6 hours. |
| Maternal blood pressure and heart rate | | • Atosiban infusion can cause ↓BP and ↑pulse.<br>• ECG monitoring should be carried out in patients with pre-existing cardiovascular disease, or in any patients exhibiting cardiac symptoms during infusion. |
| Maternal blood glucose level | | • Atosiban infusion can cause hyperglycaemia. |
| Fetal heart rate | | • To monitor for signs of distress. |
| Postpartum blood loss | Postpartum | • As an oxytocin antagonist, atosiban may facilitate increased postpartum blood loss due to uterine relaxation. |

## Additional information

| | |
|---|---|
| Common and serious undesirable effects | *Injection/infusion-related:* Local: Injection-site reactions.<br>*Other:* Nausea, vomiting, hyperglycaemia, headache, dizziness, ↑pulse, ↓BP, hot flushes, insomnia, pruritus, rash, pyrexia. |
| Pharmacokinetics | Elimination half-life is 1.7 hours. |
| Significant interactions | No significant interactions. |
| Action in case of overdose | No specific signs or symptoms reported. No known specific treatment. |
| Counselling | Small amounts of atosiban and an active metabolite have been found to be present in breast milk. No known adverse effects in neonates. |

| Risk rating: **AMBER** | Score = 3<br>Moderate-risk product: Risk-reduction strategies are recommended. |
| --- | --- |

This assessment is based on the full range of preparation and administration options described in the monograph. These may not all be applicable in some clinical situations.

## Bibliography

SPC Tractocile 7.5 mg/mL concentrate for solution for infusion (accessed 1 October 2009).
SPC Tractocile 7.5 mg/mL solution for injection (accessed 1 October 2009).

# Atropine sulfate

**600 micrograms/mL solution in ampoules and pre-filled syringes (other strengths available)**

**100 micrograms/mL and 200 micrograms/mL solution in pre-filled syringes of various sizes**

* Atropine sulfate is an antimuscarinic alkaloid with both central and peripheral actions. It has antispasmodic actions on smooth muscle and reduces salivary and bronchial secretions. It depresses the vagus and thereby increases the heart rate.
* It is used preoperatively to reduce secretions; during CPR to treat sinus bradycardia or asystole; to treat symptomatic sinus bradycardia induced by drugs or toxic substances; to prevent muscarinic effects on the heart (e.g. arrhythmias, ⏐pulse) during surgery and in combination with neostigmine or edrophonium during reversal of effect of non-depolarising muscle relaxants.

## Pre-treatment checks

* Contraindications are not applicable to the use of atropine in life-threatening emergencies (e.g. asystole).
* Atropine is contraindicated in obstruction of the bladder neck, e.g. due to prostatic hypertrophy, reflux oesophagitis, closed-angle glaucoma, myasthenia gravis (unless used to treat the adverse effects of an anticholinesterase agent), paralytic ileus, severe ulcerative colitis and obstructive disease of the GI tract.
* Caution in patients with hyperthyroidism, hepatic or renal disease or hypertension; febrile patients or when ambient temperature is high since antimuscarinics may cause an increase in temperature.
* Antimuscarinics block vagal inhibition of the SA (sinoatrial) nodal pacemaker and should thus be used with caution in patients with tachyarrhythmias, congestive heart failure or coronary heart disease.
* Parenterally administered atropine should be used cautiously in patients with chronic pulmonary disease since a reduction in bronchial secretions may lead to formation of bronchial plugs.
* Extreme caution is required in patients with autonomic neuropathy.
* Antimuscarinics decrease gastric motility, relax the lower oesophageal sphincter and may delay gastric emptying; they should therefore be used with caution in patients with gastric ulcer, oesophageal reflux or hiatus hernia associated with reflux oesophagitis, diarrhoea or GI infection.

*Biochemical and other tests (not all are necessary in an emergency situation)*

Blood pressure

Heart rate

LFTs

Renal function: U, Cr, CrCl (or eGFR)

## Dose

**Premedication**: 300–600 micrograms by IV injection immediately before induction of anaesthesia or 300–600 micrograms by SC or IM injection 30–60 minutes before induction.

**Intraoperative bradycardia**: 300–600 micrograms (larger doses in emergencies) by IV injection.

**Control of muscarinic side-effects of neostigmine or edrophonium in reversal of competitive neuromuscular block**: 600 micrograms–1.2 mg by IV injection.

**Bradycardia of acute myocardial infarction**: 500 micrograms by IV injection repeated every 3–5 minutes to a total dose of 3 mg. (If IV access cannot be obtained, consider the endotracheal route.)

**In CPR for asystole**: 3 mg as a single IV dose. (If IV access cannot be obtained, consider the intraosseous route or the endotracheal route.)

## Intravenous injection

*Preparation and administration*

1. Withdraw the required dose or select the appropriate pre-filled syringe.
2. The solution should be clear and colourless. Inspect visually for particulate matter or discoloration prior to administration and discard if present.
3. Give rapidly by IV injection (slow IV injection may cause paradoxical slowing of the heart).

## Subcutaneous injection

*Preparation and administration*

1. Withdraw the required dose or select the appropriate pre-filled syringe.
2. Give by SC injection.

## Intramuscular injection

*Preparation and administration*

1. Withdraw the required dose or select the appropriate pre-filled syringe.
2. Give by IM injection.

## Endotracheal administration

*Preparation and administration*

1. Withdraw the required dose (2–3 times the IV dose is given by this route).
2. Dilute the dose with 10 mL WFI or NaCl 0.9%.
3. Administer via the endotracheal tube.

| Technical information | |
|---|---|
| Incompatible with | Flucloxacillin, pantoprazole. |
| Compatible with | **Flush**: NaCl 0.9%<br>**Solutions**: NaCl 0.9%, Gluc 5% (with added KCl)<br>**Y-site**: Dobutamine, fentanyl, furosemide, hydrocortisone sodium succinate, meropenem, metoclopramide, midazolam, ondansetron, ranitidine, verapamil |
| pH | 3–6.5 |

*(continued)*

## Technical information (continued)

| | |
|---|---|
| Sodium content | Negligible |
| Storage | Store below 25°C in original packaging. Do not freeze. |

## Monitoring

| Measure | Frequency | Rationale |
|---|---|---|
| Clinical improvement | Periodically | • To ensure that treatment is effective. |

## Additional information

| | |
|---|---|
| Common and serious undesirable effects | *Injection-related:* Local: extravasation may cause tissue damage.<br>*Other:* ↑Pulse, cardiac dysrhythmias, coma, respiratory depression, ↑intraocular pressure, constipation, dry mouth, blurred vision, light intolerance, urinary retention. |
| Pharmacokinetics | Following IV administration, the peak increase in heart rate occurs within 2-4 minutes. After IM administration peak effects on the heart, sweating and salivation occur after ~1 hour. Elimination half-life is 2-5 hours. |
| Significant interactions | No significant interactions. |
| Action in case of overdose | *Antidote:* Diazepam may be administered to control excitement and convulsions but the risk of central nervous system depression should be considered.<br>Antiarrhythmic drugs are *not* recommended if dysrhythmias occur. |

| Risk rating: **GREEN** | Score = 1<br>Moderate-risk product: Risk-reduction strategies are recommended. |
|---|---|

This assessment is based on the full range of preparation and administration options described in the monograph. These may not all be applicable in some clinical situations.

## Bibliography

SPC Atropine sulphate injection 600 mcg in 1 mL, Hameln Pharmaceuticals Ltd (accessed 31 December 2008).
SPC IMS Atropine Injection BP Minijet (accessed 31 December 2008).

# Azathioprine

### 50-mg dry powder vials

- Azathioprine is an immunosuppressive anti-metabolite with actions similar to those of mercaptopurine, to which it is converted in the body.
- It is used to suppress rejection in organ transplant recipients and to treat a variety of chronic inflammatory and autoimmune diseases. Its effects may not be seen for several weeks after a dose.

## Pre-treatment checks

- Do not use if there is hypersensitivity to azathioprine or mercaptopurine.
- Caution in renal and hepatic impairment.

*Biochemical and other tests*

Bodyweight                                          LFTs
FBC                                                 Renal function: U, Cr, CrCl (or eGFR)

## Dose

> Azathioprine injection is alkaline and very irritant and it should only be used when the oral route is impractical; therapy should be switched back to the oral route as soon as it is tolerated.

**Consult specialist literature:** the starting and maintenance doses vary depending on the indication; e.g. in transplantation the first dose can be up to 5 mg/kg/day and maintenance doses range from 1 to 4 mg/kg/day. For autoimmune conditions maintenance doses are usually 1–3 mg/kg/day.

**Dose in renal impairment**: adjusted according to creatinine clearance,[1]

- CrCl >20–50 mL/minute: dose as in normal renal function.
- CrCl 10–20 mL/minute: 75–100% of dose for normal renal function.
- CrCl <10 mL/minute: 50–100% of dose for normal renal function.

**Dose in hepatic impairment:** use doses at the lower end of the range.

## Intermittent intravenous infusion (preferred method)

> See Special handling and Spillage below.

*Preparation and administration*

1. Reconstitute each 50-mg vial with 5 mL WFI to give a solution containing 10 mg/mL.
2. Withdraw the required dose and add to a suitable volume of NaCl 0.9% or Gluc 5% (usually 100 mL but up to 200 mL may be used).
3. The solution should be clear and colourless to pale yellow. Inspect visually for particulate matter or discoloration prior to administration and discard if present.
4. Give by IV infusion via a volumetric infusion device over 30–60 minutes.
5. Discard any unused portion in accordance with local protocols.

## Intravenous injection (avoid if possible – use only where dilution is not practicable)

See Special handling and Spillage below.

*Preparation and administration*

1. Reconstitute each 50-mg vial with 5 mL WFI to give a solution containing 10 mg/mL.
2. Withdraw the required dose and further dilute to 20 mL with NaCl 0.9%.
3. The solution should be clear and colourless to pale yellow. Inspect visually for particulate matter or discoloration prior to administration and discard if present.
4. Give by IV injection slowly over 3–5 minutes (and not less than 1 minute), taking care to avoid extravasation.
5. Follow immediately with a flush of at least 50 mL NaCl 0.9%.
6. Discard any unused portion in accordance with local protocols.

## Technical information

| Incompatible with | No information |
|---|---|
| Compatible with | Flush: NaCl 0.9%<br>Solutions: NaCl 0.9%, Gluc-NaCl, Gluc 5%<br>Y-site: No information |
| pH | Reconstituted: 10-12; more dilute infusion solutions have a lower pH. |
| Sodium content | Negligible |
| Storage | Store below 25°C in original packaging. |
| Displacement value | Negligible |
| Special handling | Follow local guidelines for the handling of cytotoxic drugs. |
| Spillage | Inactivate any spills using sodium hypochlorite 5% solution (household bleach), or sodium hydroxide solution. |
| Stability after preparation | From a microbiological point of view, should be used immediately; however:<br>Reconstituted vials may be stored at 5-8°C for 24 hours.<br>Prepared infusions may be stored at 2-8°C and infused (at room temperature) within 24 hours. |

## Monitoring

| Measure | Frequency | Rationale |
|---|---|---|
| FBC | Weekly for first 8 weeks (more frequently if there is renal/hepatic impairment), then monthly (or not more than 3-monthly) | • Bone marrow suppression can occur. |
| LFTs | | • Dose may need adjusting if hepatic function changes. |
| Renal function | | • Dose may need adjusting if renal function changes. |
| Any infection, unexpected bruising or bleeding | Counsel patient to seek medical advice if these are present | • Symptoms of bone marrow suppression. |

## Additional information

| | |
|---|---|
| Common and serious undesirable effects | Viral, fungal and bacterial infections; leucopenia; thrombocytopenia. |
| Pharmacokinetics | Elimination half-life is 4-6 hours. |
| Significant interactions | • The following may ↑azathioprine levels or effect (or ↑side-effects): allopurinol (give 25% of usual azathioprine dose), co-trimoxazole (↑risk of haematological toxicity), trimethoprim (↑risk of haematological toxicity).<br>• Azathioprine may ↓levels or effect of coumarin anticoagulants (monitor INR). |
| Action in case of overdose | No specific antidote. It is partially dialysable (although the value of this is unknown). Haematological monitoring is necessary to allow prompt treatment of any adverse effects that may develop (e.g. blood and platelet transfusion, antibiotics). |
| Counselling | Exposure to sunlight and UV light should be limited as patients taking azathioprine have ↑risk of skin cancer. Patients should wear protective clothing and use a high protection factor sunscreen. |

| Risk rating: **AMBER** | Score = 4<br>Moderate-risk product: Risk-reduction strategies are recommended. |
|---|---|

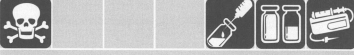

This assessment is based on the full range of preparation and administration options described in the monograph. These may not all be applicable in some clinical situations.

## Reference

1. Ashley C, Currie A, eds. *The Renal Drug Handbook*, 3rd edn. Oxford: Radcliffe Medical Press, 2009.

## Bibliography

SPC Imuran injection (accessed 2 March 2010).

# Aztreonam

**500-mg, 1-g, 2-g dry powder vials**

• Aztreonam is a synthetic monocyclic beta-lactam (monobactam) antibiotic and acts similarly to the penicillins.
• It is used to treat Gram-negative infections (including beta-lactamase-producing strains) particularly *Pseudomonas aeruginosa*, *Haemophilus influenzae* and *Neisseria meningitidis*.

## Pre-treatment checks

* Do not give in pregnancy.
* Caution in hypersensitivity to other beta-lactam antibiotics; hepatic impairment; renal impairment.

*Biochemical and other tests (not all are necessary in an emergency situation)*

FBC

LFTs

Prothrombin time in certain circumstances

Renal function: U, Cr, CrCl (or eGFR)

## Dose

**Standard dose:** 1 g by IM or IV injection or IV infusion every 6–8 hours, or 2 g by IV injection or infusion every 12 hours.

**Severe or life-threatening infections** (including systemic *Pseudomonas aeruginosa* and lung infections in cystic fibrosis): 2 g by IV injection or infusion every 6–8 hours.

**Urinary tract infections:** 500 mg–1 g by IM or IV injection or infusion every 8–12 hours.

**Gonorrhoea/cystitis:** 1 g single dose by IM injection.

**Dose in renal impairment:** adjusted according to creatinine clearance,[1]

* CrCl >30–50 mL/minute: dose as in normal renal function.
* CrCl 10–30 mL/minute: 1–2 g loading dose then maintenance of 50% of appropriate normal dose.
* CrCl <10 mL/minute: 1–2 g loading dose then maintenance of 25% of appropriate normal dose.

## Intravenous injection

*Preparation and administration*

1. Add 6–10 mL WFI to each vial. Shake immediately and vigorously.
2. Withdraw the required dose.
3. The solution should be clear and colourless to pale yellow. Inspect visually for particulate matter or discoloration prior to administration and discard if present.
4. Give by IV injection over 3–5 minutes.

## Intermittent intravenous infusion

*Preparation and administration*

1. Add 10 mL WFI to each vial. Shake immediately and vigorously.
2. Withdraw the required dose and add to a suitable volume of NaCl 0.9% or Gluc 5% (add each 1 g to at least 50 mL).
3. The solution should be clear and colourless to pale yellow. Inspect visually for particulate matter or discoloration prior to administration and discard if present.
4. Give by IV infusion over 20–60 minutes.

## Intramuscular injection (maximum dose 1 g)

*Preparation and administration*

1. Add 1.5 mL WFI or NaCl 0.9% to a 500-mg vial (use 3 mL for a 1-g vial). Shake immediately and vigorously.
2. Withdraw the required dose. The solution should be clear and colourless to pale yellow. Visually inspect for particulate matter and discoloration and discard if present.
3. Give by deep IM injection, e.g. into the upper quadrant of the gluteus maximus or the lateral part of the thigh.

## Technical information

| | |
|---|---|
| Incompatible with | Aciclovir, amphotericin B, ampicillin, ganciclovir, metronidazole, vancomycin. |
| Compatible with | **Flush**: NaCl 0.9%<br>**Solutions**: NaCl 0.9%, Gluc 5%, Gluc-NaCl, Hartmann's, Ringer's (all including added KCl)<br>**Y-site**: Amikacin, aminophylline, bumetanide, calcium gluconate, cefotaxime, ceftazidime, ceftriaxone, cefuroxime, ciprofloxacin, cisatracurium, clindamycin, co-trimoxazole, dexamethasone, dobutamine, dopamine, fluconazole, furosemide, gentamicin, granisetron, hydrocortisone sodium succinate, imipenem with cilastatin, magnesium sulfate, methylprednisolone sodium succinate, metoclopramide, piperacillin with tazobactam, propofol, ranitidine, remifentanil, sodium bicarbonate, ticarcillin with clavulanate, tobramycin |
| pH | 4.5-7.5 |
| Sodium content | Nil |
| Excipients | Contains L-arginine (may cause hypersensitivity reactions). |
| Storage | Store below 25°C in original packaging. |
| Displacement value | 0.4 mL/500 mg |
| Stability after preparation | Reconstituted vials should be used immediately.<br>From a microbiological point of view, prepared infusions should be used immediately; however, they may be stored at 2-8°C and infused (at room temperature) within 24 hours. Solutions may develop a slight pink tint on standing without potency being affected. |

## Monitoring

| Measure | Frequency | Rationale |
|---|---|---|
| Renal function | Periodically | • Transient rises in urea and creatinine occur rarely.<br>• If renal function changes a dose adjustment may be required. |
| FBC | | • Transient eosinophilia may occur in up to 11%.<br>• Occasional leucopenia, neutropenia, thrombocytopenia, pancytopenia, anaemia, leucocytosis and thrombocytosis have been reported. |
| LFTs | | • Jaundice and hepatitis have occurred.<br>• Transient ↑ALT, AST and Alk Phos may occur. |
| Prothrombin time | | • Prolongation of bleeding time and defective platelet function may occur (monitor closely if anticoagulated). |
| Signs of supra-infection or superinfection | Throughout treatment | • May result in the overgrowth of non-susceptible organisms - appropriate therapy should be commenced; treatment may need to be interrupted. |

(continued)

## Monitoring (continued)

| Measure | Frequency | Rationale |
|---------|-----------|-----------|
| Development of diarrhoea | Throughout and up to 2 months after treatment | • Development of severe, persistent diarrhoea may be suggestive of Clostridium difficile-associated diarrhoea and colitis (pseudomembranous colitis). Discontinue drug and treat. Do not use drugs that inhibit peristalsis. |

## Additional information

| | |
|---|---|
| Common and serious undesirable effects | *Immediate:* Anaphylaxis and other hypersensitivity reactions have been reported.<br>*Injection/infusion-related:* Local: Phlebitis at IV injection site, discomfort at IM injection site.<br>*Other:* Rash, pruritus, urticaria, erythema, petechiae, exfoliative dermatitis, flushing, diarrhoea, nausea, vomiting, abdominal cramps, mouth ulcer and altered taste, angioedema, bronchospasm. |
| Pharmacokinetics | Elimination half-life is 1.7 hours. |
| Significant interactions | • Aztreonam may ↑levels or effect of the following drugs (or ↑side-effects): acenocoumarol (monitor INR), warfarin (monitor INR). |
| Action in case of overdose | No reported cases of overdosage. Stop administration and give supportive therapy as appropriate. |

| | |
|---|---|
| Risk rating: **GREEN** | Score = 2<br>Lower-risk product: Risk-reduction strategies should be considered. |

This assessment is based on the full range of preparation and administration options described in the monograph. These may not all be applicable in some clinical situations.

## Reference

1. Ashley C, Currie A, eds. *The Renal Drug Handbook*, 3rd edn. Oxford: Radcliffe Medical Press, 2009.

## Bibliography

SPC Azactam for injection (accessed 1 October 2009).

# Bemiparin sodium

**2500 units/0.2 mL, 3500 units/0.2 mL pre-filled syringes**
**25 000 units/mL pre-filled syringes: 5000 units/0.2 mL, 7500 units/0.3 mL,**
**10 000 units/0.4 mL**

* Bemiparin sodium is a low-molecular-weight heparin (LMWH).
* It is used in the treatment of venous thromboembolism (VTE) i.e. pulmonary embolism (PE) and deep vein thrombosis (DVT).
* It is used for prophylaxis of VTE in surgical patients and to prevent thrombus formation in the extracorporeal circulation during haemodialysis.
* Not all products are licensed for all indications.
* Doses are expressed in terms of international anti-Factor Xa activity units.

## Pre-treatment checks

* Avoid in acute bacterial endocarditis, major bleeding or high risk of uncontrolled haemorrhage including recent haemorrhagic stroke.
* Avoid in patients with severe impairment of renal, hepatic and/or pancreatic functions.
* It is contraindicated in treatment dosage in patients undergoing locoregional anaesthesia in elective surgical procedures.
* Placement or removal of a spinal/epidural catheter should be delayed for 10–12 hours after administration of prophylactic doses, whereas patients receiving treatment doses require a 24-hour delay. Subsequent doses should be given no sooner than 4 hours after catheter removal.
* Caution with other drugs affecting haemostasis such as aspirin or clopidogrel.
* Use with extreme caution in patients with a history of heparin-induced thrombocytopenia (HIT).

*Biochemical and other tests (not all are necessary in an emergency situation)*

| | |
|---|---|
| Anti-Factor Xa activity in patients with severe renal impairment | LFTs |
| | Platelet count |
| Bodyweight (in some indications) | Renal function: U, Cr, CrCl (or eGFR) |
| Electrolytes–serum K | |

## Dose

*Prophylaxis*

**General surgery with moderate risk of VTE:** 2500 units by SC injection 2 hours before or 6 hours after surgery. On subsequent days give 2500 units every 24 hours for 7–10 days.
**Orthopaedic surgery with high risk of VTE:** 3500 units by SC injection 2 hours before or 6 hours after surgery. On subsequent days give 3500 units every 24 hours for 7–10 days.
**Prevention of extracorporeal thrombus formation during haemodialysis:** for haemodialysis of ≤4 hours duration, in patients not at risk of bleeding give 2500 units (weight <60 kg) or 3500 units (weight >60 kg) introduced into the arterial line at the start of the dialysis session.

*Treatment*

**Treatment of VTE:** give by SC injection once daily based on bodyweight as indicated in Table B1. For patients >100 kg dose is calculated on the basis of 115 units/kg and two syringes used to administer the dose. Treat for at least 5 days and until INR > 2.

**Table B1** Treatment doses of bemiparin for VTE

| | Bodyweight | | | |
|---|---|---|---|---|
| | **<50 kg** | **50–70 kg** | **70–100 kg** | **>100 kg** |
| Syringe volume | 0.2 mL | 0.3 mL | 0.4 mL | 115 units/kg - use two syringes to provide dose |
| Syringe dose | 5000 units | 7500 units | 10 000 units | |

**Dose in renal impairment**: adjusted according to creatinine clearance:[1]

- CrCl >20–50 mL/minute: dose as in normal renal function.
- CrCl 10–20 mL/minute: dose as in normal renal function for prophylaxis only.
- CrCl <10 mL/minute: dose as in normal renal function for prophylaxis only.

**Dose in hepatic impairment:** the manufacturer advises avoidance in severe hepatic impairment.

## Subcutaneous injection

*Preparation and administration*

1. Select the correct pre-filled syringe. Pre-filled syringes are ready for immediate use; do not expel the air bubble.
2. The patient should be seated or lying down.
3. Pinch up a skin fold on the abdominal wall between the thumb and forefinger and hold throughout the injection.
4. Give by deep SC injection into the thick part of the skin fold at right angles to the skin. Do not rub the injection site after administration. Alternate doses between the right and left sides.

## Arterial line injection (haemodialysis circuits)

*Preparation and administration*

1. Select the correct pre-filled syringe and expel the air bubble.
2. The solution should be clear and colourless to slightly yellowish. Inspect visually for particulate matter or discoloration prior to administration and discard if present.
3. Give over 5 seconds via a port into the arterial limb of the haemodialysis circuit.

## Technical information

| | |
|---|---|
| Incompatible with | Not relevant |
| Compatible with | **Flush**: NaCl 0.9%<br>**Solutions**: Not relevant<br>**Y-site**: Not relevant |
| pH[2] | 5–7.5 |
| Sodium content | Negligible |
| Storage | Store below 25°C in original packaging. |

## Monitoring

| Measure | Frequency | Rationale |
|---------|-----------|-----------|
| Platelet count | Twice a week | • Thrombocytopenia can occur from day 5 to day 21 of therapy.<br>• A 50%↓ in platelets is indicative of HIT and therapy should be switched to a non-heparin-derived agent. |
| Serum K | After 7 days | • Heparins inhibit the secretion of aldosterone and so may cause ↑K.<br>• Monitor in all patients with risk factors, particularly if therapy >7 days. |
| Signs of bleeding | Throughout therapy | • There is a higher risk of bleeding with prophylactic doses in low bodyweight: women (<45 kg); men (<57 kg). |
| Anti-Xa activity | Periodically – see rationale | • Not required routinely but may be considered in patients at ↑risk of bleeding or actively bleeding. |

## Additional information

| | |
|---|---|
| Common and serious undesirable effects | *Injection-related:* Local: Pain, haematoma and mild local irritation may follow the SC injection of bemiparin. Exceptional cases of skin necrosis, usually preceded by purpura or erythematous plaques - treatment must be discontinued.<br>*Other:*<br>• Common: Bleeding risk with organic lesions, invasive procedures; risk of major haemorrhage. Mild, transient, asymptomatic thrombocytopenia during the first days of therapy. Transient ↑liver transaminases.<br>• Rare: Immunoallergic thrombocytopenia with or without thrombosis. Significant ↑K in patients with diabetes or chronic renal failure. |
| Pharmacokinetics | Rapidly absorbed after SC injection (peak activity 2-3 hours) with elimination half-life of 5-6 hours. Elimination is prolonged in renal impairment and severe hepatic dysfunction. |
| Significant interactions | • The following may ↑risk of bleeding with bemiparin: aspirin, diclofenac IV (avoid combination), ketorolac (avoid combination).<br>• Glyceryl trinitrate infusion may ↓bemiparin levels or effect. |
| Action in case of overdose | *Symptoms to watch for:* Bleeding.<br>*Antidote:* Protamine sulfate may be used to ↓bleeding risk if clinically required. See Protamine sulfate monograph. |
| Counselling | Report any bleeding or bruising, and any injection-site effects. |

| | |
|---|---|
| Risk rating: **GREEN** | Score = 1<br>Lower-risk product. Risk-reduction strategies should be considered. |

This assessment is based on the full range of preparation and administration options described in the monograph. These may not all be applicable in some clinical situations.

## Reference

1. Ashley C, Currie A, eds. *The Renal Drug Handbook*, 3rd edn. Oxford: Radcliffe Medical Press, 2009.
2. Communiqué from Archimedes Pharma UK Ltd, 19 January 2010.

## Bibliography

SPC Zibor 25 000 units Anti-Xa/ml solution for injection in pre-filled syringes (accessed 27 November 2009).

SPC Zibor 2500 units (accessed 27 November 2009).

SPC Zibor 3500 units (accessed 27 November 2009).

# Benzatropine mesilate (benztropine mesylate)

**1 mg/mL solution in 2-mL ampoules**

* Benzatropine mesilate is an antimuscarinic drug.
* It is used parenterally to treat acute dystonic reactions and extra pyramidal symptoms caused by drugs.

## Pre-treatment checks

* Do not use to treat tardive dyskinesia as it is ineffective.
* Do not use in closed-angle glaucoma.
* Benzatropine may cause anhidrosis – use with caution in hot weather especially when given with other atropine-like drugs to the chronically ill, in alcoholism, those who have CNS disease and those who do manual labour in a hot environment.

*Biochemical and other tests*

None required.

## Dose

Onset of action is similar for the IM and IV routes and therefore IV administration is rarely required.

**Standard dose:** 1–2 mg by IM or IV injection. Repeat if symptoms reappear. Maximum daily dose: 6 mg.

## Intramuscular injection (preferred route)

*Preparation and administration*

1. Withdraw the required dose.
2. Give by IM injection.

## Intravenous injection

*Preparation and administration*

1. Withdraw the required dose.
2. The solution should be clear and colourless. Inspect visually for particulate matter or discoloration prior to administration and discard if present.
3. Give by IV injection.

## Technical information

| Incompatible with | Haloperidol |
|---|---|
| Compatible with | **Flush**: NaCl 0.9%<br>**Solutions**: NaCl 0.9%<br>**Y-site**: Fluconazole, metoclopramide |
| pH | 5-8 |
| Sodium content | Negligible |
| Storage | Store below 25°C in original packaging. Do not freeze. |

## Monitoring

| Measure | Frequency | Rationale |
|---|---|---|
| Reduction of extrapyramidal movements, rigidity, tremor, gait disturbances. | Post administration | • To ensure that treatment is effective. |
| Pulse | | • May cause ↑pulse. |

## Additional information

| Common and serious undesirable effects | *Common:* ↑Pulse, constipation, nausea, dry mouth, blurred vision, urinary retention. |
|---|---|
| Pharmacokinetics | Given by the IM route, onset of effect occurs within minutes. There is very little information available about its elimination half-life. |
| Significant interactions | No significant interactions are known. |
| Action in case of overdose | *Symptoms to watch for:* Agitation, restlessness and severe sleeplessness lasting 24 hours or more. Visual and auditory hallucinations have been reported. ↑Pulse has also been reported.<br>*Antidote:* Active measures such as the use of cholinergic agents or haemodialysis are unlikely to be of clinical value. If convulsions do occur they should be controlled by injections of diazepam. |

| Risk rating: **GREEN** | Score = 1<br>Lower-risk product: Risk-reduction strategies should be considered. |
|---|---|

This assessment is based on the full range of preparation and administration options described in the monograph. These may not all be applicable in some clinical situations.

## Bibliography

Cogentin PIL (2001). Merck & Co., Inc. http://www.merck.com/product/usa/pi_circulars/c/cogentin/ cogentin_pi.pdf (accessed 28 September 2010).

# Benzylpenicillin (penicillin G)

### 600-mg, 1.2-g dry powder vials

* Benzylpenicillin sodium is a penicillin.
* It is bactericidal against Gram-positive bacteria, Gram-negative cocci, some other Gram-negative bacteria, spirochaetes, and actinomycetes.
* Doses below are expressed in terms of the sodium salt.
* In some countries the dose is expressed as units:
  Benzylpenicillin sodium 600 mg $\cong$ 1 000 000 units (1 mega unit) of benzylpenicillin

## Pre-treatment checks

* Do not give if there is known hypersensitivity to penicillins and use with caution if sensitive to other beta-lactam antibiotics.

*Biochemical and other tests*

Electrolytes: serum Na, K
FBC
Renal function: U, Cr, CrCl (or eGFR)

## Dose

**Standard dose:** 600 mg–1.2 g by IM or IV injection or IV infusion every 6 hours, increased if necessary in more serious infections.

**Endocarditis** (in combination with another antibacterial if indicated): 1.2 g by IV injection or infusion every 4 hours, increased if necessary (e.g. in enterococcal endocarditis or monotherapy) to 2.4 g every 4 hours.

**Anthrax** (in combination with other antibacterials): 2.4 g by IV injection or infusion every 4 hours.

**Intrapartum prophylaxis against group B streptococcal infection:** initially 3 g by IV injection or infusion then 1.5 g every 4 hours until delivery.

**Meningococcal disease:** 2.4 g by IV injection or infusion every 4 hours.

**Dose in renal impairment:** adjusted according to creatinine clearance:[1]

* CrCl >20–50 mL/minute: dose as in normal renal function.
* CrCl 10–20 mL/minute: 600 mg–2.4 g every 6 hours depending on the severity of the infection.
* CrCl <10 mL/minute: 600 mg–1.2 g every 6 hours depending on the severity of the infection.

## Intravenous injection

*Preparation and administration*

See Special handling below.

1. Reconstitute each 600-mg vial with 5 mL WFI or NaCl 0.9% (use 10 mL for each 1.2-g vial). If planning to administer part of a 600-mg vial, use 5.6 mL WFI or NaCl 0.9%, which then gives a solution containing 100 mg/mL.

*(continued)*

2. Withdraw the required dose.
3. The solution should be clear and colourless. Inspect visually for particulate matter or discoloration prior to administration and discard if present.
4. Give by IV injection over about 5 minutes (maximum rate 300 mg/minute).

## Intermittent intravenous infusion

*Preparation and administration*

See Special handling below.

1. Reconstitute each 600-mg vial with 5 mL WFI or NaCl 0.9% (use 10 mL for each 1.2-g vial). If planning to administer part of a 600-mg vial use 5.6 mL WFI or NaCl 0.9% which then gives a solution containing 100 mg/mL.
2. Withdraw the required dose and add to a suitable volume of compatible infusion fluid (usually 100 mL NaCl 0.9%).
3. The solution should be clear and colourless. Inspect visually for particulate matter or discoloration prior to administration and discard if present.
4. Give by IV infusion over 30–60 minutes.

## Intramuscular injection (maximum dose 1.2 g)

*Preparation and administration*

See Special handling below.

1. Dissolve the contents of a 600-mg vial in 1.6 mL of WFI (use 3.2 mL for a 1.2-g vial) to give a solution containing 300 mg/mL.
2. Withdraw the required dose.
3. Give by deep IM injection. Rotate injection sites for subsequent injections.

## Technical information

| | |
|---|---|
| Incompatible with | Amphotericin, flucloxacillin, methylprednisolone sodium succinate, potassium chloride. |
| Compatible with | **Flush**: NaCl 0.9%<br>**Solutions**: NaCl 0.9%, Gluc 5% (but less stable)<br>**Y-site**: Calcium gluconate, chloramphenicol sodium succinate, clarithromycin, clindamycin phosphate, erythromycin lactobionate, furosemide, hydrocortisone sodium succinate, ranitidine, verapamil |
| pH | 5.5-7.5 |
| Sodium content | 1.7 mmol/600 mg; 3.4 mmol/1.2 g |
| Storage | Store below 25°C in original packaging. |
| Displacement value | 0.4 mL/600 mg |

*(continued)*

## Technical information (*continued*)

| | |
|---|---|
| Special handling | After contact with skin, wash immediately with water. If it contacts the eyes, rinse immediately with plenty of water; seek medical advice if discomfort persists. |
| Stability after preparation | Use reconstituted vials and prepared infusions immediately. |

## Monitoring

| Measure | Frequency | Rationale |
|---|---|---|
| Renal function, U&Es | Periodically if used for longer than 5 days | • The high Na content can cause ↓K (a K-sparing diuretic may help protect against this) and ↑Na (caution in renal failure and/or heart failure: use a non-Na-containing infusion fluid if indicated).<br>• Changes in renal function may require a dose adjustment. |
| FBC | | • ↑risk of neutropenia when given over long periods. Warning signs include fever, rash, and eosinophilia.<br>• WCC: For signs of the infection resolving. |
| Signs of supra-infection or superinfection | Throughout treatment | • May result in the overgrowth of non-susceptible organisms - appropriate therapy should be commenced; treatment may need to be interrupted. |
| Signs of hypersensitivity | | • Observe for 30 minutes after administration; if an allergic reaction occurs withdraw the drug and give appropriate treatment.<br>• Rashes, fever, serum sickness all commonly occur.<br>• Antihistamines are the treatment of choice. |
| Development of diarrhoea | Throughout and up to 2 months after treatment | • Development of severe, persistent diarrhoea may be suggestive of *Clostridium difficile*-associated diarrhoea and colitis (pseudomembranous colitis). Discontinue drug and treat. Do not use drugs that inhibit peristalsis. |

## Additional information

| | |
|---|---|
| Common and serious undesirable effects | *Immediate:* Anaphylaxis and other hypersensitivity reactions have been reported.<br>*Other:* Urticaria, fever, joint pains, rashes, angioedema, anaphylaxis, serum sickness-like reaction. Patients treated for syphilis or neurosyphilis may develop a Jarisch-Herxheimer reaction (occurs 2-12 hours after initiation of therapy - headache, fever, chills, sweating, sore throat, myalgia, arthralgia, malaise, ↑pulse and ↑BP followed by a ↓BP. Usually subsides within 12-24 hours. Corticosteroids may ↓incidence and severity). |
| Pharmacokinetics | Elimination half-life is 20–50 minutes. |
| Significant interactions | No significant interactions. |

(continued)

## Additional information (*continued*)

| | |
|---|---|
| Action in case of overdose | *Symptoms to watch for:* Large doses have been associated with seizures. *Antidote:* None, but haemodialysis may be effective. Stop administration and give supportive therapy as appropriate. |
| Counselling | Women taking the combined contraceptive pill should be should be advised to take additional precautions during and for 7 days after the course. |

| | |
|---|---|
| Risk rating: **GREEN** | Score = 2 Lower-risk product: Risk-reduction strategies should be considered. |

This assessment is based on the full range of preparation and administration options described in the monograph. These may not all be applicable in some clinical situations.

### Reference

1. Ashley C, Currie A, eds. *The Renal Drug Handbook*, 3rd edn. Oxford: Radcliffe Medical Press, 2009.

### Bibliography

SPC Crystapen injection (accessed 2/03/09).

# Betamethasone

### 4 mg/mL solution in 1-mL ampoules

- Betamethasone sodium phosphate is a corticosteroid with mainly glucocorticoid activity.
- It is used in the treatment of conditions for which systemic corticosteroid therapy is indicated (except adrenal-deficiency states). Its virtual lack of mineralocorticoid properties makes it particularly suitable for treating conditions in which water retention would be a disadvantage.
- It is also used by local injection in soft-tissue injury such as tennis elbow, tenosynovitis and bursitis.
- Doses are usually expressed in terms of the base:
  Betamethasone 1 mg ≅ 1.3 mg betamethasone sodium phosphate.

### Pre-treatment checks

- Avoid where systemic infection is present (unless specific therapy given).
- Avoid live virus vaccines in those receiving immunosuppressive doses.
- May activate or exacerbate amoebiasis or strongyloidiasis (exclude before initiating a corticosteroid in those at risk or with suggestive symptoms). Fungal or viral ocular infections may also be exacerbated.
- Caution in patients predisposed to psychiatric reactions, including those who have previously suffered corticosteroid-induced psychosis, or who have a personal or family history of psychiatric disorders.

- Do not use in the treatment of cerebral oedema associated with acute head injury or cerebrovascular accident, as it is unlikely to be of benefit and may even be harmful.

*Biochemical and other tests (not all are necessary in an emergency situation)*

Electrolytes: serum Na, K, Ca
LFTs

## Dose

**Standard dose:** 4–20 mg by IV injection repeated 3–4 times in 24 hours, or as required, depending upon the condition being treated and the patient's response. It may also be given by IM injection and IV infusion.

**Injection into soft tissue:** 4–8 mg repeated on 2–3 occasions depending upon the patient's response.

**Dose in hepatic impairment:** as betamethasone is metabolised in the liver, dosage adjustments may be necessary.

### Intravenous injection (preferred route)

*Preparation and administration*

1. Withdraw the required dose.
2. The solution should be clear and colourless. Inspect visually for particulate matter or discoloration prior to administration and discard if present.
3. Give by IV injection over 30–60 seconds.

### Intramuscular injection (less rapid response)

*Preparation and administration*

1. Withdraw the required dose.
2. Give by deep IM injection.

### Intermittent intravenous infusion

*Preparation and administration*

1. Withdraw the required dose.
2. Add to a suitable volume of compatible infusion fluid (usually 100 mL NaCl 0.9%).
3. The solution should be clear and colourless. Inspect visually for particulate matter or discoloration prior to administration and discard if present.
4. Give by IV infusion over 15–30 minutes.

| Technical information | |
| --- | --- |
| Incompatible with | No information |
| Compatible with | **Flush**: NaCl 0.9%<br>**Solutions**: NaCl 0.9%, Gluc 5%<br>**Y-site**: No information |
| pH | 8–9 |
| Sodium content | Negligible |
| Excipients | Contains sulfites (may cause allergic reactions). |

*(continued)*

## Technical information (continued)

| | |
|---|---|
| Storage | Store below 30°C in original packaging. |
| Stability after preparation | Use prepared infusions immediately. |

## Monitoring

| Measure | Frequency | Rationale |
|---|---|---|
| Serum Na, K, Ca | Throughout treatment | • May cause fluid and electrolyte disturbances. |
| Withdrawal symptoms and signs | During withdrawal and after stopping treatment | • During prolonged therapy with corticosteroids, adrenal atrophy develops and can persist for years after stopping. Abrupt withdrawal after a prolonged period can lead to acute adrenal insufficiency, ↓BP or death.<br>• The CSM has recommended that gradual withdrawal of systemic corticosteroids should be considered in patients whose disease is unlikely to relapse. Full details can be found in the BNF. |
| Signs of infection | During treatment | Prolonged courses ↑susceptibility to infections and severity of infections. Serious infections may reach an advanced stage before being recognised. |
| Signs of chickenpox | | • Unless they have had chickenpox, patients receiving corticosteroids for purposes other than replacement should be regarded as being at risk of severe chickenpox.<br>• Confirmed chickenpox requires urgent treatment; corticosteroids should not be stopped and dosage may need to be increased. |
| Exposure to measles | | • Patients should be advised to take particular care to avoid exposure to measles and to seek immediate medical advice if exposure occurs.<br>• Prophylaxis with IM normal immunoglobulin may be needed. |

## Additional information

| | |
|---|---|
| Common and serious undesirable effects | *Immediate:* Anaphylaxis and other hypersensitivity reactions have been reported.<br>*Undesirable effects that may result from short-term use* (minimise by using the lowest effective dose for the shortest time): ↑BP, Na and water retention, ↓K, ↓Ca, ↑blood glucose, peptic ulceration and perforation, psychiatric reactions, ↑susceptibility to infection, muscle weakness, tendon rupture, insomnia, ↑intracranial pressure, ↓seizure threshold, impaired healing. For undesirable effects resulting from long-term corticosteroid use, refer to the BNF. |
| Pharmacokinetics | Elimination half-life is 5.6 hours. |

(continued)

## Additional information (*continued*)

| | |
|---|---|
| Significant interactions | • The following may ↓corticosteroid levels or effect: barbiturates, carbamazepine, phenytoin, primidone, rifabutin, rifampicin.<br>• Corticosteroids may ↑levels or effect of the following drugs (or ↑side-effects): aldesleukin (avoid combination), amphotericin (risk of ↑K), anticoagulants (monitor INR), methotrexate (↑risk of blood dyscrasias).<br>• Corticosteroids may ↓levels or effect of vaccines (↓immunological response, ↑risk of infection with live vaccines). |
| Action in case of overdose | Give supportive therapy as appropriate. Following chronic overdose the possibility of adrenal suppression should be considered. |
| Counselling | Patients on long-term corticosteroid treatment should read and carry a Steroid Treatment Card. |

| Risk rating: **GREEN** | Score = 1<br>Lower-risk product: Risk-reduction strategies should be considered. |
|---|---|

This assessment is based on the full range of preparation and administration options described in the monograph. These may not all be applicable in some clinical situations.

## Bibliography

SPC Betnesol injection (accessed 1 October 2009).

# Bivalirudin

**250-mg dry powder vials**

• Bivalirudin, an analogue of the peptide hirudin, is a direct thrombin inhibitor with actions similar to lepirudin.
• It is used as an anticoagulant in patients undergoing PCI, including those with, or at risk of, HIT. It is also licensed for use in the acute coronary syndromes (ACS): unstable angina and NSTEMI.

## Pre-treatment checks

• Avoid in severe ↑BP; sub-acute bacterial endocarditis; active bleeding; bleeding disorders.
• Caution with previous exposure to lepirudin (theoretical risk from lepirudin antibodies), brachytherapy procedures, and concomitant use of drugs that ↑risk of bleeding.
• Bivalirudin may be commenced 30 minutes after discontinuation of an unfractionated heparin IV infusion, or 8 hours after discontinuation of SC LMWH.

*Biochemical and other tests (not all are necessary in an emergency situation)*

| | |
|---|---|
| ACT | FBC |
| Blood pressure | Renal function: U, Cr, CrCl (or eGFR) |
| Bodyweight | |

## Dose

**Patients undergoing PCI:** 0.75 mg/kg by IV injection followed immediately by 1.75 mg/kg/hour by IV infusion for at least the duration of the procedure. This infusion may be continued for up to 4 hours post-PCI if necessary. After the 1.75 mg/kg/hour infusion has a finished, a reduced infusion of 0.25 mg/kg/hour may be continued for 4–12 hours as clinically necessary.

**Treatment of ACS:** 0.1 mg/kg by IV injection followed by 0.25 mg/kg/hour by IV infusion. Patients who are to be medically managed may continue the infusion for up to 72 hours.

**ACS patients proceeding to PCI:** an additional 0.5 mg/kg by IV injection is given before the procedure and the infusion increased as per PCI patients above.

**ACS patients who proceed to coronary artery bypass graft (CABG) surgery off pump:** the infusion is continued until the time of surgery. An additional 0.5 mg/kg by IV injection is given just prior to surgery followed by 1.75 mg/kg/hour by IV infusion for the duration of the surgery.

**ACS patients who proceed to CABG surgery on pump:** the infusion is continued until 1 hour prior to surgery then stopped and the patient treated with unfractionated heparin.

**Dose in renal impairment:** adjusted according to creatinine clearance:

* CrCl 30–59 mL/minute: loading dose remains unchanged but the IV infusion for patients undergoing PCI (whether being treated for ACS or not) should be reduced to 1.4 mg/kg/hour.
* CrCl <30 mL/minute: do not use.

## Intravenous injection

*Preparation and administration*

1. Reconstitute each 250-mg vial with 5 mL WFI. Swirl gently until completely dissolved to give a solution containing 50 mg/mL.
2. Withdraw 5 mL from the vial and further dilute to a final volume of 50 mL with Gluc 5% or NaCl 0.9% to give a solution containing 5 mg/mL. Mix well.
3. The solution should be a clear to slightly opalescent, colourless to slightly yellow solution. Inspect visually for particulate matter or discoloration prior to administration and discard if present.
4. Withdraw the required dose (retain the remainder of the solution for IV infusion).
5. Give as a rapid IV injection.

## Continuous intravenous infusion via a syringe pump

*Preparation and administration*

1. For the initial IV infusion, use the remainder of the solution prepared for IV injection.
2. When a further supply is needed, reconstitute each 250-mg vial with 5 mL WFI. Swirl gently until completely dissolved to give a solution containing 50 mg/mL.
3. Withdraw 5 mL from the vial and make up to 50 mL in a syringe pump with Gluc 5% or NaCl 0.9%.
4. Cap the syringe and mix well to give a solution containing 5 mg/mL.
5. The solution should be a clear to slightly opalescent, colourless to slightly yellow solution. Inspect visually for particulate matter or discoloration prior to administration and discard if present.
6. Give by IV infusion at a rate appropriate to the indication.

## Technical information

| | |
|---|---|
| Incompatible with | Alteplase, amiodarone, amphotericin, diazepam, dobutamine, prochlorperazine, reteplase, streptokinase, vancomycin. |
| Compatible with | **Flush**: NaCl 0.9%<br>**Solutions**: NaCl 0.9%, Gluc 5%<br>**Y-site**: Abciximab, alfentanil, amikacin, aminophylline, ampicillin, aztreonam, bumetanide, calcium gluconate, cefotaxime, ceftazidime, ceftriaxone, ciprofloxacin, clindamycin phosphate, co-trimoxazole, dexamethasone sodium phosphate, dopamine, eptifibatide, erythromycin lactobionate, esmolol, fentanyl, fluconazole, furosemide, gentamicin, glyceryl trinitrate, hydrocortisone sodium succinate, labetalol, magnesium sulfate, methylprednisolone sodium succinate, metoclopramide, metronidazole, midazolam, noradrenaline (norepinephrine), piperacillin with tazobactam, ranitidine, ticarcillin with clavulanate, tobramycin, verapamil |
| pH | 5-6 |
| Sodium content | Negligible |
| Storage | Store below 25°C in original packaging. |
| Displacement value | Negligible |
| Stability after preparation | From a microbiological point of view should be used immediately, however:<br>• Reconstituted vials may be stored at 2-8°C for 24 hours.<br>• Prepared infusions may be stored at 2-8°C and infused (at room temperature) within 24 hours. |

## Monitoring

| Measure | Frequency | Rationale |
|---|---|---|
| ACT | Initially 5 minutes after loading dose (see also rationale) | • If the 5-minute ACT is <225 seconds, a second bolus dose of 0.3 mg/kg should be given and re-checked after a further 5 minutes.<br>• Once the ACT value is >225 seconds, no further monitoring is required provided the IV infusion is properly given. |
| Renal function | Periodically | • Changes in renal function may require an adjustment in infusion rate, but check ACT first. |
| FBC and Blood pressure | | • Unexplained ↓haematocrit, Hb or BP may indicate haemorrhage.<br>• Treatment should be stopped if bleeding is observed or suspected.<br>• Consider testing stool for occult blood. |

## Additional information

| | |
|---|---|
| Common and serious undesirable effects | *Immediate:* Anaphylaxis and other hypersensitivity reactions have been reported rarely.<br>*Other:* Minor bleeding at any site, major haemorrhage at any site (including reports with fatal outcome), bruising. |
| Pharmacokinetics | Elimination half-life is 35–40 minutes. |
| Significant interactions | • The following may ↑bivalirudin levels or effect (or ↑side-effects): thrombolytics, coumarin anticoagulants, antiplatelet drugs. |
| Action in case of overdose | No known antidote. Stop administration and give supportive therapy as appropriate. Monitor for signs of bleeding. |

| | |
|---|---|
| Risk rating: **AMBER** | Score = 5<br>Moderate-risk product: Risk-reduction strategies are recommended. |

This assessment is based on the full range of preparation and administration options described in the monograph. These may not all be applicable in some clinical situations.

### Bibliography

SPC Angiox 250 mg powder for concentrate for solution for injection or infusion (accessed 26 March 2010).

# Bumetanide

### 500 micrograms/mL solution in 4-mL ampoules

• Bumetanide is a loop diuretic with properties similar to those of furosemide.
• It may be given parenterally when the oral route is unavailable or ineffective in oedematous conditions, e.g. acute pulmonary oedema, acute and chronic renal failure.

### Pre-treatment checks

• Do not use in hypovolaemia, dehydration, severe ↓K, severe ↓Na; comatose or pre-comatose states associated with liver cirrhosis; renal failure due to nephrotoxic or hepatotoxic drugs, anuria.
• Caution in ↓BP; prostatic enlargement; impaired micturition; gout; diabetes; hepato-renal syndrome; hepatic impairment; renal impairment.
• Fluid balance and electrolytes should be carefully controlled and, in particular in patients with shock, measures should be taken to correct BP and circulating blood volume before commencing treatment.

*Biochemical and other tests*

| | |
|---|---|
| Blood glucose | LFTs |
| Blood pressure | Renal function: U, Cr, CrCl (or eGFR) |
| Electrolytes: serum Na, K, Mg | |

## Dose

**Pulmonary oedema:** initially 1–2 mg (or 500 micrograms in elderly patients) by IV injection, repeated 20 minutes later if necessary. Alternatively, give 1 mg by IM injection (or 500 micrograms in elderly patients) and adjust dose according to response.

**Persistent oedematous states:** 2–5 mg by IV infusion. In elderly patients, 500 micrograms daily may be sufficient.

## Intravenous injection (for doses up to 2 mg)

*Preparation and administration*

1. Withdraw the required dose.
2. The solution should be clear and colourless. Inspect visually for particulate matter or discoloration prior to administration and discard if present.
3. Give by IV injection over 1–2 minutes.

## Intermittent intravenous infusion (for doses above 2 mg)

*Preparation and administration*

1. Withdraw the required dose and add to a suitable volume of NaCl 0.9% or Gluc 5% (the manufacturer advises 500 mL; solutions containing up to 1 mg/10 mL have been used).
2. The solution should be clear and colourless. Inspect visually for particulate matter or discoloration prior to administration and discard if present.
3. Give by IV infusion over 30–60 minutes. Protect from direct sunlight.

## Intramuscular injection

*Preparation and administration*

1. Withdraw the required dose.
2. Give by IM injection.

## Technical information

| | |
|---|---|
| Incompatible with | Dobutamine, midazolam, milrinone. |
| Compatible with | **Flush**: NaCl 0.9%<br>**Solutions**: Gluc 5%, NaCl 0.9%, Gluc-NaCl, Hartmann's<br>**Y-site**: Aztreonam, bivalirudin, cisatracurium, clarithromycin, granisetron, piperacillin with tazobactam, propofol, remifentanil |
| pH | 7 |
| Sodium content | Negligible |
| Storage | Store below 25°C in original packaging. |
| Stability after preparation | From a microbiological point of view, should be used immediately; however, may be stored at 2–8°C and infused (at room temperature) within 24 hours. Protect from direct sunlight. Discard if discoloured, cloudy or evidence of precipitation. |

## Monitoring

| Measure | Frequency | Rationale |
|---|---|---|
| Urinary output and relief of symptoms | Throughout treatment | Response to therapy. |
| Fluid balance, serum electrolytes, and bicarbonate | Periodically | • Fluid balance should be carefully controlled. Electrolyte disturbances and metabolic alkalosis may occur. Replace if necessary. Disturbances may require temporary discontinuation of therapy.<br>• ↓K may precipitate coma (use a K-sparing diuretic to prevent this).<br>• ↑Risk of ↓Mg in alcoholic cirrhosis. |
| Renal function | | • Changes in renal function may require a different dose or rate of infusion.<br>• A marked ↑blood urea or the development of oliguria or anuria indicates severe progression of renal disease and treatment should be stopped. |
| Blood pressure | | • Potential for ↓BP and circulatory collapse resulting from rapid mobilisation of oedema fluid. |
| Blood glucose | | • Reduced serum potassium may blunt response to insulin in patients with diabetes mellitus. |

## Additional information

| | |
|---|---|
| Common and serious undesirable effects | *Injection/infusion-related:* Too rapid administration: Tinnitus and deafness.<br>*Other:* ↓Ca, ↓K, ↓Na, ↑uric acid levels, ↑blood glucose, ↓BP, dehydration, blood dyscrasias. |
| Pharmacokinetics | Plasma elimination half-life is about 1-2 hours. |
| Significant interactions | • Bumetanide may ↑risk of ototoxicity with the following drugs: aminoglycosides, polymyxins, vancomycin.<br>• ↓K due to bumetanide may ↑risk of cardiotoxicity with the following drugs: amisulpride, atomoxetine, cardiac glycosides, disopyramide, flecainide, pimozide, sertindole, sotalol.<br>• Bumetanide may cause ↓BP with the following drugs: ACE inhibitors, alpha blockers, ATII receptor antagonists<br>• Bumetanide may ↑levels (or ↑side-effects) of lithium (avoid combination or monitor levels).<br>• Bumetanide may ↓effect of lidocaine (↓K antagonises action). |
| Action in case of overdose | Treat with fluid replacement and electrolytes as necessary. |
| Counselling | Inform patient to report muscle pains/cramps and hearing disturbance. |

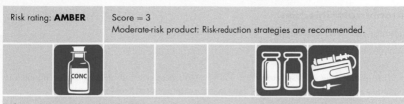

| Risk rating: **AMBER** | Score = 3<br>Moderate-risk product: Risk-reduction strategies are recommended. |

This assessment is based on the full range of preparation and administration options described in the monograph. These may not all be applicable in some clinical situations.

## Bibliography

SPC Bumetanide injection 0.5 mg/mL, solution for injection, Leo Laboratories Ltd (accessed 15 April 2010).

# Buprenorphine

### 300 micrograms/mL solution in 1-mL ampoules

- Buprenorphine hydrochloride is a strong centrally acting opioid analgesic that, at higher doses, also has an opioid antagonist effect (it may antagonise itself and other opioids). It has a lower risk of dependence than that of a pure opiate agonist such as morphine.
- It is used for the treatment of moderate to severe pain.
- Following IM injection analgesia is seen after 10 minutes and lasts for up to 6 hours (onset is quicker after IV injection).
- Doses are expressed in terms of the base:
  Buprenorphine 100 micrograms ≅108 micrograms buprenorphine hydrochloride.

### Pre-treatment checks

- Do not use in acute respiratory depression, where there is a risk of paralytic ileus, in ↑intracranial pressure and in head injury, in comatose patients and phaeochromocytoma.
- Caution in ↓BP, shock, convulsive disorders, supraventricular tachycardias, atrial flutter, chronic obstructive pulmonary disease and acute asthma attack, obstructive or inflammatory bowel diseases, biliary tract diseases, alcoholism, prostatic hyperplasia, myasthenia gravis, hypothyroidism (reduce dose), adrenocortical insufficiency (reduce dose).

*Biochemical and other tests (not all are necessary in an emergency situation)*

| | |
|---|---|
| Blood pressure and pulse | Renal function: U, Cr, CrCl (or eGFR) |
| LFTs | Respiratory rate |
| Pain score | |

### Dose

**Pain:** 300–600 micrograms every 6–8 hours as required by IM or IV injection.
**High-risk patients (i.e. risk of respiratory/CNS depression):** use half the usual adult dose.
**Dose in renal or hepatic impairment:** reduce dose or avoid.

## Intramuscular injection

*Preparation and administration*

1. Withdraw the required dose.
2. Give by deep IM injection.
3. Close monitoring of respiratory rate and consciousness is recommended for 30 minutes in patients receiving initial dose, especially elderly patients or those of low bodyweight.

## Intravenous injection

*Preparation and administration*

1. Withdraw the required dose.
2. The solution should be clear and colourless. Inspect visually for particulate matter or discoloration prior to administration and discard if present.
3. Give by IV injection over at least 2 minutes.
4. Close monitoring of respiratory rate and consciousness is recommended for 30 minutes in patients receiving initial dose, especially elderly patients or those of low bodyweight.

## Technical information

| | |
|---|---|
| Incompatible with | Diazepam, flucloxacillin, furosemide, lorazepam. |
| Compatible with | **Flush**: NaCl 0.9%<br>**Solutions**: NaCl 0.9%, Gluc 5%, Gluc-NaCl, Hartmann's<br>**Y-site**: Aztreonam, cisatracurium, granisetron, midazolam, piperacillin with tazobactam, propofol, remifentanil |
| pH | 3.5–5.5 |
| Sodium content | Nil |
| Storage | Store below 25°C in original packaging. Do not freeze. Controlled Drug. |

## Monitoring

Close monitoring of respiratory rate and consciousness is recommended for 30 minutes in patients receiving initial dose, especially elderly patients of those of low bodyweight.

| Measure | Frequency | Rationale |
|---|---|---|
| Pain score | At regular intervals | • To ensure therapeutic response. |
| Blood pressure, pulse and respiratory rate | | • ↓BP, ↓pulse, ↑pulse, palpitations and respiratory depression with ↓ oxygen saturation can occur. |
| Sedation | | • Can cause sedation and CNS depression. |

## Additional information

| | |
|---|---|
| Common and serious undesirable effects | *Immediate:* Serious hypersensitivity reactions have been reported rarely. *Other:* Nausea and vomiting (particularly initially), constipation, dry mouth, urticaria, pruritus, biliary spasm, ↑ or ↓pulse, hallucinations, euphoria, drowsiness *At higher dose:* ↑ or ↓BP, sedation, respiratory depression, muscle rigidity |
| Pharmacokinetics | Elimination half-life following IV administration is an average of 2.2 hours. Plasma level/analgesia relationship is highly variable. |
| Significant interactions | • The following may ↑buprenorphine levels or effect (or ↑side-effects): antihistamines-sedating (↑sedation), ketoconazole (↓dose), MAOIs (avoid combination and for 2 weeks after stopping MAOI), moclobemide.<br>• Buprenorphine may ↑levels or effect (or ↑side-effects) of sodium oxybate (avoid combination). |
| Action in case of overdose | *Symptoms to watch for:* ↑Sedation, respiratory depression. *Antidote:* Naloxone (see the Naloxone monograph) but may only partially reverse toxicity. Stop administration and give supportive therapy as appropriate. |
| Counselling | May cause drowsiness and dizziness, which may affect the ability to perform skilled tasks; if affected, do not drive or operate machinery, avoid alcoholic drink (the effects of alcohol are enhanced). Drink plenty of fluids to help avoid constipation. |

| | |
|---|---|
| Risk rating: **GREEN** | Score = 2<br>Lower-risk product: Risk-reduction strategies should be considered. |

This assessment is based on the full range of preparation and administration options described in the monograph. These may not all be applicable in some clinical situations.

## Bibliography

SPC Temgesic injection 1 ml (accessed 29 June 2008).

# Buserelin

**1 mg/mL solution in 5.5-mL multidose vials**

- Buserelin acetate is an analogue of gonadorelin (gonadotrophin-releasing hormone).
- In men it is used for the suppression of testosterone in the treatment of prostate cancer (Suprefact).
- In women it is used SC as an adjunct to ovulation induction with gonadotrophins in the treatment of infertility (Suprecur). It is also used intranasally in the treatment of endometriosis.
- Doses are expressed in terms of the base:
  Buserelin 1 mg ≡ 1.05 mg buserelin acetate.

## Pre-treatment checks

- Do not give if there is known hypersensitivity to LHRH or buserelin.
- Contraindicated if tumour is found to be insensitive to hormone manipulation, and in cases of undiagnosed vaginal bleeding.
- Do not use in pregnancy.
- Caution in osteoporosis or those at risk (i.e. chronic alcohol and/or tobacco use, strong family history of osteoporosis or long-term use of drugs that can reduce bone mass e.g. anticonvulsants or corticosteroids).
- Screen for depression in men.

*Biochemical and other tests*

Baseline lipid profile                     LFTs
Blood pressure                            Pregnancy test if appropriate
FBC

## Dose

**Prostate cancer:** 500 micrograms by SC injection every 8 hours for 7 days. On the eighth day the patient is changed to maintenance therapy by the intranasal route. An anti-androgen agent may be given for 5 days before until 3–4 weeks after commencement to ↓risk of disease flare, e.g. cyproterone acetate 100 mg three times daily.

**Assisted reproduction:** 200–500 micrograms by SC injection once daily is administered to down-regulate the pituitary gland. Serum estradiol levels should decline to levels similar to those in the early follicular phase in 7–21 days. Gonadotrophin is then administered following the protocol of the individual clinic.

## Subcutaneous injection

*Preparation and administration*

1. Withdraw the required dose.
2. Give by SC injection.

| Technical information | |
| --- | --- |
| Incompatible with | Not relevant |
| Compatible with | Not relevant |
| pH | Not relevant |

*(continued)*

## Technical information (continued)

| | |
|---|---|
| Sodium content | Negligible |
| Excipients | Contains benzyl alcohol. |
| Storage | Store below 25°C in original packaging. Do not freeze. Discard vials 10 days after opening. |

## Monitoring

| Measure | Frequency | Rationale |
|---|---|---|
| Blood glucose in diabetic patients | Regularly | • ↑Blood glucose levels can occur (↓glucose tolerance). |
| Monitor for signs of OHSS in women | During treatment | • When combined with gonadotrophins there is a higher risk of OHSS than with gonadotrophins alone. The stimulation cycle should be monitored carefully to identify patients at risk of developing OHSS and HCG should be withheld if necessary. <br> • Symptoms include: abdominal pain, feeling of abdominal tension, ↑abdominal girth, occurrence of ovarian cysts, nausea, vomiting, massive enlargement of the ovaries, dyspnoea, diarrhoea, oliguria, haemoconcentration, hypercoagulability. |
| Serum testosterone in men | If indicated | • Consider measurement if the anticipated clinical or biochemical response in prostate cancer has not been achieved within 4 weeks (levels <20 nanograms/dL are considered equivalent to surgical castration).[1] |
| LFTs | Periodically | • Levels of serum Alk Phos and bilirubin may be raised. |
| Blood lipid levels | | • Lipid levels can be lowered and raised. |
| FBC | | • Thrombocytopenia and leucopenia sometimes occur. |
| Blood pressure | | • ↓BP or ↑BP can occur (rarely) and may require medical intervention or withdrawal of treatment. |
| Symptoms of depression in men | | • Emotional instability is a frequent side-effect. |

## Additional information

| | |
|---|---|
| Common and serious undesirable effects | *Immediate:* Rarely anaphylaxis and other hypersensitivity reactions. <br> *Injection/infusion-related:* Local: Injection-site pain, reddening of the skin, itching. <br> *Other:* ↓BMD, hot flushes, sweating, ↓libido, breast tenderness (infrequently). <br> Women: Headaches, mood changes, depression, vaginal dryness, change in breast size. |
| Pharmacokinetics | Elimination half-life is 80 minutes. |

(continued)

## Additional information (continued)

| Significant interactions | No significant interactions. |
|---|---|
| Action in case of overdose | There is no specific antidote and treatment should be symptomatic. |
| Counselling | Buserelin may impair the ability to concentrate and react, so caution is needed if operating a vehicle or machinery. <br> Fertile women should use non-hormonal barrier methods of contraception during the entire treatment period. |

| Risk rating: **GREEN** | Score = 1 <br> Lower-risk product: Risk-reduction strategies should be considered. |
|---|---|

This assessment is based on the full range of preparation and administration options described in the monograph. These may not all be applicable in some clinical situations.

## Reference

1. Morote J *et al*. Redefining clinically significant castration levels in patients with prostate cancer receiving continuous androgen deprivation therapy. *J Urol* 2007; 178(4): 1290–1295.

## Bibliography

SPC Suprecur injection (accessed 2 March 2009).
SPC Suprefact injection (accessed 2 March 2009).

# Calcitonin (salmon)

**50 units/mL solution in 1-mL ampoules; 100 units/mL solution in 1-mL ampoules; 200 units/mL solution in 2-mL vials**

* Calcitonin (salmon) is a hormone acting mainly on bone to ↓Ca levels and inhibit bone resorption. It is prepared synthetically or by recombinant DNA technology.
* There is some confusion about terminology, but in practice the terms salcatonin, calcitonin (salmon), salmon calcitonin and calcitonin-salmon appear to be used for the same substance.
* Calcitonin (salmon) is licensed for use in the treatment of Paget's disease (of bone), in hypercalcaemia of malignancy and to prevent acute bone loss due to sudden immobilisation. It is also licensed for intranasal use in the treatment of postmenopausal osteoporosis.
* Doses are expressed in units:
  Calcitonin (salmon) 128 units ≈ 20 micrograms of freeze dried purified synthetic salmon calcitonin.

## Pre-treatment checks

* Avoid in hypocalcaemia.
* If sensitivity to calcitonin is suspected, a skin test should be conducted prior to treatment.
* Ensure that the patient is adequately hydrated before giving by IV infusion.

*Biochemical and other tests*

Electrolytes: serum Ca

## Dose

Administer at bedtime, particularly at the start of therapy, to ↓incidence of nausea or vomiting.

**Hypercalcaemia of malignancy:** initially 100 units by SC or IM injection every 6–8 hours, increasing to a maximum of 400 units every 6–8 hours after 1–2 days if necessary. In severe or emergency cases up to 10 units/kg may be given by IV infusion.

**Paget's disease:** doses range from 50 units three times a week to 100 units daily by SC or IM injection adjusted to patient's needs.

**Prevention of acute bone loss:** 100 units daily or 50 units twice daily by SC or IM injection. The dose may be reduced to 50 units daily at the start of remobilisation; maintain treatment until patient is fully mobile.

## Subcutaneous injection

*Preparation and administration*

1. Remove from refrigerator and allow injection to reach room temperature.
2. Withdraw the required dose.
3. Give by SC injection.

## Intramuscular injection

*Preparation and administration*

1. Remove from refrigerator and allow injection to reach room temperature.
2. Withdraw the required dose.
3. Give by IM injection.

## Intravenous infusion

*Preparation and administration*

1. Withdraw the required dose and add to 500 mL NaCl 0.9% (glass or hard plastic containers should not be used).
2. The solution should be clear and colourless. Inspect visually for particulate matter or discoloration prior to administration and discard if present.
3. Give by IV infusion over at least 6 hours.

## Technical information

| | |
|---|---|
| Incompatible with | Glass or hard plastic containers should not be used. |
| Compatible with | **Flush**: NaCl 0.9%<br>**Solutions**: NaCl 0.9%<br>**Y-site**: No information |
| pH | 3.9-4.5 |
| Sodium content | Negligible |
| Storage | Store in a refrigerator (2-8°C).<br>*In use:* Multidose vials may be stored at room temperature for a maximum of 1 month from first use. |
| Stability after preparation | Use prepared infusions immediately. |

## Monitoring

| Measure | Frequency | Rationale |
|---|---|---|
| Serum Ca | Daily when treatment commences then periodically | • Monitoring of effectiveness in hypercalcaemia of malignancy. |
| Markers of bone remodelling, e.g. Alk Phos or urinary hydroxyproline or deoxypyridinoline | Periodically | • Monitoring of effectiveness in Paget's disease. |

## Additional information

| | |
|---|---|
| Common and serious undesirable effects | *Immediate:* Allergic reactions including anaphylaxis and bronchospasm have been reported. Flushing of the face or upper body is not an allergic reaction but is commonly seen 10-20 minutes after administration.<br>*Injection/infusion-related:* Local: Injection-site reactions.<br>*Other:* Nausea, vomiting (may be given at bedtime to reduce incidence of nausea and vomiting), diarrhoea, abdominal pain, musculoskeletal pain, fatigue, dizziness, headache, taste disturbances. |
| Pharmacokinetics | Elimination half-life is 1-1.5 hours. Clearance is longer in end-stage renal impairment but the clinical significance of this is unknown. |

*(continued)*

| **Additional information** (*continued*) | |
|---|---|
| Significant interactions | No significant interactions. |
| Action in case of overdose | Symptoms of overdose include nausea and vomiting. Treatment should be symptomatic and supportive. |

Risk rating: **GREEN**  Score = 2
Lower-risk product: Risk-reduction strategies should be considered.

This assessment is based on the full range of preparation and administration options described in the monograph. These may not all be applicable in some clinical situations.

## Bibliography

SPC Miacalcic (accessed 6 July 2010).

# Calcitriol (1,25-dihydroxycholecalciferol)

**1 microgram/mL solution in ampoules**

* The term vitamin D is used for a range of closely related sterol compounds including alfacalcidol, calcitriol, colecalciferol and ergocalciferol. Vitamin D compounds possess the property of preventing or curing rickets.
* Calcitriol injection is indicated in the management of hypocalcaemia in patients undergoing dialysis for chronic renal failure. It has been shown to significantly reduce elevated parathyroid hormone (PTH) levels. Reduction of PTH has been shown to result in an improvement in renal osteodystrophy.

## Pre-treatment checks

* Do not give to patients with hypercalcaemia, including hypercalcaemia of malignancy.
* For treatment to be effective, patients should be receiving an adequate daily intake of calcium (dietary or prescribed).

*Biochemical and other tests*

Electrolytes: serum Ca, $PO_4$
Liver function: Alk Phos
Renal function: U, Cr

## Dose

**Hypocalcaemia in adult dialysis patients:** initially 500 nanograms ($\simeq$10 nanograms/kg) three times a week, increased if necessary in steps of 250–500 nanograms at intervals of 2–4 weeks; usual dose 0.5–3 micrograms 3 times a week.

**Moderate to severe secondary hyperparathyroidism in adult dialysis patients:** initially 0.5–4 micrograms 3 times a week, increased if necessary in steps of 250–500 nanograms at intervals of 2–4 weeks; maximum dose is 8 micrograms 3 times a week.

### Intravenous injection

*Preparation and administration*

1. Withdraw the required dose into a plastic 1-mL tuberculin syringe.
2. The solution should be a clear, colourless to yellow solution. Inspect visually for particulate matter or discoloration prior to administration.
3. Give by rapid IV injection or through the catheter at the end of dialysis.

## Technical information

| | |
|---|---|
| Incompatible with | Do not infuse with the dialysate during CAPD as there is significant absorption onto PVC bags and tubing. |
| Compatible with | **Flush**: NaCl 0.9% <br> **Solutions**: No information <br> **Y-site**: No information |
| pH | 5.9-7 |
| Sodium content | Negligible |
| Storage | Store below 25°C in original packaging but do not refrigerate. |

## Monitoring

| Measure | Frequency | Rationale |
|---|---|---|
| Hypersensitivity reactions | During and after administration | • Local or systemic allergic reactions, including anaphylaxis have been reported rarely. |
| Serum Ca and $PO_4$ | Initially weekly until dose and plasma Ca and $PO_4$ are stable, then monthly; also whenever nausea or vomiting occurs | • ↑Ca and ↑$PO_4$ can occur during treatment with pharmacological doses of compounds having vitamin D activity. <br> • Plasma $PO_4$ concentrations should be controlled to reduce the risk of ectopic calcification. |
| LFTs | Monthly | • A fall in serum Alk Phos levels often precedes the appearance of ↑Ca. |
| Ophthalmological examination | Periodically | • To check for ectopic calcification. |
| Signs/symptoms of toxicity | | • E.g. persistent constipation or diarrhoea, constant headache, loss of appetite, mental changes. |

| Additional information | |
|---|---|
| Common and serious undesirable effects | *Immediate:* Rarely hypersensitivity reactions including anaphylaxis.<br>*Injection-related:* Local: Redness at injection site.<br>*Other:* ↑Ca (persistent constipation or diarrhoea, constant headache, vertigo, loss of appetite, polyuria, thirst, sweating). |
| Pharmacokinetics | Elimination half-life is 5–8 hours. However, the metabolic effects of calcitriol continue long after the plasma level of the hormone has returned to baseline therefore plasma half-life is considered irrelevant. |
| Significant interactions | No significant interactions. |
| Action in case of overdose | Stop treatment if ↑Ca develops until plasma Ca levels return to normal (about 1 week). Restart treatment at a lower dose if appropriate. In severe ↑Ca give supportive therapy as appropriate. |
| Counselling | Advise patients to report symptoms of ↑Ca: persistent constipation or diarrhoea, constant headache, vertigo, loss of appetite, polyuria, thirst, sweating. |

| Risk rating: **GREEN** | Score = 1<br>Lower-risk product: Risk-reduction strategies should be considered. |
|---|---|

This assessment is based on the full range of preparation and administration options described in the monograph. These may not all be applicable in some clinical situations.

## Bibliography

SPC Calcijex SPC (accessed 25 January 2009).

# Calcium chloride

**10% solution in 10-mL pre-filled syringes; 13.4% solution in 10-mL ampoules**

* Calcium is the most abundant mineral in the body. It is required for bone and tooth formation and is an essential electrolyte.
* Normal range for plasma total calcium ('corrected' if necessary): 2.1–2.6 mmol/L.
* Calcium chloride may be used parenterally in cardiac resuscitation if PEA is thought to be caused by ↑K or ↓Ca or in calcium channel blocker overdose.[1]
* Calcium salts are used to treat severe acute ↓Ca or tetany and to stabilise the myocardium in severe ↑K. Calcium gluconate is generally preferred to calcium chloride in non-emergency situations because it is less irritant to veins.
* Calcium salts are also used (unlicensed) in the treatment of patients with significant clinical features of magnesium poisoning.

10% calcium chloride injection contains:     $Ca^{2+}$ 680 micromol/mL (calcium 27.3 mg/mL).

13.4% calcium chloride injection contains:     $Ca^{2+}$ 910 micromol/mL (calcium 36 mg/mL).

These preparations must not be confused with calcium gluconate injection, which has a markedly different $Ca^{2+}$ content.

## Pre-treatment checks

* Do not give to patients receiving cardiac glycosides.
* Do not use for hypocalcaemia caused by renal impairment.
* Do not use in conditions associated with hypercalcaemia and hypercalciuria (e.g. some forms of malignant disease).
* Caution in patients with impaired renal function, cardiac disease, sarcoidosis, respiratory acidosis or respiratory failure.
* In cardiac resuscitation do not administer if the patient is in ventricular failure.

*Biochemical and other tests (not all are necessary in an emergency situation)*

Blood pressure                                    Electrolytes: serum Ca
ECG                                               Renal function: Cr, CrCl (or eGFR)

## Dose

Calcium chloride must not be given IM or SC.
Calcium chloride is more irritant than calcium gluconate when given IV and is generally reserved for use in emergency situations.

**Cardiac resuscitation:** initially 6.8 mmol (10 mL of 10% injection $\equiv$ 7.5 mL of 13.4% injection) repeated as necessary. In cardiac arrest give by rapid IV injection, in the presence of spontaneous circulation give by slow IV injection.[1]
**Acute hypocalcaemia:** see the Calcium gluconate monograph.
**Hyperkalaemia as part of overall treatment regimen (K > 6.5 mmol/L or if ECG changes are present):** see the Calcium gluconate monograph.
**Magnesium toxicity:** it is essential to consult a poisons information service, e.g. Toxbase at www.toxbase.org (password or registration required), for full details of the management of magnesium toxicity.

## Intravenous injection (cardiac resuscitation)

*Preparation and administration*

Very irritant: give into the largest accessible vein if possible.

1. Either assemble the pre-filled syringe in accordance with the manufacturer's instructions or withdraw the required dose.
2. The solution should be clear and colourless. Inspect visually for particulate matter or discoloration prior to administration and discard if present.
3. Give by IV injection into a large vein at a rate appropriate to the patient's clinical condition.

## Technical information

| | |
|---|---|
| Incompatible with | Sodium bicarbonate, other bicarbonates, phosphates, tartrates and sulfates.<br>Amphotericin. |
| Compatible with | **Solutions**: NaCl 0.9%, Gluc 5%, Gluc-NaCl<br>**Y-site**: Adrenaline (epinephrine), lidocaine, milrinone, noradrenaline (norepinephrine), verapamil |
| pH | 5–8 |
| Sodium content | Negligible |
| Osmolarity (plasma osmolality = 280–300 mOsmol/L)[2] | Calcium chloride 10% $\cong$ 2040 mOsmol/L. |
| Storage | Store below 25°C in original packaging. |

## Monitoring

| Measure | Frequency | Rationale |
|---|---|---|
| ECG | During administration | • If using to treat ↑K. |
| Blood pressure | Post administration | • May ↓BP |
| Injection site | | • Injection-site reactions have occurred. |
| Serum Ca | Daily | • To ensure ↓Ca is effectively treated. |

## Additional information

| | |
|---|---|
| Common and serious undesirable effects | *Injection-related:*<br>• Ioo rapid administration: Vasodilatation, ↓BP, ↓pulse and arrhythmias, tingling sensations, taste of calcium and a sense of oppression or heat wave.<br>• Local: Irritation of skin. Extravasation may cause necrosis and sloughing of tissue. |
| Pharmacokinetics | After IV administration serum Ca will increase immediately and may return to normal values in 30–120 minutes. |
| Significant drug interactions | • The following may ↑Ca levels or effect (or ↑side-effects):<br>thiazides (↓urinary Ca excretion).<br>• Calcium chloride may ↑levels or effect of the following drugs (or ↑side-effects):<br>digoxin, digitoxin. |
| Action in case of overdose | Overdose can lead to ↑Ca. Treat initially with IV infusion of NaCl 0.9%. |

| Risk rating: **AMBER** | Score = 3<br>Moderate-risk product: Risk-reduction strategies are recommended. |
|---|---|

This assessment is based on the full range of preparation and administration options described in the monograph. These may not all be applicable in some clinical situations.

### References

1. Resuscitation Council UK. *Resuscitation Guidelines 2005*. www.resus.org.uk/pages/mediMain.htm (accessed 12 April 2010).
2. Longmore M *et al*., eds. *Oxford Handbook of Clinical Medicine*, 6th edn. Oxford: Oxford University Press, 2004.

### Bibliography

SPC Calcium Chloride Injection Minijet 10%, International Medication Systems (accessed 30 March 2010).
SPC Calcium Chloride BP sterile solution 13.4%, UCB Pharma Ltd (accessed 30 March 2010).

# Calcium folinate (calcium leucovorin)

**3 mg/mL, 7.5 mg/mL, 10 mg/mL solution in ampoules or vials (various sizes)**
* Calcium folinate is a derivative of tetrahydrofolic acid, the active form of folic acid.
* It is used as an antidote to folic acid antagonists such as methotrexate (commonly known as 'folinic acid rescue' or 'calcium leucovorin rescue') and as an adjunct to fluorouracil (FU) in the treatment of colorectal cancer.
* Doses are usually expressed in terms of folinic acid:
  Folinic acid 1 mg ≅1.08 mg anhydrous calcium folinate.

### Pre-treatment checks

* Do not give if the patient is anaemic owing to vitamin $B_{12}$ deficiency.

*Biochemical and other tests*

FBC                                              Renal function: U, Cr, CrCl (or eGFR)
LFTs                                             U&Es

### Dose

Calcium folinate **must not** be administered intrathecally.

Consult specialist literature as regimens vary greatly depending on the indication.

## Intravenous injection

*Preparation and administration*

1. In the UK vials do not require reconstitution; in the USA some products require reconstitution with WFI (volume varies with product).
2. Withdraw the required dose.
3. The solution should be clear and pale yellow. Inspect visually for particulate matter or discoloration prior to administration and discard if present.
4. Give by IV injection at a maximum rate of 160 mg/minute (due to the Ca content of the solution).

## Intermittent intravenous infusion

*Preparation and administration*

1. In the UK vials do not require reconstitution; in the USA some products require reconstitution with WFI or NaCl 0.9% (volume varies with product).
2. Withdraw the required dose and add to a suitable volume of compatible infusion fluid (usually 100–250 mL NaCl 0.9%).
3. The solution should be clear and pale yellow. Inspect visually for particulate matter or discoloration prior to administration and discard if present.
4. Give by IV infusion over (usually) 2 hours. Protect from light.

## Intramuscular injection

*Preparation and administration*

1. In the UK vials do not require reconstitution; in the USA some products require reconstitution with WFI or NaCl 0.9% (volume varies with product).
2. Withdraw the required dose.
3. Give by IM injection.

## Technical information

| | |
|---|---|
| Incompatible with | Sodium bicarbonate.<br>Amphotericin, fluorouracil, foscarnet. |
| Compatible with | **Flush**: NaCl 0.9%<br>**Solutions**: NaCl 0.9%, Gluc 5%<br>**Y-site**: Aztreonam, fluconazole, furosemide, granisetron, linezolid, metoclopramide, piperacillin with tazobactam |
| pH | 6.5–8.5 |
| Electrolyte content | Sodium: Negligible<br>Calcium: 0.2 mmol/100 mg |
| Storage | Store at 2–8°C in original packing. |
| Stability after preparation | From a microbiological point of view, should be used immediately; however, prepared infusions may be protected from light, stored at 2–8°C and infused (at room temperature) within 24 hours. |

## Monitoring

| Measure | Frequency | Rationale |
|---------|-----------|-----------|
| Serum Ca | Periodically | • Monitored if combined with FU.<br>• Supplementation should be provided if Ca levels are low. |
| Diarrhoea | During treatment | • A sign of GI toxicity when combined with FU.<br>• ↓Dose of FU until symptoms have fully disappeared. |
| Creatinine and methotrexate levels | At least daily in folinic acid rescue | • Dose of calcium folinate is dependent on these parameters in 'rescue'. |
| FBC | Weekly during first two courses of FU then once each cycle thereafter | • In combination with FU only. |
| U&Es, LFTs | Prior to each treatment for the first 3 cycles and prior to every other cycle thereafter | • In combination with FU only. |

## Additional information

| | |
|---|---|
| Common and serious undesirable effects | In combination with FU: vomiting and nausea, severe mucosal toxicity, diarrhoea with higher grades of toxicity leading to dehydration. |
| Pharmacokinetics | Elimination half-life is about 6 hours. |
| Significant interactions | No significant interactions. |
| Action in case of overdose | There have been no reports of overdose with calcium folinate. |

| Risk rating: **AMBER** | Score = 5<br>Moderate-risk product: Risk-reduction strategies are recommended. |
|---|---|

This assessment is based on the full range of preparation and administration options described in the monograph. These may not all be applicable in some clinical situations.

## Bibliography

SPC Calcium folinate 10 mg/mL injection, Hospira UK Ltd (accessed 2 March 2009).

SPC Calcium folinate 15 mg/2 mL injection, Hospira UK Ltd (accessed 2 March 2009).

SPC Calcium folinate 3 mg/mL injection, Hospira UK Ltd (accessed 2 March 2009).

SPC Lederfolin solution (Calcium leucovorin solution for injection 350mg/vial) (accessed 2 March 2009).

# Calcium gluconate

**10% solution in 10-mL ampoules**

- Calcium is the most abundant mineral in the body. It is required for bone and tooth formation and is an essential electrolyte.
- Normal range for plasma total calcium ('corrected' if necessary): 2.1–2.6 mmol/L.
- Calcium gluconate injection is used to treat severe acute ↓Ca or tetany and to stabilise the myocardium in severe ↑K.
- Calcium gluconate injection is also used (unlicensed) in the treatment of patients with significant clinical features of magnesium poisoning.
- Calcium may be used parenterally in cardiac resuscitation (more usually in the form of calcium chloride pre-filled syringes) if PEA is thought to be caused by ↑K or ↓Ca or in calcium channel blocker overdose.
- Intra-arterial calcium gluconate followed by hepatic venous sampling has been used to diagnose insulinomas (unlicensed).
- Because of the risk of aluminium exposure, calcium gluconate injection packed in small-volume glass containers should not be used for repeated or prolonged treatment in children < 18 years or in patients with renal impairment. Calcium gluconate injection packed in plastic containers may be used.[1]

10% calcium gluconate injection contains: $Ca^{2+}$ 225 micromol/mL (calcium 8.4 mg/mL).

This preparation must not be confused with calcium chloride injections, which have a markedly different $Ca^{2+}$ content.

## Pre-treatment checks

- Do not give to patients receiving cardiac glycosides.
- Do not use for hypocalcaemia caused by renal impairment.
- Do not use in conditions associated with hypercalcaemia and hypercalciuria (e.g. some forms of malignant disease) and in severe renal impairment.
- Caution in patients with mild to moderate renal impairment, cardiac disease, sarcoidosis, respiratory acidosis or respiratory failure.

*Biochemical and other tests (not all are necessary in an emergency situation)*

Renal function: U, Cr, CrCl (or eGFR)          ECG
Electrolytes: serum Ca          Bodyweight (in certain indications)

## Dose

Calcium salts are irritant and may cause tissue necrosis and sloughing if given IM or SC. Calcium chloride is more irritant than calcium gluconate when given IV although both may cause irritation and should be given with care to avoid extravasation.

**Acute hypocalcaemia:** 2.25 mmol (10 mL of 10% injection) by slow IV injection. In tetany this should be followed by 9 mmol (40 mL of 10% injection) in 500 mL NaCl 0.9% or Gluc 5% by IV infusion daily over 8–24 hours with frequent monitoring of serum Ca. Smaller volumes may be used in fluid restriction.

An alternative regimen is to give 22.5 mmol Ca (100 mL of 10% injection) in 1 L of NaCl 0.9% or Gluc 5% solution by IV infusion at an initial rate of 50 mL/hour. Adjust the rate of infusion according to 4–6 hourly plasma Ca measurements.

**Hyperkalaemia as part of overall treatment regimen (K > 6.5 mmol/L or if ECG changes are present):** give 10 mL calcium gluconate 10% by IV injection to stabilise cardiac muscle. Repeat as necessary, dependent on ECG.

**Cardiac resuscitation:** calcium chloride injection is preferred (see the Calcium chloride monograph).

**Magnesium toxicity:** it is essential to consult a poisons information service, e.g. Toxbase at www. toxbase.org (password or registration required), for full details of the management of magnesium toxicity.

## Intravenous injection

*Preparation and administration*

1. Withdraw the required dose.
2. The solution should be clear and colourless. Inspect visually for particulate matter or discoloration prior to administration and discard if present.
3. Give by slow IV injection (10 mL of 10% injection over a minimum of 3 minutes).

## Intermittent or continuous intravenous infusion

*Preparation and administration*

1. Withdraw the required dose and add to a 500–1000 mL (see information above) NaCl 0.9% or Gluc 5%. Mix well.
2. The solution should be clear and colourless. Inspect visually for particulate matter or discoloration prior to administration and discard if present.
3. Give by IV infusion over 8–24 hours depending on the dosing regimen. Adjust dose and rate according to serum Ca.
4. Prepare a fresh infusion bag at least every 24 hours.

## Technical information

| | |
|---|---|
| Incompatible with | Bicarbonates, phosphates, tartrates and sulfates. Amphotericin, dobutamine. |
| Compatible with | **Flush**: NaCl 0.9% <br> **Solutions**: NaCl 0.9%, Gluc 5%, Gluc-NaCl, Hartmann's <br> **Y-site**: No information |
| pH | 6-8.2 |
| Sodium content | Nil |
| Osmolality (plasma osmolality = 280-300 mOsmol/L)[2] | Calcium gluconate 10% $\cong$ 680 mOsmol/L. |
| Storage | Store below 25°C in original packaging. Do not freeze. |
| Stability after preparation | Use prepared infusions immediately. |

## Monitoring

| Measure | Frequency | Rationale |
|---------|-----------|-----------|
| ECG | During administration | • If using to treat ↑K. |
| Serum Ca | During therapy | • For signs of clinical improvement.<br>• Monitor every 4-6 hours if giving by continuous infusion. |
| Blood pressure | Periodically | • May ↓BP. |
| Injection site | | • Injection-site reactions have occurred. |

## Additional information

| | |
|---|---|
| Common and serious undesirable effects | *Injection/infusion-related:*<br>• Too rapid administration: nausea, vomiting, hot flushes, sweating, ↓BP and vasomotor collapse may occur.<br>• Local: Irritation. Extravasation may cause tissue damage. |
| Pharmacokinetics | After IV administration serum Ca will increase immediately and may return to normal values in 30–120 minutes. |
| Significant interactions | • The following may ↑calcium levels or effect (or ↑side-effects): thiazides (↓urinary Ca excretion).<br>• Calcium gluconate may ↑levels or effect of the following drugs (or ↑side-effects): digoxin, digitoxin. |
| Action in case of overdose | Overdose can lead to ↑Ca. Treat initially with IV infusion of NaCl 0.9%. |

| Risk rating: **AMBER** | Score = 3<br>Moderate-risk product: Risk-reduction strategies are recommended. |

This assessment is based on the full range of preparation and administration options described in the monograph. These may not all be applicable in some clinical situations.

## Reference

1. MHRA. Calcium gluconate injection in small-volume glass containers: new contraindications due to aluminium exposure risk. *Drug Safety Update*: Volume 4, Issue 1, August 2010.
2. Longmore M *et al.*, eds. *Oxford Handbook of Clinical Medicine*, 6th edn. Oxford: Oxford University Press, 2004.

## Bibliography

SPC Calcium Gluconate Injection BP, Hameln (accessed 30 March 2010).
SPC Calcium Gluconate Injection BP, Goldshield (accessed 30 March 2010).

# Calcium levofolinate (calcium levoleucovorin)

**10 mg/mL solution in 2.5-mL, 5-mL or 17.5-mL vials**

* Calcium levofolinate is the levorotatory enantiomer of calcium folinate. It is used in a similar way but generally at half the doses recommended for the racemic form.
* It is used as an antidote to folic acid antagonists such as methotrexate (commonly known as 'folinic acid rescue' or 'calcium leucovorin rescue') and as an adjunct to fluorouracil (FU) in the treatment of colorectal cancer.
* Doses are usually expressed in terms of folinic acid:
  Folinic acid 1 mg $\equiv$ 1.08 mg anhydrous calcium levofolinate.

## Pre-treatment checks

* Do not give if anaemic due to vitamin $B_{12}$ deficiency.

*Biochemical and other tests*

FBC                                         Serum creatinine
LFTs                                        U&Es

## Dose

Calcium levofolinate **must not** be administered intrathecally.

Consult specialist literature as regimens vary greatly depending on the indication.

## Intravenous injection

*Preparation and administration*

1. Withdraw the required dose.
2. The solution should be clear and pale yellow. Inspect visually for particulate matter or discoloration prior to administration and discard if present.
3. Give by IV injection at a maximum rate of 160 mg/minute (due to the Ca content of the solution).

## Intermittent intravenous infusion

*Preparation and administration*

1. Withdraw the required dose and add to a suitable volume of compatible infusion fluid (usually 100–250 mL NaCl 0.9%).
2. The solution should be clear and pale yellow. Inspect visually for particulate matter or discoloration prior to administration and discard if present.
3. Give by IV infusion over (usually) 2 hours. Protect from light.

## Intramuscular injection

*Preparation and administration*

1. Withdraw the required dose.
2. Give by IM injection.

## Technical information

| | |
|---|---|
| Incompatible with | Sodium bicarbonate.<br>Fluorouracil. |
| Compatible with | **Flush**: NaCl 0.9%<br>**Solutions**: NaCl 0.9%, Gluc 5%, Gluc-NaCl, Hartmann's<br>**Y-site**: Granisetron |
| pH[1] | 7.5-8.5 |
| Electrolyte content | Sodium: Negligible<br>Calcium: 0.2 mmol/100 mg |
| Storage | Store at 2-8°C in original packing. |
| Stability after preparation | From a microbiological point of view, should be used immediately; however, prepared infusions may be protected from light, stored at 2-8°C and infused (at room temperature) within 24 hours. |

## Monitoring

| Measure | Frequency | Rationale |
|---|---|---|
| Serum Ca | Periodically | • Monitored if combined with FU.<br>• Supplementation should be provided if Ca levels are low. |
| Diarrhoea | During treatment | • A sign of GI toxicity when combined with FU.<br>• ↓Dose of FU until symptoms have fully disappeared. |
| Creatinine and methotrexate levels | At least daily in folinic acid rescue | • Dose of calcium folinate is dependent on these parameters in 'rescue'. |
| FBC | Weekly during first two courses of FU then once each cycle thereafter | • In combination with FU only. |
| U&Es, LFTs | Prior to each treatment for the first 3 cycles and prior to every other cycle thereafter | • In combination with FU only. |

## Additional information

| | |
|---|---|
| Common and serious undesirable effects | In combination with FU: vomiting and nausea, severe mucosal toxicity, diarrhoea with higher grades of toxicity leading to dehydration. |
| Pharmacokinetics | Elimination half-life is about 6 hours. |
| Significant interactions | No significant interactions. |
| Action in case of overdose | There have been no reports of overdose with calcium levofolinate. |

| Risk rating: **AMBER** | Score = 4 Moderate-risk product: Risk-reduction strategies are recommended. |

This assessment is based on the full range of preparation and administration options described in the monograph. These may not all be applicable in some clinical situations.

## Reference

1. Correspondence with Wyeth 6 April 2009.

## Bibliography

SPC Isovorin (accessed 6 April 2009).
PIL Levofolinic acid 10 mg/ml solution for injection, Hospira UK Ltd (accessed 6 April 2009).

# Capreomycin

**1-g (1 million units) dry powder vials**
* Capreomycin sulfate is a polypeptide complex of four microbiologically active components.
* It may be used as a second-line antimycobacterial in the treatment of tuberculosis as part of a multidrug regimen when resistance to primary drugs has developed.
* Doses are expressed in terms of capreomycin base.

## Pre-treatment checks

Use with caution in patients with auditory impairment or eighth cranial nerve damage.

*Biochemical and other tests*

| | |
|---|---|
| Baseline check of auditory and vestibular function | FBC |
| Bodyweight | LFTs |
| Electrolytes: serum K, Mg | Renal function: U, Cr, CrCl (or eGFR) |

## Dose

**Standard dose:** 1 g daily by IM injection (and not more than 20 mg/kg) for 2–4 months, then 1 g 2–3 times each week.

**Dose in renal impairment**: there are two similar strategies for dosing in renal impairment:
* The manufacturer recommends doses should be adjusted according to creatinine clearance. The doses in Table C1 are calculated to achieve a mean steady-state capreomycin level of 10 micrograms/mL, at various levels of renal function.
* The British Thoracic Society recommends CrCl >50 mL/minute be dosed daily and CrCl <50 mL/minute be dosed every 48 hours. In both cases the dose should be adjusted according to the capreomycin serum concentration with a desired steady state level of 10 micrograms/mL.[1]
* If the patient is receiving haemodialysis, give the dose after a dialysis session.

**Table C1**  Capreomycin: dose adjustment according to creatinine clearance

| Creatinine clearance (mL/minute) | Dose for these dosing intervals (mg/kg) | | |
|---|---|---|---|
| | 24-hourly | 48-hourly | 72-hourly |
| 0 | 1.29 | 2.58 | 3.87 |
| 10 | 2.43 | 4.87 | 7.30 |
| 20 | 3.58 | 7.16 | 10.70 |
| 30 | 4.72 | 9.45 | 14.20 |
| 40 | 5.87 | 11.70 | |
| 50 | 7.01 | 14.00 | |
| 60 | 8.16 | | |
| 80 | 10.40 | | |
| 100 | 12.70 | | |
| 110 | 13.90 | | |

## Intramuscular injection

*Preparation and administration*

1. Reconstitute each 1-g vial with 2 mL* NaCl 0.9% or WFI.
2. Allow 2–3 minutes for complete dissolution.
3. The solution should be clear and colourless to pale straw in colour. Inspect visually for particulate matter or discoloration prior to administration and discard if present.
4. If giving a 1 g dose*, withdraw the whole vial contents and give by deep IM injection into a large muscle mass.

*If the dose required is other than 1 g the manufacturer recommends the volumes of solvent shown in Table C2 are used to enable withdrawal of the required dose.

**Table C2**  Capreomycin: Volume of diluent to give desired capreomycin concentrations

| Volume of diluent added (mL) | Final volume (mL) | Concentration of capreomycin (mg/mL) |
|---|---|---|
| 2.15 | 2.85 | 370 |
| 2.63 | 3.33 | 310 |
| 3.3 | 4.0 | 260 |
| 4.3 | 5.0 | 210 |

## Intermittent intravenous infusion (unlicensed in UK)

*Preparation and administration*

1. Reconstitute each 1-g vial with 2 mL* NaCl 0.9% or WFI.
2. Allow 2–3 minutes for complete dissolution.
3. The solution should be clear and colourless to pale straw in colour. Inspect visually for particulate matter or discoloration prior to administration and discard if present.
4. If giving a 1 g dose*, withdraw the whole vial contents and add to 100 mL NaCl 0.9%.
5. Give by IV infusion over 60 minutes.

*If the dose required is other than 1 g the manufacturer recommends the volumes of solvent shown in Table C2 are used to enable withdrawal of the required dose.

## Technical information

| | |
|---|---|
| Incompatible with | No information |
| Compatible with | **Flush**: NaCl 0.9%<br>**Solutions**: NaCl 0.9%, WFI<br>**Y-site**: No information |
| pH | 4.5-7.5 |
| Sodium content | Nil |
| Storage | Store below 25°C in original packaging.<br>Vials are for single use only: discard any unused portion. |
| Displacement value | 0.7 mL/vial |
| Stability after preparation | From a microbiological point of view, should be used immediately; however, may be stored below 25°C for 24 hours. A pale straw colour may develop which may darken over time, but this is not harmful. |

## Monitoring

| Measure | Frequency | Rationale |
|---|---|---|
| U&Es | At least monthly (more frequently in renal impairment, especially after initiation) | • Capreomycin is nephrotoxic.<br>• ↑Serum creatinine may indicate toxicity and require a dose reduction.<br>• Severe ↓K, ↓Mg and ↓Ca may occur in overdose.<br>• Proteinuria and the presence of casts, erythrocytes, and leucocytes in the urine are also indicative of nephrotoxicity. |

*(continued)*

## Monitoring (continued)

| Measure | Frequency | Rationale |
|---|---|---|
| Vestibular and auditory function | Periodically | • Ototoxicity is a potential effect of overexposure to capreomycin.<br>• Deterioration of balance or hearing may be indicative of toxic levels.<br>• Perform an audiogram if ototoxicity suspected. Some authorities suggest that an audiogram be performed every 2 months. |
| LFTs | | • Abnormal results have occurred especially if capreomycin is given in combination with other antituberculous agents that are known to cause hepatic function changes. |
| FBC | | • Leucocytosis, leucopenia and eosinophilia have been observed and rarely thrombocytopenia |
| Capreomycin serum concentration | Only if appropriate. Take sample in the middle of a dosage interval. | • May be measured to check that the desired steady-state concentration of 10 micrograms/mL is achieved, especially in renal impairment. |

## Additional information

| | |
|---|---|
| Common and serious undesirable effects | *Injection-related:* Local: Pain and induration at injection site.<br>*Other:* Hypersensitivity reactions including urticaria and rashes, leucocytosis or leucopenia, electrolyte disturbances, hearing loss with tinnitus and vertigo, neuromuscular block after large doses. |
| Pharmacokinetics | Elimination half-life is 4-6 hours; up to 55 hours in severe renal impairment. |
| Significant interactions | No significant interactions. |
| Action in case of overdose | *Symptoms to watch for:* ↓K, ↓Ca, ↓Mg and other electrolyte disturbances.<br>*Antidote:* No known antidote but haemodialysis may be effective.<br>Stop administration and give supportive therapy as appropriate. |
| Counselling | Patients should report any deterioration in balance or hearing. |

| | |
|---|---|
| Risk rating: **AMBER** | Score = 4<br>Moderate-risk product: Risk-reduction strategies are recommended. |

This assessment is based on the full range of preparation and administration options described in the monograph. These may not all be applicable in some clinical situations.

## Reference

1. British Thoracic Society Standards of Care Committee and Joint Tuberculosis Committee. Guidelines for the prevention and management of *Mycobacterium tuberculosis* infection and disease in adult patients with chronic kidney disease. *Thorax* June 2010; 65: 559–570.

## Bibliography

SPC Capreomycin injection, King Pharmaceuticals Ltd (accessed 16 July 2010).

# Carbetocin

### 100 micrograms/mL solution in 1-mL ampoules

* Carbetocin is a synthetic analogue of oxytocin, with a longer duration of action.
* It is used to prevent loss of uterine muscle tone and postpartum haemorrhage following Caesarean section under spinal or epidural anaesthesia.
* Carbetocin must **not** be used at any stage of labour before delivery of the infant, as it has a prolonged effect on the uterus that may last for several hours following a single IV injection.

## Pre-treatment checks

* Do not give during pregnancy and labour before delivery of the infant.
* Do not use for the induction of labour or in pre-eclampsia or eclampsia.
* Avoid use in serious cardiovascular disorders and in epilepsy.
* Contraindicated in hepatic and renal impairment.
* Carbetocin has some vasopressin activity (<0.025 units per 1-mL ampoule), so caution should be exercised when using in any pre-existing condition where the rapid increase of extracellular water, and associated ↓Na may be hazardous to the patient (e.g. cardiovascular disease, epilepsy, asthma, migraine, pre-eclampsia or eclampsia).

*Biochemical and other tests*

| | |
|---|---|
| Electrolytes: serum Na, K | Maternal blood pressure |
| FBC | Renal function: U, Cr, CrCl (or eGFR) |
| LFTs | |

## Dose

**Standard dose:** 100 micrograms (1 mL) by IV injection, immediately post-delivery by Caesarean section and preferably prior to removal of placenta. No further doses should be given.

## Intravenous injection

*Preparation and administration*

1. Withdraw 100 micrograms (1 mL).
2. The solution should be clear and colourless. Inspect visually for particulate matter or discoloration prior to administration and discard if present. Do not dilute prior to use.
3. Give by IV injection over 1 minute.

## Technical information

| | |
|---|---|
| Incompatible with | No information |
| Compatible with | **Flush**: NaCl 0.9%<br>**Solutions**: No information<br>**Y-site**: No information |
| pH | 3.5-4.5 |
| Sodium content | Negligible |
| Storage | Store at 2-8° C in original packaging. Do not freeze. |

## Monitoring

| Measure | Frequency | Rationale |
|---|---|---|
| Postpartum haemorrhage | Postpartum | • If carbetocin has been ineffective in controlling excessive bleeding postpartum, alternative therapy with oxytocin and/or ergometrine may be required once the cause has been determined. |
| U&Es | Daily in immediate post-Caesarean period | • Carbetocin has some vasopressin activity, and as a result can cause ↓Na.<br>• Symptomatic signs of ↓Na should also be monitored, e.g. drowsiness, listlessness, headache (all early warning signs to be monitored to prevent seizure activity and coma). |
| FBC | | • Anaemia reported in some patients receiving carbetocin. |

## Additional information

| | |
|---|---|
| Common and serious undesirable effects | Nausea, vomiting, abdominal discomfort, flushing, ↓BP, headache, tremor, pruritus, metallic taste, ↑pulse, chest pain, dyspnoea, dizziness, back pain, anaemia, sweating, chills. |
| Pharmacokinetics | Elimination half-life is 40 minutes. |
| Significant interactions | No significant interactions. |
| Action in case of overdose | Symptomatic and supportive therapy should be provided (oxygen, restricted fluid intake, diuresis, correction of electrolyte imbalances and convulsion control). |
| Counselling | Small amounts of carbetocin pass into breast milk. It is assumed that any transferred carbetocin is degraded by enzymes in the infant's digestive tract. |

| Risk rating: **GREEN** | Score = 0 Lower-risk product: Risk-reduction strategies should be considered. |
|---|---|

| | | | | | | |
|---|---|---|---|---|---|---|

This assessment is based on the full range of preparation and administration options described in the monograph. These may not all be applicable in some clinical situations.

## Bibliography

SPC Pabal 100 micrograms in 1 mL solution for injection (accessed 29 September 2009).

# Carboprost

**250 micrograms/mL solution in ampoules**

- Carboprost trometamol is a synthetic analogue of prostaglandin $F_2$ alpha (dinoprost).
- It is used to treat postpartum haemorrhage due to loss of uterine muscle tone, refractory to first-line treatments with oxytocic agents and/or ergometrine.
- Carboprost has also been used for the termination of pregnancy in the second trimester (between 13 and 20 weeks' gestation) and as a bladder instillation for the treatment of cyclophosphamide-induced haemorrhagic cystitis (both unlicensed).
- Doses are expressed in terms of the base:
  Carboprost 1 microgram ≅ 1.3 micrograms carboprost trometamol.

## Pre-treatment checks

- Contraindicated in known cardiac, pulmonary, renal or hepatic disease and in acute pelvic inflammatory disease.
- Caution in patients with asthma, diabetes, jaundice and epilepsy.

*Biochemical and other tests (not all are necessary in an emergency situation)*

Blood pressure (caution in hypo/hypertension)
FBC (caution in presence of anaemia)
Intraocular pressure (caution in patients with ↑intraocular pressure/glaucoma)

LFTs
Renal function: U, Cr, CrCl (or eGFR)

## Dose

**Postpartum haemorrhage:** 250 micrograms by deep IM injection, followed as clinically required by up to seven further 250-microgram doses at intervals of approximately 90 minutes (maximum total carboprost dose 2 mg). In severe cases, at the discretion of an expert attending clinician, the interval between doses may be reduced, but must not be less than 15 minutes.

## Intramuscular injection

*Preparation and administration*

1. Ideally, allow injection to reach room temperature before administration.
2. Withdraw the required dose.
3. Give by deep IM injection. Rotate injection sites for subsequent injections.

## Technical information

| | |
|---|---|
| Incompatible with | Not relevant |
| Compatible with | Not relevant |
| pH | 7-8 |
| Sodium content | Negligible |
| Excipients | Contains benzyl alcohol. |
| Storage | Store at 2-8°C. |

## Monitoring

| Measure | Frequency | Rationale |
|---|---|---|
| Physical signs of successful treatment | Ongoing during treatment | • Monitor patient for signs of improvement in postpartum bleeding. |
| Maternal arterial oxygen saturation and respiration | | • Recommended in patients with pre-existing cardiopulmonary disease, as carboprost may reduce maternal arterial oxygen levels and oxygen support may be required. Monitor for bronchospasm or dyspnoea. |
| Maternal temperature | | • Carboprost may induce hyperthermia, which would need symptomatic management.<br>• Consider reduced frequency or discontinuation of treatment if severe. |
| Maternal blood pressure | Ongoing during treatment | • ↑BP may occur, consider reduced frequency or discontinuation of treatment if severe. |
| Cardiac monitoring | Ongoing at discretion of clinician | • Cardiovascular collapse, although rare, is possible following treatment with carboprost. |
| FBC | During admission | • Leucocytosis has been reported: monitor WCC count. |

## Additional information

| | |
|---|---|
| Common and serious undesirable effects | *Immediate:* Bronchospasm and dyspnoea have been reported.<br>*Injection/infusion-related:* Local: Injection site erythema and pain.<br>*Other:* Nausea, vomiting, diarrhoea (pre-treatment with antiemetics and antidiarrhoeals may help), hyperthermia, flushing, ↑BP, pulmonary oedema, chills, headache, excessive sweating, dizziness. |
| Pharmacokinetics | Peak plasma concentrations attained in 20-30 minutes. Elimination half-life has not been studied. |
| Significant interactions | Carboprost may ↑effect of oxytocin. |

*(continued)*

| **Additional information** (*continued*) | |
|---|---|
| Action in case of overdose | *Symptoms to watch for:* Excessive doses may cause uterine rupture. *Antidote:* No known antidote. Stop administration and give supportive therapy as appropriate. |
| Counselling | No adverse effects to the nursing infant are anticipated. |

| Risk rating: **GREEN** | Score = 1 Lower-risk product: Risk-reduction strategies should be considered. |
|---|---|

This assessment is based on the full range of preparation and administration options described in the monograph. These may not all be applicable in some clinical situations.

## Bibliography

SPC Hemabate sterile solution (accessed 29 September 2009).

# Caspofungin

### 50-mg and 70-mg dry powder vials

- Caspofungin acetate is a semisynthetic echinocandin antifungal agent.
- It is used in the treatment of invasive aspergillosis in patients who are refractory to or intolerant of other therapy. It is also used in the treatment of invasive candidiasis and as empirical therapy for presumed fungal infections in febrile, neutropenic patients.
- Doses are expressed in terms of the base:
  Caspofungin 70 mg $\cong$ 77.7 mg caspofungin acetate.

## Pre-treatment checks

Do not give in fructose intolerance.

*Biochemical and other tests*

FBC
LFTs

## Dose

**Adults ≤80 kg**: 70 mg by IV infusion on the first day then 50 mg by IV infusion once daily.
**Adults >80 kg**: 70 mg by IV infusion once daily.
**Dose in hepatic impairment**: adjusted according to Child–Pugh score:
- Child–Pugh Class A: dose as in normal hepatic function.
- Child–Pugh Class B: 70 mg on first day then 35 mg once daily.
- Child–Pugh Class C: there is no experience of dosing in severe hepatic impairment.

## Intermittent intravenous infusion

*Preparation and administration*

Caspofungin is incompatible with Gluc solutions.

1. Allow to reach room temperature then reconstitute each vial with 10.5 mL WFI.
2. Mix gently to obtain a clear solution containing 5 mg/mL (50-mg vial) or 7 mg/mL (70-mg vial).
3. Visually inspect the infusion solution for particulate matter or discoloration – discard if present.
4. Withdraw the required dose and add to 250 mL NaCl 0.9% or Hartmann's.
5. The solution should be clear and colourless. Inspect visually for particulate matter or discoloration prior to administration and discard if present.
6. Give by IV infusion over 60 minutes.

**Fluid restriction:** 50 mg and 35 mg doses (but not 70 mg) may be given in 100 mL NaCl 0.9% or Hartmann's in fluid-restricted patients.

## Technical information

| | |
|---|---|
| Incompatible with | Caspofungin is incompatible with Gluc solutions.<br>Otherwise no information. |
| Compatible with | **Flush**: NaCl 0.9%<br>**Solutions**: NaCl 0.9%, Hartmann's<br>**Y-site**: No information |
| pH | 6.6 |
| Sodium content | Negligible |
| Excipients | Contains sucrose. |
| Storage | Store at 2–8°C in original packaging. |
| Displacement value | Not relevant. The vial contains an overage so that the final solution contains 5 mg/mL (50-mg vial) or 7 mg/mL (70-mg vial) when reconstituted as directed. |
| Stability after reconstitution | From a microbiological point of view, should be used immediately; however: Reconstituted vials may be stored at 2–8°C for 24 hours.<br>Prepared infusions may be stored at 2–8°C and infused (at room temperature) within 24 hours. Check that the solution is clear before use. |

## Monitoring

| Measure | Frequency | Rationale |
|---|---|---|
| LFTs | Periodically | • Commonly increases in AST, ALT, Alk Phos, direct and total bilirubin are observed.<br>• If the Child-Pugh score changes in hepatic impairment, a dose adjustment may be necessary. |
| U&Es | | • ↑Cr, ↓K and ↓Na occur commonly. |
| FBC | | • ↓Hb, ↓haematocrit, ↓WCC, ↓platelets and ↓neutrophils observed commonly while eosinophils are often increased.<br>• Neutrophil count is also a measure of therapeutic efficacy. |
| Urinalysis | | • ↑Red blood cells, protein and white blood cells sometimes observed in urine. |

## Additional information

| | |
|---|---|
| Common and serious undesirable effects | *Infusion-related:* Local: Phlebitis/thrombophlebitis, infused-vein complications.<br>*Other:* Anaemia, headache, ↑pulse, flushing, dyspnoea, fever, pain, chills; abdominal pain, nausea, diarrhoea, vomiting; rash, pruritus, sweating; ↓Mg, ↓Ca; low albumin, increased partial thromboplastin time, decreased total serum protein, increased prothrombin time. |
| Pharmacokinetics | Elimination half-life is 9–11 hours. |
| Significant interactions | • Ciclosporin may ↑caspofungin levels or effect (or ↑side-effects): manufacturer advises monitoring LFTs.<br>• The following may ↓caspofungin levels – consider ↑dose to 70 mg daily if inadequate clinical response occurs in patients receiving these drugs: carbamazepine, dexamethasone, efavirenz, nevirapine, phenytoin, rifampicin.<br>• Caspofungin may ↓levels or effect of tacrolimus (monitor levels). |
| Action in case of overdose | No specific antidote. Caspofungin is not dialysable. |

| | |
|---|---|
| Risk rating: **AMBER** | Score = 4<br>Moderate-risk product: Risk-reduction strategies are recommended. |

  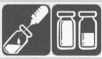

This assessment is based on the full range of preparation and administration options described in the monograph. These may not all be applicable in some clinical situations.

## Bibliography

SPC CANCIDAS (formerly Caspofungin MSD) (accessed 9 March 2010).

# Cefotaxime

### 500-mg, 1-g, 2-g dry powder vials

* Cefotaxime sodium is a third-generation cephalosporin.
* It is used in the treatment of infections due to susceptible organisms, especially serious and life-threatening infections.
* Doses are expressed in terms of cefotaxime:
  Cefotaxime 1 g ≅ 1.05 g cefotaxime sodium.

## Pre-treatment checks

* Do not give if there is known hypersensitivity to cefotaxime, cephalosporins or previous immediate hypersensitivity reaction to penicillins or any other beta-lactam antibiotic.
* Do not give in severe heart failure and in patients with an un-paced heart block.

*Biochemical and other tests*

FBC
LFTs
Renal function: U, Cr, CrCl (or eGFR)

## Dose

**Mild to moderate infections**: 1 g by IM or IV injection or IV infusion every 12 hours.
**Severe infections**: 2 g by IV injection or infusion four times daily. Higher doses up to 12 g daily in 3–4 divided doses may be required.
**Gonorrhoea**: 500 mg by IM or IV injection as a single dose.
**Bacterial meningitis:** cefotaxime is given before urgent transfer to hospital if benzylpenicillin cannot be given. Suitable doses are: adult and child over 12 years 1 g; child under 12 years 50 mg/kg. (Chloramphenicol may be used if there is a history of anaphylaxis to penicillins or cephalosporins.)
**Dose in renal impairment**: adjusted according to creatinine clearance:

* CrCl <5 mL/minute: 1 g loading dose then maintenance of 50% of appropriate normal dose.

## Intravenous injection

*Preparation and administration*

> If used in combination with an aminoglycoside (e.g. amikacin, gentamicin, tobramycin), prefer-ably administer at a different site. If this is not possible then flush the line thoroughly with a compatible solution between drugs.

1. Reconstitute each 500-mg vial with 2 mL WFI (use 4 mL for each 1-g vial; 10 mL for each 2-g vial) and shake well.
2. Withdraw the required dose.
3. The solution should be clear and straw-coloured. Inspect visually for particulate matter or discoloration prior to administration and discard if present.
4. Give by IV injection over 3–5 minutes.

## Intermittent intravenous infusion

*Preparation and administration*

> If used in combination with an aminoglycoside (e.g. amikacin, gentamicin, tobramycin), prefer-ably administer at a different site. If this is not possible then flush the line thoroughly with a compatible solution between drugs.

1. Reconstitute each 500-mg vial with 2 mL WFI (use 4 mL for each 1-g vial; 10 mL for each 2-g vial) and shake well.
2. Withdraw the required dose and add to a suitable volume of compatible infusion fluid (usually 100 mL NaCl 0.9%).
3. The solution should be clear and straw-coloured. Inspect visually for particulate matter or discoloration prior to administration and discard if present.
4. Give by IV infusion over 20–60 minutes.

## Intramuscular injection

*Preparation and administration*

1. Reconstitute each 500-mg vial with 2 mL WFI (use 4 mL for each 1-g vial; 10 mL for each 2-g vial) and shake well.
2. Withdraw the required dose.
3. Give by deep IM injection into a large muscle mass. Doses of 2 g should be distributed between two injection sites. Rotate injection sites for subsequent injections. If pain occurs, 1% lidocaine may be used for reconstitution (see the Lidocaine monograph for cautions and monitoring).

## Technical information

| | |
|---|---|
| Incompatible with | Sodium bicarbonate.<br>Amikacin, aminophylline, doxapram, fluconazole, gentamicin, pantoprazole, tobramycin, vancomycin. |
| Compatible with | **Flush**: NaCl 0.9%<br>**Solutions**: NaCl 0.9%, Gluc 5%, Gluc-NaCl, Hartmann's<br>**Y-site**: Aciclovir, aztreonam, clindamycin phosphate, granisetron, magnesium sulfate, metronidazole (in the same bag), midazolam, propofol, remifentanil, sodium fusidate, verapamil |
| pH | 5-7.5 |
| Sodium content | 2.1 mmol/g |
| Storage | Store below 25°C in original packaging. |
| Displacement value | 0.2 mL/500 mg; 0.5 mL/1 g; 1.2 mL/2 g |
| Stability after preparation | From a microbiological point of view, should be used immediately; however:<br>• Reconstituted vials may be stored at 2-8°C for 24 hours.<br>• Prepared infusions may be stored at 2-8°C and infused (at room temperature) within 24 hours. |

## Monitoring

| Measure | Frequency | Rationale |
|---|---|---|
| U&Es | Periodically, especially if for longer than 10 days | • Urea and creatinine occasionally rise. If renal function changes, a dose adjustment may be necessary. |
| LFTs | | • Transient rises in ALT, AST, Alk Phos and bilirubin may occur. |
| FBC | | • Rarely can cause thrombocytopenia, eosinophilia and neutropenia. |

*(continued)*

## Monitoring (continued)

| Measure | Frequency | Rationale |
|---|---|---|
| Development of diarrhoea | Throughout and up to 2 months after treatment | • Development of severe, persistent diarrhoea may be suggestive of *Clostridium difficile*-associated diarrhoea and colitis (pseudomembranous colitis). Discontinue drug and treat. Do not use drugs that inhibit peristalsis. |
| Signs of supra-infection or superinfection | Throughout treatment | • May result in the overgrowth of non-susceptible organisms - appropriate therapy should be commenced; treatment may need to be interrupted. |

## Additional information

| | |
|---|---|
| Common and serious undesirable effects | *Immediate:* Anaphylaxis and other hypersensitivity reactions have been reported. *Injection/infusion-related:*<br>• Too rapid administration: Arrhythmias reported when given rapidly through a central venous catheter.<br>• Local: Transient pain at injection site (change site if appropriate).<br>*Other:* Candidiasis, nausea, vomiting, abdominal pain, diarrhoea, encephalopathy (in high dose and especially in renal impairment). |
| Pharmacokinetics | Elimination half-life is about 1 hour (main metabolite: 1.3 hours). In severe renal impairment it is about 2.5 hours (main metabolite: 10 hours). |
| Significant interactions | • Cefotaxime may ↑levels or effect of the following drugs (or ↑side-effects): acenocoumarol (monitor INR), warfarin (monitor INR). |
| Action in case of overdose | *Symptoms to watch for:* Large doses have been associated with seizures. *Antidote:* There is no known antidote but haemodialysis may be effective. Stop administration and give supportive therapy as appropriate. |
| Counselling | Women taking the combined contraceptive pill should be should be advised to take additional precautions during and for 7 days after the course. |

| | |
|---|---|
| Risk rating: **GREEN** | Score = 2<br>Lower-risk product: Risk-reduction strategies should be considered. |

This assessment is based on the full range of preparation and administration options described in the monograph. These may not all be applicable in some clinical situations.

## Bibliography

SPC Cefotaxime 2 g powder for solution for injection or infusion, Wockhardt UK Ltd (accessed 2 March 2009).

SPC Cefotaxime 500 mg, 1 g powder for solution for injection or infusion, Wockhardt UK Ltd (accessed 2 March 2009).

SPC Claforan (accessed 18 January 2010).

# Cefradine (cephradine)

**500-mg, 1-g dry powder vials**
* Cefradine is a first-generation cephalosporin.
* It is used for infections of the respiratory and urinary tracts and of the skin and soft tissues, and is also used for surgical infection prophylaxis.

## Pre-treatment checks

Do not give if there is known hypersensitivity to cefradine, cephalosporins or previous immediate hypersensitivity reaction to penicillins, any other beta-lactam antibiotic or L-arginine.

*Biochemical and other tests*

FBC
LFTs
Renal function: U, Cr, CrCl (or eGFR)

## Dose

**Standard dose**: 500 mg–1 g by IM or IV injection or IV infusion every 6 hours.
**Severe infections**: up to 2 g by IV injection or infusion every 6 hours (or up to 8 g/day if giving by continuous IV infusion).
**Surgical prophylaxis**: 1–2 g by IM or IV injection at induction. Check local policies.
**Dose in renal impairment**: adjusted according to creatinine clearance:[1]
* CrCl >20–50 mL/minute: dose as in normal renal function.
* CrCl 10–20 mL/minute: dose as in normal renal function.
* CrCl <10 mL/minute: 250–500 mg every 6 hours.

## Intramuscular injection

*Preparation and administration*

1. Reconstitute each 500-mg vial with 2 mL WFI or NaCl 0.9% (use 4 mL for each 1-g vial) and shake well.
2. Withdraw the required dose.
3. Give by deep IM injection. Avoid SC injection as this has resulted in sterile abscess.

## Intravenous injection

*Preparation and administration*

1. Dissolve the contents of each 500-mg vial in 5 mL NaCl 0.9% or WFI (use 10 mL for each 1-g vial).
2. The solution should be clear and light to straw yellow. Inspect visually for particulate matter or discoloration prior to administration and discard if present.
3. Give by IV injection over 3–5 minutes.

## Intermittent intravenous infusion

*Preparation and administration*

1. Dissolve the contents of each 500-mg vial in 5 mL of a compatible solution (use 10 mL for each 1-g vial).
2. Withdraw the required dose and add to a suitable volume of compatible infusion fluid (usually 100 mL NaCl 0.9%).

3. The solution should be clear and light to straw yellow. Inspect visually for particulate matter or discoloration prior to administration and discard if present.
4. Give by IV infusion over at least 30 minutes.

**Cefradine is also licensed for continuous infusion:** if it is being given continuously, replace 5% infusions every 10 hours and 1% infusions every 12 hours with freshly prepared solutions. Protect infusion from strong light and direct sunlight.

## Technical information

| | |
|---|---|
| Incompatible with | No information |
| Compatible with | **Flush**: NaCl 0.9%<br>**Solutions**: NaCl 0.9%, Gluc 5%, WFI<br>**Y-site**: No information |
| pH | 3.5–6.0 |
| Sodium content | Nil |
| Excipients | Contains L-arginine (may cause hypersensitivity reactions). |
| Storage | Store below 25°C in original packaging. |
| Displacement value | There is an overage of cefradine in each vial.<br>• To make 100 mg/mL from a 500-mg vial, add 4.95 mL of diluent.<br>• To make 200 mg/mL from a 1-g vial, add 4.45 mL of diluent.[2] |
| Stability after preparation | From a microbiological point of view, should be used immediately; however:<br>• Reconstituted vials may be stored at 2–8°C for 12 hours.<br>• Prepared infusions may be stored at 2–8°C and infused (at room temperature) within 24 hours. |

## Monitoring

| Measure | Frequency | Rationale |
|---|---|---|
| U&Es | Periodically | • Urea and creatinine occasionally rise. If renal function changes a dose adjustment may be necessary. |
| LFTs | | • Can rarely cause ↑ AST, ALT, Alk Phos and bilirubin. |
| FBC | | • Can rarely can cause neutropenia, leucopenia and eosinophilia. |
| Development of diarrhoea | Throughout and up to 2 months after treatment | • Development of severe, persistent diarrhoea may be suggestive of Clostridium difficile-associated diarrhoea and colitis (pseudomembranous colitis). Discontinue drug and treat. Do not use drugs that inhibit peristalsis. |
| Signs of supra-infection or superinfection | Throughout treatment | • May result in the overgrowth of non-susceptible organisms - appropriate therapy should be commenced; treatment may need to be interrupted. |

## Additional information

| | |
|---|---|
| Common and serious undesirable effects | *Immediate:* Anaphylaxis and other hypersensitivity reactions have been reported.<br>*Injection/infusion-related:* Local: Thrombophlebitis following IV injection; sterile abscesses following inadvertent SC injection.<br>*Other:* Candidiasis, nausea, vomiting, glossitis, abdominal pain, diarrhoea, urticaria, pruritus. |
| Pharmacokinetics | Elimination half-life is 40 minutes. |
| Significant interactions | • Cefradine may ↑levels or effect of the following drugs (or ↑side-effects): acenocoumarol (monitor INR), warfarin (monitor INR). |
| Action in case of overdose | No reports of overdose.<br>Stop administration and give supportive therapy as appropriate. |
| Counselling | Women taking the combined contraceptive pill should be should be advised to take additional precautions during and for 7 days after the course. |

| | |
|---|---|
| Risk rating: **GREEN** | Score = 2<br>Lower-risk product: Risk-reduction strategies should be considered. |

This assessment is based on the full range of preparation and administration options described in the monograph. These may not all be applicable in some clinical situations.

### References

1. Ashley C, Currie A, eds. *The Renal Drug Handbook*, 3rd edn. Oxford: Radcliffe Medical Press, 2009.
2. Correspondence with Bristol-Myers Squibb Pharmaceuticals Ltd, 11 June 2008.

### Bibliography

SPC Velosef for injection 500 mg and 1 g (accessed 2 March 2009).

# Ceftazidime

**250-mg, 500-mg, 2-g, 3-g dry powder vials; 2-g dry powder vial with transfer needle**

- Ceftazidime pentahydrate is a semisynthetic third-generation cephalosporin.
- It is used in the treatment of susceptible infections especially those due to *Pseudomonas* spp.
- Doses are expressed in terms of ceftazidime:
  Ceftazidime 1 g ≡ 1.16 g ceftazidime pentahydrate.

## Pre-treatment checks

Do not give if there is known hypersensitivity to ceftazidime or cephalosporins, or previous immediate hypersensitivity reaction to penicillins or any other beta-lactam antibiotic.

*Biochemical and other tests*

FBC

LFTs

PT (possibly, see Monitoring)

Renal function: U, Cr, CrCl (or eGFR)

## Dose

**Standard dose**: 1 g by IM or IV injection every 8 hours or 2 g by IV injection or infusion every 12 hours.

**Severe infections**: 2 g by IV injection or infusion every 8–12 hours or 3 g every 12 hours.

**Urinary tract and less serious infections**: 500 mg–1 g by IM or IV injection every 12 hours.

**Pseudomonal lung infection in cystic fibrosis**: up to 50 mg/kg by IV injection or infusion every 8 hours.

**Surgical prophylaxis – prostatic surgery**: 1 g at induction of anaesthesia repeated if necessary when catheter removed. Check local policy.

**Dose in renal impairment**: adjusted according to creatinine clearance:[1]

* CrCl >50 mL/minute: dose as in normal renal function.
* CrCl 31–50 mL/minute: 1–2 g every 12 hours.
* CrCl 16–30 mL/minute: 1–2 g every 24 hours.
* CrCl 6–15 mL/minute: 500 mg–1 g every 24 hours.
* CrCl <5 mL/minute: 500 mg–1 g every 48 hours.

## Intravenous injection

*Preparation and administration*

If used in combination with an aminoglycoside (e.g. amikacin, gentamicin, tobramycin), preferably administer at a different site. If this is not possible then flush the line thoroughly with a compatible solution between drugs.

1. Insert the syringe needle through the vial closure and inject 5 mL WFI into each 500-mg vial; 10 mL WFI into each 1 g or 2-g vial; 15 mL WFI into each 3-g vial.
2. Remove the needle and shake to dissolve. $CO_2$ is released and a clear solution should develop in about 1–2 minutes.
3. Invert the vial and, with syringe plunger fully depressed, insert the needle through the vial closure and withdraw all the solution into the syringe. Ensure that the needle does not enter the head space.
4. Expel any small bubbles of $CO_2$ present in the syringe.
5. The solution should be clear and light yellow to amber. Inspect visually for particulate matter or discoloration prior to administration and discard if present.
6. Give by IV injection over 3–5 minutes.

## Intermittent intravenous infusion

*Preparation and administration*

If used in combination with an aminoglycoside (e.g. amikacin, gentamicin, tobramycin), preferably administer at a different site. If this is not possible then flush the line thoroughly with a compatible solution between drugs.

1. Insert the syringe needle through the vial closure and inject 10 mL WFI into each 2-g vial; 15 mL WFI into each 3-g vial.
2. Remove the needle and shake to dissolve: $CO_2$ is released and a clear solution should develop in about 1–2 minutes.
3. Withdraw the required dose and add to a suitable volume of compatible infusion fluid (usually 100 mL NaCl 0.9%). Use a minimum 50 mL for a 2-g dose; 100 mL for a 3-g dose.
4. Give by IV infusion over 20–30 minutes.

## Intramuscular injection (maximum dose 1 g)

*Preparation and administration*

1. Insert the syringe needle through the vial closure and inject 1.5 mL WFI into each 500-mg vial; 3 mL WFI into each 1-g vial.
2. Remove the needle and shake to dissolve. $CO_2$ is released and a clear solution should develop in about 1–2 minutes.
3. Invert the vial and with syringe plunger fully depressed, insert the needle through the vial closure and withdraw all the solution into the syringe. Ensure that the needle does not enter the head space.
4. Expel any small bubbles of $CO_2$ present in the syringe.
5. Give by IM injection into a large muscle such as the gluteus or the lateral aspect of the thigh. Rotate injection sites for subsequent injections. If pain occurs, 0.5–1% lidocaine may be used for reconstitution (see the Lidocaine monograph for cautions and monitoring).

## Technical information

| | |
|---|---|
| Incompatible with | Sodium bicarbonate.<br>Acetylcysteine, amikacin, amiodarone, amphotericin, cisatracurium, clarithromycin, dobutamine, erythromycin lactobionate, fluconazole, gentamicin, midazolam, pantoprazole, phenytoin sodium, propofol, tobramycin, vancomycin. |
| Compatible with | **Flush**: NaCl 0.9%<br>**Solutions**: NaCl 0.9% (also with added KCl), Gluc 5%, NaCl-Gluc, Hartmann's, Ringer's<br>**Y-site**: Aciclovir, aztreonam, dopamine, esmolol, furosemide, granisetron, isosorbide dinitrate, ketamine, labetalol, methylprednisolone sodium succinate, metronidazole (in the same bag), ondansetron, ranitidine, remifentanil, sodium valproate, tigecycline |
| pH | 6–8 |
| Sodium content | 2.3 mmol/g |
| Storage | Store below 25°C in original packaging. |
| Displacement value | There is considerable variation between brands and within brands, and whether for IM or IV use - see individual SPCs for details. |
| Stability after preparation | From a microbiological point of view, should be used immediately; however:<br>• Reconstituted vials may be stored 2–8°C for 24 hours.<br>• Prepared infusions may be stored at 2–8°C and infused (at room temperature) within 24 hours. |

## Monitoring

| Measure | Frequency | Rationale |
|---------|-----------|-----------|
| Serum ceftazidime level | If indicated | • Patients on high doses for severe infections and with renal impairment, should have a trough level ≤40 mg/L. |
| U&Es | Periodically | • Transient rises in urea and creatinine may occur. Deterioration in renal function may require a dose reduction. |
| FBC | | • Eosinophilia, thrombocytosis, leucopenia, neutropenia, and thrombocytopenia may occur. |
| LFTs | | • Transient rises in ALT, AST, GGT, Alk Phos and bilirubin may occur. |
| Prothrombin time | If indicated and in at-risk individuals | • A slight prolongation of prothrombin time occurs rarely. Patients with impaired vitamin K synthesis or low vitamin K stores, e.g. patients with chronic hepatic disease or malnutrition may need a 10-mg weekly dose of vitamin K. |
| Signs of supra-infection or superinfection | Throughout treatment | • May result in the overgrowth of non-susceptible organisms - appropriate therapy should be commenced; treatment may need to be interrupted. |
| Development of diarrhoea | Throughout and up to 2 months after treatment | • Development of severe, persistent diarrhoea may be suggestive of *Clostridium difficile*-associated diarrhoea and colitis (pseudomembranous colitis). Discontinue drug and treat. Do not use drugs that inhibit peristalsis. |

## Additional information

| | |
|---|---|
| Common and serious undesirable effects | *Immediate:* Anaphylaxis and other hypersensitivity reactions have been reported.<br>*Injection/infusion-related:* Local: Thrombophlebitis following IV injection; pain and/or inflammation after IM injection.<br>*Other:* Nausea, vomiting, abdominal pain, diarrhoea, urticaria, pruritus. |
| Pharmacokinetics | Elimination half-life is 2 hours. |
| Significant interactions | • Ceftazidime may ↑levels or effect of the following drugs (or ↑side-effects): acenocoumarol (monitor INR), warfarin (monitor INR). |
| Action in case of overdose | General symptomatic and supportive methods, together with specific measures to control any seizures. Ceftazidime can be removed by haemodialysis and haemoperfusion. |
| Counselling | Women taking the combined contraceptive pill should be should be advised to take additional precautions during and for 7 days after the course. |

| Risk rating: **AMBER** | Score = 3 Moderate-risk product: Risk-reduction strategies are recommended. | | |
|---|---|---|---|
|  |   | | |

This assessment is based on the full range of preparation and administration options described in the monograph. These may not all be applicable in some clinical situations.

## Reference

1. Ashley C, Currie A, eds. *The Renal Drug Handbook*, 3rd edn. Oxford: Radcliffe Medical Press, 2009.

## Bibliography

SPC Ceftazidime 1 g, 2 g powder for solution for injection or infusion, Wockhardt UK Ltd (accessed 3 March 2009).
SPC Fortum 500mg, 1 g, 2 g and 3 g injection (accessed 3 March 2009).
SPC Kefadim vials (accessed 3 March 2009).

# Ceftriaxone

**250-mg, 1-g, 2-g dry powder vials**
• Ceftriaxone sodium is a third-generation cephalosporin.
• It is used in the treatment of infections due to susceptible organisms, especially serious and life-threatening infections.
• Doses are expressed in terms of ceftriaxone:
 Ceftriaxone 1 g ≅ 1.19 g ceftriaxone sodium.

## Pre-treatment checks

Do not give if there is known hypersensitivity to ceftriaxone, cephalosporins or previous immediate hypersensitivity reaction to penicillins or any other beta-lactam antibiotic.

*Biochemical and other tests*

FBC                                            PT (possibly, see monitoring)
LFTs                                           Renal function: U, Cr, CrCl (or eGFR)

## Dose

**Standard dose:** 1 g by IM or IV injection daily.
**Severe infections:** 2–4 g by IV infusion daily.
**Uncomplicated gonorrhoea**: 250 mg by IM injection as a single dose.
**Surgical prophylaxis:** 1 g by IM or IV injection at induction; colorectal surgery 2 g by IM injection or IV infusion at induction. Check local policies.
**Dose in renal impairment**: adjusted according to creatinine clearance:
• CrCl ≥10 mL/minute: dose as in normal renal function.
• CrCl <10 mL/minute: maximum 2 g every 24 hours.

## Intravenous injection (doses up to 1 g)

*Preparation and administration*

Ceftriaxone is incompatible with Ca-containing solutions, e.g. Hartmann's, Ringer's.

1. Reconstitute each 1-g vial with 10 mL WFI.
2. The solution should be clear and light yellow to amber. Inspect visually for particulate matter or discoloration prior to administration and discard if present.
3. Give by IV injection over a minimum of 2–4 minutes.

## Intermittent intravenous infusion

*Preparation and administration*

Ceftriaxone is incompatible with Ca-containing solutions, e.g. Hartmann's, Ringer's.

1. Reconstitute each 1-g vial with 10 mL WFI.
2. Withdraw the required dose and add to 50–100 mL compatible infusion fluid (usually NaCl 0.9%). Alternatively, reconstitute each 2-g vial with 40 mL of compatible infusion fluid (usually NaCl 0.9%) and infuse directly from the vial.
3. The solution should be clear and light yellow to amber. Inspect visually for particulate matter or discoloration prior to administration and discard if present.
4. Give by IV infusion over at least 30 minutes.

## Intramuscular injection

*Preparation and administration*

1. Reconstitute each 250-mg vial with 1 mL lidocaine 1% (use 3.5 mL for a 1-g vial). The injection is painful if not given with lidocaine (see the Lidocaine monograph for cautions and monitoring).
2. Withdraw the required dose.
3. Aspirate before injection to avoid inadvertent intravascular injection.
4. Give by deep IM injection. Doses >1 g should be distributed between two injection sites.

## Technical information

| | |
|---|---|
| Incompatible with | Ceftriaxone is incompatible with Ca-containing solutions, e.g. Hartmann's, Ringer's. Fatalities have occurred in neonates and infants due to precipitates forming in lungs and kidneys.<br>Aminophylline, amphotericin, clindamycin phosphate, fluconazole, gentamicin, labetalol, tobramycin, vancomycin. |
| Compatible with | **Flush**: NaCl 0.9%<br>**Solutions**: Gluc 5%, NaCl 0.9%, Gluc-NaCl (all with added KCl)<br>**Y-site**: Aciclovir, amikacin, aztreonam, cisatracurium, granisetron, metronidazole, pantoprazole, propofol, remifentanil, sodium bicarbonate, tigecycline |
| pH | 6–8 |
| Sodium content | 3.6 mmol/g |
| Storage | Store below 25°C in original packaging. |

*(continued)*

## Technical information (continued)

| | |
|---|---|
| Displacement value | 0.194 mL/250 mg (Rocephin)<br>0.5 mL/g with WFI, 0.55 mL/g with lidocaine 1% (Wockhardt) |
| Stability after preparation | From a microbiological point of view, should be used immediately; however:<br>• Reconstituted vials may be stored at 2-8°C for 24 hours.<br>• Prepared infusions may be stored at 2-8°C and infused (at room temperature) within 24 hours. |

## Monitoring

| Measure | Frequency | Rationale |
|---|---|---|
| Ceftriaxone serum concentration | Regularly if treatment prolonged | • For patients with severe renal impairment and concomitant hepatic insufficiency (it is eliminated by both routes, each of which normally compensates for a deficiency in the other) and in patients receiving dialysis, serum concentration should be checked regularly and dosage adjusted if necessary.<br>• In a healthy adult the mean peak concentration is about 200 mg/L after a 1-g IV injection and about 250 mg/L 30 minutes after a 2-g infusion. |
| U&Es | Periodically | • Urea and creatinine occasionally rise. If renal function changes, a dose adjustment may be necessary. |
| FBC | | • Rarely can cause neutropenia, leucopenia, eosinophilia, thrombocytopenia, anaemia. |
| LFTs | | • Rarely ↑AST, ALT, Alk Phos and bilirubin. If this is severe and renal function is impaired, a dose reduction may be necessary. |
| Prothrombin time | If indicated and in at-risk individuals | • A slight prolongation of prothrombin time occurs rarely. Patients with impaired vitamin K synthesis or ↓vitamin K stores, e.g. patients with chronic hepatic disease or malnutrition, may need a 10-mg weekly dose of vitamin K. |
| Development of signs and symptoms of gallbladder disease | Throughout treatment | • The drug can precipitate in the gallbladder. Discontinuation and conservative management should be considered if this occurs. |
| Signs of supra-infection or superinfection | Throughout treatment | • The drug may result in the overgrowth of non-susceptible organisms - appropriate therapy should be commenced; treatment may need to be interrupted. |
| Development of diarrhoea | Throughout and up to 2 months after treatment | • Development of severe, persistent diarrhoea may be suggestive of *Clostridium difficile*-associated diarrhoea and colitis (pseudomembranous colitis). Discontinue drug and treat. Do not use drugs that inhibit peristalsis. |

## Additional information

| Common and serious undesirable effects | *Immediate:* Anaphylaxis and other hypersensitivity reactions have been reported.<br>*Injection/infusion-related:* Local: Phlebitis and pain following IV injection.<br>*Other:* Nausea, vomiting, abdominal pain, diarrhoea, urticaria, pruritus. |
|---|---|
| Pharmacokinetics | Elimination half-life is 5.8-8.7 hours. |
| Significant interactions | • Ceftriaxone may ↑levels or effect of the following drugs (or ↑side-effects): acenocoumarol (monitor INR), warfarin (monitor INR). |
| Action in case of overdose | There is no specific antidote; treatment should be symptomatic. |
| Counselling | Women taking the combined contraceptive pill should be should be advised to take additional precautions during and for 7 days after the course. |

Risk rating: **GREEN**  Score = 2
Lower-risk product: Risk-reduction strategies should be considered.

This assessment is based on the full range of preparation and administration options described in the monograph. These may not all be applicable in some clinical situations.

## Bibliography

SPC Ceftriaxone 1 g, 2 g powder for solution for injection (Wockhardt UK Ltd) (accessed 3 March 2009).
SPC Rocephin 250mg, 1 g and 2 g vials (accessed 3 March 2009).

# Cefuroxime

### 250-mg, 750-mg, 1.5-g dry powder vials

• Cefuroxime sodium is a second-generation cephalosporin.
• It is used in the treatment of susceptible infections causing lower respiratory tract infections (including pneumonia), serious skin and skin structure infections, genitourinary tract infections, bone and joint infections, septicaemia and meningitis.
• Doses are expressed in terms of cefuroxime:
Cefuroxime 1 g ≅ 1.05 g cefuroxime sodium.

## Pre-treatment checks

Do not give if there is known hypersensitivity to cefuroxime, cephalosporins or previous immediate hypersensitivity reaction to penicillins or any other beta-lactam antibiotic.

*Biochemical and other tests*

FBC

LFTs

Prothrombin time (possibly, see monitoring)

Renal function: U, Cr, CrCl (or eGFR)

## Dose

**Standard dose:** 750 mg by IM or IV injection or IV infusion every 6–8 hours.

**Severe infections:** 1.5 g by IV injection or infusion every 6–8 hours.

**Gonorrhoea**: 1.5 g as a single dose by IM injection (divided between two sites). An oral dose of 1 g probenecid may also be given (to slow the rate of tubular secretion of cefuroxime).

**Surgical prophylaxis:** 1.5 g by IV injection at induction; up to three further doses of 750 mg may be given by IM or IV injection every 8 hours for high-risk procedures. Check local policies.

**Meningitis:** 3 g by IV injection or infusion every 8 hours.

**Dose in renal impairment**: adjusted according to creatinine clearance:

- CrCl >50 mL/minute: dose as in normal renal function.
- CrCl 20–50 mL/minute: 750 mg–1.5 g every 8 hours.
- CrCl 10–20 mL/minute: 750 mg–1.5 g every 8–12 hours.
- CrCl <10 mL/minute: 750 mg–1.5 g every 12–24 hours.

## Intravenous injection

*Preparation and administration*

1. Reconstitute each 750-mg vial with 6–10 mL WFI (use 15–20 mL for each 1.5-g vial) and shake gently.
2. Withdraw the required dose.
3. The solution should be clear and colourless to brownish yellow. Inspect visually for particulate matter or discoloration prior to administration and discard if present.
4. Give by IV injection over 3–5 minutes.

## Intermittent intravenous infusion

*Preparation and administration*

1. Reconstitute each 750-mg vial with 6–10 mL WFI (use 15–20 mL for each 1.5-g vial) and shake gently.
2. Withdraw the required dose and add to 50–100 mL of compatible infusion fluid (usually NaCl 0.9%).
3. The solution should be clear and colourless to brownish yellow. Inspect visually for particulate matter or discoloration prior to administration and discard if present.
4. Give by IV infusion over 30 minutes.

## Intramuscular injection (doses up to 750 mg)

*Preparation and administration*

1. Add 3 mL WFI to each 750-mg vial and shake gently to produce a colourless to slightly yellow suspension.
2. Withdraw the required dose.
3. Give by IM injection into a large muscle such as the gluteus or the lateral aspect of the thigh. Doses >750 mg should be distributed between two injection sites.

## Technical information

| | |
|---|---|
| Incompatible with | Sodium bicarbonate.<br>Amikacin, ciprofloxacin, cisatracurium, clarithromycin, fluconazole, gentamicin, midazolam, pantoprazole, ranitidine, tobramycin, vancomycin. |
| Compatible with | **Flush**: NaCl 0.9%<br>**Solutions**: NaCl 0.9%, Gluc 5%, Gluc-NaCl, Hartmann's, Ringer's (all including added KCl)<br>**Y-site**: Aciclovir, clindamycin phosphate, flucloxacillin, furosemide, granisetron, linezolid, metronidazole (in the same bag), ondansetron, propofol, remifentanil, vecuronium bromide |
| pH | 5.5–8.5 |
| Sodium content | 1.8 mmol/750 mg |
| Storage | Store below 25°C in original packaging. |
| Displacement value | 0.2 mL/250 mg; 0.8 mL/750 mg; 1.5 mL/1.5 g |
| Stability after preparation | From a microbiological point of view, should be used immediately; however:<br>• Reconstituted vials may be stored at 2–8°C for 24 hours.<br>• Prepared infusions may be stored at 2–8°C and infused (at room temperature) within 24 hours. |

## Monitoring

| Measure | Frequency | Rationale |
|---|---|---|
| U&Es | Periodically | • Transient rises in urea and creatinine may occur. Deterioration in renal function may require a dose reduction. |
| FBC | | • Can cause neutropenia, eosinophilia and rarely leucopenia, anaemia, ↓haematocrit and thrombocytopenia. |
| LFTs | | • Transient rises in AST, ALT, Alk Phos and bilirubin may occur. |
| Signs of supra-infection or superinfection | Throughout treatment | • May result in the overgrowth of non-susceptible organisms – appropriate therapy should be commenced; treatment may need to be interrupted. |
| Development of diarrhoea | Throughout and up to 2 months after treatment | • Development of severe, persistent diarrhoea may be suggestive of *Clostridium difficile*-associated diarrhoea and colitis (pseudomembranous colitis). Discontinue drug and treat. Do not use drugs that inhibit peristalsis. |
| Prothrombin time | If indicated and in at-risk individuals | • A slight prolongation of PT occurs rarely. Patients with impaired vitamin K synthesis or low vitamin K stores, e.g. patients with chronic hepatic disease or malnutrition may need a 10-mg weekly dose of vitamin K. |

## Additional information

| | |
|---|---|
| Common and serious undesirable effects | *Immediate:* Anaphylaxis and other hypersensitivity reactions have been reported. *Injection/infusion-related:* Local: Thrombophlebitis following IV injection; pain and/or inflammation after IM injection. *Other:* Nausea, vomiting, abdominal pain, diarrhoea, urticaria, pruritus. |
| Pharmacokinetics | Elimination half-life is 80 minutes. |
| Significant interactions | • Cefuroxime may ↑levels or effect of the following drugs (or ↑side-effects): acenocoumarol (monitor INR), warfarin (monitor INR). |
| Action in case of overdose | In overdose cerebral irritation and seizures may occur (use anticonvulsant therapy if indicated). Cefuroxime can be removed by haemodialysis or peritoneal dialysis. |
| Counselling | Women taking the combined contraceptive pill should be should be advised to take additional precautions during and for 7 days after the course. |

| | |
|---|---|
| Risk rating: **GREEN** | Score = 2 Lower-risk product: Risk-reduction strategies should be considered. |

This assessment is based on the full range of preparation and administration options described in the monograph. These may not all be applicable in some clinical situations.

## Bibliography

SPC Cefuroxime sodium injection, Flynn Pharma Ltd (accessed 3 March 2009).
SPC Zinacef injection (accessed 3 March 2009).
SPC Cefuroxime, Sandoz (accessed 21 January 2010).

# Chloramphenicol

### 1-g dry powder vials

- Chloramphenicol sodium succinate is a potent broad-spectrum antibiotic.
- It is used in typhoid, meningitis caused by *Haemophilus influenzae* and other serious infections caused by other sensitive bacteria. However, the risk of life-threatening adverse effects, particularly bone-marrow aplasia, has severely limited the clinical usefulness of chloramphenicol.
- It should **not** be used in the treatment of any infection for which a less-toxic antibiotic is appropriate.
- Doses are expressed in terms of base:
  Chloramphenicol 1 g ≅ 1.4 g chloramphenicol sodium succinate.

## Pre-treatment checks

- Do not give if there is known hypersensitivity and/or toxic reaction to chloramphenicol.
- Do not give in acute porphyria.

*Biochemical and other tests*

FBC
LFTs
Renal function: U, Cr, CrCl (or eGFR)

## Dose

**Standard dose**: 12.5 mg/kg by IV injection or infusion every 6 hours.

**Severe infection, e.g. septicaemia or meningitis**: 25 mg/kg by IV injection or infusion every 6 hours, provided dose is reduced as soon as clinically indicated.

To prevent relapse treatment should be continued until apyrexial for 4 days in rickettsial diseases and for 8–10 days in typhoid fever.

**Dose in renal impairment**: dose as in normal renal function.[1]

**Dose in hepatic impairment**: an initial 1-g loading dose is given followed by 500 mg every 6 hours for an adult (with dose adjustment depending on plasma levels).[2]

## Intravenous injection (preferred method)

*Preparation and administration*

1. Reconstitute each 1-g vial with 9.2 mL WFI, NaCl 0.9% or Gluc 5% to give a solution containing 100 mg/mL.
2. Withdraw the required dose.
3. The solution should be clear and colourless. Inspect visually for particulate matter or discoloration prior to administration and discard if present.
4. Give by IV injection over 1 minute.

## Intravenous infusion

*Preparation and administration*

1. Reconstitute each 1-g vial with 9.2 mL WFI, NaCl 0.9% or Gluc 5% to give a solution containing 100 mg/mL.
2. Withdraw the required dose and add to a suitable volume of compatible infusion fluid (usually 100 mL NaCl 0.9%).
3. The solution should be clear and colourless. Inspect visually for particulate matter or discoloration prior to administration and discard if present.
4. Give by IV infusion over 10 minutes.

## Intramuscular injection
## (not recommended – absorption can be slow and unpredictable)

*Preparation and administration*

1. Reconstitute each 1-g vial with 1.7 mL WFI, NaCl 0.9% or Gluc 5% to give a solution containing 400 mg/mL.
2. Withdraw the required dose.
3. Give by deep IM injection.

## Technical information

| | |
|---|---|
| Incompatible with | Fluconazole, phenytoin sodium, prochlorperazine, vancomycin. |
| Compatible with | **Flush**: NaCl 0.9%<br>**Solutions**: NaCl 0.9%, Gluc 5%, Gluc-NaCl, Hartmann's, Ringer's<br>**Y-site**: Aciclovir, amikacin, aminophylline, ampicillin, benzylpenicillin, calcium gluconate, colistimethate sodium, dopamine, esmolol, foscarnet, hydrocortisone sodium succinate, labetalol, magnesium sulfate, methylprednisolone sodium succinate, metronidazole, phytomenadione, ranitidine, sodium bicarbonate, verapamil |
| pH | 6.4-7 |
| Sodium content | 3.14 mmol/g |
| Storage | Store below 25°C in original packaging. |
| Displacement value | 0.8 mL/vial |
| Stability after reconstitution | From a microbiological point of view, should be used immediately; however:<br>• Reconstituted vials may be stored at room temperature for 24 hours.<br>• Prepared infusions may be stored at room temperature and given within 24 hours. |

## Monitoring

| Measure | Frequency | Rationale |
|---|---|---|
| FBC | Every 2 days | • Can cause severe bone marrow depression leading to reticulocytopenia, leucopenia, thrombocytopenia, anaemia and other haematological abnormalities. More common with high dose, prolonged therapy or repeated courses.<br>• Discontinue therapy immediately if these occur. |
| LFTs | No specific periodicity but may be apt with FBC | • Changes in hepatic function (bilirubin is the best indicator) may require a dose adjustment. |
| U&Es | | • Changes in renal function may require a dose adjustment. |
| Chloramphenicol plasma concentration | Every 2-3 days (usually only required in elderly patients and in hepatic impairment) | • A trough level is taken just before a dose and should be 5-15 mg/L.<br>• A peak level is taken 1 hour after the dose has been given and should be 15-25 mg/L.<br>For meaningful interpretation of results the laboratory request form must state:<br>• The time the previous dose was given.<br>• The time the blood sample was taken. |

*(continued)*

## Monitoring (continued)

| Measure | Frequency | Rationale |
|---------|-----------|-----------|
| Signs of supra-infection or superinfection | Throughout treatment | • May result in the overgrowth of non-susceptible organisms - appropriate therapy should be commenced; treatment may need to be interrupted. |
| Signs of optic or peripheral neuritis | | • More common in high doses. If these symptoms occur discontinue therapy immediately. |
| Development of diarrhoea | Throughout and up to 2 months after treatment | • Development of severe, persistent diarrhoea may be suggestive of *Clostridium difficile*-associated diarrhoea and colitis (pseudomembranous colitis). Discontinue drug and treat. Do not use drugs that inhibit peristalsis. |

## Additional information

| | |
|---|---|
| Common and serious undesirable effects | Dryness of the mouth, nausea and vomiting, diarrhoea, urticaria. Optic neuritis with blurring or temporary loss of vision, peripheral neuritis, headache and depression. Blood disorders including reversible and irreversible aplastic anaemia (with reports of resulting leukaemia), erythema multiforme. |
| Pharmacokinetics | Elimination half-life is 1.6-3.3 hours (up to 7 hours in end-stage kidney disease). |
| Significant interactions | • The following may ↓chloramphenicol levels or effect: barbiturates, primidone.<br>• Chloramphenicol may ↑levels or effect of the following drugs (or ↑side-effects): ciclosporin, coumarin anticoagulants, phenytoin (↑risk of toxicity), sulfonylureas, tacrolimus.<br>• Chloramphenicol may ↑risk of agranulocytosis with clozapine (and other drugs likely to cause agranulocytosis). |
| Action in case of overdose | *Symptoms to watch for:* Abdominal distension, vomiting, respiratory difficulty, pale cyanotic skin, ↓BP, metabolic acidosis.<br>*Antidote:* No known antidote. Stop administration and give supportive therapy as appropriate. |

| | |
|---|---|
| Risk rating: **AMBER** | Score = 3<br>Moderate-risk product: Risk-reduction strategies are recommended. |

This assessment is based on the full range of preparation and administration options described in the monograph. These may not all be applicable in some clinical situations.

## References

1. Ashley C, Currie A, eds. *The Renal Drug Handbook*, 3rd edn. Oxford: Radcliffe Medical Press, 2009.
2. Kasten MJ. Clindamycin, metronidazole, and chloramphenicol. *Mayo Clin Proc* 1999; 74(8): 825–833.

## Bibliography

SPC Kemicetine succinate injection (accessed 3 March 2009).

# Chlorphenamine maleate (chlorpheniramine maleate)

**10 mg/mL solution in 1-mL ampoules**

* Chlorphenamine maleate is a sedating antihistamine that causes a moderate degree of sedation; it also has antimuscarinic activity.
* It is indicated for acute urticaria, control of allergic reactions to insect bites and stings, angioedema, drug and serum reactions, desensitisation reactions, hay fever, vasomotor rhinitis, severe pruritus of non-specific origin.
* It may be given IV as an adjunct in the emergency treatment of anaphylactic shock.

## Pre-treatment checks

* Avoid in patients taking monoamine oxidase inhibitors up to 14 days previously because of ↑risk of extrapyramidal side-effects.
* Use with caution in asthma, bronchitis or bronchiectasis as it may thicken secretions.
* Use with care in narrow-angle glaucoma, prostatic hypertrophy, urinary retention and pyloroduodenal obstruction because of its antimuscarinic effects.
* Use with care in epilepsy as it may ↓convulsive threshold.
* Chlorphenamine is thought to be safe in acute porphyria.

*Biochemical and other tests*

None required.

## Dose

**Standard dose**: 10 mg by SC, IM or IV injection repeated up to four times in 24 hours if required (maximum 40 mg in 24 hours).
**Dose in hepatic impairment:** avoid in severe liver disease; may cause ↑sedation.

## Intravenous injection

*Preparation and administration*

1. Withdraw the required dose. May be diluted to 10 mL with NaCl 0.9% to facilitate slow administration.
2. Give by slow IV injection over 1 minute.
3. Flush with 5 mL NaCl 0.9%.

## Intramuscular injection

*Preparation and administration*

1. Withdraw the required dose.
2. Give by IM injection into a large muscle such as the gluteus or lateral aspect of the thigh.

## Subcutaneous injection

*Preparation and administration*

1. Withdraw the required dose.
2. Give by SC injection.

## Technical information

| | |
|---|---|
| Incompatible with | Noradrenaline (norepinephrine) |
| Compatible with | **Flush**: NaCl 0.9%<br>**Solutions**: NaCl 0.9%, Gluc 5%, Gluc-NaCl, Hartmann's, Ringer's<br>**Y-site**: No information |
| pH | 4–5.2 |
| Sodium content | Negligible |
| Storage | Store below 25°C in original packaging. |

## Monitoring

| Measure | Frequency | Rationale |
|---|---|---|
| Blood pressure | Post IV injection | • ↓BP may follow rapid IV injection. |

## Additional information

| | |
|---|---|
| Common and serious undesirable effects | *Injection-related:*<br>• Too rapid administration: Transient ↓BP, paradoxical CNS stimulation.<br>• Local: Stinging or burning at the site of injection.<br>*Other:* Drowsiness, headache, psychomotor impairment, urinary retention, dry mouth, blurred vision |
| Pharmacokinetics | In adults with normal renal and hepatic function, the half-life of chlorphenamine ranges from 2 to 43 hours. The duration of action is reported as 4–6 hours. |
| Significant interactions | • Chlorphenamine may ↑side-effects of the following drugs: MAOIs (↑risk of EPSE; avoid within 14 days), opioid analgesics (↑sedation). |
| Action in case of overdose | *Symptoms to watch for:* ↑drowsiness.<br>*Antidote:* No known antidote; stop administration and give supportive therapy as appropriate. |
| Counselling | May cause drowsiness; if affected do not drive or operate machinery.<br>Do not drink alcohol for a few hours after injection. |

| Risk rating: **GREEN** | Score = 0 Lower-risk product: Risk-reduction strategies should be considered. |
|---|---|

| | | | | | | | |
|---|---|---|---|---|---|---|---|
| | | | | | | | |

This assessment is based on the full range of preparation and administration options described in the monograph. These may not all be applicable in some clinical situations.

## Bibliography

SPC Chlorphenamine, Link Pharmaceuticals (accessed 3 July 2008).

# Chlorpromazine hydrochloride

**25 mg/mL solution in 2-mL ampoules**

- Chlorpromazine hydrochloride is a phenothiazine antipsychotic with a wide range of actions. It is a dopamine inhibitor; it has antiemetic activity; it has muscle relaxant properties; and it inhibits the heat-regulating centre.
- It is used to treat schizophrenia and other psychoses. By IM injection it is used to manage severely disturbed, agitated or violent behaviour.
- It is also used for intractable hiccup and to treat nausea and vomiting associated with terminal illness. It has been used to facilitate the induction of hypothermia because it prevents shivering and causes vasodilatation.
- In all cases the injection is intended for short-term treatment until the oral route is available.

## Pre-treatment checks

- Do not give to patients with known bone marrow depression.
- Avoid using in patients with renal or hepatic impairment, Parkinson disease, hypothyroidism, cardiac failure, phaeochromocytoma, myasthenia gravis and prostatic hypertrophy.
- Use with caution in patients with a history of narrow-angle glaucoma or agranulocytosis.

*Biochemical and other tests (not all are necessary in an emergency situation)*

| | |
|---|---|
| Blood pressure | LFTs |
| ECG | Renal function: U, Cr, CrCl (or eGFR) |

## Dose

**For acute relief of symptoms in schizophrenia, other psychoses, anxiety and agitation:** 25–50 mg by deep IM injection every 6 to 8 hours.

**For intractable hiccups:** 25–50 mg by deep IM injection every 6–8 hours. If this is ineffective, 25–50 mg may be given by slow IV infusion.

**For induction of hypothermia to prevent shivering:** 25–50 mg by deep IM injection every 6–8 hours.

**For nausea and vomiting associated with terminal illness:** 25 mg by deep IM injection then 25–50 mg every 3–4 hours until vomiting stops. Transfer to oral therapy as soon as possible.

## Intramuscular injection

*Preparation and administration*

See Special handling below.
Take care to avoid inadvertent SC administration as it is extremely irritant.

1. Withdraw the required dose.
2. Give by deep IM injection into large muscle such as the gluteal muscle. If irritation at the injection site is a problem the injection may be diluted with NaCl 0.9%.
3. Patient should remain supine for 30 minutes after administration.

## Intermittent intravenous infusion

*Preparation and administration*

See Special handling below.

1. Withdraw the required dose and add to 500 mL–1L NaCl 0.9%.
2. The solution should be clear and colourless to very pale yellow. Inspect visually for particulate matter or discoloration prior to administration and discard if present.
3. Give by slow IV infusion. Patient should remain supine during administration.

## Technical information

| | |
|---|---|
| Incompatible with | Amphotericin, aztreonam, furosemide, linezolid, piperacillin with tazobactam, remifentanil, tigecycline. |
| Compatible with | **Flush**: NaCl 0.9%<br>**Solutions**: NaCl 0.9%<br>**Y-site**: Cisatracurium, fluconazole, granisetron, hydrocortisone sodium succinate, ondansetron, propofol |
| pH | 5–6.5 |
| Sodium content | Negligible |
| Excipients | Contains sulfites (may cause allergic reactions). |
| Storage | Store below 25°C in original packaging. A slight yellowish discoloration does not indicate loss of potency - markedly discoloured solutions should not be used. |
| Special handling | Handle solutions with care to avoid risk of contact sensitisation. |
| Stability after preparation | Prepared infusions should be used immediately. |

## Monitoring

| Measure | Frequency | Rationale |
|---|---|---|
| Blood pressure | First 30 minutes and periodically thereafter if required. | • Patient should remain lying down for 30 minutes after injection and BP should be monitored as ↓BP may occur. |
| Pulse | | • May cause ↑pulse. |
| Injection site | Post administration | • May be painful and may cause nodule formation. |
| EPSE | | • May cause extrapyramidal side-effects. |
| Therapeutic improvement | Periodically | • Reduction in nausea and vomiting, hiccups or improvement in symptoms of psychotic illness schizophrenia or mania. |
| LFTs | Periodically if on long-term treatment | • Stop treatment if jaundice develops. |

## Additional information

| | |
|---|---|
| Common and serious undesirable effects | *Immediate:* EPSEs, ↓BP, ↑pulse, drowsiness.<br>*Other:* neuroleptic malignant syndrome.<br>Other adverse effects may be experienced on long-term therapy. |
| Pharmacokinetics | Half-life is approximately 30 hours but elimination of chlorpromazine metabolites may be very prolonged. |
| Significant interactions | • The following may ↑chlorpromazine levels or effect (or ↑side-effects): anaesthetics-general (↑risk of ↓BP), antidepressants- tricyclic, artemether with lumefantrine (avoid combination), propranolol, ritonavir, sibutramine (avoid combination).<br>• Chlorpromazine may ↑levels of propranolol.<br>• Chlorpromazine may ↓ effect of levodopa.<br>• Chlorpromazine may ↑risk of ventricular arrhythmias with the following drugs:<br>amiodarone (avoid combination), antidepressants-tricyclic, atomoxetine, disopyramide, droperidol (avoid combination), methadone, moxifloxacin (avoid combination), pentamidine isetionate, pimozide (avoid combination), sotalol.<br>• Chlorpromazine ↓convulsive threshold and may ↓effect of the following drugs:<br>barbiturates, carbamazepine, ethosuximide, oxcarbazepine, phenytoin, primidone, valproate. |
| Action in case of overdose | Treatment is supportive and symptomatic.<br>• Severe dystonic reactions may be treated with 5-10 mg procyclidine or 20-40 mg orphenadrine.<br>• Convulsions may be treated with IV diazepam.<br>• Neuroleptic malignant syndrome should be treated with cooling. Dantrolene sodium may be required.<br>• Do not give adrenaline. |
| Counselling | Patients on long-term chlorpromazine should avoid exposure to direct sunlight as they may develop photosensitisation. |

| Risk rating: **GREEN** | Score – 1<br>Lower-risk product: Risk-reduction strategies should be considered. |
|---|---|

This assessment is based on the full range of preparation and administration options described in the monograph. These may not all be applicable in some clinical situations.

## Bibliography

SPC Largactil (accessed 2 October 2007).

# Ciclosporin (cyclosporine, cyclosporin)

**50 mg/mL solution in 1-mL and 5-mL ampoules**

* Ciclosporin is an immunosuppressant that appears to act on lymphocytes (mainly helper T-cells), with little effect on bone marrow.
* It is usually given orally, often with corticosteroids and other immunosuppressants, in organ and tissue transplantation for the management or prophylaxis of graft rejection. It is also used in severe forms of atopic dermatitis, psoriasis, rheumatoid arthritis and nephrotic syndrome.
* The IV form is used for patients who cannot tolerate the oral form post surgery or in whom oral absorption may be impaired during episodes of GI disturbance. Patients should be switched to oral therapy as soon as is practical.

## Pre-treatment checks

* Do not give if hypersensitive to polyethoxylated castor oils.
* Caution in acute porphyria.
* Consult product literature for indication-specific cautions.

*Biochemical and other tests*

Blood pressure
Electrolytes: serum K, Mg
LFTs

Lipid profile
Renal function: U, Cr, CrCl (or eGFR)

## Dose

For existing patients switched from maintenance to IV dosing:
IV dose ≡ maintenance oral dose divided by 3.

**Organ transplantation, bone marrow transplantation/prevention and GVHD:** 3 mg/kg/day, from the day before transplantation to 2 weeks until oral maintenance therapy begins. The dose may be lower if given concomitantly with other immunosuppressant therapy.

**Refractory ulcerative colitis** (unlicensed): 2 mg/kg daily dose adjusted according to blood ciclosporin concentration and response.

## Intermittent intravenous infusion

*Preparation and administration*

PVC containers (e.g. Viaflex bags) should not be used as phthalate leaching can occur.

1. Withdraw the required dose and add to a suitable volume of compatible infusion fluid (usually NaCl 0.9%). Ensure that each 50 mg is diluted in 20–100 mL.
2. The solution should be clear and colourless to faintly brown-yellow. Inspect visually for particulate matter or discoloration prior to administration and discard if present.
3. Give by IV infusion over 2–6 hours using a syringe or volumetric pump. Observe for at least 30 minutes after starting infusion and at frequent intervals thereafter.

## Technical information

| | |
|---|---|
| Incompatible with | PVC containers (e.g. Viaflex bags) should not be used as phthalate leaching can occur.<br>Amphotericin, drotrecogin alfa (activated), magnesium sulfate, pantoprazole. |
| Compatible with | **Flush**: NaCl 0.9%<br>**Solutions**: NaCl 0.9%, Gluc 5%<br>**Y-site**: Linezolid, micafungin, propofol |
| pH | 6.0-7.0 |
| Sodium content | Nil |
| Excipients | Contains ethanol (may interact with metronidazole, possible religious objections).<br>Contains polyoxyl castor oils (have been associated with severe anaphylactic reactions). |
| Storage | Store below 30°C in original packaging. Do not freeze. |
| Stability after preparation | From a microbiological point of view, should be used immediately; however, infusions prepared in glass containers may be stored at room temperature and infused within 12 hours. |

## Monitoring

| Measure | Frequency | Rationale |
|---|---|---|
| Blood pressure | Regularly initially then monthly | • ↑BP may develop (treat with antihypertensive drugs as appropriate).<br>• Frequency of monitoring may vary with the indication. |
| U&Es | Weekly for first few weeks then 3-monthly | • Serum Cr and urea may rise (dose adjustment may be necessary).<br>• ↑K can occur especially with other drugs likely to raise potassium (corrective action may be necessary). |

*(continued)*

## Monitoring (continued)

| Measure | Frequency | Rationale |
|---|---|---|
| LFTs | Monthly for 3 months then 3-monthly | • Bilirubin and liver enzymes may rise.<br>• Dose adjustment may be necessary. |
| Serum magnesium | Intermittently | • Clearance of Mg is enhanced (if ↓Mg occurs, treat by supplementation). |
| Lipid profile | 6-monthly | • A reversible increase in lipids can occur (compare with baseline measure). |
| Symptoms of infection | Throughout treatment | • Immunosuppression predisposes patients to infection. |
| Ciclosporin level | 3 or 4 times weekly during early post transplantation then monthly by 6-12 months post transplantation or if considered necessary.<br>NB: Clearly state time elapsed since last dose given on blood sample. | • There is debate as to whether measurement is necessary; some authorities state desired trough concentrations:<br>  • 1 month post transplant: not less than 150 nanograms/mL<br>  • 3 months post transplant: 250-300 nanograms/mL<br>• Others state that measuring a level 2 hours after a dose ($C_2$) is more appropriate. For adult renal transplant recipients desired $C_2$ concentrations are:<br>  • 1 month post transplant: 1.5-2 micrograms/mL<br>  • 2 months post transplant: 1.5 micrograms/mL<br>  • 3 months post transplant: 1.3 micrograms/mL<br>  • 4-6 months post transplant: 1.1 micrograms/mL<br>  • 7-12 months post transplant: 0.9 micrograms/mL<br>  • >12 months post transplant: 0.8 micrograms/mL<br>• For adult liver transplant recipients desired $C_2$ concentrations are:<br>  • 0-6 months post transplant: 1 micrograms/mL<br>  • 6-12 months post transplant: 0.8 micrograms/mL<br>  • >12 months post transplant: 0.6 micrograms/mL |

## Additional information

| | |
|---|---|
| Common and serious undesirable effects | *Immediate:* Severe anaphylactoid reactions have been reported (reputedly due to polyoxyl castor oil content).<br>*Other:* Hyperlipidaemia, hyperuricaemia, ↑K, ↓Mg, tremor, headache, paraesthesia, ↑BP, anorexia, nausea, vomiting, abdominal pain, diarrhoea, gingival hyperplasia, hepatic dysfunction, hypertrichosis (gonk-like hair), muscle cramps, myalgia, renal dysfunction, fatigue. |
| Pharmacokinetics | Elimination half-life is 19 hours. |

(continued)

## Additional information (*continued*)

| | |
|---|---|
| Significant interactions | • The following may ↑ciclosporin levels or effect (or ↑side-effects): atazanavir, carvedilol, chloramphenicol, chloroquine, cimetidine, clarithromycin, colchicine, danazol, daptomycin (preferably avoid combination), diltiazem, doxorubicin, doxycycline, erythromycin, ezetimibe, fluconazole, grapefruit juice, hydroxychloroquine, indinavir, itraconazole, ketoconazole, lercanidipine (avoid combination), macrolides, methotrexate, methylprednisolone (risk of convulsions with high doses), metoclopramide, miconazole, nelfinavir, posaconazole, progestogens, quinupristin/ dalfopristin, ritonavir, rosuvastatin (avoid combination), saquinavir, tacrolimus (avoid combination), telithromycin, verapamil, voriconazole. <br> • The following may cause ↑K with ciclosporin: ACE inhibitors, aldosterone antagonists, angiotensin-II receptor antagonists, potassium salts, potassium-sparing diuretics. <br> • The following may ↑risk of nephrotoxicity with ciclosporin: aminoglycosides, amphotericin, colchicine, melphalan, polymyxins, quinolones, sulfonamides, trimethoprim, vancomycin. <br> • The following may ↓ciclosporin levels or effect: carbamazepine, barbiturates, bosentan (avoid combination), efavirenz, modafinil, octreotide, phenytoin, primidone, rifampicin, St John's wort (avoid combination), sulfadiazine, sulfinpyrazone, trimethoprim. <br> • Ciclosporin may ↑levels or effect of the following drugs (or ↑side-effects): aliskiren (avoid combination), bosentan (avoid combination), caspofungin (monitor LFTs), diclofenac (halve diclofenac dose), digoxin, NSAIDs, saquinavir, sitaxentan (avoid combination), statins, vaccines-live attenuated (avoid combination). <br> • Injectable preparation contains ethanol: may interact with disulfiram and metronidazole. |
| Action in case of overdose | Treatment should be symptomatic with general supportive measures. Monitor BP and cardiac rhythm. Ciclosporin is not dialysable and not cleared by charcoal haemoperfusion. |
| Counselling | Do not take oral form with grapefruit or grapefruit juice. <br> Avoid excessive exposure to UV light including sunlight. |

| Risk rating: **AMBER** | Score = 5 <br> Moderate-risk product: Risk-reduction strategies are recommended. |
|---|---|

This assessment is based on the full range of preparation and administration options described in the monograph. These may not all be applicable in some clinical situations.

## Bibliography

SPC SANDIMMUN concentrate for solution for infusion 50 mg/mL [ciclosporin] (accessed 3 March 2009).

# Cidofovir

**75 mg/mL concentrate for infusion in 5-mL vials**
* Cidofovir is a nucleoside analogue that is active against herpes viruses.
* It is used in the treatment of cytomegalovirus (CMV) retinitis in patients with AIDS for whom other drugs are inappropriate.

Cidofovir is toxic and personnel must be adequately protected during handling and administration – consult product literature.

## Pre-treatment checks
* Do not give if there is known hypersensitivity to cidofovir or probenecid.
* Avoid if CrCl ≤55 mL/minute or proteinuria ≥100 mg/dL (≥2+).
* Do not use with other potentially nephrotoxic drugs.
* Caution in diabetes mellitus (↑risk of ocular hypotony).
* To minimise the risk of nephrotoxicity, ensure that probenecid is co-prescribed and that patient is adequately hydrated with IV fluids.

*Biochemical and other tests*

Intraocular pressure | Renal function: U, Cr, CrCl (or eGFR)
LFTs | Urine dipstick for protein

## Dose

Cidofovir must only be given as an IV infusion and must never be given as a direct intraocular injection.
Cidofovir is nephrotoxic. Acute renal failure has been reported after only one or two doses, and there have been fatalities. To minimise potential nephrotoxicity the patient must be pre-treated with oral probenecid and IV NaCl 0.9% hydration before each dose.

**Induction dose**: 5 mg/kg by IV infusion once weekly for 2 weeks (with probenecid and IV fluids, see below).
**Maintenance dose** (beginning 2 weeks after completion of induction): 5 mg/kg by IV infusion once every 2 weeks (with probenecid and IV fluids, see below).
**Probenecid co-treatment by mouth (preferably after food to ↓nausea/vomiting)**: 2 g 3 hours before cidofovir infusion followed by 1 g at 2 hours and 1 g at 8 hours after the end of cidofovir infusion (total probenecid 4 g). The use of an antiemetic may be necessary if nausea/vomiting are a problem.
**Prior hydration by IV infusion**: give NaCl 0.9% 1 L over 1 hour immediately before each cidofovir infusion. If tolerated, an additional 1 L may be given over 1–3 hours, starting at the same time as the cidofovir infusion or immediately afterwards.
**Dose in renal impairment:**
* CrCl >55 mL/minute: dose as in normal renal function.
* CrCl ≤ 55 mL/minute: manufacturer advises avoid.

## Intermittent intravenous infusion

*Preparation and administration*

Cidofovir infusion should be prepared in a CIVAS unit.
See Special handling and Spillage below.

1. The solution should be clear and colourless. Inspect visually for particulate matter or discoloration prior to administration and discard if present.
2. Ensure that prophylactic probenecid and hydration have been given.
3. Give the entire volume by IV infusion via a volumetric infusion device over 60 minutes. The infusion must be given at a constant rate. To minimise the risk of nephrotoxicity, the dose must be infused over a minimum of 60 minutes.
4. Ensure further prophylactic probenecid and hydration (if appropriate) are given.

## Technical information

| | |
|---|---|
| Incompatible with | No information |
| Compatible with | **Flush**: NaCl 0.9%<br>**Solutions**: NaCl 0.9%<br>**Y-site**: No information |
| pH | 7.4 |
| Sodium content | 2.5 mmol per 5 mL vial |
| Storage | Store below 30°C in original packaging. Do not refrigerate or freeze.<br>Use opened vials immediately and discard any unused solution. |
| Special handling | Should be prepared in a CIVAS unit in a laminar flow cabinet and be administered only by clinicians suitably experienced in the care of AIDS patients. |
| Spillage | If cidofovir contacts the skin or mucosa, wash thoroughly with water. Excess solution and all other materials used in the preparation and administration should be placed in a leak-proof, puncture-proof container for disposal and in accordance with local policy. |
| Stability after preparation | From a microbiological point of view, prepared infusions should be used immediately; however, the preparation may be stored at 2–8°C and infused (at room temperature) within 24 hours (or as guided by CIVAS unit). |

## Monitoring

| Measure | Frequency | Rationale |
|---|---|---|
| Serum creatinine and urine protein | Within 24 hours prior to each dose of cidofovir | • Proteinuria is an early and sensitive indicator of cidofovir-induced nephrotoxicity.<br>• If serum creatinine increases by 44 micromol/L (500 micrograms/dL) above baseline, or if persistent proteinuria ≥2+ develops, therapy should be stopped and IV hydration commenced.<br>• If following hydration, a ≥2+ proteinuria is still observed, cidofovir therapy should be discontinued.<br>• In the USA a reduction of the maintenance dose to 3 mg/kg is permitted for increases in serum creatinine of 300–400 micrograms/dL above baseline. |
| WCC including differential neutrophil count | Prior to each dose of cidofovir | • Reversible neutropenia sometimes occurs, which may resolve spontaneously whether or not the cidofovir is stopped.<br>• Filgrastim (G-CSF) has been used in some patients. |

*(continued)*

## Monitoring (continued)

| Measure | Frequency | Rationale |
|---------|-----------|-----------|
| Ophthalmological examination (intraocular pressure, visual acuity, and symptoms of uveitis/iritis) | Regularly | • Iritis/uveitis occur commonly, which may respond to a topical corticosteroid (with or without a cycloplegic drug).<br>• Discontinue cidofovir if there is no response to topical corticosteroid or if the condition worsens, or if iritis/uveitis recurs after successful treatment.<br>• Intraocular pressure may decrease by up to 50% from pre-treatment baseline. |
| Development of hypersensitivity reaction to probenecid | Throughout treatment | • If rash, fever or chills occur, consider prophylactic or therapeutic use of an antihistamine and/or paracetamol. |

## Additional information

| | |
|---|---|
| Common and serious undesirable effects | Neutropenia, iritis/uveitis; ↓intraocular pressure, dyspnoea; pneumonia, nausea, vomiting, alopecia, proteinuria; ↑creatinine, asthenia; fever, death; infection. Rash and fever may also commonly present due to probenecid. |
| Pharmacokinetics | Elimination half-life is 2.5 hours (major metabolite 17 hours). |
| Significant interactions | • Cidofovir therapy may ↑levels or effect of the following drugs (or ↑side-effects):<br>Zidovudine should be temporarily stopped or dose reduced by 50% on days when cidofovir is administered (probenecid ↓clearance of zidovudine).<br>Potentially nephrotoxic drugs should be stopped at least 7 days before starting cidofovir, e.g. aminoglycosides, amphotericin, foscarnet, pentamidine, vancomycin or NSAIDs. |
| Action in case of overdose | Monitor renal function. Give prophylactic probenecid and vigorous hydration for 3 7 days. |
| Counselling | Men should use barrier contraceptive methods during and for 3 months after treatment with cidofovir.<br>Women should not become pregnant during and for 1 month after treatment. |

| Risk rating: **RED** | Note: Risk adjusted to RED - this scoring system does not account for the extra safety requirements for handling this product.<br>Must be prepared in a CIVAS unit. |
|---|---|

This assessment is based on the full range of preparation and administration options described in the monograph. These may not all be applicable in some clinical situations.

## Bibliography

SPC Vistide (accessed 9 March 2009).

# Ciprofloxacin

**2 mg/mL solution in 50-mL, 100-mL, 200-mL infusion bottles**
* Ciprofloxacin lactate is a fluorinated quinolone antibacterial.
* It is active against both Gram-positive and Gram-negative bacteria with particular activity against Gram-negatives: *Salmonella, Shigella, Campylobacter, Neisseria* and *Pseudomonas*.
* Ciprofloxacin is rapidly and well absorbed from the GI tract following oral dosing, so the IV route should be used only when the oral route is unavailable.
* Doses are expressed in terms of the base:
  Ciprofloxacin 200 mg ≅ 254 mg ciprofloxacin lactate.

## Pre-treatment checks

* Do not give if there is known hypersensitivity to ciprofloxacin or other quinolone antibacterials.
* Use with caution in G6PD deficiency.
* Ciprofloxacin lowers seizure threshold and should be used cautiously in patients with a history of convulsions.
* Patients must be adequately hydrated and asked to drink fluids liberally. Excessive urine alkalinity should be avoided to limit the risk of crystalluria.

*Biochemical and other tests*

FBC                                                    Renal function: U, Cr, CrCl (eGFR)
LFTs

## Dose

Patients must be adequately hydrated and asked to drink fluids liberally.

**Standard dose**: 200–400 mg twice daily (depending on severity of infection).
**Serious infections:** in cases of very serious, life-threatening or recurrent infections 400 mg three times daily has been used.
**Pseudomonal lower respiratory tract infection in cystic fibrosis:** 400 mg twice daily.
**Anthrax (treatment and post-exposure prophylaxis):** 400 mg twice daily (length of course depends on route of infection).
**Urinary tract infections:** 100 mg twice daily.
**Gonorrhoea:** 100 mg as a single dose.
**Dose in renal impairment**: adjusted according to creatinine clearance:[1]
* CrCl >20–50 mL/minute: dose as in normal renal function.
* CrCl 10–20 mL/minute: 50–100% of normal dose.
* CrCl <10 mL/minute: 50% of normal dose.

## Intermittent intravenous infusion

*Preparation and administration*

Infusion into a large vein minimises patient discomfort.

1. Select the correct size of infusion bottle.
2. The infusion is pre-prepared for use. It should be clear and colourless to slightly yellow. Inspect visually for particulate matter or discoloration prior to administration and discard if present.
3. Give by IV infusion over 30 minutes for 200 mg (60 minutes for 400 mg). Infusion into a large vein minimises patient discomfort.

## Technical information

| | |
|---|---|
| Incompatible with | Sodium bicarbonate.<br>Aminophylline, amoxicillin, amphotericin, ampicillin, ceftazidime, cefuroxime, clindamycin phosphate, co-amoxiclav, dexamethasone sodium phosphate, drotrecogin alfa (activated), flucloxacillin, furosemide, hydrocortisone sodium succinate, magnesium sulfate, methylprednisolone sodium succinate, pantoprazole, phenytoin sodium, propofol, teicoplanin, ticarcillin with clavulanate. |
| Compatible with | **Flush**: NaCl 0.9%<br>**Solutions**: NaCl 0.9%, Gluc 5%, Gluc-NaCl, Hartmann's, Ringer's (all with added KCl)<br>**Y-site**: Amikacin, atracurium, aztreonam, calcium gluconate, cisatracurium, clarithromycin, digoxin, dobutamine, dopamine, fluconazole, gentamicin, granisetron, linezolid, metoclopramide, metronidazole, midazolam, noradrenaline (norepinephrine), ranitidine, remifentanil, tigecycline, tobramycin, verapamil |
| pH | 3.5-4.5 |
| Sodium content | 15.4 mmol/100 mL |
| Storage | Store below 25°C in original packaging. Do not refrigerate or freeze (crystals may form, which will re-dissolve at room temperature without affecting potency).<br>Use opened vials immediately and discard any unused solution. |

## Monitoring

| Measure | Frequency | Rationale |
|---|---|---|
| Temperature | Minimum daily | • For clinical signs of fever declining. |
| Renal function | Periodically | • If renal function changes, a dose adjustment may be necessary. Urea and creatinine usually increase.<br>• The manufacturer recommends twice-weekly creatinine measurement if the patient is on concomitant ciclosporin. |
| FBC | | • Eosinophilia is common; leucopenia, neutropenia, anaemia, pancytopenia and thrombocytopenia may also occur.<br>• WCC for signs of the infection resolving. |
| LFT | | • ALT, AST, often rise transiently; Alk Phos, GGT and bilirubin rise less commonly. |
| Sensitivity testing of infection | Periodically in prolonged therapy | • To ensure that microorganism remains sensitive to therapy.<br>• Especially critical with *Pseudomonas aeruginosa* and *Staphylococcus aureus*. |
| Blood glucose concentration | ↑ frequency in diabetic patients | • Symptomatic hyperglycaemia and/or hypoglycaemia have been reported requiring closer monitoring<br>• If signs or symptoms of glucose disturbances develop therapy should be reviewed. |

*(continued)*

## Monitoring (continued)

| Measure | Frequency | Rationale |
|---|---|---|
| Signs of CNS disorders | Throughout treatment | • Use with caution in patients with epilepsy or tendency to spasms, previous seizures, vascular disorders in the brain, alterations in brain structure or stroke.<br>• If self-destructive behaviour is demonstrated or if seizures occur, discontinue treatment. |
| Signs of tendon damage (including rupture) | | • If tendinitis is suspected, discontinue immediately; the affected limb should not be exerted and should be made non-weight-bearing.<br>• Most likely in elderly patients or with concomitant corticosteroids. |
| Symptoms of neuropathy | | • Due to axonal polyneuropathy and may be irreversible, although incidence is rare.<br>• Discontinue if such symptoms occur, e.g. pain, burning, tingling, numbness; or deficits in light touch, pain, temperature, position sense, vibratory sensation, motor strength. |
| Signs of supra-infection or superinfection | | • May result in the overgrowth of non-susceptible organisms - appropriate therapy should be commenced; treatment may need to be interrupted. |
| Development of diarrhoea | Throughout and up to 2 months after treatment | • Development of severe, persistent diarrhoea may be suggestive of *Clostridium difficile*-associated diarrhoea and colitis (pseudomembranous colitis). Discontinue drug and treat. Do not use drugs that inhibit peristalsis. |

## Additional information

| | |
|---|---|
| Common and serious undesirable effects | *Infusion-related:* Local: Infusion-site phlebitis.<br>*Other:* Nausea, diarrhoea, vomiting, abdominal pain; rash, occasionally dizziness and light-headedness; rarely can cause hypoglycaemia in elderly diabetic patients - monitor blood glucose. |
| Pharmacokinetics | Elimination half-life is 3–6 hours. |
| Significant interactions | • Ciprofloxacin may ↑levels or effect of the following drugs (or ↑side-effects): agomelatine (avoid combination), artemether with lumefantrine (avoid combination), ciclosporin (↑risk of nephrotoxicity), coumarin anticoagulants (monitor INR), duloxetine (avoid combination), NSAIDs (↑risk of seizures), theophylline (↑risk of seizures; ↑levels - reduce dose or monitor).<br>• Ciprofloxacin may ↓levels or effect of antiepileptic drugs (↓seizure threshold). |
| Action in case of overdose | Treat symptomatically. Ensure adequate hydration to prevent crystalluria. Monitor renal function. |
| Counselling | The patient should drink fluids liberally.<br>A rash may develop on exposure to strong sunlight and ultraviolet rays, e.g. sunlamps, solariums - patients should avoid unnecessary exposure. |

| Risk rating: **GREEN** | Score = 0<br>Lower-risk product: Risk-reduction strategies should be considered. |
|---|---|

| | | | | | | |
|---|---|---|---|---|---|---|

This assessment is based on the full range of preparation and administration options described in the monograph. These may not all be applicable in some clinical situations.

## Reference

1. Ashley C, Currie A, eds. *The Renal Drug Handbook*, 3rd edn. Oxford: Radcliffe Medical Press, 2009.

## Bibliography

SPC Ciproxin infusion (accessed 9 March 2009).

# Clarithromycin

**500-mg dry powder vials**

- Clarithromycin is a macrolide antibacterial with a broad, mainly bacteriostatic action against many Gram-positive and, to a lesser extent, some Gram-negative bacteria, as well as some 'atypicals'.
- It is used to treat infections caused by susceptible organisms, e.g. community-acquired pneumonia and skin and soft-tissue infections.

## Pre-treatment checks

- Contraindicated in patients with known hypersensitivity to macrolide antibiotics.
- Avoid in acute porphyria.
- Caution if predisposition to QT interval prolongation (including electrolyte disturbances, concomitant use of drugs that prolong QT interval).

*Biochemical and other tests (not all are necessary in an emergency situation)*

| | |
|---|---|
| LFTs | Temperature |
| Renal function: U, Cr, CrCl (or eGFR) | WCC |
| Signs of infection | |

## Dose

**Standard dose:** 500 mg by IV infusion every 12 hours.

**Dose in renal impairment**: adjusted according to creatinine clearance:[1]

- CrCl >30–50 mL/minute: dose as in normal renal function.
- CrCl 10–30 mL/minute: 250–500 mg every 12 hours.
- CrCl <10 mL/minute: 250–500 mg every 12 hours (vomiting may be a problem).

## Intermittent intravenous infusion

*Preparation and administration*

Clarithromycin must not be given by direct IV or IM injection.
Give by IV infusion into a large proximal vein to reduce pain.

1. Reconstitute each 500-mg vial with 10 mL WFI.
2. Withdraw the required dose and add to a suitable volume of compatible infusion fluid to give a solution containing approximately 2 mg/mL (e.g. add 500 mg to 250 mL NaCl 0.9%).
3. The solution should be clear and colourless. Inspect visually for particulate matter or discoloration prior to administration and discard if present.
4. Give by IV infusion into a large proximal vein over 60 minutes.

**Fluid restriction:** concentrations up to 5 mg/mL have been given via a central line.

## Technical information

| | |
|---|---|
| Incompatible with | Aminophylline, ceftazidime, cefuroxime, flucloxacillin, furosemide, heparin sodium, phenytoin sodium. |
| Compatible with | **Flush**: NaCl 0.9%<br>**Solutions**: Gluc 5% (with added KCl), NaCl 0.9%, Gluc-NaCl, Hartmann's, Ringer's<br>**Y-site**: Ampicillin, atracurium, benzylpenicillin, bumetanide, cimetidine, ciprofloxacin, co-amoxiclav, dobutamine, dopamine, gentamicin, metoclopramide, metronidazole, ranitidine, ticarcillin with clavulanate, vancomycin, vecuronium bromide, verapamil |
| pH | 5 |
| Sodium content | Negligible |
| Storage | Store below 30°C in original packaging. |
| Displacement value | Negligible |
| Stability after preparation | From a microbiological point of view, should be used immediately; however:<br>• Reconstituted vials may be stored at 2-8°C for 24 hours.<br>• Prepared infusions (2 mg/mL) may be stored at 2-8°C and infused (at room temperature) within 24 hours. |

## Monitoring

| Measure | Frequency | Rationale |
|---|---|---|
| Physical signs of infection | Daily | • Monitor patient response (e.g. FBC, normalisation of observations) for signs of infection resolution - consider review to oral clarithromycin as appropriate. |
| Injection site | At regular intervals | • Local tenderness and inflammation, phlebitis, pain at the injection site. |

*(continued)*

## Monitoring (continued)

| Measure | Frequency | Rationale |
|---------|-----------|-----------|
| Renal function | Weekly | • Dose may need adjusting if renal function changes. |
| LFTs | | • Toxicity - patients should be monitored for elevations of serum hepatic enzymes.<br>• Caution required in hepatic impairment.<br>• Hepatic dysfunction including cholestatic jaundice has been reported. |
| Signs of hypersensitivity | Throughout treatment | • In case of hypersensitivity reactions. |
| Signs of supra-infection or superinfection | | • May result in the overgrowth of non-susceptible organisms - appropriate therapy should be commenced; treatment may need to be interrupted. |
| Development of diarrhoea | Throughout and up to 2 months after treatment | • Development of severe, persistent diarrhoea may be suggestive of *Clostridium difficile*-associated diarrhoea and colitis (pseudomembranous colitis). Discontinue drug and treat. Do not use drugs that inhibit peristalsis. |

## Additional information

| | |
|---|---|
| Common and serious undesirable effects | *Immediate:* Anaphylaxis has been reported rarely.<br>*Infusion-related:* Local: Pain, thrombophlebitis, extravasation (↑ if administration too rapid).<br>*Other:* GI disturbances, antibiotic-associated colitis, urticaria, rashes, angioedema, reversible hearing loss after large doses, chest pain, arrhythmias, stomatitis, glossitis |
| Pharmacokinetics | Elimination half-life is 3–7 hours (main metabolite: 5–9 hours). Metabolism may become saturated at higher doses. |
| Significant interactions | • ↑Risk of ventricular arrhythmias with pimozide (avoid combination).<br>• The following may ↑clarithromycin levels or effect (or ↑side-effects): ritonavir (CrCl 30–60 mL/minute the dose of clarithromycin should be ↓by 50%; for CrCl <30 mL/minute the dose of clarithromycin should be ↓ by 75%).<br>• Clarithromycin may ↑levels or effect of the following drugs (or ↑side-effects): artemether/lumefantrine (avoid combination), carbamazepine, ciclosporin, cilostazol (avoid combination), clozapine (possible ↑risk of convulsions), colchicine, coumarins (monitor INR), disopyramide, eletriptan (avoid combination), ergotamine (avoid combination), methysergide (avoid combination), midazolam, mizolastine (avoid combination), reboxetine (avoid combination), rifabutin (↑risk of uveitis, ↓rifabutin dose), simvastatin (↑risk of myopathy, avoid combination), sirolimus, tacrolimus, theophylline (monitor levels), verapamil, vinblastine (avoid combination). |
| Action in case of overdose | No known antidote; stop administration and give supportive therapy as appropriate. |
| Counselling | Potential for drug interactions; explain short-term alterations in co-prescribing, e.g. withholding statins or theophylline. |

| Risk rating: **AMBER** | Score = 3<br>Moderate-risk product: Risk-reduction strategies are recommended. |
|---|---|

This assessment is based on the full range of preparation and administration options described in the monograph. These may not all be applicable in some clinical situations.

## Reference

1. Ashley C, Currie A, eds. *The Renal Drug Handbook*, 3rd edn. Oxford: Radcliffe Medical Press, 2009.

## Bibliography

SPC: Klaricid IV, Abbott Laboratories Ltd (accessed 24 October 2007).

# Clindamycin

### 150 mg/mL solution in 2-mL, 4-mL ampoules

- Clindamycin phosphate is a semisynthetic antibiotic that is a derivative of lincomycin (a lincosamide).
- It has primarily bacteriostatic action against Gram-positive aerobes and a wide range of anaerobic bacteria.
- Doses are expressed in terms of the base:
  Clindamycin 1 g ≅1.2 g clindamycin phosphate.

## Pre-treatment checks

- Do not give if there is known hypersensitivity to clindamycin or lincomycin.
- Avoid in acute porphyria and do not give in diarrhoeal states.

*Biochemical and other tests*

FBC
LFTs
Renal function: U, Cr, CrCl (or eGFR)

## Dose

**Serious infections**: give every 6–12 hours by IM injection or IV infusion to provide a total daily dose of 600 mg–2.7 g daily.

**Life threatening infections**: up to 1.2 g by IV infusion every 6 hours.

**Dose in renal impairment**: dose as in normal renal function. However, prolonged half-life may necessitate dose reduction.[1]

## Intramuscular injection (maximum dose 600 mg)

*Preparation and administration*

1. Withdraw the required dose.
2. Give by deep IM injection.

## Intermittent intravenous infusion

*Preparation and administration*

1. Withdraw the required dose and add to a suitable volume of compatible infusion fluid (usually 100 mL NaCl 0.9%). The final concentration of the drug should be no more than 18 mg/mL.
2. The solution should be clear and colourless. Inspect visually for particulate matter or discoloration prior to administration and discard if present.
3. Give by IV infusion at a **maximum** rate of 30 mg/minute (e.g. 300 mg over 15 minutes; 600 mg over 30 minutes; 900 mg over 45 minutes; 1.2 g over 60 minutes).

## Technical information

| | |
|---|---|
| Incompatible with | Clindamycin phosphate is incompatible with natural rubber closures. Aminophylline, ampicillin, calcium gluconate, ceftriaxone, ciprofloxacin, doxapram, drotrecogin alfa (activated), fluconazole, magnesium sulfate, phenytoin sodium, ranitidine, tramadol. |
| Compatible with | **Flush**: NaCl 0.9%<br>**Solutions**: NaCl 0.9%, Gluc 5%, Gluc-NaCl (all including added KCl)<br>**Y-site**: Aciclovir, amikacin, aztreonam, benzylpenicillin, cefotaxime, ceftazidime, cefuroxime, cisatracurium, esmolol, gentamicin, granisetron, hydrocortisone sodium succinate, labetalol, methylprednisolone sodium succinate, metoclopramide, metronidazole, midazolam, ondansetron, piperacillin with tazobactam, propofol, remifentanil, sodium bicarbonate, tobramycin, verapamil |
| pH | 5.5-7 |
| Sodium content | Negligible |
| Excipients | Contains benzyl alcohol. |
| Storage | Store below 25°C in original packaging. Do not refrigerate or freeze (crystals may form, which will re-dissolve at room temperature without affecting potency). |
| Stability after preparation | From a microbiological point of view, should be used immediately; however, prepared infusions may be stored at 2-8°C and infused (at room temperature) within 24 hours. |

## Monitoring

| Measure | Frequency | Rationale |
|---|---|---|
| Renal function | Periodically if treatment prolonged | • Manufacturer's recommendation. |
| LFTs | | • Jaundice and deranged LFTs have occasionally been reported. |
| FBC | | • Leucopenia, eosinophilia, and thrombocytopenia have occasionally been reported |

*(continued)*

## Monitoring (continued)

| Measure | Frequency | Rationale |
|---------|-----------|-----------|
| Development of diarrhoea | Throughout and up to 3 weeks after treatment | • Development of severe, persistent diarrhoea may be suggestive of *Clostridium difficile*-associated diarrhoea and colitis (pseudomembranous colitis). Discontinue drug and treat. Do not use drugs that inhibit peristalsis. |
| Signs of supra-infection or superinfection | Throughout treatment | • May result in the overgrowth of non-susceptible organisms - appropriate therapy should be commenced; treatment may need to be interrupted. |

## Additional information

| | |
|---|---|
| Common and serious undesirable effects | *Immediate:* Anaphylactoid and other hypersensitivity reactions have been reported.<br>*Injection/infusion-related:* Local: Pain, induration, abscess after IM injection; thrombophlebitis after IV injection.<br>*Other:* Diarrhoea (see monitoring above), abdominal discomfort, oesophagitis, oesophageal ulcers, taste disturbances, nausea, vomiting, jaundice, rashes. |
| Pharmacokinetics | Elimination half-life is 2-3 hours. |
| Significant interactions | • Clindamycin ↑effect of the following drugs: non-depolarising muscle relaxants, suxamethonium. |
| Action in case of overdose | No known antidote; stop administration and give supportive therapy as appropriate. |

| Risk rating: **AMBER** | Score = 3<br>Moderate-risk product: Risk-reduction strategies are recommended. |
|---|---|

This assessment is based on the full range of preparation and administration options described in the monograph. These may not all be applicable in some clinical situations.

### Reference

1. Ashley C, Currie A, eds. *The Renal Drug Handbook*, 3rd edn. Oxford: Radcliffe Medical Press, 2009.

### Bibliography

SPC Dalacin C Phosphate (accessed 9 March 2009).

# Clodronate sodium (sodium clodronate, disodium clodronate)

**60 mg/mL solution in 5-mL ampoules**

* Sodium clodronate is a bisphosphonate with properties similar to those of the other bisphosphonates. It inhibits bone resorption but appears to have less effect on bone mineralisation.
* It is used in the treatment of severe ↑Ca associated with malignancy (TIH).
* Doses are expressed as sodium clodronate.

## Pre-treatment checks

* Do not give to patients already receiving other bisphosphonates.
* Osteonecrosis of the jaw can occur: consider dental examination and preventive dentistry prior to *planned* treatment in patients with risk factors (e.g. cancer, chemotherapy, radiotherapy, corticosteroids, poor oral hygiene). Avoid invasive dental procedures during treatment if possible.
* Give cautiously to patients who have had previous thyroid surgery (increased risk of ↓Ca)
* Contraindicated in pregnancy. Women of child-bearing potential should take contraceptive precautions during *planned* treatment.
* Hydrate patient adequately before, during and after infusions (up to 4 L may be given over 24 hours but over-hydration should be avoided; risk of cardiac failure).

*Biochemical and other tests*

Electrolytes: serum Na, K, Ca, $PO_4$, Mg
Renal function: U, Cr, CrCl (or eGFR)

## Dose

The patient must be adequately hydrated using NaCl 0.9% before dosing.

**Tumour-induced hypercalcaemia (TIH):** single infusion of 1500 mg or as multiple infusions of 300 mg daily. The dose given is not dependent on the patient's serum Ca concentration.

* For single infusions, a significant fall in serum Ca is usually seen 24–48 hours after administration and normalisation within 3–7 days. For multiple infusions, these are repeated daily until normocalcaemia is achieved, or for a maximum of 7 days
* Dose may be repeated in patients not achieving clinically acceptable serum Ca levels by either method. The duration of the response varies.
* Treatment can be repeated whenever ↑Ca recurs. Alternatively, oral treatment may be given daily if appropriate.

**Dose in renal impairment:** adjusted according to creatinine clearance (see Table C3).
It seems wise to give the dose as smaller multiple infusions – no guidance exists for dose adjustment for large single infusions.

**Table C3** Clodronate sodium dose adjustment in renal impairment

| Creatinine clearance (or eGFR) (mL/minute) | Recommended dose reduction | Recommended daily dose (mg) | Equivalent volume of concentrate (mL) |
|---|---|---|---|
| >80 | Standard dose | 300 mg | 5 mL |
| 50-80 | Reduce by 25% | 225 mg | 3.75 mL |
| 10-50 | Reduce by 25-50% | 150-225 mg | 2.5-3.75 mL |
| <10 | Not recommended | Not recommended | Not recommended |

## Single intravenous infusion

*Preparation and administration*

Clodronate sodium is incompatible with Hartmann's and Ringer's (which contain Ca).

1. Withdraw 1500 mg (5 × 5-mL ampoules) and add to 500 mL of either NaCl 0.9% or Gluc 5%.
2. The solution should be clear and colourless. Inspect visually for particulate matter or discoloration prior to administration and discard if present.
3. Give by IV infusion over 4 hours.

## Multiple intravenous infusions

*Preparation and administration*

Clodronate sodium is incompatible with Hartmann's and Ringer's (which contain Ca).

1. Withdraw the required dose and add to 500 mL of either NaCl 0.9% or Gluc 5%.
2. The solution should be clear and colourless. Inspect visually for particulate matter or discoloration prior to administration and discard if present.
3. Give by IV infusion over at least 2 hours.

## Technical information

| Incompatible with | Clodronate sodium is incompatible with Hartmann's and Ringer's (which contain Ca). |
|---|---|
| Compatible with | **Flush**: NaCl 0.9%<br>**Solutions**: NaCl 0.9%, Gluc 5%<br>**Y-site**: No information |
| pH | 3-4.5 |
| Sodium content | Negligible |
| Storage | Store below 25°C in original packaging. |
| Stability after preparation | From a microbiological point of view, should be used immediately; however, prepared infusions should be infused within 12 hours of preparation. |

## Monitoring

| Measure | Frequency | Rationale |
|---------|-----------|-----------|
| Fluid balance | Frequently during therapy | • Hydration ↑Ca diuresis.<br>• Hydration reduces decline in renal function and ↓formation of calcium renal calculi. |
| U&E, CrCl (or eGFR) | Prior to each dose and periodically post dose | • ↓Renal function has been reported during bisphosphonate therapy - may require ↓dose or cessation of therapy. |
| Serum Ca, PO₄, Mg | | • Stop treatment if ↓Ca develops.<br>• Serum Ca determines if further treatment is required.<br>• PO₄ and Ca share common control systems. Disruption to Ca metabolism affects PO₄ levels.<br>• ↓Mg occurs commonly during treatment. |

## Additional information

| | |
|---|---|
| Common and serious undesirable effects | *Immediate:* Angioedema and bronchospasm have been reported.<br>*Other:* Renal dysfunction, transient proteinuria immediately after IV infusion, reversible ↑parathyroid hormone, lactic acid dehydrogenase, transaminase and alkaline phosphatase, asymptomatic ↓Ca has been noted infrequently; symptomatic ↓Ca is rare, pruritus, urticaria, exfoliative dermatitis, jaw osteonecrosis (see above). |
| Pharmacokinetics | The half-life for elimination from plasma is 2 hours but a second phase with a half-life of 13 hours has been identified (<10% of total urinary excretion takes place during this phase). The substance which is bound to bone is excreted more slowly at a rate corresponding to bone turnover. |
| Significant drug interactions | Clodronate sodium may ↑levels or effect (or ↑side-effects) of estramustine. |
| Action in case of overdose | *Symptoms to watch for:* Clinically significant ↓Ca (paraesthesia, tetany, ↓BP).<br>*Antidote:* Calcium gluconate infusion (see the Calcium gluconate monograph). Stop administration and give supportive therapy as appropriate. Monitor serum Ca, PO₄, Mg, K. |
| Counselling | Not known to affect the patient's ability to drive or use machinery.<br>Maintain fluid intake during the hours post infusion.<br>Inform of symptoms of ↓Ca (paraesthesia, tetany, muscle cramps, confusion).<br>Advise patients with risk factors for osteonecrosis of the jaw (see pre-treatment checks) not to undergo invasive dental procedures during treatment. |

| | |
|---|---|
| Risk rating: **AMBER** | Score = 3<br>Moderate-risk product: Risk-reduction strategies are recommended. |

This assessment is based on the full range of preparation and administration options described in the monograph. These may not all be applicable in some clinical situations.

## Bibliography

SPC Bonefos concentrate (accessed 10/02/09).

# Clonazepam

### 1 mg/mL solution in ampoules with 1-mL diluent ampoules (WFI)

*   Clonazepam is a benzodiazepine with marked antiepileptic properties.
*   It is used for the treatment of epilepsy and myoclonus. By the IV route it has a fast onset of action and may be used in the management of status epilepticus.
*   Oral antiepileptic agents should be instituted as soon as the oral route becomes available and is clinically indicated.

### Pre-treatment checks

*   Do not use in respiratory depression; acute pulmonary insufficiency; sleep apnoea syndrome; marked neuromuscular respiratory weakness including unstable myasthenia gravis.
*   Caution in elderly or debilitated patients, respiratory disease, spinal or cerebellar ataxia; history of alcohol or drug abuse, depression or suicidal ideation; avoid sudden withdrawal; myasthenia gravis (avoid if unstable); acute porphyria; hepatic impairment; renal impairment; pregnancy and breast feeding.
*   Ensure that resuscitation equipment is available.

*Biochemical and other tests (not all are necessary in an emergency situation)*

Blood pressure
LFTs
Renal function: U, Cr, CrCl (or eGFR)

### Dose

**Standard dose:** 1 mg by slow IV injection or intermittent IV infusion. The dose may be repeated if required.
**Continuous IV infusion:** the BNF advises that IV infusion is potentially hazardous (particularly if prolonged), calling for close and constant observation, and is best carried out in specialist centres with intensive care facilities. Prolonged infusion may lead to accumulation and delayed recovery.
**Dose in hepatic impairment**: reduce dose and avoid if severe.

### Intravenous injection

*Preparation and administration*

Give slowly into a large vein to reduce risk of thrombophlebitis.

1.  Withdraw the required dose and dilute with an equal volume of WFI (supplied) to give a concentration of 0.5 mg/mL.
2.  The solution should be clear and colourless to slightly greenish yellow. Inspect visually for particulate matter or discoloration prior to administration and discard if present.
3.  Give by IV injection into a large vein of the antecubital fossa at a maximum rate of 0.5 mg/minute. (There is a risk of thrombophlebitis if smaller veins or faster rates are used.)

**Intermittent intravenous infusion**

*Preparation and administration*

1. Withdraw the required dose and add to a suitable volume of compatible infusion fluid to give a maximum concentration of 3 mg in 250 mL, e.g. add 1 mg to 100 mL NaCl 0.9%.
2. The solution should be clear and colourless to slightly greenish yellow. Inspect visually for particulate matter or discoloration prior to administration and discard if present.
3. Give by IV infusion at a maximum rate of 0.5 mg/minute via volumetric infusion device.

## Technical information

| | |
|---|---|
| Incompatible with | Sodium bicarbonate |
| Compatible with | **Flush**: NaCl 0.9%<br>**Solutions**: NaCl 0.9%, Gluc 5%, Gluc-NaCl<br>**Y-site**: Nil |
| pH | 3.8 |
| Sodium content | Nil |
| Excipients | Contains benzyl alcohol, ethanol, propylene glycol (adverse effects seen if renal elimination is impaired and may interact with disulfiram and metronidazole). |
| Storage | Store below 30°C in original packaging. |
| Stability after preparation | Use diluted injection immediately.<br>Use prepared infusions immediately. Complete the infusion within 2 hours if PVC containers are used, or 12 hours if glass bottles are used. |

## Monitoring

| Measure | Frequency | Rationale |
|---|---|---|
| Seizure frequency and severity | At regular intervals | • Monitor for reduction in the frequency and severity to ensure therapeutic effect. |
| Injection site | | • Thrombophlebitis may occur (rarely). |
| Respiration, blood pressure and EEG (where available) | Continuously through administration | • ↑Drowsiness and CNS depression may occur.<br>• ↓BP or apnoea may occur (rarely). |
| Full blood count | Periodically | • May cause blood dyscrasias.<br>• Withdraw therapy if spontaneous bruising or bleeding occurs. |
| LFTs | | • Altered LFTs may occur. |

## Additional information

| | |
|---|---|
| Common and serious undesirable effects | *Injection/infusion-related:* Local: Thrombophlebitis and thrombus formation (particularly if a small vein is used).<br>*Other:* Drowsiness, fatigue, dizziness, disorientation, muscle hypotonia, restlessness, confusion, amnesia. |
| Pharmacokinetics | Elimination half-life is 20–60 hours (average 30 hours). |
| Significant interactions | • The following may ↑clonazepam levels or effect (or ↑side-effects): olanzapine IM (↓BP, ↓pulse, respiratory depression), ritonavir.<br>• Clonazepam may ↑levels or effect (or ↑side-effects) of sodium oxybate (avoid combination).<br>• Injectable preparation contains ethanol and propylene glycol: may interact with disulfiram and metronidazole. |
| Action in case of overdose | *Symptoms to watch for:* ↑Sedation, respiratory depression, ↓BP.<br>*Antidote:* Flumazenil (use with caution in patients with a history of seizures, head injury or chronic benzodiazepine use including for the control of epilepsy). Stop administration and give supportive therapy as appropriate. |
| Counselling | May cause transient drowsiness - if affected do not drive or operate machinery. Advise women of child-bearing potential to use adequate contraception. |

**Risk rating: AMBER**  Score = 3
Moderate-risk product: Risk-reduction strategies are recommended.

This assessment is based on the full range of preparation and administration options described in the monograph. These may not all be applicable in some clinical situations.

## Bibliography

SPC Rivotril ampoules (accessed 14/07/08)

# Clonidine hydrochloride

**150 micrograms/mL solution in 1-mL ampoules**
• Clonidine hydrochloride acts in the CNS to reduce peripheral resistance, renal vascular resistance, heart rate and BP; it also has effects on spinal alpha$_2$-adrenoceptors.
• It may be used IV in management of hypertensive crises but has largely been superseded by drugs with an improved side-effect profile.

- Clonidine has been given (unlicensed) by the epidural and intrathecal routes for the management of pain.
- It has also been given IV (unlicensed) for the management of severe agitation (often that associated with substance withdrawal) in the critical care setting.

## Pre-treatment checks

- Avoid in patients with severe bradyarrhythmia resulting from either sick sinus syndrome or AV block of second or third degree; unsafe in patients with porphyria.
- Use with caution in patients with cerebrovascular or coronary insufficiency, with a history of depression, Raynaud disease or other peripheral vascular occlusive disease, mild to moderate bradyarrhythmia.

*Biochemical and other tests*

Blood pressure
Pulse

## Dose

**Hypertensive emergency:** 150–300 micrograms by IV injection or infusion. Maximum 750 micrograms in 24 hours. Reduce dose gradually to avoid withdrawal ↑BP.

## Intravenous infusion

*Preparation and administration*

1. Withdraw the required dose and add to a suitable volume of NaCl 0.9% (e.g. 50–100 mL).
2. The solution should be clear and colourless. Inspect visually for particulate matter or discoloration prior to administration and discard if present.
3. Give by IV infusion over 10–15 minutes. Avoid faster administration as this may cause a transient ↑BP.

## Intravenous injection

*Preparation and administration*

1. Withdraw the required dose. May be diluted to 10 mL with NaCl 0.9% to facilitate slow administration.
2. The solution should be clear and colourless. Inspect visually for particulate matter or discoloration prior to administration and discard if present.
3. Give by slow IV injection over 10–15 minutes. Avoid faster administration as this may cause a transient ↑BP.

## Technical information

| Incompatible with | Midazolam |
|---|---|
| Compatible with | **Flush**: NaCl 0.9%<br>**Solutions**: NaCl 0.9% (including added KCl), Gluc 5%<br>**Y-site**: Adrenaline (epinephrine), aminophylline, dobutamine, dopamine, fentanyl, glyceryl trinitrate, magnesium sulfate, noradrenaline (norepinephrine) |
| pH | 4–4.5 |
| Sodium content | Negligible |

*(continued)*

## Technical information (*continued*)

| | |
|---|---|
| Storage | Store below 30°C in original packaging. |
| Stability after preparation | From a microbiological point of view, should be used immediately; however, prepared infusions may be stored at 2-8°C and infused (at room temperature) within 24 hours. |

## Monitoring

| Measure | Frequency | Rationale |
|---|---|---|
| Blood pressure | Every 30 minutes initially | • Response to IV therapy is maximal after 60 minutes.<br>• ↓BP is common after epidural use. |
| Heart rate | | • ↓Pulse may occur after IV and epidural use. |

## Additional information

| | |
|---|---|
| Common and serious undesirable effects | *Injection/infusion-related:* Too rapid administration: Transient ↑BP.<br>*Other:* Severe ↓BP, ↓pulse, dizziness, sedation, headache, nausea, vomiting, constipation, salivary gland pain, fatigue, Raynaud's phenomenon. Systemic effects also occur after epidural use and patients should be closely monitored, particularly during the first few days of therapy. |
| Pharmacokinetics | Duration of antihypertensive effect is 3-7 hours after IV injection. Elimination half-life is 10-20 hours and up to 41 hours in severe renal impairment. |
| Significant interactions | • The following may ↑clonidine effect (or ↑side-effects): beta-blockers including eye drops (risk of withdrawal ↑BP), methylphenidate (avoid combination).<br>• The following may ↓ clonidine levels or effect: antidepressants-tricyclic (also risk of withdrawal ↑BP). |
| Action is case of overdose | *Symptoms to watch for:* Severe ↓BP, ↓pulse.<br>*Antidote:* Stop administration and give supportive therapy as appropriate. Atropine may be required to counter ↓pulse, IV fluids and ephedrine may be used for ↓BP. |
| Counselling | Dizziness and constipation may be experienced. |

| | |
|---|---|
| Risk rating: **AMBER** | Score = 4<br>Moderate-risk product: Risk-reduction strategies are recommended. |

This assessment is based on the full range of preparation and administration options described in the monograph. These may not all be applicable in some clinical situations.

## Bibliography

SPC Catapres ampoules 150 micrograms in 1 mL solution for injection (accessed 29 September 2009).

# Co-amoxiclav (amoxicillin sodium-clavulanate)

**600-mg and 1.2-g dry powder vials**

- Co-amoxiclav is a mixture of the amino penicillin amoxicillin and the beta-lactamase inhibitor clavulanic acid, which synergistically enhances the spectrum of the amoxicillin.
- It should be reserved for bacterial infections likely to be caused by amoxicillin-resistant beta-lactamase-producing strains.
- Co-amoxiclav doses below are expressed as the combined total mass (mg) of the two constituents: Co-amoxiclav 1.2 g ≡ amoxicillin 1 g (as sodium salt) with clavulanate 200 mg (as potassium salt). Co-amoxiclav doses may also be expressed as individual mass (mg) of amoxicillin/clavulanate.

## Pre-treatment checks

- Do not give if there is known hypersensitivity to penicillins or previous history of penicillin associated jaundice/hepatic dysfunction.
- Maintain adequate hydration with high doses.

*Biochemical and other tests*

FBC
LFTs
Renal function: U, Cr, CrCl (or eGFR)

## Dose

**Standard dose**: 1.2 g by IV injection or infusion every 8 hours increased to 1.2 g every 6 hours in more serious infections.

**Surgical prophylaxis**: 1.2 g by IV injection at induction and for high-risk procedures (e.g. colorectal surgery); 2–3 further doses of 1.2 g may be given every 8 hours. Check local policies.

**Dose in renal impairment**: adjusted according to creatinine clearance:[1]

- CrCl >30–50 mL/minute: dose as in normal renal function.
- CrCl 10–30 mL/minute: 1.2 g every 12 hours.
- CrCl <10 mL/minute: 1.2 g every 12 hours or 1.2 g loading dose then 600 mg every 8 hours.

## Intravenous injection

*Preparation and administration*

Co-amoxiclav is incompatible with Gluc 5% (but may be injected into drip tubing over 3–4 minutes).

If used in combination with an aminoglycoside (e.g. amikacin, gentamicin, tobramycin), preferably administer at a different site. If this is not possible then flush the line thoroughly with a compatible solution between drugs.

1. Add 10 mL WFI to a 600-mg vial (use 20 mL for a 1.2-g vial) then shake vigorously.
2. Withdraw the required dose.
3. The solution should be clear. Inspect visually for particulate matter or discoloration prior to administration and discard if present.
4. Give by IV injection over 3–4 minutes.

## Intermittent intravenous infusion

*Preparation and administration*

Co-amoxiclav is incompatible with Gluc 5%
If used in combination with an aminoglycoside (e.g. amikacin, gentamicin, tobramycin), preferably administer at a different site. If this is not possible then flush the line thoroughly with a
compatible solution between drugs.

1. Add 10 mL WFI to a 600-mg vial (use 20 mL for a 1.2-g vial) and shake vigorously.
2. Withdraw the required dose and add 600 mg to 50 mL NaCl 0.9%; 1.2 g to 100 mL NaCl 0.9%.
3. The solution should be clear. Inspect visually for particulate matter or discoloration prior to
   administration and discard if present.
4. Give by IV infusion over 30–40 minutes.

## Technical information

| | |
|---|---|
| Incompatible with | Co-amoxiclav is incompatible with Gluc 5% (but may be injected into drip tubing over 3-4 minutes). <br> Sodium bicarbonate. <br> Amikacin, ciprofloxacin, gentamicin, midazolam, metronidazole, tobramycin. |
| Compatible with | **Flush**: NaCl 0.9% <br> **Solutions**: NaCl 0.9%, WFI <br> **Y-site**: Clarithromycin |
| pH | 8-10 |
| Electrolyte content | 3 mmol sodium and 1 mmol potassium/1.2-g vial |
| Storage | Store below 25°C in original packaging. |
| Displacement value | 0.5 mL/600-mg vial; 0.9 mL/1.2-g vial |
| Stability after preparation | Use reconstituted vials and prepared infusions immediately (within 20 minutes). |

## Monitoring

| Measure | Frequency | Rationale |
|---|---|---|
| LFTs | Periodically | • Cholestatic jaundice occurs rarely but may be severe and may not present for several weeks after treatment. It is more common in patients above the age of 65 years and in men. <br> • The risk of acute liver toxicity is about 6 times greater with co-amoxiclav than with amoxicillin <br> • Transient ↑AST and ↑ALT may occur. |
| CrCl | | • If renal function changes, a dose adjustment may be necessary. |
| Prothrombin time | | • Prolongation of bleeding time and defective platelet function may occur (monitor closely if anticoagulated). |
| FBC | | • Transient leucopenia, thrombocytopenia, haemolytic anaemia, neutropenia may occur. |

*(continued)*

## Monitoring (continued)

| Measure | Frequency | Rationale |
|---|---|---|
| Patency of bladder catheters | Regularly in affected patients | • May precipitate in catheters at high doses. |
| Signs of supra-infection or superinfection | Throughout treatment | • May result in the overgrowth of non-susceptible organisms – appropriate therapy should be commenced; treatment may need to be interrupted. |
| Development of diarrhoea | Throughout and up to 2 months after treatment | • Development of severe, persistent diarrhoea may be suggestive of *Clostridium difficile*-associated diarrhoea and colitis (pseudomembranous colitis). Discontinue drug and treat. Do not use drugs that inhibit peristalsis. |

## Additional information

| | |
|---|---|
| Common and serious undesirable effects | *Immediate:* Anaphylaxis and other hypersensitivity reactions have been reported.<br>*Other:* Diarrhoea, nausea, urticaria, maculopapular rashes (often appearing > 7 days after commencing treatment), fever, joint pains and angioedema. |
| Pharmacokinetics | Elimination half-life is about 1 hour for both constituents (amoxicillin 10-15 hours; clavulanic acid 3-4 hours in anuria). |
| Significant interactions | No significant interactions. |
| Action in case of overdose | *Symptoms to watch for:* Large doses have been associated with seizures.<br>*Antidote:* None but haemodialysis may be effective.<br>Stop administration and give supportive therapy as appropriate. |
| Counselling | During administration of high doses of amoxicillin maintain adequate fluid intake and urinary output to reduce the possibility of amoxicillin crystalluria. Women taking the combined contraceptive pill should be should be advised to take additional precautions during and for 7 days after the course. |

Risk rating: **GREEN**　　Score = 2
Lower-risk product: Risk-reduction strategies should be considered.

This assessment is based on the full range of preparation and administration options described in the monograph. These may not all be applicable in some clinical situations.

## Reference

1. Ashley C, Currie A, eds. *The Renal Drug Handbook*, 3rd edn. Oxford: Radcliffe Medical Press, 2009.

## Bibliography

SPC Co-amoxiclav for injection 500/100 mg and 1000/200 mg, Wockhardt UK Ltd (accessed 9 March 2009).
SPC Augmentin intravenous (accessed 9 March 2009).

# Codeine phosphate

**60 mg/mL solution in 1-mL ampoules**

- Codeine phosphate is an opioid analgesic.
- It is used IM for the treatment of mild to moderate pain. It is much less potent than morphine: 60 mg codeine phosphate IM has the analgesic effect of 5 mg morphine sulfate IM in most individuals.
- Some patients may be ultra-rapid metabolisers of codeine due to a CYP2D6 polymorphism. Rapid conversion of codeine to morphine results in higher serum morphine levels and may result in toxicity at moderate dosing levels. Conversely, poor metabolisers may not obtain adequate analgesia.
- Codeine produces less euphoria and sedation than morphine but is still subject to misuse.

## Pre-treatment checks

- Do not use in acute respiratory depression, where there is a risk of paralytic ileus, in raised intracranial pressure and in head injury, in comatose patients and in phaeochromocytoma.
- Caution in ↓BP, shock, convulsive disorders, supraventricular tachycardias, atrial flutter, chronic obstructive pulmonary disease and acute asthma attack, obstructive or inflammatory bowel diseases, biliary tract diseases, alcoholism, prostatic hyperplasia, myasthenia gravis, hypothyroidism (reduce dose), adrenocortical insufficiency (reduce dose).
- Caution in elderly patients – use lower doses; initial dose should not exceed 25 mg.
- As codeine reduces peristalsis, increases tone in the bowel and can ↑colonic pressure; it should not be used in diverticulitis, after bowel surgery or in those with acute colitis.
- Ensure that resuscitation equipment and naloxone are available.

*Biochemical and other tests*

| | |
|---|---|
| Blood pressure and pulse | Renal function: U, Cr, CrCl (or eGFR) |
| LFTs | Respiratory rate |
| Pain score | |

## Dose

Codeine phosphate should not be given IV: anaphylaxis may occur.

**Standard adult dose:** 30–60 mg by IM injection every 4 hours when required.
**Elderly patients:** reduced doses are recommended.
**Dose in renal impairment:** reduce doses or avoid.
**Dose in hepatic impairment:** avoid or reduce dose.

## Intramuscular injection

*Preparation and administration*

1. Withdraw the required dose.
2. Give by deep IM injection.

## Technical information

| | |
|---|---|
| Incompatible with | Not relevant |
| Compatible with | Not relevant |
| pH | 3–6 |
| Sodium content | Negligible |
| Storage | Store below 25°C in original packaging. Do not refrigerate or freeze. The solution may darken on storage – do not use if it is darker than pale straw. Controlled Drug. |

## Monitoring

| Measure | Frequency | Rationale |
|---|---|---|
| Pain score | At regular intervals | • To ensure therapeutic response. |
| Blood pressure, heart rate and respiratory rate | | • ↓BP, ↓pulse, ↑pulse, palpitations and respiratory depression with decreased oxygen saturation can occur. |
| Sedation | | • Can cause sedation and CNS depression. |
| Monitor for side-effects and toxicity | | • Can cause side-effects such as constipation, which may need treatment. |
| Monitor breast-fed babies | Frequently | • Ultra-rapid metabolisers can have higher levels of the active metabolite morphine in breast milk resulting in ↑adverse effects in the baby and potential toxicity. |

## Additional information

| | |
|---|---|
| Common and serious undesirable effects | *Immediate:* Anaphylaxis can occur after IV use.<br>*Common:* Nausea and vomiting (particularly initially), constipation, dry mouth, urticaria, pruritus, biliary spasm, ↑ or ↓pulse, hallucinations, euphoria, drowsiness.<br>*At higher doses:* ↓BP, sedation, respiratory depression, muscle rigidity. |
| Pharmacokinetics | After IM injection, peak plasma concentrations occur in about 30 minutes and the elimination half-life is approximately 3 hours. |
| Significant interactions | • The following may ↑codeine levels or effect (or ↑side-effects): antihistamines-sedating (↑sedation), MAOIs (avoid combination and for 2 weeks after stopping MAOI), moclobemide.<br>• Codeine may ↑levels or effect (or ↑side-effects) of sodium oxybate (avoid combination). |
| Action in case of overdose | *Symptoms to watch for:* ↑Sedation, respiratory depression.<br>*Antidote:* Naloxone (see the Naloxone monograph).<br>Stop administration and give supportive therapy as appropriate. |

*(continued)*

**Additional information** (continued)

| Counselling | May cause drowsiness that may affect the ability to perform skilled tasks; if affected do not drive or operate machinery, avoid alcoholic drink (effects of alcohol enhanced).<br>Drink plenty of fluids to help avoid constipation. |

| Risk rating: **GREEN** | Score =2<br>Lower-risk product: Risk-reduction strategies should be considered. |

This assessment is based on the full range of preparation and administration options described in the monograph. These may not all be applicable in some clinical situations.

## Bibliography

SPC Codeine Phosphate BP injection 60 mg in 1 mL, Martindale Pharma (received 17 April 2009).

# Co-fluampicil (flucloxacillin with ampicillin)

**500-mg dry powder vials**

- Co-fluampicil is a compound preparation of two penicillins (ampicillin and flucloxacillin) both present as their sodium salts.
- In practice it is used for the treatment of mixed infections, particularly where beta-lactamase-producing staphylococci are involved or suspected.
- Co-fluampicil doses are expressed below as the combined total mass of the two constituents:
  Co-fluampicil 500 mg ≡ flucloxacillin 250 mg (as sodium salt) with ampicillin 250 mg (as sodium salt).

## Pre-treatment checks

- Do not give if there is known hypersensitivity to penicillins or beta-lactam antibiotics and to patients with a history of flucloxacillin-associated jaundice/hepatic dysfunction.
- Caution in erythematous rashes common in glandular fever, cytomegalovirus infection, and acute or chronic lymphocytic leukaemia.

*Biochemical and other tests*

Electrolytes: serum Na                      LFTs
FBC                                         Renal function: U, Cr, CrCl (or eGFR)

## Dose

**Standard dose**: 500 mg every 6 hours (may be doubled in severe infections).

**Dose in renal impairment:** There is no guidance on dose reduction in renal impairment, so this product may be unsuitable in these circumstances.

## Intravenous injection

*Preparation and administration*

> See Special handling below.
> If used in combination with an aminoglycoside (e.g. amikacin, gentamicin, tobramycin), prefer-ably administer at a different site. If this is not possible then flush the line thoroughly with a compatible solution between drugs.

1. Add 10 mL WFI to each vial and shake vigorously.
2. Withdraw the required dose.
3. The solution should be clear and colourless. Inspect visually for particulate matter or discolor-ation prior to administration and discard if present.
4. Give by IV injection over 3–4 minutes.

## Intermittent intravenous infusion

*Preparation and administration*

> See Special handling below.
> If used in combination with an aminoglycoside (e.g. amikacin, gentamicin, tobramycin), prefer-ably administer at a different site. If this is not possible then flush the line thoroughly with a compatible solution between drugs.

1. Add 10 mL WFI to each vial and shake vigorously.
2. Withdraw the required dose and add to a suitable volume of compatible infusion fluid (usually 100 mL NaCl 0.9%).
3. The solution should be clear and colourless. Inspect visually for particulate matter or discolor-ation prior to administration and discard if present.
4. Give by IV infusion over 30–60 minutes.

## Intramuscular injection

*Preparation and administration*

> See Special handling below.

1. Add 1.5 mL WFI to each vial and shake vigorously.
2. Withdraw the required dose.
3. Give by deep IM injection. Rotate injection sites for subsequent injections.

## Technical information

| | |
|---|---|
| Incompatible with | Co-fluampicil is incompatible with Hartmann's.<br>Sodium bicarbonate.<br>Adrenaline (epinephrine), amikacin, amiodarone, amphotericin, benzylpenicillin, calcium gluconate, ciprofloxacin, cisatracurium, clarithromycin, diazepam, dobutamine, dopamine, erythromycin lactobionate, fluconazole, gentamicin, hydralazine, hydrocortisone sodium succinate, metoclopramide, midazolam, ofloxacin, ondansetron, tobramycin, verapamil. |
| Compatible with | **Flush**: NaCl 0.9%<br>**Solutions**: NaCl 0.9%, Gluc 5%, Gluc-NaCl<br>**Y-site**: No information |
| pH | 8.0-10.0 |

*(continued)*

## Technical information (continued)

| | |
|---|---|
| Sodium content | 1.3 mmol/500 mg |
| Storage | Store below 25°C in original packaging. |
| Displacement value | 0.4 mL/500 mg |
| Special handling | Avoid skin contact as may cause sensitisation. |
| Stability after preparation | Reconstituted vials and infusions prepared in Gluc 5% or Gluc-NaCl should be used immediately.<br>From a microbiological point of view, infusions prepared in NaCl 0.9% should be used immediately; however, they may be stored at 2–8°C and infused (at room temperature) within 24 hours. |

## Monitoring

| Measure | Frequency | Rationale |
|---|---|---|
| Renal function | Periodically, especially if treatment prolonged | • There is no guidance on dose reduction in renal impairment, so this product may be unsuitable in these circumstances.<br>• Electrolyte disturbances may occur (high Na content). |
| FBC | | • Transient leucopenia, thrombocytopenia, haemolytic anaemia, neutropenia may occur. |
| Prothrombin time | | • Prolongation of bleeding time and defective platelet function may occur (monitor closely if anticoagulated). |
| LFTs | | • Moderate ↑AST and ↑ALT have been reported (rarely).<br>• Flucloxacillin-induced hepatitis and cholestatic jaundice can occur up to 2 months post treatment. Effects can last several months and are not related to either dose or route of administration. Older patients and those receiving more than two weeks treatment are at higher risk. |
| Signs of supra-infection or superinfection | Throughout treatment | • May result in the overgrowth of non-susceptible organisms - appropriate therapy should be commenced; treatment may need to be interrupted. |
| Development of rash | | • A maculopapular rash sometimes occurs (often appearing more than 7 days after commencing treatment) which may or may not be related to a hypersensitivity reaction. In practice clinicians most often discontinue if this occurs.<br>• It should preferably not be given to patients with infectious mononucleosis since they are especially susceptible to ampicillin-induced skin rashes. |

(continued)

## Monitoring (continued)

| Measure | Frequency | Rationale |
|---------|-----------|-----------|
| Development of diarrhoea | Throughout and up to 2 months after treatment | • Development of severe, persistent diarrhoea may be suggestive of *Clostridium difficile*-associated diarrhoea and colitis (pseudomembranous colitis). Discontinue drug and treat. Do not use drugs that inhibit peristalsis. |

## Additional information

| | |
|---|---|
| Common and serious undesirable effects | *Immediate:* Anaphylaxis and other hypersensitivity reactions have been reported. *Injection/infusion-related:* Local: Phlebitis following IV infusion. *Other:* Diarrhoea, urticaria, fever, joint pains, rashes, maculopapular rashes (often appearing >7 days after commencing treatment), angioedema, anaphylaxis, serum sickness-like reaction, nausea, vomiting and diarrhoea (pseudomembranous reported rarely). Patients treated for syphilis or neurosyphilis may develop a Jarisch-Herxheimer reaction (occurs 2-12 hours after initiation of therapy - headache, fever, chills, sweating, sore throat, myalgia, arthralgia, malaise, ↑pulse and ↑BP followed by a ↓BP. Usually subsides within 12-24 hours. Corticosteroids may ↓incidence and severity). |
| Pharmacokinetics | Elimination half-life is about 1 hour. |
| Significant interactions | No significant interactions. |
| Action in case of overdose | *Symptoms to watch for:* Large doses have been associated with seizures. *Antidote:* None; ampicillin (but not flucloxacillin) may be removed by haemodialysis. Stop administration and give supportive therapy as appropriate. |
| Counselling | Women taking the combined contraceptive pill should be advised to take additional precautions during and for 7 days after the course. |

| Risk rating: **GREEN** | Score = 2 Lower-risk product: Risk-reduction strategies should be considered. |
|---|---|

This assessment is based on the full range of preparation and administration options described in the monograph. These may not all be applicable in some clinical situations.

## Bibliography

SPC Magnapen vials for injection (accessed 10 March 2009).

# Colistimethate sodium (colistin sulfomethate sodium)

**500 000-unit, 1 million- and 2 million-unit dry powder vials**
* Colistimethate sodium is the anionic form of colistin, a polymyxin antibacterial.
* Because of its toxicity it is used in the treatment of severe Gram-negative infections where there is resistance to other antibacterials.
* It may also used by inhalation in the management of respiratory infections, particularly in patients with cystic fibrosis.
* Doses are expressed in international units (IU) in the UK but as milligrams of colistin in the USA:
  Colistimethate sodium 1 mg ≡ 12 500 units.
  Colistin base 1 mg ≡ 30 000 units.

## Pre-treatment checks

* Do not give if there is known hypersensitivity to colistimethate sodium or to polymyxin B and in patients with myasthenia gravis.
* Caution in acute porphyria.

*Biochemical and other tests*

Renal function: U, Cr, CrCl (or eGFR)

## Dose

Dosing schedules in the USA differ and the IM route may also be used.

**Bodyweight under 60 kg**: give every 8 hours by IV infusion to provide a total daily dose of 50 000–75 000 units/kg.
**Bodyweight over 60 kg:** 1–2 million units every 8 hours by IV infusion up to a maximum of 6 million units in 24 hours.
**Dose in renal impairment**: dose is adjusted according to CrCl and then further adjusted according to blood levels and evidence of toxicity. Doses here are for bodyweight >60 kg.
* CrCl >20–50 mL/minute: dose as in normal renal function.
* CrCl 10–20 mL/minute: 1 million units every 12–18 hours.
* CrCl <10 mL/minute: 1 million units every 18–24 hours.

**Nebulisation:** 1–2 million units twice daily.

## Intermittent intravenous infusion (preferred route)

*Preparation and administration*

1. Reconstitute each vial with 10 mL WFI or NaCl 0.9%. The vial should be gently swirled to avoid frothing.
2. Withdraw the required dose and add to a suitable volume of compatible infusion fluid (usually 100 mL NaCl 0.9%).
3. The solution should be clear and colourless. Inspect visually for particulate matter or discoloration prior to administration and discard if present.
4. Give by IV infusion over 30 minutes.

## Intravenous injection (in patients with a totally implantable venous access device [TIVAD] only)

*Preparation and administration*

1. Reconstitute each vial with 10 mL WFI or NaCl 0.9%. The vial should be gently swirled to avoid frothing.
2. The solution should be clear and colourless. Inspect visually for particulate matter or discoloration prior to administration and discard if present.
3. Withdraw the required dose and give by IV injection over a minimum of 5 minutes.

## Nebulisation

*Preparation and administration*

Nebulisation should take place in a well-ventilated room; the output from the nebuliser should be vented to the open air or a filter may be fitted.

1. Dissolve the powder for the required dose in 2–4 mL NaCl 0.9% or WFI.
2. The solution will be slightly hazy and may froth if shaken.
3. Give by nebuliser: a jet or ultrasonic nebuliser is preferred.

## Technical information

| | |
|---|---|
| Incompatible with | Erythromycin lactobionate, hydrocortisone sodium succinate. |
| Compatible with | **Flush**: NaCl 0.9%<br>**Solutions**: NaCl 0.9%, Gluc 5%, Gluc-NaCl, Hartmann's<br>**Y-site**: Amikacin, benzylpenicillin, chloramphenicol sodium succinate, ranitidine |
| pH | 6.5-8.5 |
| Sodium content | Negligible |
| Storage | Store below 25°C in original packaging.<br>Vials are single use only - discard unused portion. |
| Displacement value | Negligible |
| Special handling | See notes above under administration by nebulisation. |
| Stability after reconstitution | NB: Drug concentration increases with storage time above 24 hours and has resulted in severe toxicity.<br>From a microbiological point of view, should be used immediately; however:<br>• Reconstituted vials may be stored at 2-8°C for 24 hours.<br>• Prepared infusions may be stored at 2-8°C and infused (at room temperature) within 24 hours.<br>Nebulisation solutions should be used immediately. |

## Monitoring

| Measure | Frequency | Rationale |
|---------|-----------|-----------|
| Serum colistimethate concentration | When clinically indicated - see Rationale | • Serum level estimations are recommended especially in renal impairment, in neonates and in cystic fibrosis patients.<br>• Peak plasma concentration should be taken about 30 minutes after IV injection or infusion.<br>• The therapeutic range is 10-15 mg/L (125-200 units/mL). |
| Renal function | Periodically | • Dose adjustment may be needed if renal function changes.<br>• ↑Incidence of adverse effects if a higher than intended dose is given compounding the potential nephrotoxic effects of the drug. These usually resolve on discontinuation. |
| Signs of neurotoxicity | Throughout treatment | • Reducing the dose may alleviate these symptoms. |
| Hypersensitivity or skin rash | | • Withdraw treatment if these occur. |
| Signs of supra-infection or superinfection | | • May result in the overgrowth of non-susceptible organisms - appropriate therapy should be commenced; treatment may need to be interrupted. |
| Development of diarrhoea | Throughout and up to 2 months after treatment | • Development of severe, persistent diarrhoea may be suggestive of *Clostridium difficile*-associated diarrhoea and colitis (pseudomembranous colitis). Discontinue drug and treat. Do not use drugs that inhibit peristalsis. |
| Bronchospasm | Throughout nebulisation | • May be prevented or treated with beta$_2$-agonists, but may require withdrawal of treatment if bothersome. |

## Additional information

| | |
|---|---|
| Common and serious undesirable effects | *Immediate:* Hypersensitivity reactions have been reported, including rash<br>*Injection/infusion-related:* Local: Injection-site reactions.<br>*Other:* Neurotoxicity (especially at high doses), nephrotoxicity. Inhalation may cause sore throat, sore mouth, cough, bronchospasm. |
| Pharmacokinetics | Elimination half-life is 2-3 hours (2 hours in cystic fibrosis). |
| Significant interactions | • Colistimethate may ↑levels or effect of the following drugs (or ↑side-effects): ciclosporin (↑risk of nephrotoxicity), diuretics-loop (↑risk of ototoxicity), muscle relaxants-non depolarising, platinum compounds (↑risk of nephrotoxicity and ototoxicity), suxamethonium.<br>• Colistimethate may ↓levels or effect of the following drugs: neostigmine, pyridostigmine. |
| Action in case of overdose | No specific antidote; manage by supportive treatment. Overdose can result in neuromuscular blockade leading to muscular weakness, apnoea, possible respiratory arrest; also acute renal failure. |
| Counselling | Patients using nebulised solutions at home should be advised to administer them immediately after reconstitution. |

| Risk rating: **GREEN** | Score = 2 Lower-risk product: Risk-reduction strategies should be considered. |
| --- | --- |

This assessment is based on the full range of preparation and administration options described in the monograph. These may not all be applicable in some clinical situations.

## Bibliography

SPC Colomycin injection (accessed 10 March 2009).
SPC Promixin 1 MIU powder for solution for injection (accessed 10 March 2009).
SPC Promixin 1 MIU powder for nebuliser solution (accessed 10 March 2009).

# Co-trimoxazole (trimethoprim-sulfamethoxazole)

**96 mg/mL solution in 5-mL ampoules**

* Co-trimoxazole contains a 5 : 1 ratio of sulfamethoxazole to trimethoprim (i.e. 80 mg : 16 mg/mL), each of which act synergistically at different points of the folate metabolic pathway.
* Its main use IV is in the management of *Pneumocystis* pneumonia, toxoplasmosis and nocardiasis.
* Because of the risk of serious side-effects, co-trimoxazole should only be considered for other infections where there is good bacteriological evidence of sensitivity to co-trimoxazole and good reason to prefer this combination to a single antibacterial.
* Doses in this monograph are expressed in terms of the total combined mass (mg) of the two constituents. (Doses in the USA are usually expressed in terms of the trimethoprim component.)

## Pre-treatment checks

* Do not give if there is known hypersensitivity to sulfonamides, trimethoprim, co-trimoxazole or any of the excipients and in acute porphyria.
* Use with caution in asthma and G6PD-deficiency.

*Biochemical and other tests*

Electrolytes: serum K, Na
FBC including folate

LFTs
Renal function: U, Cr, CrCl (or eGFR)

## Dose

**Standard dose**: 960 mg (10 mL) by IV infusion every 12 hours.
**Severe infections**: 1.44 g (15 mL) by IV infusion every 12 hours.
**Treatment of *Pneumocystis jiroveci (P. carinii)* infections**: give every 6–12 hours by IV infusion to provide a total daily dose of 120 mg/kg. Switch to oral dosing (at the same dose) as soon as possible. Treat for 14–21 days.

**Dose in renal impairment**: adjusted according to creatinine clearance:

* CrCl >30–50 mL/minute: dose as in normal renal function.
* CrCl 15–30 mL/minute: 480 mg every 12 hours.
* CrCl <15 mL/minute: not recommended unless haemodialysis facilities are available.

## Intermittent intravenous infusion

*Preparation and administration*

1. Withdraw the required dose and add to a suitable volume of compatible infusion fluid (NaCl 0.9% or Gluc 5%). Manufacturer recommends that 5 mL be added to 125 mL; 10 mL to 250 mL; 15 mL to 500 mL.*
2. Shake thoroughly then visually inspect for turbidity or crystallisation and discard if present.
3. Give by IV infusion over 90 minutes. If turbidity or crystallisation develops during the infusion the mixture should be discarded.

*An alternative source reports doses <40 mL being added to 500 mL Gluc 5% and doses >40 mL being added to 1 L NaCl 0.9%. The resultant mixture is given by IV infusion over 90–120 minutes and observed closely for signs of turbidity.[1]

**Fluid restriction**: add each 5-mL ampoule to 75 mL Gluc 5% and give by IV infusion over no more than 60 minutes.

## Technical information

| Incompatible with | Cisatracurium, fluconazole, foscarnet, linezolid, midazolam, pantoprazole, verapamil. |
|---|---|
| Compatible with | **Flush**: NaCl 0.9%<br>**Solutions**: Gluc 5%, Gluc-NaCl, NaCl 0.9%<br>**Y-site**: Aciclovir, atracurium, aztreonam, esmolol, granisetron, labetalol, magnesium sulfate, piperacillin with tazobactam, remifentanil, vecuronium |
| pH | 10 |
| Sodium content | 1.7 mmol/5 mL |
| Excipients | Contains ethanol (may interact with metronidazole, possible religious objections).<br>Contains propylene glycol (adverse effects seen if renal elimination is impaired and may interact with disulfiram and metronidazole).<br>Contains sulfites (may cause hypersensitivity reactions). |
| Storage | Store below 30°C in original packaging. |
| Stability after preparation | Use prepared infusions immediately. Do not refrigerate. Crystallisation or turbidity may develop at any time; inspect during infusion and discard if present. |

## Monitoring

| Measure | Frequency | Rationale |
|---|---|---|
| Plasma concentration of sulfamethoxazole | At intervals of 2-3 days in renal impairment | • In samples taken 12 hours after administration, if the sulfamethoxazole concentration exceeds 150 micrograms/mL then interrupt treatment until the value falls below 120 micrograms/mL. |

*(continued)*

## Monitoring (continued)

| Measure | Frequency | Rationale |
|---------|-----------|-----------|
| Plasma concentration of trimethoprim | In treatment of *P. jiroveci* pneumonia to confirm therapeutic dose | • The aim is to obtain a peak plasma or serum trimethoprim concentration $\geq 5$ micrograms/mL. |
| FBC | Monthly if long term | • Should not be given to patients with serious haematological disorders.<br>• Folate deficiency may develop (treat with folinic acid 5-10 mg daily until normal haematopoiesis is restored). |
| LFTs | Periodically | • Contraindicated in patients showing marked liver parenchymal damage (very rarely causes potentially fatal cholestatic jaundice and hepatic necrosis).<br>• Very rarely causes ↑ALT, AST, bilirubin. |
| Renal function and serum Na and K | Periodically, but more frequently if known renal impairment | • Contraindicated in severe renal insufficiency where repeated measurements of the plasma concentration cannot be performed.<br>• Adequate urinary output should be maintained at all times.<br>• Monitor closely patients at risk of ↑K or ↓Na. |
| Development of a rash | Throughout treatment | • Discontinue at the first sign of a rash.<br>• Although very rare, fatalities have occurred due to, e.g. Stevens-Johnson syndrome, toxic epidermal necrolysis, photosensitivity. |

## Additional information

| | |
|---|---|
| Common and serious undesirable effects | *Infusion-related:* Local: Pain, local irritation, inflammation, and rarely thrombophlebitis may occur with IV use especially if extravasation occurs.<br>*Other:* Candidal overgrowth, headache, nausea, vomiting, diarrhoea, rash (see Monitoring above) |
| Pharmacokinetics | Elimination half-life of trimethoprim is 6-17 hours; that of sulfamethoxazole is 8-11 hours. |
| Significant Interactions | • Co-trimoxazole may ↑levels or side-effects of the following drugs: amiodarone (↑risk of ventricular arrhythmias – avoid combination), azathioprine (↑haematological toxicity), ciclosporin (↑risk of nephrotoxicity), clozapine (↑risk of agranulocytosis), coumarin anticoagulants (monitor INR), mercaptopurine (↑haematological toxicity), methenamine (↑risk of crystalluria), methotrexate (↑haematological toxicity), phenytoin (monitor levels, ↑antifolate effect), pyrimethamine (↑antifolate effect).<br>• Co-trimoxazole may ↓levels or effect of ciclosporin.<br>• Injectable preparation contains ethanol and propylene glycol; may interact with disulfiram and metronidazole. |
| Action in case of overdose | *Symptoms to watch for:* Nausea, vomiting, dizziness and confusion.<br>*Antidote:* No known antidote but haemodialysis may be effective.<br>Stop administration and give supportive therapy as appropriate. |
| Counselling | The development of rash, sore throat, fever, pallor, arthralgia, cough, shortness of breath, purpura, or jaundice may be an early sign of a serious adverse reaction. |

| Risk rating: **AMBER** | Score = 3 Moderate-risk product: Risk-reduction strategies are recommended. |
|---|---|

This assessment is based on the full range of preparation and administration options described in the monograph. These may not all be applicable in some clinical situations.

### Reference

1. Pharmacy Department UCLH. *Injectable Medicines Administration Guide*, 2nd edn. London: Blackwell, 2007.

### Bibliography

SPC Septrin for infusion (accessed 10 March 2009).

# Cyanocobalamin (vitamin B$_{12}$)

**1 mg/mL solution in ampoules**

- Vitamin B$_{12}$, a water-soluble vitamin, occurs in the body in various forms including cyanocobalamin. Deficiency may occur in strict vegetarians, in patients with malabsorption syndromes or metabolic disorders, or in patients following gastrectomy or extensive ileal resection. Deficiency results in megaloblastic anaemias, demyelination and other neurological damage.
- Cyanocobalamin is no longer the vitamin B$_{12}$ form of choice for therapy as hydroxocobalamin is retained in the body for longer and maintenance therapy therefore involves less frequent administration.
- Vitamin B$_{12}$ preparations are used to treat pernicious anaemia, for prophylaxis and treatment of other macrocytic anaemias associated with vitamin B$_{12}$ deficiency. Only hydroxocobalamin is used to treat tobacco amblyopia and Leber's optic atrophy (use of cyanocobalamin may allow these optic atrophies to degenerate further).
- Hydroxocobalamin or cyanocobalamin may be used diagnostically as part of the Schilling test to assess absorption of vitamin B$_{12}$ if absence of intrinsic factor is suspected.

### Pre-treatment checks

- Do not use for the treatment of megaloblastic anaemia of pregnancy unless a definite diagnosis of vitamin B$_{12}$ deficiency has been established.
- Contraindicated in Leber disease and tobacco amblyopia.

*Biochemical and other tests*

Electrolytes: serum K (cardiac arrhythmias secondary to ↓K during initial therapy have been reported – correct if necessary).
FBC.
Folate (to ensure that folate deficiency is not a contributory/causative factor).
A baseline assessment of neurological function is useful to assess impact of treatment in cases of vitamin B$_{12}$ deficiency anaemia with neurological complications.

## Dose

The IV route is not recommended as most of the dose is lost in the urine.

**Pernicious anaemia and other macrocytic anaemias without neurological involvement:** initially 250–1000 micrograms by IM injection on alternate days for 1–2 weeks then 250 micrograms once weekly until the blood count has normalised, then 1 mg monthly.

**Pernicious anaemia and other macrocytic anaemias with neurological involvement:** initially 1 mg by IM injection on alternate days as long as improvement is occurring then 1 mg monthly.

**Prophylaxis of macrocytic anaemias associated with vitamin B$_{12}$ deficiency:** 250 micrograms–1 mg monthly.

**Schilling test:** involves use of IM vitamin B$_{12}$ as part of the test.

### Intramuscular injection

*Preparation and administration*

1. Withdraw the required dose.
2. Give by IM injection.

## Technical information

| Incompatible with | Not relevant |
|---|---|
| Compatible with | Not relevant |
| pH | 4.5-7 |
| Sodium content | Negligible |
| Storage | Store below 25°C in original packaging. |

## Monitoring

| Measure | Frequency | Rationale |
|---|---|---|
| Serum K | Daily for first 48 hours, then consider 2-3 times weekly during acute phase | • If ↓K occurs, correct potassium levels, consider withdrawing cyanocobalamin and monitor cardiac function. |
| Neurological function | Ongoing through treatment | • Vitamin B$_{12}$ deficiency anaemias with neurological complications require dosing to continue until no further neurological improvement is seen. Inadequate treatment may manifest as a decline in neurological function. |

*(continued)*

## Monitoring (continued)

| Measure | Frequency | Rationale |
|---------|-----------|-----------|
| Mean cell volume (MCV) | Once weekly during acute phase of treatment | • Vitamin $B_{12}$ anaemia is characterised by macrocytosis, therefore response to treatment can be judged by cell size reducing to normal range. |
| Haemoglobin | | • Monitor level of Hb to assess response to treatment. |
| Reticulocyte and erythrocyte count | | • Generation of new reticulocytes and erythrocytes supports a diagnosis and treatment of vitamin $B_{12}$ deficiency anaemia. |
| WCC and platelets | Once weekly during acute phase of treatment if baseline abnormal | • Production may be affected in megaloblastic anaemia. |
| Physical assessment of patient | Ongoing | • Assess patient symptoms to assess relief of typical anaemic presentation, in addition to more specific symptoms of vitamin $B_{12}$ deficiency (glossitis, angular stomatitis, diarrhoea, altered bowel habit, mild jaundice, and neuropathy). |

## Additional information

| | |
|---|---|
| Common and serious undesirable effects | Hypersensitivity reactions (rash, pruritus, rarely anaphylaxis); pyrexia; chills; hot flushes; dizziness; malaise; nausea; diarrhoea; acneiform and bullous eruptions. |
| Pharmacokinetics | Most of SC or IM dose is excreted within 8 hours of administration. Tissue stores of vitamin $B_{12}$ may take years to dissipate, with a wide amount of inter-subject variability. |
| Significant interactions | Vitamin $B_{12}$ assay: anti-metabolites and most antibiotics invalidate vitamin $B_{12}$ assays by microbiological techniques. |
| Action in case of overdose | Treatment unlikely to be needed in case of overdose. |

| Risk rating: **GREEN** | Score = 0 <br> Lower-risk product: Risk-reduction strategies should be considered. |
|---|---|

This assessment is based on the full range of preparation and administration options described in the monograph. These may not all be applicable in some clinical situations.

## Bibliography

SPC Cytamen, UCB Pharma Ltd (accessed 4 April 2010).

# Cyclizine

### 50 mg/mL solution in 1-mL ampoules

- Cyclizine lactate is an antihistamine with antimuscarinic activity and mild sedative effects.
- It is used as an antiemetic in the management of nausea and vomiting including postoperatively and after radiotherapy (especially for breast cancer since cyclizine does not ↑prolactin levels). It may also be used to treat vomiting and attacks of vertigo associated with Ménière's disease and other vestibular disturbances.
- At lower doses cyclizine increases the lower oesophageal sphincter tone, thereby reducing the risk of regurgitation and aspiration.
- Cyclizine lactate may also be given (unlicensed) by SC infusion in palliative care to treat nausea and vomiting.
- Doses of parenteral cyclizine lactate are similar to cyclizine hydrochloride doses given orally.

## Pre-treatment checks

- Caution in patients with glaucoma, obstructive disease of the GI tract, hepatic disease, severe heart failure, epilepsy and males who may have prostatic hypertrophy.
- Avoid in patients with porphyria.

*Biochemical and other tests (not all are necessary in an emergency situation)*

Blood pressure
LFTs

## Dose

**Prevention and treatment of nausea and vomiting**: 50 mg up to three times a day by IM or IV injection.

**Preoperatively in patients undergoing emergency surgery**: 25 mg by IV injection to reduce risk of aspiration of gastric contents during induction of general anaesthesia.

**Prevention of postoperative nausea and vomiting (PONV)**: administer first dose of cyclizine by slow IV injection 20 minutes before the anticipated end of surgery.

## Intramuscular injection

*Preparation and administration*

1. Withdraw the required dose.
2. Give by IM injection.

## Intravenous injection

*Preparation and administration*

1. Withdraw the required dose. It may be diluted with an equal volume of WFI to facilitate slow administration.
2. The solution should be clear and colourless. Inspect visually for particulate matter or discoloration prior to administration and discard if present.
3. Give by IV injection over 3–5 minutes.

## Technical information

| | |
|---|---|
| Incompatible with | Benzylpenicillin |
| Compatible with | **Flush**: WFI or NaCl 0.9%<br>**Solutions**: WFI, Gluc 5% (via Y-site), less stable in NaCl 0.9%<br>**Y-site**: Stability is dependent upon concentrations |
| pH | 3.3-3.7 |
| Sodium content | Nil |
| Storage | Store below 25°C in original packaging. |

## Monitoring

| Measure | Frequency | Rationale |
|---|---|---|
| Improvement in nausea and vomiting or dizziness | Periodically | • For signs of clinical improvement. |
| Blood pressure | 4-hourly until within normal range | • May cause ↓BP. |

## Additional information

| | |
|---|---|
| Common and serious undesirable effects | *Immediate:* Anaphylaxis and other hypersensitivity reactions have been reported.<br>*Injection/infusion-related:*<br>• Too rapid administration: Transient paralysis has been reported.<br>• Local: Injection-site reactions including vein tracking, erythema, pain, thrombophlebitis and blisters.<br>*Other:* Drowsiness, urticaria, rash, headache, dryness of the mouth, nose and throat, blurred vision, ↑pulse, urinary retention, constipation, restlessness, nervousness, insomnia and auditory and visual hallucinations. |
| Pharmacokinetics | Elimination half-life is 20 hours. |
| Significant interactions | • Cyclizine may ↑sedative effect of opioid analgesics and other sedating medicines. |
| Action in case of overdose | Stop administration and give supportive therapy as appropriate. |
| Counselling | Cyclizine has abuse potential - euphoric and hallucinatory effects. This can be particularly dangerous if it is taken with large amounts of alcohol. |

| Risk rating: **GREEN** | Score = 1<br>Lower-risk product: Risk-reduction strategies should be considered. |

This assessment is based on the full range of preparation and administration options described in the monograph. These may not all be applicable in some clinical situations.

## Bibliography

SPC Valoid (accessed 7 July 2008).

# Dalteparin sodium

**10 000 units/mL solution in 1-mL ampoules and 1-mL graduated pre-filled syringes**
**12 500 units/mL solution in 0.2-mL pre-filled syringes**
**25 000 units/mL solution in 0.2-mL, 0.3-mL, 0.4-mL, 0.5-mL, 0.6-mL and 0.72-mL pre-filled syringes**
**25 000 units/mL solution in 4-mL multidose vials**

* Dalteparin sodium is an antithrombotic low-molecular-weight heparin (LMWH).
* It is used in the prophylaxis and treatment of VTE including the extended treatment of patients with solid tumours, the treatment of ACS and also for the prevention of thrombus formation in the extracorporeal circulation during haemodialysis.
* Not all preparations are licensed for all indications.
* Doses are expressed in terms of international anti-Factor Xa activity units:
Dalteparin sodium 1 mg $\cong$ 110–210 units of anti-Factor Xa activity.

## Pre-treatment checks

* Avoid in acute bacterial endocarditis, major bleeding or high risk of uncontrolled haemorrhage including recent haemorrhagic stroke.
* Dalteparin in treatment dosage is contraindicated in patients undergoing locoregional anaesthesia in elective surgical procedures.
* Placement or removal of a spinal/epidural catheter should be delayed for 10–12 hours after administration of prophylactic doses, whereas patients receiving higher doses (1.5 mg/kg once daily) require a 24 hours delay. Subsequent doses should be given no sooner than 4 hours after catheter removal.
* Caution with other drugs affecting haemostasis, such as aspirin or clopidogrel.
* Use with extreme caution in patients with a history of HIT.
* Patients with severe renal or hepatic impairment may need a reduced dose (or at least closer monitoring of ADRs).

*Biochemical and other tests (not all are necessary in an emergency situation)*

Bodyweight (in certain indications)    Platelet count
Electrolytes: serum K                  Renal function: U, Cr, CrCl (or eGFR)
LFTs

## Dose

*Prophylaxis*

**General surgery with moderate risk of VTE:** 2500 units by SC injection 1–2 hours before the procedure and thereafter 2500 units by SC injection once daily until the patient is mobile.
**General surgery with high risk of VTE:** 5000 units by SC injection the evening before the surgical procedure and 5000 units on subsequent evenings. Alternatively, 2500 units by SC injection 1–2 hours before the procedure followed by 2500 units by SC injection after 8–12 hours. Thereafter give 5000 units by SC injection once daily until mobile.
**Prolonged thromboprophylaxis in hip replacement surgery:** 5000 units by SC injection the evening before the surgical procedure and 5000 units on subsequent evenings. Dosing may be continued for up to 5 weeks after hip replacement surgery.
**Medical patients (high risk of VTE):** 5z000 units by SC injection once daily.

**Prevention of extracorporeal thrombus formation during haemodialysis:**
- For dialysis sessions <4 hours give 5000 units by IV injection at the start of dialysis.
- For dialysis sessions >4 hours give 30–40 units/kg by IV injection at the start of dialysis followed by 10–15 units/kg/hour by IV infusion. In patients at high risk of bleeding or in acute renal failure give 5–10 units/kg by IV injection followed by 4–5 units/kg/hour by IV infusion.

*Treatment*

**Treatment of VTE:** give by SC injection once daily based on bodyweight as indicated in Table D1 (approximately 200 units/kg). Treat for at least 5 days and until INR > 2.

In patients at high risk of bleeding, give 100 units/kg by SC injection twice daily. Ampoules or multidose vials may be used to facilitate dosing.

**Table D1**  Treatment of VTE and treatment for the first 30 days of cancer-related VTE

| Bodyweight (kg) | Syringe to use |
| --- | --- |
| <46 | 7500 units (0.3 mL) |
| 46-56 | 10 000 units (0.4 mL) |
| 57-68 | 12 500 units (0.5 mL) |
| 69-82 | 15 000 units (0.6 mL) |
| ≥83 | 18 000 units (0.72 mL) |

**Cancer-related VTE:** give by SC injection once daily based on bodyweight as indicated in Table D1 (approximately 200 units/kg) for the first 30 days. Then give by SC injection once daily based on bodyweight as indicated in Table D2 (approximately 150 units/kg) for a further 5 months or longer depending on individual risk.

See product literature for dose in chemotherapy-induced thrombocytopenia.

**Table D2**  Treatment for months 2 to 6 of cancer-related VTE

| Bodyweight (kg) | Syringe to use |
| --- | --- |
| ≤56 | 7500 units (0.3 mL) |
| 57-68 | 10 000 units (0.4 mL) |
| 69-82 | 12 500 units (0.5 mL) |
| 83-98 | 15 000 units (0.6 mL) |
| ≥99 | 18 000 units (0.72 mL) |

**Treatment of ACS:** give 120 units/kg by SC injection every 12 hours (maximum 10 000 units every 12 hours) for up to 8 days until clinically stable. See Table D3.

If treatment is required beyond 8 days, reduce the dose to either 5000 units (women <80 kg, men <70 kg) or 7500 units (women ≥80 kg, men ≥70 kg) every 12 hours for no more than 45 days.

**Table D3** Treatment of ACS (for up to 8 days)

| Bodyweight | | Prescribed dose (Anti-Factor Xa units) | Injection volume (mL) |
|---|---|---|---|
| kg | Stones/lb | | |
| 40 | 6/4 | 4 800 | 0.48 |
| 45 | 7/1 | 5 400 | 0.54 |
| 50 | 7/12 | 6 000 | 0.60 |
| 55 | 8/9 | 6 600 | 0.66 |
| 60 | 9/6 | 7 200 | 0.72 |
| 65 | 10/3 | 7 800 | 0.78 |
| 70 | 11/0 | 8 400 | 0.84 |
| 75 | 11/11 | 9 000 | 0.90 |
| 80 | 12/8 | 9 600 | 0.96 |
| ≥85 | ≥ 13/5 | 10 000 | 1.00 |

**Dose in renal impairment:** adjusted according to creatinine clearance:[1]
- CrCl >20–50 mL/minute: dose as in normal renal function.
- CrCl 10–20 mL/minute: dose as in normal renal function for prophylaxis only. For treatment doses either monitor anti-Factor Xa levels or use unfractionated heparin.
- CrCl <10 mL/minute: dose as in normal renal function for prophylaxis only. For treatment doses either monitor anti-Factor Xa levels or use unfractionated heparin.

**Dose in hepatic impairment:** the manufacturer advises to avoid in severe hepatic impairment.

## Subcutaneous injection

*Preparation and administration*

1. Select the correct pre-filled syringe. Pre-filled syringes are ready for immediate use; do not expel the air bubble. If necessary expel any excess dalteparin to give the required dose.
2. If using multidose vials or ampoules, withdraw the required dose using a needle suitable for SC administration.
3. The patient should be seated or lying down.
4. Pinch up a skin fold on the abdominal wall between the thumb and forefinger and hold throughout the injection.
5. Give by deep SC injection into the thick part of the skin fold at right angles to the skin. Do not rub the injection site after administration. Alternate doses between the right and left sides.

## Intravenous injection (haemodialysis only)

*Preparation and administration*

1. Withdraw the required dose.
2. The solution should be clear and colourless to pale straw in colour. Inspect visually for particulate matter or discoloration prior to administration.
3. Give as a rapid IV injection.

## Intravenous infusion via a syringe pump (haemodialysis only)

*Preparation and administration*

1. Withdraw the required dose and make up to a suitable volume with NaCl 0.9% or Gluc 5% for administration via syringe pump.
2. Cap the syringe and mix well.
3. The solution should be clear and colourless to pale straw in colour. Inspect visually for particulate matter or discoloration prior to administration.
4. Give by IV infusion at the prescribed rate via a syringe pump.

## Technical information

| | |
|---|---|
| Incompatible with | No information |
| Compatible with | **Flush**: NaCl 0.9%<br>**Solutions**: NaCl 0.9%, Gluc 5%<br>**Y-site**: No information |
| pH | 5–7.5 |
| Sodium content | Negligible |
| Excipients | Multidose vials contain benzyl alcohol. |
| Storage | Pre-filled syringes: store below 25°C<br>Multidose vials and ampoules: store below 30°C.<br>*In use:* Vials should be stored below 30°C and contents used within 14 days of first use. |
| Stability after preparation | From a microbiological point of view, prepared infusions should be used immediately; however, the preparation is known to be stable at room temperature for up to 24 hours. |

## Monitoring

| Measure | Frequency | Rationale |
|---|---|---|
| Platelets | Alternate days from day 5 to day 21 | • Thrombocytopenia can occur in this period of therapy.<br>• A 50%↓ in platelets is indicative of HIT and therapy should be switched to a non-heparin-derived agent. |
| Serum K | After 7 days | • Heparins ↓secretion of aldosterone and so may cause ↑K (especially in chronic kidney disease).<br>• K should be monitored in all patients with risk factors, particularly those receiving dalteparin for >7 days. |
| Bleeding | Throughout treatment | • Low bodyweight: In women <45 kg and men <57 kg there is a higher risk of bleeding with prophylactic dalteparin doses. |
| Anti-Xa activity | If indicated | • Not required routinely but may be considered in patients at ↑risk of bleeding or actively bleeding. |

## Additional information

| | |
|---|---|
| Common and serious undesirable effects | *Immediate:* Anaphylaxis has been reported rarely. <br> *Injection/infusion-related:* Local: Pain, haematoma and mild local irritation may follow SC injection. <br> *Other:* Risk of bleeding with organic lesions, invasive procedures, asymptomatic thrombocytopenia during the first days of therapy, clinically significant ↑K in patients with diabetes or chronic renal failure. |
| Pharmacokinetics | Rapidly absorbed after SC injection (peak activity 3-4 hours) with elimination half-life of 3-5 hours. Elimination after IV injection is about 2 hours. Elimination is prolonged in renal impairment and severe hepatic dysfunction. |
| Significant interactions | • The following may ↑risk of bleeding with dalteparin: <br>   aspirin, diclofenac IV (avoid combination), ketorolac (avoid combination). <br> • Glyceryl trinitrate infusion may ↓dalteparin levels or effect. |
| Action in case of overdose | Symptoms to watch for: Bleeding. <br> *Antidote:* Protamine sulfate may be used to ↓bleeding risk if clinically required. See the Protamine sulfate monograph. |
| Counselling | Report any bleeding or bruising. <br> Report injection-site effects. |

| Risk rating: **GREEN** | Score = 1 <br> Lower-risk product. Risk-reduction strategies should be considered. |
|---|---|

This assessment is based on the full range of preparation and administration options described in the monograph. These may not all be applicable in some clinical situations.

## Reference

1. Ashley C, Currie A, eds. *The Renal Drug Handbook*, 3rd edn. Oxford: Radcliffe Medical Press, 2009.

## Bibliography

SPC Fragmin – Surgical and Medical Thromboprophylaxis, Pharmacia Ltd (accessed 2 September 2009).

SPC Fragmin – Treatment of VTE, Pharmacia Ltd (accessed 2 September 2009).

SPC Fragmin – Unstable Angina, Pharmacia Ltd (accessed 2 September 2009).

SPC Fragmin – Extended Treatment in Oncology, Pharmacia Ltd (accessed 2 September 2009).

SPC Fragmin – Haemodialysis/Haemofiltration, Pharmacia Ltd (accessed 2 September 2009).

# Danaparoid sodium

**750 anti-Factor Xa units/0.6 mL solution in ampoules**

* Danaparoid sodium is a low-molecular-weight heparinoid with actions similar to heparin.
* Provided there is no evidence of cross-reactivity, danaparoid may be used in the treatment of VTE in patients who have previously had, or who develop, HIT.
* It may be also be used for the prevention of VTE in patients undergoing general or orthopaedic surgery.
* Doses are expressed in terms of international anti-Factor Xa activity units:
  Danaparoid 1 mL $\cong$ 1250 units of anti-Factor Xa activity.

## Pre-treatment checks

* There are a number of contraindications:
  * Treatment of DVT: do not use locoregional anaesthesia in surgical procedures.
  * Severe haemorrhagic diathesis, e.g. haemophilia and idiopathic thrombocytopenic purpura, unless the patient also has HIT and no alternative antithrombotic treatment is available.
  * Haemorrhagic stroke in the acute phase.
  * Uncontrollable active bleeding state.
  * Severe renal and/or hepatic insufficiency, unless the patient also has HIT and no alternative antithrombotic treatment is available.
  * Severe uncontrolled hypertension.
  * Active gastroduodenal ulcer, unless it is the reason for operation.
  * Diabetic retinopathy.
  * Acute bacterial endocarditis.
  * A positive in-vitro aggregation test for the heparin-induced antibody in the presence of danaparoid in patients with a history of HIT.
  * Hypersensitivity to sulfites.
* Use with caution in moderate impairment of renal and/or hepatic function.

*Biochemical and other tests*

Bodyweight
Plasma cross-reactivity in plasma for patients with history of HIT (if test is available)
Renal function: U, Cr, CrCl (or eGFR)

## Dose

*Prophylaxis*

**VTE prophylaxis in general or orthopaedic surgery:** 750 anti-Factor Xa units (0.6 mL) by SC injection twice daily until the patient is mobile. Danaparoid should be started preoperatively; the last preoperative dose being given a minimum of 1–4 hours before surgery.

*Treatment*

**Treatment of VTE in HIT:** an initial dose is given by IV injection based on bodyweight:
* <55 kg: 1250 anti-Factor Xa units (1 mL).
* 55–90 kg: 2500 anti-Factor Xa units (2 mL).
* >90 kg: 3750 anti-Factor Xa units (3 mL).

This is followed by an IV infusion given at a rate of 400 units/hour for 2 hours, then 300 units/hour for 2 hours, then a maintenance infusion of 200 units/hour for 5 days.

**Dose in renal impairment:** adjusted according to creatinine clearance:[1]
- CrCl >20–50 mL/minute: dose as in normal renal function.
- CrCl 10–20 mL/minute: use with caution.
- CrCl <10 mL/minute: use with caution. Reduce second and subsequent doses for VTE prophylaxis.

**Dose in hepatic impairment:** use with caution in moderate hepatic impairment.

## Subcutaneous injection

*Preparation and administration*

1. Withdraw the required dose.
2. The patient should be seated or lying down.
3. Pinch up a skin fold on the abdominal wall between the thumb and forefinger and hold throughout the injection.
4. Give by deep SC injection into the thick part of the skin fold at right angles to the skin. Do not rub the injection site after administration. Alternate doses between the right and left sides.

## Intravenous injection

*Preparation and administration*

1. Withdraw the required dose.
2. The solution should be clear and colourless. Inspect visually for particulate matter or discoloration prior to administration and discard if present.
3. Give by rapid IV injection.

## Intravenous infusion via a syringe pump

*Preparation of a 200 anti-Factor Xa units/mL infusion with a total volume of 22.5 mL (other concentrations and volumes may be used)*

1. Withdraw 4500 units (3.6 mL $\equiv$ 6 × 0.6-mL ampoules) of danaparoid injection solution into a syringe.
2. Withdraw 18.9 mL of compatible diluent into a 30-mL syringe.
3. Add the danaparoid injection to the diluent, cap the syringe, and mix well.
4. The solution should be clear and colourless. Inspect visually for particulate matter or discoloration prior to administration and discard if present.

*Administration*

1. Give by IV infusion via syringe pump at 2 mL/hour for 2 hours, then 1.5 mL/hour for 2 hours then continue at 1 mL/hour.
2. Prepare a fresh syringe at least every 24 hours.

| Technical information | |
|---|---|
| Incompatible with | No information |
| Compatible with | **Flush**: NaCl 0.9%<br>**Solutions**: NaCl 0.9%, Gluc 5%, Gluc-NaCl<br>**Y-site**: No information |
| pH | 7 |
| Sodium content | Negligible |
| Excipients | Contains sulfites (may cause hypersensitivity reactions). |

*(continued)*

## Technical information (continued)

| Storage | Store below 30°C in original packaging. Do not freeze. |
|---|---|
| Stability after preparation | Use prepared infusions immediately. |

## Monitoring

| Measure | Frequency | Rationale |
|---|---|---|
| Platelet count (patients with history of HIT) | Daily | • To rule out cross-reactivity (↓platelets). |
| Anti-Xa activity | | • Not routinely necessary; consider in renal insufficiency and patients >90 kg. |
| Signs and symptoms of neurologic impairment (peridural or spinal anaesthesia) | Continuously | • If danaparoid is administered in the context of peridural or spinal anaesthesia, extreme vigilance and frequent monitoring must be exercised to detect any signs and symptoms of neurologic impairment, such as back pain, sensory and motor deficits (numbness and weakness in lower limbs) and bowel or bladder dysfunction.<br>• Attending staff should be trained to detect such signs and symptoms.<br>• There is a risk epidural or spinal haematoma could occur resulting in prolonged or permanent paralysis. The risk is increased by the prolonged use of these routes, by the concomitant use of drugs affecting haemostasis, e.g. NSAIDs, and by traumatic or repeated puncture. |

## Additional information

| Common and serious undesirable effects | *Immediate:* Generalised hypersensitivity reactions have been reported, also allergy to sulfite content in asthma<br>*Injection/infusion-related:*<br>• Too rapid administration:<br>• Local: Bruising and/or pain at injection sites<br>*Other:* ↑Risk of bleeding, skin rashes, thrombocytopenia in <10% of patients with history of HIT, altered LFTs. |
|---|---|
| Pharmacokinetics | Danaparoid is well absorbed after SC injection. The elimination half-lives of anti-Factor Xa and anti-Factor IIa (anti-thrombin) activities are about 25 and 7 hours, respectively. Excretion is via the urine. |
| Significant interactions | No significant interactions. |
| Action in case of overdose | Supportive therapy as appropriate. Protamine sulfate only partially neutralises the anticoagulant effect of danaparoid and cannot be relied on to reverse bleeding associated with overdosage. |
| Counselling | Report bleeding episodes.<br>Report any signs of neurological impairment with concurrent spinal anaesthesia. |

| Risk rating: **AMBER** | Score = 4 Moderate-risk product: Risk-reduction strategies are recommended. |
|---|---|

This assessment is based on the full range of preparation and administration options described in the monograph. These may not all be applicable in some clinical situations.

## Reference

1. Ashley C, Currie A, eds. *The Renal Drug Handbook*, 3rd edn. Oxford: Radcliffe Medical Press, 2009.

## Bibliography

SPC Orgaran, Organon Laboratories Ltd (accessed 31 March 2010).

# Dantrolene sodium

**20-mg dry powder vials**

- Dantrolene sodium is a muscle relaxant acting directly on skeletal muscle, thus reducing muscle contractility in response to excitation.
- It is used IV to treat malignant hyperthermia. It has also been used in the USA both orally and IV to pretreat individuals prior to surgery who are at risk of developing malignant hyperthermia.

## Pre-treatment checks

As soon as the malignant hyperthermia syndrome is recognised, stop all anaesthetic agents.

*Biochemical and other tests (not all are necessary in an emergency situation)*

Bodyweight
LFTs – do not give to patients with active liver disease

## Dose

**Malignant hyperthermia:** 1 mg/kg given by rapid IV injection. Repeat as necessary up to a cumulative maximum of 10 mg/kg. Clinical experience has shown that the average dose required is 2.5 mg/kg. The manufacturers note that a 70-kg man may require approximately 36 vials (to give 10 mg/kg) and that such a volume could be administered in approximately $1^1/_2$ hours.

**Prophylaxis of malignant hyperthermia (unlicensed):** in the USA, pretreatment with either 1–2 mg/kg orally four times daily for 1–2 days prior to surgery or 2.5 mg/kg by IV infusion over 60 minutes starting approximately 75 minutes before anaesthesia. Further doses are given during anaesthesia if signs of malignant hyperthermia develop.

## Intravenous injection

*Preparation and administration*

Dantrolene sodium is incompatible with NaCl 0.9%, Gluc 5%.
Use of a central line is preferable if possible because of the high pH.

1. Add 60 mL WFI to each 20-mg vial and shake the vial until the solution is clear. The resultant solution contains dantrolene sodium 0.333 mg/mL.
2. Withdraw the required dose.
3. The solution should be clear and colourless to orange. Inspect visually for particulate matter or discoloration prior to administration and discard if present.
4. Give by rapid IV injection. Use of a central line is preferable if possible because of the high pH.

## Intermittent intravenous infusion

*Preparation and administration*

Dantrolene sodium is incompatible with NaCl 0.9%, Gluc 5%.
Use of a central line is preferable if possible because of the high pH.

1. Add 60 mL WFI to vial and shake the vial until the solution is clear. The resultant solution contains dantrolene sodium 0.333 mg/mL.
2. Transfer the required volume of reconstituted solution into an appropriate sized empty sterile IV plastic bag for administration.
3. The solution should be clear and colourless to orange. Inspect visually for particulate matter or discoloration prior to administration and discard if present.
4. Give by IV infusion over 60 minutes. Use of a central line is preferable because of the high pH.

## Technical information

| | |
|---|---|
| Incompatible with | Dantrolene sodium is incompatible with NaCl 0.9%, Gluc 5%. |
| Compatible with | **Flush**: WFI<br>**Solutions**: WFI<br>**Y-site**: No information but likely to be unstable |
| pH | 9.5 |
| Sodium content | Negligible |
| Storage | Store below 30°C in original packaging. The powder may have a mottled orange/white appearance or be in the form of loose aggregates; this does not affect the stability of the product. |
| Displacement value | Negligible |
| Stability after preparation | From a microbiological point of view, should be used immediately; however, reconstituted vials may be stored at 15-30°C for 6 hours. Do not refrigerate. Prepared infusions should be used immediately. |

## Monitoring

| Measure | Frequency | Rationale |
|---------|-----------|-----------|
| LFTs | Periodically | • If abnormal results are found, treatment should generally be stopped. |

## Additional information

| | |
|---|---|
| Common and serious undesirable effects | *Infusion-related:*<br>• Too rapid administration: Side-effects tend to occur at the start of treatment but are often short lived and can be controlled by adjusting the dose.<br>• Local: extravasation may cause tissue damage.<br><br>*Other:* Drowsiness, dizziness, fatigue, weakness and general malaise. Rarely diarrhoea may develop and be severe enough to require cessation of treatment. If diarrhoea recurs on restarting dantrolene then the treatment should be stopped permanently. |
| Pharmacokinetics | Elimination half-life is 5–9 hours. |
| Significant interactions | • Dantrolene may ↑levels or effect of the following drugs (or ↑side-effects): calcium channel blockers (↑risk cardiovascular depression and ↑K), vecuronium (↑neuromuscular block). |
| Action in case of overdose | Stop administration and give supportive therapy as appropriate. |

| Risk rating: **RED** | Score = 7<br>High-risk product: Risk-reduction strategies are required to minimise these risks. |
|---|---|

This assessment is based on the full range of preparation and administration options described in the monograph. These may not all be applicable in some clinical situations.

### Bibliography

SPC Dantrium (accessed 20 January 2009).

# Daptomycin

**350-mg, 500-mg dry powder vials**

• Daptomycin is a cyclic lipopeptide antibacterial.
• It is used to treat complicated skin and soft-tissue infections (cSSTI) caused by resistant Gram-positive bacteria, and right-sided infective endocarditis (RIE) due to *Staphylococcus aureus*.

## Pre-treatment checks

Culture and sensitivity confirmation if used for RIE.

*Biochemical tests*

| | |
|---|---|
| Bodyweight | LFTs |
| CK | Renal function: U, Cr, CrCl (or eGFR) |
| FBC | |

## Dose

**cSSTI without concurrent *S. aureus* bacteraemia:** 4 mg/kg once every 24 hours for 7–14 days or until the infection is resolved.

**cSSTI with concurrent *S. aureus* bacteraemia:** 6 mg/kg once every 24 hours in accordance with the perceived risk of complications in the patient (duration may be longer than 14 days).

**Known or suspected RIE due to *S. aureus*:** 6 mg/kg once every 24 hours. The duration is determined by whichever official guideline is being followed.

**Dose in renal impairment:** adjusted according to creatinine clearance:[1]

* CrCl 30–50 mL/minute: dose as in normal renal function.
* CrCl <30 mL/minute: 4 mg/kg every 48 hours.

**Dose in hepatic impairment:** no dose adjustment necessary in mild to moderate impairment (Child–Pugh Class A or B) but insufficient experience is available with Child–Pugh Class C, therefore caution should be exercised.

## Intermittent intravenous infusion

*Preparation and administration*

Daptomycin is incompatible with Gluc solutions.

1. Reconstitute each 350-mg vial with 7 mL NaCl 0.9% (use 10 mL for each 500-mg vial). Inject through the rubber stopper and aim at the wall of the vial.
2. Gently rotate to fully wet the powder then leave to stand for 10 minutes.
3. Gently swirl the vial (do not shake) for a few minutes until a clear solution has developed. The reconstituted solution contains 50 mg/mL.
4. The solution should be clear and yellow to light brown. Inspect visually for particulate matter or discoloration prior to administration and discard if present.
5. Invert the vial to allow the solution to drain towards the stopper. Withdraw the required dose by slowly pulling the syringe plunger all the way to end of the syringe to remove the entire vial contents.
6. Expel air, large bubbles and any excess solution to obtain the required dose and add to a suitable volume of NaCl 0.9% (usually 50 mL).
7. Give by IV infusion over 30 minutes.

## Intravenous injection

*Preparation and administration*

Daptomycin is incompatible with Gluc solutions.

1. Reconstitute each 350-mg vial with 7 mL NaCl 0.9% (use 10 mL for each 500-mg vial). Inject through the rubber stopper and aim at the wall of the vial.
2. Gently rotate to fully wet the powder then leave to stand for 10 minutes.
3. Gently swirl the vial (do not shake) for a few minutes until a clear solution has developed. The reconstituted solution contains 50 mg/mL.

(continued)

4. The solution should be clear and yellow to light brown. Inspect visually for particulate matter or discoloration prior to administration and discard if present.
5. Invert the vial to allow the solution to drain towards the stopper. Withdraw the required dose by slowly pulling the syringe plunger all the way to end of the syringe to remove the entire vial contents.
6. Expel air, large bubbles and any excess solution to obtain the required dose.
7. Give by IV injection over 2 minutes.

## Technical information

| Incompatible with | Daptomycin is incompatible with Gluc solutions. |
|---|---|
| Compatible with | **Flush**: NaCl 0.9%<br>**Solutions**: NaCl 0.9%<br>**Y-site** (but only if prepared in NaCl 0.9%): Aztreonam, ceftazidime, ceftriaxone, dopamine, fluconazole, levofloxacin |
| pH[1] | 4.0-5.0 |
| Sodium content[2] | Negligible |
| Storage | Store at 2-8°C in original packaging.<br>Vials are single use only - discard unused portion. |
| Displacement value | Negligible |
| Stability after preparation | From a microbiological point of view, should be used immediately, however:<br>• Reconstituted vials may be stored at 2-8°C for 24 hours. Discard unused portion.<br>• Prepared infusions may be stored at 2-8°C and infused (at room temperature) within 24 hours. |

## Monitoring

| Measure | Frequency | Rationale |
|---|---|---|
| Plasma CK | At least weekly | • ↑CK levels associated with muscular pains and/or weakness and cases of myositis, myoglobinaemia and rhabdomyolysis have been reported (very rarely).<br>• In patients at greater risk - e.g. baseline level >5 times ULN, severe renal impairment, taking statins - the monitoring frequency should be 2-3 times a week.<br>• Monitor every 2 days if unexplained muscle pain, tenderness, weakness or cramps develop.<br>• If there is unexplained muscle pain and a marked increase to >5 times ULN, discontinue daptomycin. |
| Renal function | Periodically | • If renal function changes a dose adjustment may be necessary. |
| LFTs | | • ↑ALT, ↑AST and ↑Alk Phos occur commonly. |
| FBC | | • Thrombocythaemia, anaemia and eosinophilia occasionally occur. |

*(continued)*

## Monitoring (continued)

| Measure | Frequency | Rationale |
|---------|-----------|-----------|
| Signs of peripheral neuropathy | Throughout treatment | • Paraesthesias occur uncommonly but consider discontinuing therapy if this develops. |
| Signs of supra-infection or superinfection | | • May result in the overgrowth of non-susceptible organisms - appropriate therapy should be commenced; treatment may need to be interrupted. |
| Development of diarrhoea | Throughout and up to 2 months after treatment | • Development of severe, persistent diarrhoea may be suggestive of *Clostridium difficile*-associated diarrhoea and colitis (pseudomembranous colitis). If needed, discontinue drug and treat. Do not use drugs that inhibit peristalsis. |

## Additional information

| | |
|---|---|
| Common and serious undesirable effects | *Immediate:* Anaphylaxis and other hypersensitivity reactions have rarely been reported. Also wheezing, systemic flushing.<br>*Injection/infusion-related:* Local: Infusion-site reactions.<br>*Other:* Fungal infections, headache, nausea, vomiting, diarrhoea, rash, ↑pulse, metallic taste. |
| Pharmacokinetics | Elimination half-life is 7–11 hours (>27 hours if CrCl <30 mL/minute). |
| Significant interactions | • ↑Risk of myopathy with the following (preferably avoid combination): ciclosporin, fibrates, statins.<br>• Daptomycin may affect the following tests:<br>PT and INR (take blood sample immediately before daptomycin dose). |
| Action in case of overdose | *Antidote:* No known antidote, but haemodialysis or peritoneal dialysis may clear daptomycin slowly. Stop administration and give supportive therapy as appropriate. |

| | |
|---|---|
| Risk rating: **AMBER** | Score =4<br>Moderate-risk product: Risk-reduction strategies are recommended. |

This assessment is based on the full range of preparation and administration options described in the monograph. These may not all be applicable in some clinical situations.

## Reference

1. Ashley C, Currie A, eds. *The Renal Drug Handbook*, 3rd edn. Oxford: Radcliffe Medical Press, 2009.
2. Correspondence from Novartis, February 2008.

## Bibliography

SPC Cubicin powder for concentrate for solution for infusion accessed (16 March 2009).

# Desferrioxamine mesilate (desferoxamine mesylate)

**500-mg or 2-g dry powder vials**

- Desferrioxamine is a chelating agent that has a high affinity for ferric iron. When given by injection it forms a stable water-soluble iron-complex (ferrioxamine) that can be excreted in the urine and in bile. It can also chelate aluminium.
- It increases the excretion of iron from the body and is used in acute iron poisoning and also in conditions associated with chronic iron overload such as iron storage disorders and in conditions requiring repeated blood transfusions.
- As desferrioxamine can also chelate aluminium, it has also been used to reduce aluminium overload in patients with end-stage renal failure on maintenance dialysis. However, it may exacerbate aluminium-related encephalopathy and precipitate seizures.
- Theoretically 100 mg desferrioxamine could chelate 8.5 mg of ferric iron, and 4.1 mg of aluminium.

## Pre-treatment checks

- Not recommended for use in pregnancy or lactation, and has been found to be teratogenic in animal studies (especially in the first trimester). The risks and benefits of treatment should be assessed before considering chelation therapy in pregnancy or lactation.
- Check that the patient does not have a history of desferrioxamine mesilate intolerance before administration.

*Biochemical and other tests*

Baseline audiological review.

Baseline neurological assessment in patients with aluminium-related encephalopathy.

Baseline ophthalmic assessment (visual field measurements, funduscopy, colour vision testing using pseudoisochromatic plates and the Farnsworth D-15 colour test, slit lamp investigation and visual evoked potential studies).

Baseline U&Es (may require dose adjustment in renal impairment; treatment of aluminium overload may result in ↓Ca).

Bodyweight.

Coma and shock indicate severe poisoning. Urgent treatment is required. Death may occur at this stage.

Serum aluminium level (in diagnosis and treatment of aluminium overload in end-stage renal failure).

Serum ferritin (in chronic iron overload).

Serum iron taken at about 4 hours after ingestion is the best laboratory measure of severity of overdose:

<3 mg/L (55 micromol/L) – mild toxicity

3–5 mg/L (55–90 micromol/L) – moderate toxicity

>5 mg/L (90 micromol/L) – severe toxicity.

## Dose

It is essential to consult a poisons information service, e.g. Toxbase at www.toxbase.org (password or registration required) for full details of the management of acute iron toxicity.

**Acute iron poisoning (in addition to other supportive measures as appropriate):** 15 mg/kg/hour by continuous IV infusion, reduced after 4–6 hours. Maximum dose is usually 80 mg/kg in 24 hours.

Alternatively, if IV infusion is not possible, give 2 g by IM injection as a single dose. (In the USA, 1 g is given by IM injection followed by 500 mg at intervals of 4–12 hours up to a maximum of 6 g daily depending on clinical response.)

**Chronic iron overload:** usually 20–60 mg/kg/day by SC infusion 3–7 times per week. 24-hour urinary iron excretion should be monitored daily initially. Higher doses should only be used if likely benefit outweighs risks. Desferrioxamine may also be given by IV infusion during blood transfusion.

**Diagnosis of iron storage disease and certain anaemias:** 500 mg by IM injection. Urine is then collected for 6 hours and its iron content is determined. Excretion of 1–1.5 mg (18–27 micromoles) of iron is suggestive of iron overload; values >1.5 mg (27 micromoles) can be regarded as pathological.

**Diagnosis of aluminium overload in end-stage renal failure:** recommended in patients with serum aluminium levels >60 nanograms/mL associated with serum ferritin levels >100 nanograms/mL. Baseline serum aluminium level is determined immediately before haemodialysis. During the last 60 minutes of the haemodialysis session, desferrioxamine 5 mg/kg is given by slow IV infusion. Before the next haemodialysis session a second blood sample is taken. An increase in serum aluminium above baseline of >150 nanograms/mL is suggestive of aluminium overload; a negative test does not eliminate the possibility of aluminium overload.

**Treatment of aluminium overload in end-stage renal failure:** indicated if the patient is symptomatic owing to organ impairment, or if aluminium level is consistently >60 nanograms/mL associated with a positive desferrioxamine test (see above). Usual dose in all patients is 5 mg/kg once weekly. This is given by IV infusion in haemodialysis/haemofiltration, or by the intraperitoneal route, IM injection, SC infusion or IV infusion in CAPD or CCPD patients. Regimens are dependent on test results – see product literature for details.

**Dose in renal impairment:** dose as in normal renal function but elimination of chelated metals may be impaired in severe renal impairment – haemodialysis is advised.

## Continuous intravenous infusion

Used for acute iron poisoning and where SC infusions are not feasible in chronic conditions.

*Preparation and administration*

1. Dissolve each 500-mg vial in 5 mL WFI (or 2-g vial in 20 mL WFI) to make a 10% solution (100 mg/mL).
2. Withdraw the required dose and add to a convenient volume of NaCl 0.9% or Gluc 5%. Mix well.
3. The solution should be clear and pale yellow. Inspect visually for particulate matter or discoloration prior to administration and discard if present.
4. Give by IV infusion at a rate not exceeding 15 mg/kg/hour reducing to 5 mg/kg/hour as soon as there is clinical improvement.
5. Care should be taken when flushing the line to avoid the sudden infusion of residual desferrioxamine which may be present in the dead space of the line, as this may lead to flushing, ↓BP and acute collapse.
6. 24-hour urinary iron excretion should be measured regularly where intensive IV chelation is required, and the dose adjusted accordingly.

## Subcutaneous infusion

*Preparation and administration*

1. Dissolve each 500-mg vial in 5 mL WFI (or 2-g vial in 20 mL WFI) to make a 10% solution (100 mg/mL).
2. Withdraw the required dose into a suitable syringe. This may then be further diluted with a convenient volume of NaCl 0.9% or Gluc 5%.
3. Give by SC infusion over 8–12 hours taking care not to insert the needle too close to the dermis. It may be possible to further ↑iron excretion by infusing the same daily dose over a 24-hour period.

## Intraperitoneal administration

*Preparation and administration*

1. Dissolve each 500-mg vial in 5 mL WFI to make a 10% solution (100 mg/mL).
2. Withdraw the required dose and add to an appropriate volume of dialysis fluid.
3. The solution should be clear and pale yellow. Inspect visually for particulate matter or discoloration prior to administration and discard if present.
4. Give intraperitoneally whilst patient is on CAPD or CCPD usually prior to last exchange of the day.

## Intramuscular injection (relatively ineffective – use only when SC infusion are not feasible)

*Preparation and administration*

1. Dissolve each 500-mg vial in 5 mL WFI (or 2-g vial in 20 mL WFI) to make a 10% solution.
2. Withdraw the required dose.
3. Give by IM injection.

## Technical information

| | |
|---|---|
| Incompatible with | Heparin sodium |
| Compatible with | **Flush**: NaCl 0.9%<br>**Solutions**: NaCl 0.9%, Gluc 5%, Gluc-NaCl, WFI<br>**Y-site**: Blood products (given as close to the infusion site as possible) |
| pH | 3.7–4.5 |
| Sodium content | Nil |
| Storage | Store below 25°C in original packaging. Use opened vials immediately. |
| Displacement value | Negligible |
| Stability after preparation | From a microbiological point of view, should be used immediately; however:<br>• Reconstituted vials may be stored below 25°C for 24 hours (do not refrigerate).<br>• Prepared infusions should be used immediately. |

## Monitoring

| Measure | Frequency | Rationale |
|---|---|---|
| U&Es | At least every 3 months during therapy | • Caution in renal impairment as metal complexes are eliminated renally. Dialysis will ↑elimination.<br>• Renal impairment has been reported.<br>• Treatment of aluminium toxicity with desferrioxamine can cause ↓Ca and aggravation of hyperparathyroidism. |
| FBC | | • Thrombocytopenia and pancytopenia reported in a small number of cases. |

*(continued)*

## Monitoring (continued)

| Measure | Frequency | Rationale |
| --- | --- | --- |
| Ophthalmic review | Every 3 months during therapy | • Visual disturbances reported, especially when using high doses of desferrioxamine or in patients with low ferritin levels.<br>• Discontinue treatment, effects may be reversible. If clinically indicated following risk-benefit assessment, treatment can be restarted at lower doses with intensive ophthalmic review throughout treatment. |
| Audiological review | | • Disturbances in hearing reported, especially when using high doses of desferrioxamine or in patients with low ferritin levels.<br>• By keeping the ratio of the mean daily dose (mg/kg of desferrioxamine) divided by the serum ferritin (microgram/L) below 0.025 the risk of audiometric abnormalities may be reduced in thalassaemia patients.<br>• Discontinue treatment; effects may be reversible. If clinically indicated following risk-benefit assessment, treatment can be restarted at lower doses with intensive audiological review throughout treatment. |
| Urinary iron excretion | Regularly through therapy | • To assess degree of iron chelation in order to tailor dose regimen. |
| Respiratory function | Ongoing during therapy | • Pulmonary complications, including fatal acute respiratory distress syndrome, have been reported in cases of long-term or high-dose therapy. |
| Cardiac function | As clinically indicated | • When desferrioxamine used in conjunction with ascorbic acid (vitamin C) - see significant drug interactions below. |

## Additional information

| | |
| --- | --- |
| Common and serious undesirable effects | *Immediate:* Anaphylaxis and angioedema have very rarely been reported.<br>*Infusion-related:*<br>• Too rapid administration: Shock (flushing, ↓BP, collapse and urticaria), acute transient loss of vision, aphasia, agitation, headache, nausea, ↓pulse, ↓BP, acute renal impairment<br>• Local: Swelling, erythema, pruritus, eschar/crust, vesicles, local oedema, burning<br>*Other:* Childhood growth retardation (↑risk at doses >40 mg/kg) Rarely: disturbances in vision and hearing, renal impairment, neurological disturbances, thrombocytopenia, acute respiratory distress syndrome, arthralgia, myalgia, headache, urticaria, nausea, vomiting, diarrhoea, pyrexia, dizziness. |

(continued)

## Additional information *(continued)*

| | |
|---|---|
| Pharmacokinetics | Elimination half-life is 3–6 hours. |
| Significant interactions | • The following may ↑desferrioxamine levels or effect (or ↑side-effects): ascorbic acid (oral doses of up to 200 mg daily may ↑iron complex excretion – which may impair cardiac function. The combination should not be used in the first month of therapy).<br>• Desferrioxamine may ↑levels or effect (or ↑side-effects) of prochlorperazine (prolonged unconsciousness reported; avoid combination).<br>• Gallium-67 imaging results may be distorted due to rapid excretion of the desferrioxamine-bound radiolabel. Discontinuation of desferrioxamine 48 hours before scintigraphy is recommended.<br>• Desferrioxamine may affect the estimation of total iron-binding capacity. |
| Action in case of overdose | *Symptoms to watch for:* ↑Pulse, ↓BP and GI disturbances. Rapid IV injection may cause acute transient loss of vision, aphasia, agitation, headache, nausea, ↓pulse, ↓BP and acute renal impairment.<br>*Antidote:* No known antidote, but haemodialysis may be effective. Stop administration and give supportive therapy as appropriate. |
| Counselling | May colour the urine reddish-brown.<br>CNS effects such as dizziness or impaired vision/hearing may affect the ability to drive or use machinery.<br>Compliance is a major issue with long-term treatment – invest time in counselling and planning to facilitate concordance and compliance.<br>Report any signs of infection. |

| Risk rating: **AMBER** | Score = 4<br>Moderate-risk product: Risk-reduction strategies are recommended. |
|---|---|

This assessment is based on the full range of preparation and administration options described in the monograph. These may not all be applicable in some clinical situations.

## Bibliography

SPC Desferal lyophilised powder (accessed 2 May 2010).
SPC Desferrioxamine mesilate 500 mg and 2 g powder for injection (accessed 2 May 2010).
Toxbase at www.toxbase.org (accessed 2 May 2010).

# Desmopressin acetate (DDAVP)

**4 micrograms/mL solution in 1-mL ampoules**

* Desmopressin is a synthetic analogue of vasopressin. It has greater antidiuretic activity and a more prolonged action than vasopressin. It also stimulates factor VIII and plasminogen activator activity in the blood, but has little pressor activity. In its injectable form it is used:
  * To diagnose cranial diabetes insipidus; assess renal concentration capacity; to test for fibrinolytic response.
  * To treat cranial diabetes insipidus; to increase Factor VIII:C and Factor VIII:Ag in patients with mild to moderate haemophilia or von Willebrand disease undergoing surgery or following trauma; to treat headache resulting from lumbar puncture.
* Doses are expressed in terms of desmopressin acetate:
  Desmopressin acetate 1 microgram ≅ desmopressin 0.903 microgram.

## Pre-treatment checks

* Do not use in habitual and psychogenic polydipsia.
* Caution in hypertension, heart disease, cardiac insufficiency and other conditions requiring treatment with diuretic agents.
* Desmopressin does not reduce prolonged bleeding time in thrombocytopenia.

*Diagnostic testing*

* When used for diagnostic purposes, fluid intake must be limited to that required to satisfy thirst, and must not exceed 500 mL from 1 hour before until 8 hours after administration.

*Haemostatic use*

* Do not give in unstable angina pectoris, decompensated cardiac insufficiency or von Willebrand disease Type IIB (where administration may result in pseudo thrombocytopenia).
* For haemophilia and von Willebrand disease, if the patient has not previously received desmopressin treatment, assay Factor VIII levels prior to the start of treatment.

*Biochemical and other tests*

Bodyweight (in some indications)
Baseline blood pressure and pulse

Baseline plasma osmolarity *or* baseline bodyweight (to enable monitoring of fluid balance)
Electrolytes: Serum Na, K

## Dose

**For existing diabetes insipidus patients switched from maintenance to parenteral dosing:**

* Intranasal 10 micrograms ≅ parenteral 1 microgram.
* Oral 100 micrograms ≅ parenteral 1 microgram.

**Treatment of cranial diabetes insipidus:** 1–4 micrograms once daily by SC or IM injection or IV infusion (see above for conversion from other routes).
**Diagnosis of cranial diabetes insipidus:** 2 micrograms by SC or IM injection. Limit fluid intake (see above). Failure to produce concentrated urine after water deprivation, followed by the ability to do so after the administration of desmopressin, confirms a diagnosis of cranial diabetes insipidus. Failure to concentrate after the administration suggests nephrogenic diabetes insipidus.

**Renal function testing:** 2 micrograms by SC or IM injection should elicit urine concentrations > 700 mOsmol/kg in the period of 5–9 hours following the dose. The bladder should be emptied at the time the dose is given. Limit fluid intake (see above).

**Fibrinolytic response testing:** 0.4 micrograms/kg bodyweight by IV infusion. Take a venous blood sample 20 minutes after the infusion. In patients with a normal response the sample should show fibrinolytic activity of euglobulin clot precipitate on fibrin plates of $\geq$240 mm$^2$.

**Mild to moderate haemophilia and von Willebrand disease:** 0.4 micrograms/kg bodyweight by IV infusion. Give the dose immediately prior to surgery or following trauma.

If results from a previous administration of desmopressin are not available then take blood pre-dose and 20 minutes post-dose for assay of Factor VIII levels. The increase in Factor VIII levels is dependent on basal levels and is normally 2–5 times the pre-treatment levels.

Give further doses every 12 hours for as long as cover is required. Continue to monitor Factor VIII levels as some patients have shown a diminishing response to successive doses.

For surgical patients, unless contraindicated, give tranexamic acid orally from 24 hours beforehand until healing is complete.

**Post lumbar puncture headache due to dural puncture:** 4 micrograms by SC or IM injection. Repeat after 24 hours if necessary. Alternatively, 4 micrograms can be given prophylactically immediately prior to lumbar puncture and 24 hours later.

## Subcutaneous injection

*Preparation and administration*

1. Withdraw the required dose.
2. Give by SC injection.

## Intramuscular injection

*Preparation and administration*

1. Withdraw the required dose.
2. Give by IM injection.

## Intravenous infusion

*Preparation and administration*

1. Withdraw the required dose and add to 50 mL NaCl 0.9%.
2. The solution should be clear and colourless. Inspect visually for particulate matter or discoloration prior to administration and discard if present.
3. Give by IV infusion over 20 minutes.

| Technical information | |
|---|---|
| Incompatible with | No information |
| Compatible with | **Flush**: NaCl 0.9%<br>**Solutions**: NaCl 0.9%<br>**Y-site**: No information |
| pH | 4 |
| Sodium content | Negligible |
| Storage | Store at 4-8°C. |
| Stability after preparation | Use prepared infusions immediately. |

## Monitoring

| Measure | Frequency | Rationale |
|---|---|---|
| Blood pressure and pulse | Continuously during IV infusion; periodically during repeated doses by other routes | • Vasodilatation may occur during IV infusion (↓BP, ↑pulse and facial flushing). Decrease infusion rate if adverse effects are observed.<br>• ↑BP has also been reported. |
| Signs of hypersensitivity | During and immediately post dose | • Allergic reactions have been reported rarely. |
| Fluid balance | Frequently during treatment | • Fluid overload may occur with repeated doses.<br>• Monitor fluid intake/output closely and check for fluid accumulation either by monitoring bodyweight or by determining plasma sodium or osmolality.<br>• Fluid intake must be reduced and treatment interrupted if there is a gradual increase of the bodyweight, or serum sodium $<130$ mmol/L, or plasma osmolality $<270$ mOsmol/kg. |
| Factor VIII in patients who have not previously received desmopressin | Pre dose and 20 minutes post dose | • To check adequacy of response in haemophilia and von Willebrand disease. |
| Fibrinolytic response | 20 minutes after dose | • To check response. |

## Additional information

| | |
|---|---|
| Common and serious undesirable effects | *Immediate:* Severe general allergic reactions have been reported rarely.<br>*Injection/infusion-related:* Too rapid administration: vasodilatation, ↓BP, ↑pulse, facial flushing (↓infusion rate).<br>*Other:* Allergic skin reactions, water intoxication, headache, stomach pain, nausea. |
| Pharmacokinetics | When given IV desmopressin exhibits biphasic pharmacokinetics, with half-lives of about 8 minutes and 75 minutes, respectively, for the two phases. |
| Significant interactions | No significant interactions. |
| Action in case of overdose | *Symptoms to watch for:* ↑Risk of water retention and/or ↓Na i.e. water intoxication. Restrict fluid intake and manage symptomatically. |
| Counselling | For diagnostic tests, limit fluid intake to a maximum of 500 mL from 1 hour before until 8 hours after administration. |

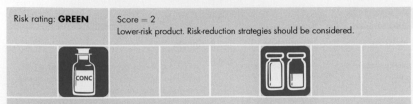

Risk rating: **GREEN**    Score = 2
Lower-risk product. Risk-reduction strategies should be considered.

This assessment is based on the full range of preparation and administration options described in the monograph. These may not all be applicable in some clinical situations.

**Bibliography**

SPC DDAVP/Desmopressin injection (accessed 3 February 09).

# Dexamethasone

**4 mg/mL solution in 1-mL ampoules and 2-mL vials; 24 mg/mL solution in 5-mL vials**

* Dexamethasone sodium phosphate is a corticosteroid with mainly glucocorticoid activity.
* It is used in the treatment of conditions for which systemic corticosteroid therapy is indicated (except adrenal-deficiency states). Its virtual lack of mineralocorticoid properties makes it particularly suitable for treating conditions in which water retention would be a disadvantage such as cerebral oedema associated with cerebral neoplasm.
* It is used parenterally when a rapid effect is required in emergencies, e.g. cerebral oedema, and also when the oral route is temporarily unavailable or inappropriate.
* It may also be given by intra-articular, intrasynovial, intralesional or soft-tissue injection for various inflammatory conditions.
* Doses below are expressed in terms of dexamethasone phosphate:
  Dexamethasone phosphate 1 mg $\cong$ 1.1 mg dexamethasone sodium phosphate.
  NB: Some manufacturers state the strength of their products in terms of dexamethasone:
  Dexamethasone 3.3 mg $\equiv$ 4 mg dexamethasone phosphate $\equiv$ 4.3 mg dexamethasone sodium phosphate.

## Pre-treatment checks

* Avoid where systemic infection is present (unless specific therapy given).
* Avoid live virus vaccines in those receiving immunosuppressive doses.
* May activate or exacerbate amoebiasis or strongyloidiasis (exclude before initiating a corticosteroid in those at risk or with suggestive symptoms). Fungal or viral ocular infections may also be exacerbated.
* Caution in patients predisposed to psychiatric reactions, including those who have previously suffered corticosteroid-induced psychosis, or who have a personal or family history of psychiatric disorders.

*Biochemical and other tests (not all are necessary in an emergency situation)*

Bodyweight in certain indications
Electrolytes: serum Na, K

## Dose

**Standard dose:** 0.5–24 mg daily by IM or IV injection/infusion; doses vary depending on the condition being treated.

**Cerebral oedema associated with malignancy:** initially 10 mg by IV injection followed by 4 mg IM every 6 hours as required for 2–4 days. This should be gradually reduced and stopped or an oral maintenance dose may be necessary. Much higher doses are also licensed for use in acute life-threatening cerebral oedema.

**Adjunctive treatment of bacterial meningitis (unlicensed):** 10 mg by IV injection every 6 hours for 4 days (starting before or with first dose of antibacterial treatment).

**Intra-articular, intrasynovial or soft-tissue injection:**

*   Large joints: 2–4 mg; small joints: 0.8–1 mg; bursas: 2–3 mg; tendon sheaths: 0.4–1 mg; soft tissue infiltration: 2–6 mg; ganglia: 1–2 mg.
*   Injections may be repeated every 3–5 days (e.g. for bursas) or every 2–3 weeks (for joints).

## Intravenous injection

*Preparation and administration*

1.  Withdraw the required dose.
2.  The solution should be clear and colourless. Inspect visually for particulate matter or discoloration prior to administration and discard if present.
3.  Give by IV injection over a minimum of 3 minutes (may be diluted with NaCl 0.9% or Gluc 5% to facilitate slow administration.)

## Intermittent intravenous infusion

*Preparation and administration*

1.  Withdraw the required dose and add to 100 mL of compatible infusion fluid (usually NaCl 0.9%).
2.  The solution should be clear and colourless. Inspect visually for particulate matter or discoloration prior to administration and discard if present.
3.  Give by IV infusion over 15 minutes.

## Intramuscular injection

*Preparation and administration*

1.  Withdraw the required dose.
2.  Give by deep IM injection into the gluteal muscle.

## Other routes

*Preparation and administration*

1.  Withdraw the required dose
2.  Inject into the affected area.
    *   In tenosynovitis care should be taken to inject into the tendon sheath rather than into the substance of the tendon.
    *   After intra articular injections treatment failure is usually the result of not entering the joint space.

## Technical information

| | |
|---|---|
| Incompatible with | Ciprofloxacin, midazolam, vancomycin. |
| Compatible with | **Flush**: NaCl 0.9%<br>**Solutions**: NaCl 0.9% Gluc 5%, Hartmann's, Ringer's (all with added KCl)<br>**Y-site**: Aciclovir, amikacin, aminophylline, aztreonam, cisatracurium, fentanyl, flucloxacillin, fluconazole, foscarnet, granisetron, levofloxacin, linezolid, meropenem, metoclopramide, ondansetron, piperacillin with tazobactam, propofol, ranitidine, verapamil |

*(continued)*

## Technical information (continued)

| | |
|---|---|
| pH | 7-8.5 |
| Sodium content | Negligible |
| Storage | Store below 25°C in original packaging. Do not freeze. |
| Stability after preparation | From a microbiological point of view, should be used immediately; however, prepared infusions may be stored at 2-8°C and infused (at room temperature) within 24 hours. |

## Monitoring

| Measure | Frequency | Rationale |
|---|---|---|
| Symptoms | Following intra-articular injection | • Marked ↑pain accompanied by local swelling, further restriction of joint motion, fever, and malaise are suggestive of septic arthritis. |
| Serum Na, K, Ca | Throughout treatment | • May cause fluid and electrolyte disturbances. |
| Withdrawal symptoms and signs | During withdrawal and after stopping treatment | • During prolonged therapy with corticosteroids, adrenal atrophy develops and can persist for years after stopping. Abrupt withdrawal after a prolonged period can lead to acute adrenal insufficiency, ↓BP or death.<br>• The CSM has recommended that gradual withdrawal of systemic corticosteroids should be considered in patients whose disease is unlikely to relapse. Full details can be found in the BNF. |
| Signs of infection | During treatment | • Prolonged courses ↑susceptibility to infections and severity of infections. Serious infections may reach an advanced stage before being recognised. |
| Signs of chickenpox | | • Unless they have had chickenpox, patients receiving corticosteroids for purposes other than replacement should be regarded as being at risk of severe chickenpox.<br>• Confirmed chickenpox requires urgent treatment; corticosteroids should not be stopped and dosage may need to be increased. |
| Exposure to measles | | • Patients should be advised to take particular care to avoid exposure to measles and to seek immediate medical advice if exposure occurs.<br>• Prophylaxis with IM normal immunoglobulin may be needed. |

## Additional information

| | |
|---|---|
| Common and serious undesirable effects | *Immediate:* Anaphylaxis and other hypersensitivity reactions have been reported.<br>*Undesirable effects that may result from short-term use* (minimise by using the lowest effective dose for the shortest time): ↑BP, Na and water retention, ↓K, ↓Ca, ↑blood glucose, peptic ulceration and perforation, psychiatric reactions, ↑susceptibility to infection, muscle weakness, tendon rupture, insomnia, ↑intracranial pressure, ↓seizure threshold, impaired healing.<br>For undesirable effects resulting from long-term corticosteroid use refer to the BNF. |
| Pharmacokinetics | Elimination half-life is 3.5-4.5 hours (biological half-life 36-54 hours). |
| Significant interactions | • The following may ↓corticosteroid levels or effect:<br>  barbiturates, carbamazepine, phenytoin, primidone, rifabutin, rifampicin.<br>• Corticosteroids may ↑levels or effect of the following drugs (or ↑side-effects): anticoagulants (monitor INR), methotrexate (↑risk of blood dyscrasias). If using amphotericin IV monitor fluid balance and K level closely.<br>• Corticosteroids may ↓levels or effect vaccines (↓immunological response, ↑risk of infection with live vaccines). |
| Action in case of overdose | Give supportive therapy as appropriate. Following chronic overdose the possibility of adrenal suppression should be considered. |
| Counselling | Patients on long-term corticosteroid treatment should read and carry a Steroid Treatment Card.<br>After intra-articular injection the patient should be warned not to overwork the affected joint. |

| | |
|---|---|
| Risk rating: **GREEN** | Score = 2<br>Lower-risk product: Risk-reduction strategies should be considered. |

This assessment is based on the full range of preparation and administration options described in the monograph. These may not all be applicable in some clinical situations.

## Bibliography

SPC Dexamethasone 4.0mg/mL injection, Organon Laboratories Ltd (accessed 29 September 2009).
SPC Dexamethasone sodium phosphate 4 mg/1 mL injection, Hospira UK Ltd (accessed 29 September 2009).

# Dexrazoxane

**500-mg dry powder vials**

* Dexrazoxane hydrochloride is a cytoprotective agent which is hydrolysed to an active metabolite that chelates iron within cells.
* It is used (as Cardioxane) to reduce the cardiotoxicity of doxorubicin and other anthracyclines. It actively chelates iron within cells, thus preventing the formation of the anthracycline–iron complex that is thought to cause cardiotoxicity.
* It is also use (as Savene) in the management of anthracycline extravasation, where its action is to inhibit the enzyme topoisomerase II.

## Pre-treatment checks

*Biochemical and other tests (not all are necessary in an emergency situation)*

| | |
|---|---|
| Baseline ECG | FBC |
| Baseline LVEF | LFTs |
| Body surface area | Renal function: U, Cr, CrCl (or eGFR) |

## Dose

**Prevention of anthracycline-induced cardiotoxicity (Cardioxane):** the dose is calculated by multiplying the doxorubicin-equivalent dose by 20 or the epirubicin-equivalent dose by 10 (e.g. a dose of $1000\,mg/m^2$ dexrazoxane is given when doxorubicin is given at a dose of $50\,mg/m^2$ or epirubicin is given at a dose of $100\,mg/m^2$).

In the USA, the doxorubicin dose is multiplied by 10 and the manufacturer recommends that initiation is delayed until patients have received a cumulative doxorubicin hydrochloride dose of $300\,mg/m^2$ as one study suggested potential interference with antineoplastic efficacy.

**Anthracycline extravasation (Savene):** days 1 and 2: $1000\,mg/m^2$; day 3: $500\,mg/m^2$.

For a body surface area of $>2\,m^2$ a single dose should not exceed 2000 mg.

The first infusion should be initiated as soon as possible and within the first 6 hours after extravasation. Treatment on the remaining days should start at the same hour as on the first day. If there is a chance of extravasation by drugs other than anthracyclines through the same IV access (e.g. vincristine, mitomycin, vinorelbine) then Savene will **not** be effective for these drugs.

**Dose in renal impairment:** in patients with creatinine clearance <40 mL/minute the Cardioxane dose should be reduced by 50%. There is no experience of such reduced doses in the treatment of extravasation therefore use of Savene in renal impairment is not recommended.

**Dose in hepatic impairment:** the dosage ratio for Cardioxane remains the same. Savene has not been studied in patients with hepatic impairment.

## Intermittent intravenous infusion (Cardioxane)

See Special handling below.

*Preparation and administration*

1. Dissolve the contents of each vial in 25 mL WFI. This may take a few minutes with gentle shaking. If the colour immediately on reconstitution is **not** colourless to yellow, discard.
2. Withdraw the required dose and further dilute each 500 mg with 25–100 mL of Hartmann's (larger volumes are preferred as the infused solution is then less acidic).

3. The solution should be clear and colourless to yellow. Inspect visually for particulate matter or discoloration prior to administration and discard if present.
4. Give by IV infusion over 15 minutes approximately 30 minutes prior to anthracycline dose.

## Intermittent intravenous infusion (Savene)

See Special handling below.

*Preparation and administration*

1. Remove cooling measures such as ice packs from the affected area at least 15 minutes before administration to allow sufficient blood flow.
2. Reconstitute each vial with 25 mL WFI to give a concentration of 20 mg/mL. The reconstituted solution is slightly yellow.
3. Withdraw the required dose of dexrazoxane and add to the 500 mL of the Savene diluent provided.
4. The solution should be clear and colourless to yellow. Inspect visually for particulate matter or discoloration prior to administration and discard if present.
5. Give by IV infusion over 1–2 hours into a large vein in an area other than the one affected by the extravasation.

## Technical information

| | |
|---|---|
| Incompatible with | No information, but do not mix dexrazoxane with other drugs during infusion. |
| Compatible with | **Flush**: NaCl 0.9%<br>**Solutions**: Hartmann's (for Savene use diluent supplied)<br>**Y-site**: No information |
| pH | 1.6 for reconstituted vials which becomes less acidic upon dilution. |
| Sodium content | Cardioxane: Nil<br>Savene: Diluent contains 70 mmol/500 mL |
| Storage | Store below 25°C in original packaging. |
| Displacement value | Negligible |
| Special handling | Dexrazoxane should not be handled by pregnant staff and it is recommended that gloves and other protective clothing are worn to prevent skin contact. Any contact with skin or mucous membranes should be washed immediately and thoroughly with water. |
| Stability after preparation | Reconstituted vials should be used immediately.<br>From a microbiological point of view, prepared infusions should be used immediately; however, they may be stored at 2-8°C and infused (at room temperature) within 4 hours. |

## Monitoring

| Measure | Frequency | Rationale |
|---|---|---|
| FBC | During each course of therapy | • Dexrazoxane and the chemotherapeutic regimen have myelosuppressive effects. |
| LFTs | | • ↑ALT, ↑AST and ↑bilirubin occur only rarely. |
| Renal function and serum Na and K | | • Dose may need reducing if renal impairment develops.<br>• 500 mL of Savene diluent contains 2.5 mmol K and 70 mmol Na.<br>• Patients at risk of ↑K or on low-sodium diets should be closely monitored. |
| Cardiac function:<br>• left-ventricular ejection fraction (LVEF)<br>• symptoms of congestive cardiac failure<br>• ECG changes | If symptoms warrant concern | • Dexrazoxane does not eliminate the risk of cardiotoxicity.<br>• Declines from baseline in LVEF of 10-20% or greater or declines in LVEF to 5% or more below the lower limit of normal for the organisation may indicate anthracycline toxicity.<br>• Symptoms of congestive heart failure such as shortness of breath, basilar rales, S3 gallop, paroxysmal nocturnal dyspnoea, orthopnoea, dyspnoea on exertion or cardiomegaly may indicate anthracycline toxicity.<br>• If the absolute QRS voltage of the 6 limb leads decreases by greater than 30%, the anthracycline should be discontinued. |
| Symptoms of thromboembolic disease | If symptoms warrant concern | • Combination of dexrazoxane with chemotherapy may ↑risk of thromboembolism. |

## Additional information

| | |
|---|---|
| Common and serious undesirable effects | *Infusion-related:* Local: Injection-site pain, phlebitis, erythema, swelling, induration.<br>*Other:* The following may be due to concurrent cytotoxic therapy: nausea, vomiting, dyspepsia, abdominal pain, diarrhoea, stomatitis, dry mouth, anorexia, dizziness, syncope, asthenia, paraesthesia, tremor, fatigue, drowsiness, pyrexia; myalgia; bone-marrow suppression, conjunctivitis; alopecia, pruritus, peripheral oedema. |
| Pharmacokinetics | Elimination half-life is 2-4 hours. |
| Significant interactions | • Dexrazoxane may ↑levels or effect of the following drugs (or ↑side-effects): live attenuated vaccines including yellow fever vaccine (avoid combination), oral anticoagulants (↑monitoring), phenytoin (avoid combination), dimethyl sulfoxide (avoid combination).<br>• Caution with ciclosporin and tacrolimus (excessive immunosuppression carries risk of lymphoproliferative disease). |

*(continued)*

| **Additional information** (*continued*) | |
|---|---|
| Action in case of overdose | *Antidote:* There is no known antidote.<br>Stop administration and give supportive therapy as appropriate. |
| Counselling | Both sexually active men and women should use effective methods of contraception during treatment. Additionally, men should use contraception for at least 3 months after treatment has ceased. |

| Risk rating: **AMBER** | Score = 5<br>Moderate-risk product: Risk-reduction strategies are recommended. |
|---|---|

This assessment is based on the full range of preparation and administration options described in the monograph. These may not all be applicable in some clinical situations.

## Bibliography

SPC Cardioxane 500 mg powder for solution for infusion (accessed 16 March 2009).
SPC Savene 20 mg/mL powder for concentrate and diluent for solution for infusion. www.savene.com/multimedia/SaveneSPC28July2006v2.pdf (accessed 16 March 2009).

# Dextran 70

**Dextran 70 6% in NaCl 7.5% solution in 250-mL infusion bag**

* Dextran 70 is a colloidal plasma substitute that contains large molecules that do not readily leave the intravascular space, where they exert osmotic pressure to maintain circulatory volume. It exerts a colloidal osmotic pressure similar to that of plasma proteins and in comparison with crystalloids, smaller volumes are required to produce the same expansion of blood volume.
* It is used in the initial treatment of hypovolaemia with ↓BP induced by traumatic injury (after primary stabilisation of respiration and bleeding)

## Pre-treatment checks (not all are necessary in an emergency situation)

As this product is often used in acute, emergency settings, e.g. ambulance crews attending stab victims, it is probable that these pre-treatment checks will not be feasible in most instances.

* Caution in those patients likely to develop circulatory overload such as congestive cardiac failure, renal failure and pulmonary oedema.

- Caution also in those patients at risk of liver disease and bleeding disorders (NB: the amount of dextran 70 contained in a 250-mL dose is not likely to affect haemostasis, since changes in haemostatic variables only occur at doses above 1.5 g/kg bodyweight. Aggressive fluid resuscitation can, however, dilute blood clotting factors to such an extent that a bleeding diathesis occurs).
- Hypertonic solutions should be used with caution in patients with diabetes mellitus having severe hyperglycaemia with hyperosmolality.

*Biochemical and other tests (not all are necessary in an emergency situation)*

Blood pressure
Electrolytes: serum Na, K
FBC

Hydration status
Renal function: U, Cr

## Dose

**Initial treatment of hypovolaemia with hypotension induced by traumatic injury**: 250 mL followed immediately by the administration of appropriate isotonic replacement fluids, dosed according to the needs of the patient.

## Intravenous infusion

*Preparation and administration*

1. The infusion is pre-prepared for use. It should be clear and colourless. Inspect visually for particulate matter or discoloration prior to administration and discard if present.
2. Give the full dose by rapid IV infusion over 2–5 minutes.
3. Discard any unused portion. Do not reconnect partially used infusion containers.
4. Follow immediately by the administration of appropriate isotonic replacement fluids.

| Technical information | |
|---|---|
| Incompatible with | No information |
| Compatible with | **Flush**: NaCl 0.9%<br>**Solutions**: Not relevant<br>**Y-site**: Not relevant |
| pH | 3.5-7 |
| Sodium content | 250 mL contains approximately 320 mmol of Na and Cl. |
| Osmolarity<br>(Plasma osmolality =<br>280-300 mOsmol/L)[1] | Rescue flow ≅ 2500 mOsmol/L. |
| Storage | No special precautions for storage |

## Monitoring

| Measure | Frequency | Rationale |
|---|---|---|
| Renal function, serum Na and K, and acid-base balance | Throughout treatment | • Close monitoring is required at all times as the patient's condition is likely to be unstable.<br>• All aspects of fluid and volume replacement need to be taken into account.<br>• Dehydration should be corrected as soon as possible and adequate amounts of fluid provided daily. |
| Urine output | | • Monitor for oliguria or renal failure. |
| FBC and coagulation screen | | • Adequate haematocrit should be maintained and not allowed to fall below 25-30%, early signs of bleeding complications should be observed for.<br>• Dilutional effects upon coagulation should be avoided.<br>• Coagulation factor deficiencies should be corrected. |
| Haemorrhage | | • ↑Risk with aggressive fluid resuscitation and ↑perfusion pressures. |
| Signs of anaphylaxis | | • Severe anaphylaxis has occurred, early signs of which are severe ↓BP, respiratory or cardiac arrest. |
| CVP (and signs of circulatory overload) | | • Monitoring of CVP during the initial period of infusion will aid the detection of fluid overload. |
| Serum osmolarity | | • Hyperosmolarity can occur particularly with hypertonic solutions and in diabetic patients. |

## Additional information

| | |
|---|---|
| Common and serious undesirable effects | *Immediate:* Hypersensitivity reactions may occur such as fever, nasal congestion, joint pains, urticaria, ↓BP, bronchospasm, and rarely, severe anaphylactoid reactions.<br>*Other transient:* ↑Bleeding time. Nausea and vomiting. |
| Pharmacokinetics | Elimination half-life is 6-8 hours. After infusion of 250 mL, serum Na increases by 9-12 mmol and returns to normal in less than 4 hours. |
| Significant interactions | • Dextran may affect the following tests:<br>blood cross-matching, biochemical measurements (glucose, bilirubin, or protein). |
| Action in case of overdose | *Symptoms to watch for:* ↑Na may occur with hypertonic solutions.<br>*Antidote:* Give supportive therapy as appropriate. |

| Risk rating: **GREEN** | Score = 2<br>Lower-risk product: Risk-reduction strategies should be considered. |
|---|---|

This assessment is based on the full range of preparation and administration options described in the monograph. These may not all be applicable in some clinical situations.

## Reference

1. Longmore M *et al.*, eds. *Oxford Handbook of Clinical Medicine*, 6th edn. Oxford: Oxford University Press, 2004.

## Bibliography

SPC RescueFlow solution for infusion, Vitaline Pharmaceuticals UK Ltd (accessed 6 May 2010).

# Diamorphine hydrochloride (diacetylmorphine hydrochloride, heroin)

### 5-mg and 10-mg dry powder in ampoules

* Diamorphine hydrochloride is a potent opioid analgesic. It is more potent than morphine with a faster onset and shorter duration of action. It is also more water-soluble, which is useful in palliative care as high doses can be given in a relatively small volume.
* It is used parenterally for the treatment of severe acute pain and may also be used to relieve dyspnoea in acute pulmonary oedema.
* Diamorphine may also be given by SC infusion in to control pain in palliative care.

### Pre-treatment checks

* Do not use in acute respiratory depression, where there is a risk of paralytic ileus, in raised intracranial pressure and in head injury, in comatose patients, in acute abdomen, in delayed gastric emptying, in chronic constipation, in cor pulmonale, in acute porphyria and in phaeochromocytoma.
* Caution in ↓BP, shock, convulsive disorders, supraventricular tachycardias, atrial flutter, chronic obstructive pulmonary disease and acute asthma attack, obstructive or inflammatory bowel diseases, biliary tract diseases, alcoholism, prostatic hyperplasia, myasthenia gravis, hypothyroidism (reduce dose), adrenocortical insufficiency (reduce dose).
* Caution in toxic psychosis, pancreatitis, severe diarrhoea and CNS depression.
* Ensure that resuscitation equipment and naloxone are available especially for IV administration.

*Biochemical and other tests (not all are necessary in an emergency situation)*

| | |
|---|---|
| Blood pressure and pulse | Renal function: U, Cr, CrCl (or eGFR) |
| Pain score | Respiratory rate |

## Dose

Doses above those stated must not be given to opioid naive patients.

**Acute pain:** 5 mg by SC or IM injection or 1.25–2.5 mg by slow IV injection every 4 hours when required (dose may be increased up to 10 mg for heavier patients with ↑muscle mass).

**Chronic pain:** 5–10 mg by SC or IM injection regularly every 4 hours adjusted according to requirements. Initial dose is dependent on previous opioid exposure.

**Myocardial infarction:** 5 mg by slow IV injection, then a further 2.5–5 mg if required. Halve the dose in elderly or frail patients.

**Acute pulmonary oedema:** 2.5–5 mg by slow IV injection.

**Dose in renal impairment:** reduce dose or avoid.

**Dose in hepatic impairment:** reduce dose or avoid.

### Subcutaneous injection

*Preparation and administration*

Check that you have selected the correct strength of ampoule. High-strength ampoules, i.e. 30-mg, 100-mg and 500-mg, are available for use in palliative care. These are not suitable for use in acute situations.

1. Reconstitute the ampoule with 1 mL WFI.
2. Withdraw the required dose.
3. Give by SC injection.
4. Close monitoring of respiratory rate and consciousness is recommended for 30 minutes in patients receiving the initial dose, especially elderly patients or those of low bodyweight.

### Intramuscular injection

*Preparation and administration*

Check that you have selected the correct strength of ampoule. High-strength ampoules, i.e. 30-mg, 100-mg and 500-mg, are available for use in palliative care. These are not suitable for use in acute situations.

1. Reconstitute the ampoule with 1 mL WFI.
2. Withdraw the required dose.
3. Give by IM injection.
4. Close monitoring of respiratory rate and consciousness is recommended for 30 minutes in patients receiving the initial dose, especially elderly patients or those of low bodyweight.

### Intravenous injection

*Preparation and administration*

Check that you have selected the correct strength of ampoule. High-strength ampoules, i.e. 30-mg, 100-mg and 500-mg, are available for use in palliative care. These are not suitable for use in acute situations.

1. Reconstitute the ampoule with 1 mL WFI.
2. Withdraw the required dose. It may be further diluted with NaCl 0.9% or Gluc 5% to facilitate slow administration.

*(continued)*

3. The solution should be clear and colourless. Inspect visually for particulate matter or discoloration prior to administration and discard if present.
4. Give by slow IV injection at a maximum rate of 1 mg/minute.
5. Close monitoring of respiratory rate and consciousness is recommended for 30 minutes in patients receiving the initial dose, especially elderly patients or those of low bodyweight.

## Technical information

| Incompatible with | Stability is dependent upon concentrations. |
|---|---|
| Compatible with | **Flush**: NaCl 0.9%<br>**Solutions**: Gluc 5% (preferred), NaCl 0.9%<br>**Y-site**: Flucloxacillin, furosemide, metoclopramide, midazolam |
| pH | 3.8-4.4 |
| Sodium content | Nil |
| Storage | Store below 25°C in original packaging. Controlled Drug. |
| Displacement volume | Negligible |
| Stability after preparation | From a microbiological point of view, should be used immediately; however, prepared infusions may be stored at 2-8°C and infused (at room temperature) within 24 hours. |

## Monitoring

Close monitoring of respiratory rate and consciousness is recommended for 30 minutes in patients receiving initial dose, especially elderly patients or those of low bodyweight.

| Measure | Frequency | Rationale |
|---|---|---|
| Pain or dyspnoea | At regular intervals | • To ensure therapeutic response. |
| Blood pressure, pulse and respiratory rate | | • ↓BP, ↑ or ↓pulse, palpitations and respiratory depression can occur. |
| Sedation | | • May cause sedation. |
| Monitor for side-effects and toxicity | | • May cause side-effects such as nausea and constipation, which may need treating. |

## Additional information

| Common and serious undesirable effects | *Immediate:* Anaphylaxis has been reported following IV injection.<br>*Common:* Nausea and vomiting (particularly initially), constipation, dry mouth, urticaria, pruritus, biliary spasm, ↑ or ↓pulse, hallucinations, euphoria, drowsiness.<br>*At higher doses:* ↓BP, sedation, respiratory depression, muscle rigidity. |
|---|---|
| Pharmacokinetics | Peak analgesic response: 10-20 minutes by IV injection; 30-70 minutes by IM injection.<br>Duration of action is 3-4 hours.<br>Elimination half-life is 2-3 minutes (active metabolites: 2-3 hours). |

*(continued)*

## Additional information (continued)

| | |
|---|---|
| Significant interactions | • The following may ↑diamorphine levels or effect (or ↑side-effects) of: antihistamines-sedating (↑sedation), MAOIs (avoid combination and for 2 weeks after stopping MAOI), moclobemide.<br>• Diamorphine may ↑levels or effect (or ↑side-effects) of sodium oxybate (avoid combination). |
| Action in case of overdose | *Symptoms to watch for:* ↑Sedation, respiratory depression.<br>*Antidote:* naloxone (see the Naloxone monograph).<br>Stop administration and give supportive therapy as appropriate. |
| Counselling | May cause drowsiness which may affect the ability to perform skilled tasks; if affected do not drive or operate machinery, avoid alcoholic drink (effects of alcohol are enhanced).<br>Inform the patient of possible side-effects: see above.<br>Drink plenty of fluids if appropriate to help avoid constipation. |

Risk rating: **AMBER**     Score = 3
Moderate-risk product: Risk-reduction strategies are recommended.

This assessment is based on the full range of preparation and administration options described in the monograph. These may not all be applicable in some clinical situations.

## Bibliography

SPC Diamorphine Hydrochloride injection BP 100 mg, Auralis (accessed 30 May 2009).

SPC Diamorphine Hydrochloride BP for injection 10 mg and 30 mg, Novartis Vaccines (accessed 30 May 2009).

SPC Diamorphine Injection BP 5 mg, 10 mg, 30 mg, 100 mg, and 500 mg, Wockhardt UK Ltd (accessed 30 May 2009).

# Diazepam emulsion

**5 mg/mL emulsion in 2-mL ampoules**

Diazepam emulsion contains diazepam dissolved in the oil phase of an oil in water emulsion and should not be confused with diazepam solution (see the Diazepam solution monograph).

* Diazepam is a long-acting benzodiazepine with anxiolytic, anticonvulsant and central muscle relaxant properties.
* Diazepam emulsion is used to provide sedation prior to procedures such as endoscopy, as a pre-medication before general anaesthesia, to control acute muscle spasms (e.g. from poisoning) or convulsions (status epilepticus) and to manage severe acute anxiety or agitation.

## Pre-treatment checks

* Avoid in acute porphyria or respiratory depression.
* Caution in patients with pulmonary insufficiency or myasthenia gravis.
* Caution in patients with impaired renal and hepatic function (avoid in severe hepatic impairment).

*Biochemical and other tests (not all are necessary in an emergency situation)*

Bodyweight                              Renal function: U, Cr, CrCl (or eGFR)
LFTs                                    Respiratory rate

## Dose

**Sedation prior to minor surgical or dental procedures:** 100–200 micrograms/kg by IV injection. Usual adult dose 10–20 mg.
**Premedication:** 100–200 micrograms/kg by IV injection.
**Status epilepticus and convulsions due to poisoning:** 10 mg by slow IV injection, repeated if necessary after 10 minutes. Once the seizure is controlled, recurrence may be prevented by a slow IV infusion (maximum total dose 3 mg/kg over 24 hours). Reduce dose on prolonged use to ↓risk of accumulation and CNS depression.
**Severe acute anxiety, acute muscle spasm (including tetanus) and acute states of excitement, delirium tremens:** 10 mg by IV injection repeated after 4 hours if necessary.

### Intravenous injection

*Preparation and administration*

Diazepam emulsion is incompatible with NaCl 0.9% (but may be injected into drip tubing containing NaCl 0.9%).

1. Withdraw the required dose.
2. The preparation is a milky white emulsion. Inspect visually for particulate matter or discoloration prior to administration and discard if present.
3. Give by slow IV injection (maximum rate 5 mg/minute) into a large vein to avoid thrombosis.

### Continuous intravenous infusion

*Preparation and administration*

Diazepam emulsion is incompatible with NaCl 0.9%.

1. Withdraw the required dose (bearing in mind that the prepared infusion is only stable for a maximum of 6 hours).
2. Add to a suitable volume of compatible infusion fluid (usually Gluc 5%) to give a final concentration in the range 100–400 micrograms/mL (i.e. 2–8 mL of diazepam emulsion per 100 mL). Mix well.
3. The preparation is a milky white emulsion. Inspect visually for particulate matter or discoloration prior to administration and discard if present.
4. Give by IV infusion via a volumetric infusion device or syringe pump at an appropriate rate.
5. Prepare a fresh infusion at least every 6 hours if required.

## Technical information

| | |
|---|---|
| Incompatible with | Diazepam emulsion is incompatible with NaCl 0.9% (but may be injected into drip tubing containing NaCl 0.9%). |
| Compatible with | **Flush**: Gluc 5%, NaCl 0.9%<br>**Solutions**: Gluc 5%, Gluc 10%, Intralipid 10%, Intralipid 20%<br>**Y-site**: No information |
| pH | 8 |
| Sodium content | Negligible |
| Excipients | Contains fractionated soy bean oil, fractionated egg phospholipids. |
| Storage | Store below 25°C in original packaging. Do not freeze. |
| Stability after preparation | Use prepared infusions immediately and discard 6 hours after preparation. |

## Monitoring

| Measure | Frequency | Rationale |
|---|---|---|
| Respiratory rate | Baseline and at regular intervals | • To ensure that severe respiratory depression does not occur. |
| Clinical improvement | Post administration | • To ensure that treatment is effective. |
| FBC | With long-term therapy | • May cause blood dyscrasias. |
| LFTs | | • Liver enzymes may be elevated. |

## Additional information

| | |
|---|---|
| Common and serious undesirable effects | *Immediate:* Anaphylaxis and other hypersensitivity reactions have been reported.<br>*Injection/infusion-related:* Local: Thrombophlebitis, painless erythematous rash round the site of injection, which has resolved in 1-2 days.<br>*Other:* Sedation, drowsiness, unsteadiness, ataxia, urticaria. |
| Pharmacokinetics | The elimination half-life of diazepam is 24-48 hours but its action is further prolonged by the longer elimination half-life (2-5 days) of the main active metabolite, desmethyldiazepam. |
| Significant interactions | • The following may ↑diazepam levels or effect (or ↑side-effects): olanzapine IM (↓BP, ↓pulse, respiratory depression), ritonavir.<br>• Diazepam may ↑levels or effect (or ↑side-effects) of sodium oxybate (avoid combination). |
| Action in case of overdose | *Symptoms to watch for:* ↑sedation, respiratory depression, ↓BP.<br>*Antidote:* Flumaxenil (use with caution in patients with a history of seizures, head injury or chronic benzodiazepine use including for the control of epilepsy). (See Flumazenil monograph.)<br>Stop administration and give supportive therapy as appropriate. |

*(continued)*

## Additional information (continued)

| | |
|---|---|
| Counselling | If applicable the patient should be accompanied home by a responsible adult and should not drive or operate machinery for 24 hours. |

| Risk rating: **AMBER** | Score = 4<br>Moderate-risk product: Risk-reduction strategies are recommended. |
|---|---|

This assessment is based on the full range of preparation and administration options described in the monograph. These may not all be applicable in some clinical situations.

## Bibliography

SPC Diazemuls (accessed 21 May 2008).

# Diazepam solution

**5 mg/mL solution in 2-mL ampoules**

Diazepam solution contains diazepam dissolved in an aqueous medium and should not be confused with diazepam emulsion (see the Diazepam emulsion monograph).

* Diazepam is a long-acting benzodiazepine with anxiolytic, anticonvulsant and central muscle relaxant properties.
* It is used parenterally to provide sedation prior to procedures such as endoscopy, to control acute muscle spasms (e.g. from poisoning) or convulsions (status epilepticus) and to manage severe acute anxiety or agitation.

## Pre-treatment checks

* Avoid in acute porphyria, respiratory depression.
* Caution in patients with pulmonary insufficiency or myasthenia gravis.
* Caution in patients with impaired renal and hepatic function (avoid in severe hepatic impairment).

*Biochemical and other tests (not all are necessary in an emergency situation)*

Bodyweight                                    Renal function: U, Cr, CrCl (or eGFR)
LFTs                                          Respiratory rate

## Dose

**Sedation prior to minor surgical or dental procedures:** 100–200 micrograms/kg by IV injection. Usual adult dose 10–20 mg.

**Status epilepticus and convulsions due to poisoning:** 10 mg by slow IV injection, repeated if necessary after 10 minutes. Once the seizure is controlled, recurrence may be prevented by a slow IV infusion (maximum total dose 3 mg/kg over 24 hours). Reduce the dose on prolonged use to ↓risk of accumulation and CNS depression.

**Severe acute anxiety, acute muscle spasm (including tetanus) and acute states of excitement, delirium tremens:** 10 mg by IV injection repeated after 4 hours if necessary.

## Intravenous injection

*Preparation and administration*

1. Withdraw the required dose.
2. The solution should be clear and colourless to pale yellow. Inspect visually for particulate matter or discoloration prior to administration and discard if present.
3. Give by slow IV injection (maximum rate 5 mg/minute) into a large vein to avoid thrombosis.

## Intramuscular injection (use only if oral or IV route not possible)

*Preparation and administration*

1. Withdraw the required dose.
2. Give by IM injection.

## Continuous intravenous infusion

**Not recommended.** Diazepam emulsion (see separate monograph) is the preferred preparation for IV infusion because it forms a more stable preparation and is also less irritant to veins. It can therefore be given in more concentrated infusion solutions, thus facilitating the administration of higher doses.

PVC containers and giving sets should not be used – more than 50% of the dose may be adsorbed. Glass or polyethylene should be used in preference.

*Preparation and administration*

1. Withdraw the required dose of diazepam solution (bearing in mind that stability data are limited and that several shorter infusions would be better than a single 24-hour infusion).
2. Add each 10 mg to at least 200 mL NaCl 0.9% or Gluc 5%. Mix well.
3. The solution should be clear and colourless to pale yellow. Inspect visually for particulate matter or discoloration prior to administration and discard if present.
4. Give by continuous IV infusion via a volumetric infusion device.

## Technical information

| | |
|---|---|
| Incompatible with | PVC containers and giving sets should not be used - more than 50% of the dose may be adsorbed. Glass or polyethylene should be used in preference. Potassium chloride. Amphotericin, atracurium, cisatracurium, dobutamine, flucloxacillin, foscarnet, furosemide, heparin sodium, linezolid, meropenem, Pabrinex, propofol, remifentanil, vecuronium bromide. |
| Compatible with | **Flush**: NaCl 0.9% <br> **Solutions**: NaCl 0.9%, Gluc 5% <br> **Y-site**: No information |
| pH | 6.2-6.9 |

(continued)

## Technical information (*continued*)

| | |
|---|---|
| Sodium content | Negligible |
| Excipients | Contains benzyl alcohol, ethanol and propylene glycol (adverse effects seen if renal elimination is impaired and may interact with disulfiram and metronidazole). |
| Storage | Store below 25°C in original packaging. The solution should be colourless to pale yellow. Discoloured solutions are degraded and should not be used. |
| Stability after preparation | If diazepam solution must be given by infusion (but see information above), use prepared infusions immediately. Stability is dependent on container, fluid, concentration and giving set and is difficult to predict. |

## Monitoring

| Measure | Frequency | Rationale |
|---|---|---|
| Respiratory rate | Baseline and at regular intervals | • To ensure that severe respiratory depression does not occur. |
| Clinical improvement | Post administration | • To ensure that treatment is effective. |
| FBC | With long-term therapy | • May cause blood dyscrasias. |
| LFTs | | • Liver enzymes may be elevated. |

## Additional information

| | |
|---|---|
| Common and serious undesirable effects | *Immediate:* Anaphylaxis and other hypersensitivity reactions have been reported.<br>*Injection/infusion-related:* Local: Thrombophlebitis, painless erythematous rash round the site of injection, which has resolved in 1-2 days.<br>*Other:* Sedation, drowsiness, unsteadiness, ataxia, urticaria. |
| Pharmacokinetics | The elimination half-life of diazepam is 24-48 hours but its action is further prolonged by the longer half-life (2-5 days) of the main active metabolite, desmethyldiazepam. |
| Significant interactions | • The following may ↑diazepam levels or effect (or ↑side-effects): olanzapine IM (↓BP, ↓pulse, respiratory depression), ritonavir.<br>• Diazepam may ↑levels or effect (or ↑side-effects) of sodium oxybate (avoid combination).<br>Injectable preparation contains ethanol and propylene glycol: may interact with disulfiram and metronidazole. |
| Action in case of overdose | *Symptoms to watch for:* ↑Sedation, respiratory depression, ↓BP.<br>*Antidote:* Flumazenil (use with caution in patients with a history of seizures, head injury or chronic benzodiazepine use including for the control of epilepsy). (See Flumazenil monograph.)<br>Stop administration and give supportive therapy as appropriate. |
| Counselling | If applicable, the patient should be accompanied home by a responsible adult and should not drive or operate machinery for 24 hours. |

| Risk rating: **AMBER** | Score = 3 Moderate-risk product: Risk-reduction strategies are recommended. |
| --- | --- |

This assessment is based on the full range of preparation and administration options described in the monograph. These may not all be applicable in some clinical situations.

## Bibliography

SPC Diazepam 5 mg/mL solution for injection, Wockhardt UK Ltd (accessed 21 May 2008).

# Diazoxide

### 15 mg/mL solution in 20-mL ampoules

- Diazoxide is a benzothiadizine analogue and is related structurally to the thiazide diuretics.
- It has been used in the management of hypertensive emergencies when first-line drugs such as sodium nitroprusside or hydralazine are ineffective or unsuitable. Adverse effects are pronounced and the BNF identifies the drug as less suitable for use.
- IV injection produces a prompt reduction in BP by relaxing smooth muscle in the peripheral arterioles. Cardiac output is increased as BP is reduced; coronary and cerebral blood flow are maintained. Renal blood flow is increased after an initial decrease.

### Pre-treatment checks

- Diazoxide is not recommended for use in ↑BP due to mechanical abnormality, e.g. aortic coarctation or AV shunt.
- Caution in patients in whom retention of Na and water or abrupt reductions in BP may be hazardous, e.g. those with impaired cardiac or cerebral circulation.

*Biochemical and other tests*

Bodyweight
Blood pressure

Electrolytes: serum Na
Renal function: U, Cr, CrCl (or eGFR)

### Dose

**Standard dose:** 1–3 mg/kg by rapid IV injection up to a maximum single dose of 150 mg; may be repeated after 5–15 minutes if required. Repeated administration at 4–24 hour intervals is generally sufficient to maintain BP below pre-treatment levels. Oral antihypertensive agents should replace therapy as soon as adequate BP control has been achieved.

**Dose in renal impairment:** use with caution if CrCl <10 mL/minute.

## Intravenous injection

See Spillage precautions below.

*Preparation and administration*

1. Withdraw the required dose.
2. The solution should be clear and colourless. Inspect visually for particulate matter or discoloration prior to administration and discard if present.
3. The patient should be lying down.
4. Give by rapid IV injection over no more than 30 seconds (slow administration reduces the antihypertensive response). Use a cannula for administration, taking care to avoid extravasation.
5. Patients should remain supine during, immediately following and, preferably, for at least 1 hour after IV dosing.

## Technical information

| | |
|---|---|
| Incompatible with | Not relevant |
| Compatible with | **Flush**: NaCl 0.9%<br>**Solutions**: Diazoxide injection should not be diluted<br>**Y-site**: Not relevant |
| pH | 11.6 |
| Sodium content | Negligible |
| Storage | Store below 30°C in original packaging. Darkened solutions may be sub potent and should not be used. |
| Spillage | Solution is alkaline; use protective measures. |

## Monitoring

| Measure | Frequency | Rationale |
|---|---|---|
| Blood pressure | Continuous initially, reducing to every 15–30 minutes | • Monitor response; maximum hypotensive effects generally occur within less than 5 minutes. BP usually rises rapidly over the next 10–20 minutes, followed by a more gradual increase as pretreatment levels are approached.<br>• The initial goal of therapy is to ↓mean arterial BP by no more than 25% within minutes to 1 hour, followed by further reduction if stable toward 160/100–110 mmHg within the next 2–6 hours, avoiding excessive declines in pressure that could precipitate renal, cerebral, or coronary ischaemia.<br>• In ambulatory patients, standing BP should also be measured before monitoring of the patient is completed. |
| Injection site | Half hourly | • If diazoxide injection leaks into SC tissue, the area should be treated with warm compresses or other palliative measures. Seek advice. |

*(continued)*

## Monitoring (continued)

| Measure | Frequency | Rationale |
|---------|-----------|-----------|
| Renal function, serum Na and hydration status | At least daily | • Water and Na retention may occur especially after repeated doses and co-administration of diuretic, e.g. furosemide may be required. |
| Blood glucose | | • Hyperglycaemia; may be severe in patients with pre-existing carbohydrate metabolic disorders. Consider use of oral hypoglycaemic agents or insulin. |
| Serum uric acid (in patients with history of hyperuricaemia of gout) | If therapy >24 hours | • May cause hyperuricaemia. |
| ECG and CNS | If symptoms warrant | • Myocardial and/or cerebral ischaemia, which are usually transient, may occur in patients receiving IV diazoxide and may lead to thrombosis.<br>• Myocardial ischaemia may be manifested by angina, atrial and/or ventricular arrhythmias, and marked ECG changes. |

## Additional information

| | |
|---|---|
| Common and serious undesirable effects | *Injection/infusion-related:* Local: Extravasation causes tissue damage. *Other:* Reflex ↑pulse, ↓BP, hyperglycaemia, Na and water retention. Single doses of 300 mg have been associated with angina and with myocardial and cerebral infarction. |
| Pharmacokinetics | Plasma elimination half-life ranges from about 20–45 hours but values of up to 60 hours have been reported and may be prolonged in renal impairment.<br>A response usually occurs within 5 minutes and usually persists for up to 4 hours. Plasma half-life is at least 3 times longer than the hypotensive action, so accumulation is likely. |
| Significant interactions | No significant interactions. |
| Action in case of overdose | Give supportive therapy as appropriate. |
| Counselling | Patients should be warned to expect pain or a feeling of warmth along the injected vein and to report severe sensations. |

| Risk rating: **GREEN** | Score = 1<br>Lower-risk product. Risk-reduction strategies should be considered. |
|---|---|

This assessment is based on the full range of preparation and administration options described in the monograph. These may not all be applicable in some clinical situations.

## Bibliography

SPC Eudemine injection (accessed 20 April 2010).

# Diclofenac sodium

**25 mg/mL solution in 3-mL ampoules; 37.5 mg/mL solution in 2-mL ampoules (Dyloject)**

There are different formulations of diclofenac injectable: not all products are licensed for all indications or all routes (check product literature).

* Diclofenac sodium is a non-steroidal anti-inflammatory drug (NSAID).
* The injection form is used to treat acute pain and for treatment or prevention of postoperative pain. Maximum duration of parenteral treatment is 48 hours; oral or rectal therapy should be instituted as soon as possible if necessary.
* Parenteral administration gives rise to a 2-fold increase in bioavailability compared with oral and rectal administration as it avoids first-pass metabolism; the active substance is 99.7% protein bound.

## Pre-treatment checks

* Avoid in patients with active peptic ulceration, history of recurrent ulceration, or GI bleeding or perforation related to previous NSAID therapy, patients with severe heart failure, patients who have had asthma induced by aspirin or other NSAIDs, nasal polyps, angioedema or urticaria.
* Do not give to patients with severe hepatic or renal failure.
* In addition if using the IV route do not give:
  * If the patient is already taking a NSAID or anticoagulant (including low-dose heparin).
  * If the patient has a history of haemorrhagic diathesis, a history of confirmed or suspected cerebrovascular bleeding.
  * In operations associated with a high risk of haemorrhage.
  * When there is a history of asthma.
  * In moderate or severe renal impairment (serum creatinine >160 micromol/L).
  * In hypovolaemia or dehydration from any cause.

*Biochemical and other tests (not all are necessary in an emergency situation)*

| | |
|---|---|
| Blood pressure | LFTs |
| FBC | Renal function: U, Cr, CrCl (or eGFR) |

## Dose

The total daily dose of diclofenac is 150 mg by any route.

**For acute exacerbations of pain and postoperative pain:** 75 mg by IM injection once daily (twice daily in severe pain) for a maximum of 48 hours.
**For renal colic:** 75 mg by IM injection repeated once after 30 minutes if required.

**IV use in acute postoperative pain:**

- *Voltarol and Goldshield preparations (IV* **injection** *only):* 75 mg by IV infusion over 30–120 minutes, repeated after 4–6 hours if necessary to a maximum dose of 150 mg in 24 hours. Alternatively, give 25–50 mg by IV infusion over 15–60 minutes followed by a continuous IV infusion of 5 mg/hour up to a maximum dose of 150 mg in 24 hours.
- *Dyloject (IV* **injection** *only):* 75 mg by IV injection, repeated after 4–6 hours if necessary to a maximum dose of 150 mg in 24 hours. Alternatively, give 25–50 mg by IV injection followed by additional IV injections up to a maximum dose of 150 mg in 24 hours.

**Dose in renal impairment**: adjusted according to creatinine clearance:[1]

- CrCl >20–50 mL/minute: dose as in normal renal function.
- CrCl 10–20 mL/minute: dose as in normal renal function but avoid if possible.
- CrCl <10 mL/minute: dose as in normal renal function but only use if end-stage renal failure on dialysis.

## Intramuscular injection

*Preparation and administration*

1. Withdraw the required dose.
2. Give by deep IM injection into the upper outer quadrant of the gluteal muscle, taking care to avoid the sciatic nerve and also inadvertent SC injection. If a second injection is required, use the alternate buttock.

## Intermittent or continuous intravenous infusion

For dilution of Voltarol and Goldshield products, NaCl 0.9% or Gluc 5% must be buffered with sodium bicarbonate before use (see below). Dyloject is not licensed for use by IV infusion.

*Preparation and administration*

1. Select an infusion bag containing 100–500 mL of NaCl 0.9% or Gluc 5% and add 0.5 mL sodium bicarbonate 8.4% or 1 mL sodium bicarbonate 4.2% to buffer the solution. Mix well.
2. Withdraw the required dose of diclofenac and add to the previously buffered infusion fluid. Mix well.
3. The solution should be clear and colourless to faintly yellow. Inspect visually for particulate matter or discoloration prior to administration and discard if present.
4. Give by IV infusion over 30–120 minutes or continuously depending upon indication.

## Intravenous injection

Dyloject brand only.

*Preparation and administration*

1. Withdraw the required dose.
2. The solution should be clear and colourless. Inspect visually for particulate matter or discoloration prior to administration and discard if present.
3. Give by IV injection over 5–60 seconds.

| Technical information | |
|---|---|
| Incompatible with | No information |
| Compatible with | **Flush**: NaCl 0.9%<br>**Solutions**: NaCl 0.9%, Gluc 5%<br>**Y-site**: No information but likely to be unstable |

*(continued)*

## Technical information (*continued*)

| | |
|---|---|
| pH[2] | Voltarol 7.8-9.0 |
| Sodium content[2] | Negligible |
| Excipients | 25 mg/mL product (i.e. not Dyloject):<br>• Contains benzyl alcohol.<br>• Contains propylene glycol (adverse effects seen in ↓renal function, may interact with disulfiram and metronidazole).<br>• Contains sulfites (may cause hypersensitivity reactions). |
| Storage | Store below 30°C in original packaging. |
| Stability after preparation | Use prepared infusions immediately. |

## Monitoring

| Measure | Frequency | Rationale |
|---|---|---|
| Pain | Postoperatively or post treatment | • To ensure that treatment is effective. |
| Injection site | Post injection | • Phlebitis, injection-site reactions have occurred. |
| Blood pressure | Postoperative | • May cause ↑BP. |
| FBC, U&Es, LFTs | Periodically | • If on long-term NSAID treatment. |

## Additional information

| | |
|---|---|
| Common and serious undesirable effects | *Immediate:* Anaphylaxis and other hypersensitivity reactions may occur.<br>*Injection-related:* Local: Pain, induration, abscesses and tissue necrosis at site of IM injection. Thrombophlebitis following IV use.<br>*Other:* GI side-effects, skin reactions, oedema, ↑BP, cardiac failure, headache, dizziness, vertigo, ↑ALT and AST. |
| Pharmacokinetics | Elimination half-life is 1-2 hours. |
| Significant interactions | • The following may ↑risk of bleeding with diclofenac: antidepressants-SSRIs, aspirin, dabigatran, erlotinib, ketorolac, NSAIDs, venlafaxine.<br>• Diclofenac may ↑levels or effect of the following drugs (or ↑side-effects): ciclosporin (↑risk of nephrotoxicity), coumarin anticoagulants (monitor INR), lithium (monitor levels), methotrexate (↑toxicity, avoid combination), phenindione (monitor INR), phenytoin (monitor levels), quinolones (↑risk of seizures), sulfonylureas.<br>• Ciclosporin may ↑diclofenac levels or effect (or ↑side-effects): halve diclofenac dose. |
| Action in case of overdose | Give supportive therapy as appropriate. |

| Risk rating: **AMBER** | Score = 3<br>Moderate-risk product: Risk-reduction strategies are recommended. |
|---|---|

This assessment is based on the full range of preparation and administration options described in the monograph. These may not all be applicable in some clinical situations.

## Reference

1. Ashley C, Currie A, eds. *The Renal Drug Handbook*, 3rd edn. Oxford: Radcliffe Medical Press, 2009.
2. Personal communiqué, Novartis Pharmaceuticals UK Ltd,17 June 2009.

## Bibliography

SPC Voltarol ampoules (accessed 19 February 2010).
SPC Dyloject 75 mg/2 mL solution for injection (accessed 19 February 2010).

# Dicobalt edetate (cobalt edetate, cobalt EDTA)

### 300 mg/20 mL (1.5%) solution in 20-mL ampoules

- Dicobalt edetate is a specific antidote for cyanide poisoning. Its use arises from the property of cobalt salts to form a relatively non-toxic stable ion-complex with cyanide.

Dicobalt edetate is toxic and potentially fatal in the absence of cyanide poisoning. Use only if poisoning is confirmed and is moderate to severe (see below). It should only be given when the patient is tending to lose, or has lost, consciousness. It must never be used as a precautionary measure.

## Pre-treatment checks

- Must only be used in cases of confirmed severe cyanide poisoning. There is a reciprocal antidote action between cyanide and cobalt. Thus in the absence of cyanide, dicobalt edetate injection itself is toxic. If the patient is fully conscious, it is unlikely that the extent of poisoning warrants the use of dicobalt edetate injection.
- It is important to be aware whether any cyanide antidote therapy has been given in the pre-hospital setting since repeat doses of some antidotes can cause serious side-effects.

*Biochemical and other tests*

Nil

## Doses of cyanide poisoning antidotes[1] (see relevant entries)

It is essential to consult a poisons information service, e.g. Toxbase at www.toxbase.org (password or registration required) for full details of the management of cyanide toxicity.

**Mild poisoning** (nausea, dizziness, drowsiness, hyperventilation, anxiety):
* Observe.
* Give 12.5 g sodium thiosulfate (50 mL of 25% or 25 mL of 50% solution) IV over 10 minutes.

**Moderate poisoning** (reduced conscious level, vomiting, convulsions, ↓BP): as well as other supportive measures:
*If dicobalt edetate is available:*
* Give 300 mg (20 mL) of 1.5% dicobalt edetate solution IV over 1 minute.
* Follow immediately with 50 mL Gluc 50%.

*If dicobalt edetate is not available:*
* Give 12.5 g sodium thiosulfate (50 mL of 25% or 25 mL of 50% solution) IV over 10 minutes.

**Severe poisoning** (coma, fixed dilated pupils, cardiovascular collapse, respiratory failure, cyanosis):
*If dicobalt edetate is available:*
As well as other supportive measures:
* Give 300 mg (20 mL) of 1.5% dicobalt edetate solution IV over 1 minute.
* Follow immediately with 50 mL Gluc 50%.
* If there is only a partial response to dicobalt edetate 300 mg, or the patient relapses after recovery, give a further dose of dicobalt edetate 300 mg. If a second dose of dicobalt edetate is given, there is ↑risk of cobalt toxicity but only if the diagnosis is not cyanide poisoning.

*If dicobalt edetate is not available:*
As well as other supportive measures:
* Give 300 mg (10 mL) of 3% sodium nitrite solution IV over 5–20 minutes.
* Follow with 12.5 g sodium thiosulfate (50 mL of 25% or 25 mL of 50% solution) IV over 10 minutes.
* A further dose of sodium thiosulfate 12.5 g IV over 10 minutes may then be given.
* A second dose of sodium nitrite should **not** be given because of the risk of excessive methaemoglobinaemia.

## Intravenous injection

*Preparation and administration*

1. Withdraw the required dose.
2. The solution should be clear and rose-violet coloured. Inspect visually for particulate matter or discoloration prior to administration and discard if present.
3. Give by IV injection over 1 minute.
4. Administer Gluc 50% and sodium thiosulfate as specified above.

| Technical information | |
|---|---|
| Incompatible with | Not relevant |
| Compatible with | Not relevant |
| pH | 4–7.5 |
| Sodium content | Nil |
| Storage | Store below 25°C in original packaging. |

## Monitoring

| Measure | Frequency | Rationale |
|---------|-----------|-----------|
| Signs of hypersensitivity | Throughout treatment | • May cause anaphylactoid reactions, particularly in overdose (or in the absence of cyanide). <br> • Rashes may occur. |
| Blood pressure and pulse | | • ↓BP with compensatory ↑pulse may be seen. |
| ECG | | • Cardiac irregularities may be seen, particularly in overdose. |

## Additional information

| | |
|---|---|
| Common and serious undesirable effects | *Immediate:* Anaphylactic reactions including facial and laryngeal oedema (facilities for intubation and resuscitation should be immediately available). *Other:* ↓BP, compensatory ↑pulse and cardiac abnormalities; vomiting. |
| Pharmacokinetics | IV infusion of dicobalt edetate injection is likely to result in rapid distribution in the extracellular fluid compartment. Excretion is entirely via the kidneys within 24 hours. |
| Significant interactions | No information available. |
| Action in case of overdose | Give intensive supportive therapy as appropriate. |

| | |
|---|---|
| Risk rating: **GREEN** | Score = 1 <br> Lower-risk product: Risk-reduction strategies should be considered. |

This assessment is based on the full range of preparation and administration options described in the monograph. These may not all be applicable in some clinical situations.

## Reference

1. Toxbase at www.toxbase.org (accessed 1 May 2010).

## Bibliography

SPC Dicobalt edetate injection 300 mg (Cambridge Laboratories), Alliance Pharmaceuticals (accessed 19 January 2009).

# Digoxin

**250 micrograms/mL solution in 2-mL ampoules**

- Digoxin is a cardiac glycoside which increases force of myocardial contraction and reduces conduction through the AV node.
- It is used to treat cardiac failure and is used in the management of supraventricular arrhythmias, particularly chronic atrial flutter and fibrillation.
- The IV route may be used to administer an emergency loading dose in atrial fibrillation or flutter but often oral loading is effective.
- It may also be given IV where the enteral route is temporarily unavailable.

## Pre-treatment checks

- Avoid in intermittent complete heart block, second-degree AV block; supraventricular arrhythmias associated with accessory conducting pathways, e.g. Wolff–Parkinson–White syndrome; ventricular tachycardia or fibrillation; hypertrophic cardiomyopathy (unless concomitant atrial fibrillation and heart failure – but with caution).
- Avoid if ↓K or ↓Mg (risk of digoxin toxicity). A reduction in serum potassium concentration from 3.5 to 3.0 mmol/L is accompanied by an increase in sensitivity to digoxin of about 50% and digoxin toxicity may be present despite the serum digoxin concentration being in the apparent therapeutic range.[1]
- Caution following recent MI; sick sinus syndrome; thyroid disease and pregnancy.
- Reduce the dose in elderly patients and in renal impairment.
- Withhold for 24 hours before elective cardioversion.

*Biochemical and other tests (not all are necessary in an emergency situation)*

| | |
|---|---|
| Electrolytes: serum K | Renal function: U, Cr, CrCl (or eGFR) |
| Heart rate | TFTs |

## Dose

> The IM and SC routes should not be used because absorption is erratic and pain and tissue damage are problematic.

**Emergency loading dose for atrial fibrillation or flutter:** 0.75–1 mg by IV infusion over at least 2 hours. The dose may alternatively be given in divided doses, each over 10 to 20 minutes, with about 50% of the total dose given initially and additional fractions (usually 25%) given at intervals of 6 to 8 hours if still indicated. Reconsider or reduce dose if treated with digoxin within previous 2 weeks. Commence oral maintenance therapy on the following day adjusted according to age, lean bodyweight and renal function.

**Maintenance dose:** variable but usually in the range 50–200 micrograms by IV infusion once daily. If the patient is already maintained on digoxin convert directly from previous oral maintenance dose (see below).

> **For existing patients switched from oral maintenance to parenteral dosing:**
>
> When switching from oral to IV the dose should be reduced by about 30% and to a measurable volume, e.g.
> 62.5 microgram tablet ≅ 50 micrograms by IV infusion.

125 microgram tablet ≅ 75 micrograms by IV infusion.
250 microgram tablet ≅ 150 micrograms by IV infusion.

Consider checking levels 7–10 days after a change in route, particularly in the treatment of AF.

**Dose in renal impairment:** consider reducing maintenance dose and monitoring levels if CrCl <50 mL/minute.

## Intravenous infusion

*Preparation and administration*

1. Withdraw the required dose and add to a suitable volume of NaCl 0.9% or Gluc 5% (usually 100 mL but must be at least 4 times the injection volume). Mix well.
2. The solution should be clear and colourless. Inspect visually for particulate matter or discoloration prior to administration and discard if present.
3. Give by IV infusion via a volumetric infusion device usually over a minimum of 2 hours. For loading doses only, where a fraction is to be given, this may be infused over 10 to 20 minutes.

## Technical information

| | |
|---|---|
| Incompatible with | Amiodarone, amphotericin, fluconazole, foscarnet, insulin (soluble), propofol. |
| Compatible with | **Flush**: NaCl 0.9%<br>**Solutions**: NaCl 0.9%, Gluc 5%, Hartmann's (all including added KCl)<br>**Y-site**: Bivalirudin, ciprofloxacin, cisatracurium, linezolid, meropenem, midazolam, remifentanil |
| pH | 6.7–7.3 |
| Sodium content | Negligible |
| Excipients | Contains ethanol (may interact with metronidazole, possible religious objections).<br>Contains propylene glycol (adverse effects seen in ↓renal function, may interact with disulfiram and metronidazole). |
| Storage | Store below 25°C in original packaging. |
| Stability after preparation | From a microbiological point of view, should be used immediately; however, prepared infusions may be stored at 2–8°C and infused (at room temperature) within 24 hours. |

## Monitoring

| Measure | Frequency | Rationale |
|---|---|---|
| Heart rate | Prior to loading doses and if at risk of ↓pulse | • Ventricular rate should not be allowed to fall below 60 bpm except in exceptional circumstances, e.g. concomitant beta-blocker. |
| ECG | Continuously | • In patients with or at risk of arrhythmia. |
| Blood pressure | As per usual observations | • Risk of ↓BP. |

*(continued)*

## Monitoring (continued)

| Measure | Frequency | Rationale |
|---------|-----------|-----------|
| Serum K | Daily (see rationale) | • In patients at risk of ↓K (↑risk of toxicity - approximately 50% ↑sensitivity to the drug if serum K ≤3 mmol/L). |
| Serum digoxin concentration | If there are signs or symptoms of toxicity. If drug interaction is suspected. If renal function changes. | • A blood sample should be taken a minimum of 6 hours after dosing to ensure that a false peak is not measured during the distribution phase.<br>• Therapeutic range for heart failure: 0.9-1.5 micrograms/L (1.2-1.9 nanomol/L).<br>• Therapeutic range for atrial fibrillation: 1.5-2.0 micrograms/L (1.9-2.6 nanomol/L).<br>• Toxic effects become frequent above 2.5 micrograms/L (3.2 nanomol/L). |

## Additional information

| | |
|---|---|
| Common and serious undesirable effects | *Infusion-related:* Too rapid administration: heart block, life-threatening arrhythmias, death.<br>*Other:* ↓Pulse, arrhythmias, nausea, vomiting, diarrhoea, dizziness, blurred or yellow vision, skin rashes. |
| Pharmacokinetics | Elimination half-life is 20-50 hours; longer in renal impairment. |
| Significant interactions | • The following may ↑digoxin levels or effect (or ↑side-effects): amiodarone (halve dose of digoxin), chloroquine, ciclosporin, diltiazem, hydroxychloroquine, itraconazole, lercanidipine, nicardipine, nifedipine, propafenone, quinine, spironolactone (may also interfere with digoxin assay), St John's wort (avoid combination), verapamil (also ↑risk of AV block and ↓pulse).<br>• The following may ↑digoxin toxicity as may cause ↓K: acetazolamide, amphotericin, diuretics-loop, diuretics-thiazide.<br>• Injectable preparation contains ethanol and propylene glycol: may interact with disulfiram and metronidazole. |
| Action in case of overdose | *Symptoms to watch for:* In massive overdose progressive ↑K occurs (fatal unless reversed), arrhythmias.<br>*Antidote:* Life-threatening overdose may be treated with digoxin-specific antibody fragments (see Digoxin-specific antibody fragments monograph). Stop administration of digoxin and give supportive therapy as appropriate. |
| Counselling | Possibility of nausea and visual disturbance. |

| | |
|---|---|
| Risk rating: **AMBER** | Score = 4<br>Moderate-risk product: Risk reduction strategies are recommended |

This assessment is based on the full range of preparation and administration options described in the monograph. These may not all be applicable in some clinical situations.

## References

1. Aronson JK, Hardman M. *ABC of monitoring drug therapy: digoxin. BMJ.* 305: 1149–1152.

## Bibliography

SPC Lanoxin injection, Aspen Europe GmbH (accessed 31 March 2010).

# Digoxin-specific antibody fragments (Digibind, F(ab))

**38-mg dry powder vials**

* Digoxin specific antibody fragments are derived from sheep immunised to digoxin.
* Treatment with Digibind is generally reserved for life-threatening digoxin or digitoxin toxicity where conventional treatments (i.e. drug withdrawal and correction of electrolyte abnormalities) are insufficient.
* Each 38-mg vial of Digibind renders 500 micrograms of digoxin or digitoxin pharmacologically inactive.

> Standard digoxin serum assays cannot be used to determine free, pharmacologically active digoxin after administration of Digibind because these also detect F(ab)-bound digoxin.

## Pre-treatment checks

* Previous exposure: Although allergic reactions have been reported rarely, patients known to be allergic to sheep protein and patients who have previously received digoxin-specific antibody fragments are likely to be at greater risk of developing an allergic reaction.
* If your laboratory calculates digoxin levels as nanomol/L, multiply that figure by 0.78 to convert to micrograms/L (nanograms/mL).
* Erroneous calculations may result from inaccurate estimates of the amount of digitalis ingested or absorbed or from non-steady-state serum digitalis concentrations. Inaccurate serum digitalis concentration measurements are a possible source of error; this is especially so for very high values, since most digoxin assay kits are not designed to measure values >5 nanograms/mL.

*Biochemical and other tests (not all are necessary in an emergency situation)*

| | |
|---|---|
| Digoxin plasma concentration | ECG |
| Electrolytes: serum K | Bodyweight |

## Dose

> It is essential to consult a poisons information service, e.g. Toxbase at www.toxbase.org (password or registration required) for full details of the management of cardiac glycoside toxicity.

The dose is given in multiples of whole vials (rounding up) and is dependent on the amount of cardiac glycoside to be neutralised.

**Acute ingestion of an <u>unknown</u> amount of cardiac glycoside where serum concentration is <u>not</u> available:** 10 vials can be administered followed by an additional 10 vials if clinically indicated. This amount will be adequate to treat life-threatening ingestion in most adults.

**Acute ingestion of <u>known</u> amount of cardiac glycoside:** use the following formula to calculate number of vials needed. See Table D4 for a rough guide to dose likely to be needed.

Dose (number of vials) = Total body load (mg)* × 2

*Total body load is *either* (dose in mg of digoxin × 0.8) *or* dose in mg digitoxin.

**Table D4** Estimated dose of Digibind to treat acute ingestion of a known quantity of digoxin

| Number of 250-microgram digoxin tablets (80% bioavailability assumed) | Digibind dose (number of vials) |
|---|---|
| 25 | 10 |
| 50 | 20 |
| 75 | 30 |
| 100 | 40 |
| 150 | 60 |
| 200 | 80 |

**Toxicity during chronic therapy where serum concentration is not available:** 6 vials will usually be adequate to reverse toxicity.

**Toxicity during chronic therapy where serum concentration is available:**

**For digoxin toxicity:** if serum concentration is known, use the following formulas to calculate number of vials needed. See Table D5 for a rough guide to dose likely to be needed.

*Converting units:* nanomol/L × 0.78 = micrograms/L (or nanograms/mL).

$$\text{Dose (number of vials)} = \frac{\text{Serum \textbf{digoxin} concentration (nanograms/mL)} \times \text{bodyweight (kg)}}{100}$$

**For digitoxin toxicity:**

$$\text{Dose (number of vials)} = \frac{\text{Serum \textbf{digitoxin} concentration (nanograms/mL)} \times \text{bodyweight (kg)}}{1000}$$

## Intravenous infusion (preferred method)

*Preparation and administration*

1. Reconstitute each vial with 4 mL WFI and mix gently.
2. Withdraw the contents from the required number of vials and add to a convenient volume of NaCl 0.9% (usually 100 mL).
3. The solution should be clear and colourless. Inspect visually for particulate matter or discoloration prior to administration and discard if present.
4. Give by IV infusion over 30 minutes; through a 0.22-micron filter (if available) to remove any undissolved aggregates.

**Table D5** Estimated of number vials of Digibind required for a known serum digoxin concentration

| Bodyweight (kg) | Serum digoxin concentration | | | | | | |
| --- | --- | --- | --- | --- | --- | --- | --- |
| | nanograms/mL: 1 | 2 | 4 | 8 | 12 | 16 | 20 |
| | micrograms/L: 1 | 2 | 4 | 8 | 12 | 16 | 20 |
| | nanomol/L: 1.28 | 2.56 | 5.12 | 10.24 | 15.36 | 20.48 | 25.6 |
| | Number of vials | | | | | | |
| 40 | 0.5 | 1 | 2 | 3 | 5 | 7 | 8 |
| 60 | 0.5 | 1 | 3 | 5 | 7 | 10 | 12 |
| 70 | 1 | 2 | 3 | 6 | 9 | 11 | 14 |
| 80 | 1 | 2 | 3 | 7 | 10 | 13 | 16 |
| 100 | 1 | 2 | 4 | 8 | 12 | 16 | 20 |

## Intravenous injection (if cardiac arrest seems imminent)

*Preparation and administration*

1. Reconstitute each vial with 4 mL WFI and mix gently.
2. Withdraw the contents from the required number of vials.
3. The solution should be clear and colourless. Inspect visually for particulate matter or discoloration prior to administration and discard if present.
4. Give by IV injection over 5 minutes.

| Technical information | |
|---|---|
| Incompatible with | No information |
| Compatible with | **Flush**: NaCl 0.9%<br>**Solutions**: NaCl 0.9%<br>**Y-site**: No information but likely to be unstable |
| pH | 6-8 |
| Sodium content | 0.5 mmol/vial |
| Storage | Store at 2-8°C in original packaging. |
| Displacement value | Not relevant |
| Stability after preparation | The product should be used promptly after preparation. However, reconstituted vials may be stored at 2-8°C for up to 4 hours if necessary. |

| Monitoring | | |
|---|---|---|
| **Measure** | **Frequency** | **Rationale** |
| Signs of clinical improvement | Shortly after administration | • If after several hours toxicity has not adequately reversed or appears to recur, re-administration at a dose guided by clinical judgement may be required. |
| Serum K | Every 1-3 hours until serum K is stabilised | • Severe digitalis intoxication can cause life-threatening ↑K concentration by shifting K from within the cells.<br>• When the effect of digitalis is reversed by immune F(ab), K returns to the cells causing ↓serum K.<br>• ↓K may develop rapidly and cautious supplementation may be required. |
| ECG | Continuous for 24 hours | • Monitor for arrhythmias.<br>• Elimination of the antibody fragment-digoxin complex may be markedly delayed in severe renal impairment and prolonged monitoring may be required in such patients. |

## Additional information

| | |
|---|---|
| Common and serious undesirable effects | *Injection-related:* Too rapid administration: Although rare, allergic reactions are thought to be more likely with rapid dosing. |
| Pharmacokinetics | Elimination half-life is about 16–20 hours. Extended in renal impairment. Signs and symptoms of digitalis intoxication should begin to improve within 30 minutes of administration. |
| Significant interactions | None known. |
| Action in case of overdose | Supportive therapy as appropriate. |
| Counselling | Consider advice regarding future therapy with digoxin. |

Risk rating: **RED**     Score = 7
High-risk product: Risk-reduction strategies are required to minimise these risks.

This assessment is based on the full range of preparation and administration options described in the monograph. These may not all be applicable in some clinical situations.

## Bibliography

SPC Digibind, GlaxoSmithKline UK (accessed 31 August 2009).

# Dihydrocodeine tartrate

**50 mg/mL solution in 1-mL ampoules**

* Dihydrocodeine is an opioid analgesic.
* It is used for moderate to severe pain. It is less potent than morphine: dihydrocodeine 30 mg IM has the approximate analgesic effect of morphine sulfate 10 mg IM.

## Pre-treatment checks

* Do not use in acute respiratory depression, where there is a risk of paralytic ileus, in raised intracranial pressure and in head injury, in comatose patients and phaeochromocytoma.
* Caution in ↓BP, shock, convulsive disorders, supraventricular tachycardias, atrial flutter, chronic obstructive pulmonary disease and acute asthma attack, obstructive or inflammatory bowel diseases, biliary tract diseases, alcoholism, prostatic hyperplasia, myasthenia gravis, hypothyroidism (reduce dose), adrenocortical insufficiency (reduce dose).
* Caution in elderly patients – use lower doses; initial dose should not exceed 25 mg.
* Caution also in pancreatitis and severe cor pulmonale.
* Ensure resuscitation equipment and naloxone are available especially for IV administration.

*Biochemical and other tests*

Blood pressure and pulse
LFTs
Pain score

Renal function: U, Cr, CrCl (or eGFR)
Respiratory rate

## Dose

**Standard dose:** up to 50 mg by IM or deep SC injection every 4–6 hours when required.
**Elderly patients:** reduce initial dose then adjust dose to response.
**Dose in hepatic impairment:** reduce dose or avoid.
**Dose in renal impairment:** reduce dose or avoid.

## Subcutaneous injection

*Preparation and administration*

1. Withdraw the required dose.
2. Give by deep SC injection.
3. Close monitoring of respiratory rate and consciousness is recommended for 30 minutes in patients receiving an initial dose, especially elderly patients or those of low bodyweight.

## Intramuscular injection

*Preparation and administration*

1. Withdraw the required dose.
2. Give by deep IM injection.
3. Close monitoring of respiratory rate and consciousness is recommended for 30 minutes in patients receiving an initial dose, especially elderly patients or those of low bodyweight.

| Technical information | |
|---|---|
| Incompatible with | Not relevant |
| Compatible with | Not relevant |
| pH | 3–4.5 |
| Sodium content | Negligible |
| Excipients | Contains sulfites (may cause allergic reactions). |
| Storage | Store below 30°C in original packaging. |

## Monitoring

Close monitoring of respiratory rate and consciousness is recommended for 30 minutes in patients receiving an initial dose, especially elderly patients or those of low bodyweight.

| Measure | Frequency | Rationale |
|---------|-----------|-----------|
| Pain score | At regular intervals | • To ensure therapeutic response. |
| Blood pressure, heart rate and respiratory rate | | • ↓BP, ↓pulse, ↑pulse, palpitations and respiratory depression with decreased oxygen saturation can occur. |
| Sedation | | • Can cause sedation and CNS depression. |
| Monitor for side-effects and toxicity | | • Can cause side-effects such constipation, which may need treatment. |

## Additional information

| | |
|---|---|
| Common and serious undesirable effects | *Common:* Nausea and vomiting (particularly initially), constipation, dry mouth, urticaria, pruritus, biliary spasm, ↑ or ↓pulse, hallucinations, euphoria, drowsiness, histamine release (caution in asthmatics). <br> *At higher doses:* ↓BP, sedation, respiratory depression, muscle rigidity. |
| Pharmacokinetics | Half-life is 3.5-5 hours. |
| Significant drug interactions | • The following may ↑dihydrocodeine levels or effect (or ↑side-effects): antihistamines-sedating (↑sedation), MAOIs (avoid combination and for 2 weeks after stopping MAOI), moclobemide. <br> • Dihydrocodeine may ↑levels or effect (or ↑side-effects) of sodium oxybate (avoid combination). |
| Overdose | *Symptoms to watch for:* ↑Sedation, respiratory depression. <br> *Antidote:* Naloxone (see Naloxone monograph). <br> Stop administration and give supportive therapy as appropriate. |
| Counselling | May cause drowsiness; if affected do not drive or operate machinery, avoid alcoholic drinks (the effects of alcohol are enhanced). <br> Drink plenty of fluids if appropriate to reduce likelihood of constipation. |

| | |
|---|---|
| Risk rating: **GREEN** | Score = 2 <br> Lower-risk product: Risk-reduction strategies should be considered. |

 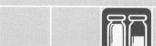

This assessment is based on the full range of preparation and administration options described in the monograph. These may not all be applicable in some clinical situations.

# Dimercaprol
# (British Anti-Lewisite, BAL)

**100 mg/2 mL solution in ampoules**

* Dimercaprol is a chelator that combines with various metal ions.
* It is used in the treatment of acute poisoning by certain heavy metals: arsenic, mercury, gold, bismuth, antimony and possibly thallium. It has also been used with sodium calcium edetate in acute lead poisoning particularly acute lead encephalopathy.
* The sulfhydryl groups on dimercaprol compete with endogenous sulfhydryl groups on proteins such as enzymes to combine with these metals. The dimercaprol–metal complex formed is readily excreted by the kidney. The aim of treatment is to provide an excess of dimercaprol in body fluids until the excretion of the metal is complete.

Do not use in iron, cadmium or selenium poisoning as the dimercaprol–metal complexes formed are more toxic than the metals themselves.

## Pre-treatment checks

* Do not use in patients with peanut allergy as the injection contains arachis oil.
* Do not use in patients with an allergy to soya.
* Avoid use in impaired hepatic function unless due to arsenic poisoning.
* Use with care in patients with ↑BP or impaired renal function.

*Biochemical and other tests*

Blood pressure

Bodyweight

LFTs

Renal function: U, Cr, CrCl (or eGFR)

## Dose

It is essential to consult a poisons information service, e.g. Toxbase at www.toxbase.org (password or registration required) for full details of the management of heavy metal toxicity.

**Standard dose:** 2.5–3 mg/kg bodyweight by IM injection every 4 hours for 2 days; then 2–4 times daily on the third day; then 1–2 times daily for 10 days or until recovery.

* Prophylactic or therapeutic administration of parenteral antihistamine or ephedrine 30 mg may prevent or relieve many of the mild adverse effects of dimercaprol.
* Side-effects may also be reduced by giving injections at least 4 hours apart.

## Intramuscular injection

Contains arachis oil – should not be given in peanut allergy.
See Special handling below.

*Preparation and administration*

1. Withdraw the required dose.
2. Give by deep IM injection. Rotate injection sites for subsequent injections.

## Technical information

| | |
|---|---|
| Incompatible with | Not relevant |
| Compatible with | Not relevant |
| pH | Not relevant |
| Sodium content | Nil |
| Excipients | Contains arachis oil. Do not use in peanut allergy. |
| Storage | Store below 25°C in original packaging. |
| Special handling | For disposal: React with weak aqueous solution (up to 15%) of calcium hypochlorite. Leave for 24 hours. Neutralise and discharge to drain with copious quantities of water. |

## Monitoring

| Measure | Frequency | Rationale |
|---|---|---|
| Temperature | After the initial injection | • Any abnormal reaction (e.g. pyrexia) occurring after the initial injection of dimercaprol should be assessed before continuing treatment. |
| Blood pressure | 15–20 minutes post dose | • Dimercaprol (particularly at the higher dosage levels) may cause ↑BP and ↑pulse.<br>• BP usually returns to normal within 2 hours. |
| Renal function | Daily during therapy | • Discontinue or continue with extreme caution if acute renal failure develops during therapy. |
| Monitor for general side-effects | Regularly during therapy | • See list below. |

## Additional information

| | |
|---|---|
| Common and serious undesirable effects | *Injection-related:* Local: Local injection-site pain and gluteal abscess has occasionally been encountered (more common if not given by deep IM injection).<br>*Other:* Side-effects are frequent, particularly at the higher dosage levels, but nearly always reversible:<br>• Elevation of BP accompanied by ↑pulse, nausea and possibly vomiting.<br>• Burning sensation of the lips, mouth, throat and eyes, salivation and lacrimation, conjunctivitis, rhinorrhoea.<br>• Muscle pain and spasm, abdominal pain.<br>• Headache, tingling of the hands and other extremities, a feeling of constriction in the chest and throat, sweating of the forehead and hands. |
| Pharmacokinetics | After IM injection, maximum plasma concentrations of dimercaprol may be attained within 1 hour. It is rapidly metabolised and the metabolites and dimercaprol-metal chelates are excreted in the urine and bile. Elimination is essentially complete within 4 hours of a single dose. |

*(continued)*

| **Additional information** (*continued*) | |
|---|---|
| Significant interactions | • Toxic complexes formed with iron may ↑dimercaprol side-effects: Iron therapy should be deferred until at least 24 hours after the last dose of dimercaprol.<br>• Dimercaprol interferes with accumulation of iodine by the thyroid gland, and iodine-131 thyroid uptake may be decreased if this test is performed during or immediately following dimercaprol therapy. |
| Action in case of overdose | *Antidote:* Treatment with a parenteral antihistamine or ephedrine 30 mg may reduce symptoms. |

| Risk rating: **AMBER** | Score = 3<br>Moderate-risk product: Risk-reduction strategies are recommended. |
|---|---|

This assessment is based on the full range of preparation and administration options described in the monograph. These may not all be applicable in some clinical situations.

**Bibliography**

SPC Dimercaprol Injection BP, Sovereign Medical (accessed 1 May 2010).
Toxbase at www.toxbase.org (accessed 1 May 2010).

# Dipyridamole

**5 mg/mL solution in 2-mL ampoules**
• Dipyridamole is a coronary vasodilator and inhibits platelet aggregation.
• It is used IV as an alternative to exercise stress in thallium-201 myocardial imaging.
• Risks associated with IV dosing need to be balanced against the risk of exercise stress.

**Pre-treatment checks**
• Do not use in dysrhythmias, second/third-degree atrioventricular block or sick sinus syndrome (unless controlled by pacemaker); systolic BP <90 mmHg, recent unexplained syncope (within 4 weeks), recent TIAs.
• Do not use in severe coronary artery disease, recent ACS, left ventricular outflow obstruction, haemodynamic instability; asthma; myasthenia gravis.
• Oral dipyridamole therapy must be discontinued for 24 hours prior to IV dosing.

- Caution in pre-existing first-degree heart block.
- Parenteral aminophylline should be readily available for relieving adverse effects such as bronchospasm or severe chest pain.

*Biochemical and other tests*

Bodyweight

Blood pressure

ECG

Electrolytes: serum Na, K

## Dose

**Standard dose:** 567 micrograms/kg by IV infusion over 4 minutes (at approximately 142 micrograms/kg/minute). Thallium-201 should be injected within 3–5 minutes following the 4-minute infusion.

**Dose calculation:**

$$\text{Total dose in mL} = \frac{567 \times \text{bodyweight (kg)}}{5000}$$

## Intravenous infusion via a syringe pump

*Preparation and administration*

1. Withdraw the required total dose.
2. Dilute to at least 3 times the original volume of dipyridamole injection with NaCl 0.9% or Gluc 5%, i.e. total volume 20–50 mL.
3. Cap the syringe and mix well.
4. The solution should be clear and pale yellow. Inspect visually for particulate matter or discoloration prior to administration and discard if present.
5. Give by IV infusion over 4 minutes using a syringe pump.

## Technical information

| Incompatible with | No information |
|---|---|
| Compatible with | **Flush**: NaCl 0.9%<br>**Solutions**: NaCl 0.9%, Gluc 5%<br>**Y-site**: No information |
| pH | 2.2-3.2 |
| Sodium content | Nil |
| Storage | Store below 25°C in original packaging. Do not freeze. |
| Stability after preparation | Use prepared infusions immediately. |

## Monitoring

| Measure | Frequency | Rationale |
|---------|-----------|-----------|
| ECG | Continuously for 10–15 minutes | • ECG changes (most commonly ST-T changes), arrhythmias. |
| Blood pressure and heart rate | | • Risk of haemodynamic instability. |
| Respiratory function and chest pain | | • Potential for bronchoconstriction and ischaemia.<br>• Parenteral aminophylline may be used to relieve these adverse effects.<br>• However, if the clinical condition of a patient with an adverse effect permits a 1-minute delay in the administration of IV aminophylline, thallium-201 may be injected and allowed to circulate for 1 minute before the injection of aminophylline. This will allow initial thallium perfusion imaging to be performed before reversal of the pharmacological effects of dipyridamole.<br>• Give aminophylline by slow IV injection at a dose of 75–100 mg, repeated if necessary.<br>• If aminophylline does not relieve chest pain symptoms within a few minutes, sublingual glyceryl trinitrate may be given. |
| Cannulation site | During infusion and for 1 hour after | • Risk of extravasation and tissue damage. |

## Additional information

| | |
|---|---|
| Common and serious undesirable effects | *Immediate:* Severe ↓BP and hot flushes. Anaphylactoid and other hypersensitivity reactions, e.g. bronchospasm, angioedema, rash and urticaria have been reported.<br>*Infusion-related:* Local: Injection-site pain.<br>*Other:* Cardiac death, cardiac arrest, MI (rarely fatal), chest pain/angina pectoris, ECG changes, arrhythmias, syncope and cerebrovascular events. Also abdominal pain, vomiting, diarrhoea, nausea, dizziness, headache, paraesthesia, myalgia. |
| Pharmacokinetics | Elimination half-life is 9–13 hours. |
| Significant interactions | • The following may ↓dipyridamole levels or effect:<br>caffeine (avoid for 24 hours before test), theophylline (avoid for 24 hours before test).<br>• Dipyridamole may ↑levels or effect of the following drugs (or ↑side-effects): adenosine, antihypertensives.<br>• Dipyridamole may ↓levels or effect of cholinesterase inhibitors (potentially aggravating myasthenia gravis). |
| Action in case of overdose | *Antidote:* No known antidote; stop administration and give supportive therapy as appropriate. |
| Counselling | Report chest pain, wheezing and infusion-site pain.<br>Bitter taste may be experienced. |

| Risk rating: **AMBER** | Score = 5<br>Moderate-risk product: Risk-reduction strategies are recommended. |
|---|---|

This assessment is based on the full range of preparation and administration options described in the monograph. These may not all be applicable in some clinical situations.

## Bibliography

SPC Persantin ampoules, Boehringer Ingelheim Limited (accessed 20 April 2010).

# Disodium folinate (sodium folinate)

### 50 mg/mL solution in 2-mL, 8-mL and 18-mL vials

* Disodium folinate is a derivative of tetrahydrofolic acid, the active form of folic acid.
* It is used as an antidote to folic acid antagonists such as methotrexate (commonly known as 'folinic acid rescue' or 'folinate rescue') and as an adjunct to fluorouracil (FU) in the treatment of colorectal cancer.
* Doses are usually expressed in terms of folinic acid:
  Folinic acid 1 mg $\cong$ 1.09 mg of disodium folinate.

## Pre-treatment checks

* Do not give if the patient is anaemic owing to vitamin $B_{12}$ deficiency.

*Biochemical tests*

Electrolytes: serum Na, K, Ca
FBC

LFTs
Renal function: U, Cr, CrCl (or eGFR)

## Dose

Disodium folinate must not be administered intrathecally.

Consult specialist literature as regimens vary greatly depending on the indication.

## Intravenous injection

*Preparation and administration*

1. Withdraw the required dose.
2. The solution should be clear and slightly yellow. Inspect visually for particulate matter or discoloration prior to administration and discard if present.
3. Give by IV injection over 1 minute.

## Intermittent intravenous infusion

*Preparation and administration*

1. Withdraw the required dose and add to a convenient volume of NaCl 0.9%.
2. The solution should be clear and colourless to slightly yellow. Inspect visually for particulate matter or discoloration prior to administration and discard if present.
3. Give by IV infusion over 1–2 hours.

| Technical information | |
|---|---|
| Incompatible with | No information |
| Compatible with | **Flush**: NaCl 0.9%<br>**Solutions**: NaCl 0.9%<br>Additives: Fluorouracil<br>**Y-Site**: No information |
| pH | 6.8-8.0 |
| Sodium content | 0.21-0.33 mmol/mL |
| Storage | Store at 2-8°C in original packaging. |
| Stability after preparation | From a microbiological point of view, should be used immediately; however, prepared infusions may be stored at 2-8°C and infused (at room temperature) within 24 hours. |

| Monitoring | | |
|---|---|---|
| **Measure** | **Frequency** | **Rationale** |
| Creatinine and methotrexate levels | At least daily in folinic acid rescue | • The dose of disodium folinate is dependent on these parameters in "rescue". |
| FBC | Weekly during first two courses of FU then once each cycle thereafter | • Monitored if in combination with FU only. |
| Renal function, LFTs | Prior to each treatment for the first 3 cycles and prior to every other cycle thereafter | |
| Diarrhoea | During treatment | • A sign of GI toxicity when combined with FU.<br>• ↓Dose of FU until symptoms have fully disappeared. |
| Serum calcium concentration | Periodically | • Monitored if combined with FU.<br>• Supplementation should be provided if calcium levels are low. |

| Additional information | |
|---|---|
| Common and serious undesirable effects | *Immediate:* Pyrexial reactions, anaphylaxis and urticaria have been reported rarely.<br>*Other:* In combination with FU: vomiting and nausea, severe mucosal toxicity, diarrhoea with higher grades of toxicity leading to dehydration. |
| Pharmacokinetics | Elimination half-life is about 6 hours. |
| Significant interactions | • Folinate may ↓levels or effect of the following drugs:<br>  possible ↓efficacy of folic acid antagonists, e.g. co-trimoxazole,<br>  pyrimethamine; phenobarbital, primidone, phenytoin may have ↓efficacy<br>  (possible ↑seizures). |
| Action in case of overdose | If overdose occurs in combination with FU, the overdosage instructions for FU should be followed. |

**Risk rating: AMBER**

Score = 3
Moderate-risk product: Risk-reduction strategies are recommended.

This assessment is based on the full range of preparation and administration options described in the monograph. These may not all be applicable in some clinical situations.

## Bibliography

SPC Sodiofolin 50 mg/mL, solution for injection (accessed 5 April 2009).

# Disodium levofolinate (sodium levofolinate)

### 50 mg/mL solution in 1-mL, 4-mL and 9-mL vials

- Disodium levofolinate is a derivative of tetrahydrofolic acid, the active form of folic acid.
- It is used as an antidote to folic acid antagonists such as methotrexate (commonly known as 'levofolinic acid rescue' or 'levofolinate rescue') and as an adjunct to fluorouracil (FU) in the treatment of colorectal cancer.
- Doses are usually expressed in terms of folinic acid:
  Folinic acid 1 mg ≅ 1.09 mg of disodium levofolinate.

### Pre-treatment checks

Do not give if the patient is anaemic owing to vitamin $B_{12}$ deficiency.

*Biochemical and other tests*

| | |
|---|---|
| Electrolytes: serum Na, K, Ca | LFTs |
| FBC | Renal function: U, Cr |

## Dose

> Disodium levofolinate must not be administered intrathecally.

Consult specialist literature as regimens vary greatly depending on the indication.

### Intravenous injection

*Preparation and administration*

1. Withdraw the required dose.
2. The solution should be clear and slightly yellow. Inspect visually for particulate matter or discoloration prior to administration and discard if present.
3. Give by IV injection over 1 minute.

### Intermittent intravenous infusion

*Preparation and administration*

1. Withdraw the required dose and add to a convenient volume of NaCl 0.9% or Gluc 5%.
2. The solution should be clear and colourless to slightly yellow. Inspect visually for particulate matter or discoloration prior to administration and discard if present.
3. Give by IV infusion over 2 hours.

## Technical information

| | |
|---|---|
| Incompatible with | No information |
| Compatible with | **Flush**: NaCl 0.9%<br>**Solutions**: NaCl 0.9%, Gluc 5%<br>Additives: Fluorouracil<br>**Y-Site**: No information |
| pH[1] | 6.8-8.0 |
| Sodium content[1] | Approximately 2-3 mmol/9-mL vial |
| Storage | Store at 2-8°C in original packaging. |
| Stability after preparation | From a microbiological point of view, should be used immediately; however, prepared infusions may be stored at 2-8°C and infused (at room temperature) within 24 hours. |

## Monitoring

| Measure | Frequency | Rationale |
|---|---|---|
| Creatinine and methotrexate levels | At least daily in folinic acid rescue | • Dose of disodium levofolinate is dependent on these parameters in 'rescue'. |

*(continued)*

## Monitoring (continued)

| Measure | Frequency | Rationale |
|---|---|---|
| Renal function, LFTs | Prior to each treatment for the first 3 cycles and prior to every other cycle thereafter | • Monitored if in combination with FU only. |
| Diarrhoea | During treatment | • A sign of gastrointestinal toxicity when combined with FU.<br>• Reduce the dose of FU until symptoms have fully disappeared. |
| Serum calcium concentration | Periodically | • Monitored if combined with FU.<br>• Supplementation should be provided if calcium levels are low. |

## Additional information

| | |
|---|---|
| Common and serious undesirable effects | *Immediate:* Pyrexial reactions, anaphylaxis and urticaria have been reported rarely.<br>*Other:* In combination with FU, vomiting and nausea, severe mucosal toxicity, diarrhoea with higher grades of toxicity leading to dehydration. |
| Pharmacokinetics | Elimination half-life is about 6 hours. |
| Significant interactions | • Levofolinate may ↓levels or effect of the following drugs:<br>possible ↓efficacy of folic acid antagonists, e.g. co-trimoxazole, pyrimethamine; phenobarbital, primidone, phenytoin may have ↓efficacy (possible ↑seizures). |
| Action in case of overdose | If overdose occurs in combination with FU, the over-dosage instructions for FU should be followed. |

Risk rating: **AMBER**    Score = 3
Moderate-risk product: Risk-reduction strategies are recommended.

This assessment is based on the full range of preparation and administration options described in the monograph. These may not all be applicable in some clinical situations.

## Reference

1. Correspondence with Medac UK, 08 April 2009.

## Bibliography

SPC Levofolinic acid 50 mg/mL solution for injection or infusion, Medac UK (accessed 6 April 2009).

# Disopyramide

**10 mg/mL solution in 5-mL ampoules**

- Disopyramide phosphate is a class Ia antiarrhythmic drug, with effects similar to those of procainamide. It also has antimuscarinic and negative inotropic properties.
- It is used only in management of life-threatening arrhythmias.
- Doses are expressed in terms of the base:
  Disopyramide 10 mg $\cong$ 12.88 mg disopyramide phosphate.

## Pre-treatment checks

- Avoid in severe heart failure, second- and third-degree heart block and sinus node dysfunction (unless a pacemaker is fitted) and cardiogenic shock.
- Caution in ventricular fibrillation or torsade de pointes, atrial flutter or atrial tachycardia with partial block, bundle branch block, heart failure.
- Caution in prostatic enlargement and susceptibility to angle-closure glaucoma.

*Biochemical and other tests (not all are necessary in an emergency situation)*

Bodyweight                                    LFTs
ECG                                           Renal function: U, Cr, CrCl (or eGFR)
Electrolytes: serum K

## Dose

The maximum dose by all routes is 800 mg in 24 hours.

**Standard dose:** give 2 mg/kg (maximum 150 mg) by IV injection. Arrhythmia usually resolves within 15 minutes. If successful continue with oral therapy. The IV dose can be repeated cautiously if the arrhythmia recurs (maximum dose 300 mg or 4 mg/kg within the first hour).

**Serious arrhythmias or inability to take oral medication:** give 2 mg/kg (maximum 150 mg) by IV injection followed by 20–30 mg/hour (or 400 micrograms/kg/hour) by IV infusion up to a maximum of 800 mg in 24 hours.

## Intravenous injection

*Preparation and administration*

1. Withdraw the required dose.
2. The solution should be clear and colourless. Inspect visually for particulate matter or discoloration prior to administration and discard if present.
3. Give by IV injection over 5 minutes (maximum 30 mg/minute).

## Intravenous infusion

*Preparation and administration*

1. Withdraw the required dose.
2. The solution should be clear and colourless. Inspect visually for particulate matter or discoloration prior to administration and discard if present.
3. Add to a convenient volume of NaCl 0.9% or Gluc 5%.
4. Give by IV infusion via a volumetric pump.

## Technical information

| | |
|---|---|
| Incompatible with | No information |
| Compatible with | **Flush**: NaCl 0.9%<br>**Solutions**: NaCl 0.9%, Gluc 5%, Ringer's, Hartmann's<br>**Y-site**: No information |
| pH | 4.5 |
| Sodium content | Nil |
| Excipients | Contains benzyl alcohol. |
| Storage | Store below 25°C in original packaging. |
| Stability after preparation | No information |

## Monitoring

| Measure | Frequency | Rationale |
|---|---|---|
| ECG | Continuously | • Observe the QT interval and QRS duration: discontinue if these increase by >25%.<br>• If arrhythmias develop: discontinue. |
| Blood pressure | Every 30 minutes | • If ↓BP occurs: discontinue. This is more likely in patients with cardiomyopathy or uncompensated congestive heart failure. |
| Renal function | Daily | • ↓K increases risk of arrhythmia. |
| Blood glucose | | • Hypoglycaemia has been reported; although rare it may be severe. |

## Additional information

| | |
|---|---|
| Common and serious undesirable effects | Anticholinergic effects such as dysuria, acute urinary retention (more likely in patients with prostatic enlargement), disorders of accommodation, diplopia, dry mouth. |
| Pharmacokinetics | Elimination half-life is 4–10 hours. Increased in renal impairment, cardiac and hepatic disease. |

*(continued)*

## Additional information (*continued*)

| | |
|---|---|
| Significant interactions | • The following may ↑disopyramide levels or effect (or ↑side-effects): clarithromycin, erythromycin, itraconazole (avoid combination), ranolazine (avoid combination), ritonavir.<br>• The following may ↓disopyramide levels or effect: rifabutin, rifampicin.<br>• ↑Risk of cardiotoxicity with drugs causing ↓K: acetazolamide, diuretics-loop, diuretics-thiazide.<br>• ↑Risk of ventricular arrhythmias with the following: amiodarone (avoid combination), amisulpride (avoid combination), antidepressants-tricyclic, arsenic trioxide, artemether with lumefantrine (avoid combination), atomoxetine, droperidol (avoid combination), haloperidol (avoid combination), ivabradine, ketoconazole (avoid combination), mizolastine (avoid combination), moxifloxacin (avoid combination), phenothiazines, pimozide (avoid combination), sertindole (avoid combination), sotalol (avoid combination), sulpiride, tolterodine, verapamil, zuclopenthixol (avoid combination). |
| Action in case of overdose | No specific antidote. Give supportive therapy as appropriate. |

| | |
|---|---|
| Risk rating: **AMBER** | Score = 5<br>Moderate-risk product: Risk-reduction strategies are recommended. |

This assessment is based on the full range of preparation and administration options described in the monograph. These may not all be applicable in some clinical situations.

### Bibliography

SPC Rythmodan injection, Sanofi-Aventis (accessed 14 June 2010).

# Dobutamine

#### 12.5 mg/mL solution in 20-mL ampoules

* Dobutamine hydrochloride is a cardiac stimulant producing a positive inotropic effect on the myocardium that results in ↑cardiac output (↑myocardial contractility, ↑stroke volume). Its use requires intensive haemodynamic monitoring and ideally should be confined to the critical care setting.
* It is used to provide positive inotropic support in treatment of cardiac decompensation due to depressed contractility; in cardiogenic shock (heart failure with severe ↓BP) and in septic shock in combination with dopamine.

- It may also be used in cardiac stress testing if the patient cannot undergo a period of exercise or if the exercise yields no useful information (dobutamine stress echocardiography).
- Doses are expressed in terms of the base:
  Dobutamine 1 microgram ≅ 1.12 micrograms dobutamine hydrochloride.

## Pre-treatment checks

- Do not use in mechanical obstruction of ventricular filling and/or outflow, hypovolaemia.
- Consult product literature for full details of exclusions to use in stress echocardiography.
- Consider the risk of sulfite sensitivity in patients with asthma.
- Inadequate circulating blood volume should be restored prior to treatment with dobutamine.

*Biochemical and other tests (not all are necessary in an emergency situation)*

Bodyweight
Electrolytes: serum K

## Dose

**Inotropic effect**: initiate at 2.5 micrograms/kg/minute by IV infusion into a central or large peripheral vein. This can be gradually increased to 10 micrograms/kg/minute as necessary according to heart rate, BP, cardiac output and urine output.

- Doses of 0.5–40 micrograms/kg/minute may be required.
- Discontinue treatment gradually.

**Cardiac stress testing**: initially 5 micrograms/kg/minute for 3–8 minutes increasing by 5 micrograms/kg/minute every 3–8 minutes, up to a usual maximum of 20 micrograms/kg/minute (occasionally up to 40 micrograms/kg/minute may be required).

## Continuous intravenous infusion via a syringe pump

The concentration used is dependent on the patient's dosage and fluid requirements but the final concentration must be no greater than 5 mg/mL. A concentration of 1 mg/mL has been recommended for cardiac stress testing.
Administer into a central or large peripheral vein.

*Preparation of a 5 mg/mL solution*

1. Withdraw 250 mg (20 mL) of the concentrate and make up to 50 mL in a syringe pump with Gluc 5% or NaCl 0.9%.
2. Cap the syringe and mix well to give a solution containing 5 mg/mL (5000 micrograms/mL).
3. The solution should be clear and no more than faintly pink in colour. Inspect visually for particulate matter or discoloration prior to administration and discard if present.

*Administration*

1. Give by IV infusion via a syringe pump at an initial rate of 2.5 micrograms/kg/minute.
2. Adjust dose according to clinical response.
3. Prepare a fresh syringe every 24 hours.

**Calculation of infusion rate:**

$$\text{Infusion rate (mL/hour)} = \frac{\text{Weight (kg)} \times \text{required rate (micrograms/minute)} \times 60}{\text{Concentration of prepared infusion (micrograms/mL)}}$$

See Table D6 below for a dosage chart detailing pre-calculated infusion rates for each bodyweight using a 5 mg/mL (5000 micrograms/mL) solution.

## Technical information

| | |
|---|---|
| Incompatible with | Sodium bicarbonate.<br>Aciclovir, alteplase, aminophylline, amphotericin, bumetanide, calcium gluconate, ceftazidime, digoxin, doxapram, drotrecogin alfa, flucloxacillin, foscarnet, furosemide, heparin sodium, insulin (soluble), micafungin, midazolam, pantoprazole, phenytoin sodium, phytomenadione, piperacillin with tazobactam. |
| Compatible with | **Flush**: NaCl 0.9%<br>**Solutions**: Gluc 5%, NaCl 0.9%, Gluc-NaCl, Hartmann's<br>**Y-site**: Adrenaline (epinephrine), atracurium, ciprofloxacin, cisatracurium, clarithromycin, dopamine, fentanyl, fluconazole, glyceryl trinitrate, granisetron, linezolid, noradrenaline (norepinephrine), propofol, ranitidine, remifentanil, tigecycline, tirofiban, vecuronium, verapamil |
| pH | 2.5-5.5 |
| Sodium content | Negligible |
| Storage | Store below 25°C in original packaging. |
| Excipients | Contains sulfites (which may cause allergic reactions). |
| Stability after preparation | From a microbiological point of view, should be used immediately; however, prepared infusions may be stored at 2-8°C and infused (at room temperature) within 24 hours. |

## Monitoring

| Measure | Frequency | Rationale |
|---|---|---|
| ECG | Continuously | • Monitoring for heart rate and arrhythmias. |
| Blood pressure | | • ↓BP requiring ↓dose or discontinuation. |
| Urine output | Hourly | • Response to therapy. |
| Blood glucose | At least 12-hourly | • May see ↑insulin requirements in patients with diabetes mellitus. |
| Serum K | Daily | • K levels may be altered by therapy. |
| Response to therapy | After 72 hours | • Tolerance may develop after 72 hours of therapy. |

## Additional information

| | |
|---|---|
| Common and serious undesirable effects | Injection/infusion-related:<br>• Too rapid administration: ↑Pulse, ↑ or ↓BP, dysrhythmias, extrasystoles, anginal pain, palpitations.<br>• Local: Phlebitis at injection site.<br>*Other:* headache, bronchoconstriction, eosinophilia, ↓platelet aggregation with prolonged therapy, nausea, urinary urgency. |
| Pharmacokinetics | Serum half-life is 2-3 minutes. |

*(continued)*

## Additional information (*continued*)

| | |
|---|---|
| Significant interactions | Risk of hypertensive crisis with the following: Beta-blockers (also ↓pulse), MAOIs, moclobemide, rasagiline. |
| Action in case of overdose | Effects are reduced rapidly on ↓dose or discontinuation. Treat anginal episodes with a nitrate. Severe ventricular arrhythmia may require IV lidocaine or propranolol. (See individual monographs.) |
| Counselling | Headache, nausea, urinary urgency may occur. |

| | |
|---|---|
| Risk rating: **AMBER** | Score = 5 Moderate-risk product: Risk-reduction strategies are recommended. |

This assessment is based on the full range of preparation and administration options described in the monograph. These may not all be applicable in some clinical situations.

## Bibliography

SPC Dobutamine 5 mg/mL, solution for infusion, Hameln Pharmaceuticals Ltd. (accessed 30 April 2009).
SPC Dobutamine concentrate 250 mg/20 mL, Hameln Pharmaceuticals Ltd (accessed 30 April 2009).

**Table D6** Dobutamine rate of infusion using dobutamine 250 mg made up to 50 mL in a 50-mL syringe pump (5000 micrograms/mL)

| Weight in kg | Infusion rate (micrograms/kg/minute) | | | | | | | | | | |
| --- | --- | --- | --- | --- | --- | --- | --- | --- | --- | --- | --- |
| | 1 | 2.5 | 5 | 7.5 | 10 | 15 | 20 | 25 | 30 | 35 | 40 |
| | Rate of infusion (mL/hour) | | | | | | | | | | |
| 40 | 0.5 | 1.2 | 2.4 | 3.6 | 4.8 | 7.2 | 9.6 | 12.0 | 14.4 | 16.8 | 19.2 |
| 45 | 0.5 | 1.4 | 2.7 | 4.1 | 5.4 | 8.1 | 10.8 | 13.5 | 16.2 | 18.9 | 21.6 |
| 50 | 0.6 | 1.5 | 3.0 | 4.5 | 6.0 | 9.0 | 12.0 | 15.0 | 18.0 | 21.0 | 24.0 |
| 55 | 0.7 | 1.7 | 3.3 | 5.0 | 6.6 | 9.9 | 13.2 | 16.5 | 19.8 | 23.1 | 26.4 |
| 60 | 0.7 | 1.8 | 3.6 | 5.4 | 7.2 | 10.8 | 14.4 | 18.0 | 21.6 | 25.2 | 28.8 |
| 65 | 0.8 | 2.0 | 3.9 | 5.9 | 7.8 | 11.7 | 15.6 | 19.5 | 23.4 | 27.3 | 31.2 |
| 70 | 0.8 | 2.1 | 4.2 | 6.3 | 8.4 | 12.6 | 16.8 | 21.0 | 25.2 | 29.4 | 33.6 |
| 75 | 0.9 | 2.3 | 4.5 | 6.8 | 9.0 | 13.5 | 18.0 | 22.5 | 27.0 | 31.5 | 36.0 |
| 80 | 1.0 | 2.4 | 4.8 | 7.2 | 9.6 | 14.4 | 19.2 | 24.0 | 28.8 | 33.6 | 38.4 |
| 85 | 1.1 | 2.6 | 5.1 | 7.7 | 10.2 | 15.3 | 20.4 | 25.5 | 30.6 | 35.7 | 40.8 |
| 90 | 1.1 | 2.7 | 5.4 | 8.1 | 10.8 | 16.2 | 21.6 | 27.0 | 32.4 | 37.8 | 43.2 |
| 95 | 1.2 | 2.9 | 5.7 | 8.6 | 11.4 | 17.1 | 22.8 | 28.5 | 34.2 | 39.9 | 45.6 |
| 100 | 1.2 | 3.0 | 6.0 | 9.0 | 12.0 | 18.0 | 24.0 | 30.0 | 36.0 | 42.0 | 48.0 |
| 110 | 1.4 | 3.3 | 6.6 | 9.9 | 13.2 | 19.8 | 26.4 | 33.0 | 39.6 | 46.2 | 52.8 |
| 120 | 1.5 | 3.6 | 7.2 | 10.8 | 14.4 | 21.6 | 28.8 | 36.0 | 43.2 | 50.4 | 57.6 |
| 130 | 1.6 | 3.9 | 7.8 | 11.7 | 15.6 | 23.4 | 31.2 | 39.0 | 46.8 | 54.6 | 62.4 |
| 140 | 1.7 | 4.2 | 8.4 | 12.6 | 16.8 | 25.2 | 33.6 | 42.0 | 50.4 | 58.8 | 67.2 |

# Dopamine hydrochloride

**40 mg/mL and 160 mg/mL solution in 5-mL ampoules**
**40 mg/mL solution in 5-mL and 10-mL vials**
**400 mg (1.6 mg/mL) and 800 mg (3.2 mg/mL) solution in 250-mL infusion bags**

* Dopamine hydrochloride is a cardiac stimulant producing a positive inotropic effect on the myocardium that results in ↑cardiac output (↑myocardial contractility, ↑stroke volume). Its use requires intensive haemodynamic monitoring and ideally should be confined to the critical care setting.
* It is used to treat acute ↓BP or shock and ↓cardiac output associated with MI, septicaemia, trauma and renal failure; persistent ↓BP after open heart surgery; maintaining urine output. In many centres its use has been superseded by dopexamine.

## Pre-treatment checks

* Do not use in phaeochromocytoma, hyperthyroidism, uncorrected atrial or ventricular tachyarrhythmias, ventricular fibrillation.
* An inadequate circulating blood volume should be restored prior to treatment with dopamine.

*Biochemical and other tests*

Bodyweight
Electrolytes: serum Na, K
Renal function: U, Cr, CrCl (or eGFR)

## Dose

**Inotropic effect:** initiate at 2–5 micrograms/kg/minute by IV infusion into a central or large peripheral vein. This can be gradually increased by up to 5–10 micrograms/kg/minute according to BP, cardiac output and urine output. Up to 20–50 micrograms/kg/minute may be required in seriously ill patients.

* Dose cautiously in patients with shock following MI.
* Discontinue treatment gradually.

## Continuous intravenous infusion

The concentration used is dependent on the patient's dosage and fluid requirements. Concentrations greater than 3.2 mg/mL must be given via a central line.

*Preparation of a 1.6 mg/mL (1600 micrograms/mL) solution*

Ideally use a pre-prepared infusion bag containing 400 mg/250 mL.
Alternatively:

1. Withdraw 400 mg of the dopamine concentrate into a syringe (see Table D7).
2. Withdraw an equal volume of fluid from a 250-mL bag of NaCl 0.9% or Gluc 5% and discard.
3. Add the dopamine concentrate to the prepared infusion bag and mix well. This gives a solution containing 1.6 mg/mL (1600 micrograms/mL).

*Preparation of a 3.2 mg/mL (3200 micrograms/mL) solution*

Ideally use a pre-prepared infusion bag containing 800 mg/250 mL.
Alternatively:

1. Withdraw 800 mg of the dopamine concentrate into a syringe (see Table D7).
2. Withdraw an equal volume of fluid from a 250-mL bag of NaCl 0.9% or Gluc 5% and discard.
3. Add the dopamine concentrate to the prepared infusion bag and mix well. This gives a solution containing 3.2 mg/mL (3200 micrograms/mL).

### Table D7

| Strength of concentrate (mg/mL) | Volume (mL) containing dopamine 200 mg | Volume (mL) containing dopamine 400 mg | Volume (mL) containing dopamine 800 mg |
|---|---|---|---|
| 40 | 5 | 10 | 20 |
| 160 | 1.25 | 2.5 | 5 |

*Administration*

1. The solution should be clear and almost colourless (the concentrate may have a pale straw colour). Inspect visually for particulate matter or discoloration prior to administration and discard if present.
2. Give by IV infusion via a volumetric infusion device into a large vein at an initial rate of 2–5 micrograms/kg/minute.
3. Adjust the dose according to clinical response.
4. Prepare a fresh infusion bag every 24 hours.

## Continuous intravenous infusion via a syringe pump

For administration via a central line only.

*Preparation of a 4 mg/mL (4000 micrograms/mL) solution*

1. Withdraw 200 mg of the concentrate and make up to 50 mL in a syringe pump with NaCl 0.9%, Gluc 5% or Hartmann's.
2. Cap the syringe and mix well to give a solution containing 4 mg/mL (4000 micrograms/mL).
3. The solution should be clear and almost colourless (the concentrate may have a pale straw-colour). Inspect visually for particulate matter or discoloration prior to administration and discard if present.

*Administration*

1. Give by IV infusion via a syringe pump into a central line at an initial rate of 2–5 micrograms/kg/minute.
2. Adjust the dose according to clinical response.
3. Prepare a fresh syringe every 24 hours.

**Calculation of infusion rate:**

$$\text{Infusion rate (mL/hour)} = \frac{\text{Weight (kg)} \times \text{required rate (micrograms/minute)} \times 60}{\text{Concentration of prepared infusion (micrograms/mL)}}$$

See Tables D8, D9 and D10 below for dosage charts detailing pre-calculated infusion rates for each bodyweight using 1.6 mg/mL (1600 micrograms/mL), 3.2 mg/mL (3200 micrograms/mL) and 4 mg/mL (4000 micrograms/mL) solutions.

## Technical information

| | |
|---|---|
| Incompatible with | Sodium bicarbonate.<br>Aciclovir, amphotericin, ampicillin, alteplase, benzylpenicillin (penicillin G), furosemide, gentamicin, insulin (soluble). |
| Compatible with | **Flush**: NaCl 0.9%<br>**Solutions**: NaCl 0.9%, Gluc 5%, Gluc-NaCl, Hartmann's<br>**Y-site**: Adrenaline (epinephrine), aminophylline, atracurium, aztreonam, ceftazidime, chloramphenicol sodium succinate, ciprofloxacin, cisatracurium, clarithromycin, dobutamine, fentanyl, fluconazole, foscarnet, glyceryl trinitrate, granisetron, hydrocortisone sodium succinate, linezolid, meropenem, methylprednisolone sodium succinate, metronidazole, micafungin, midazolam, noradrenaline (norepinephrine), ondansetron, pantoprazole, piperacillin with tazobactam, propofol, ranitidine, remifentanil, streptokinase, tigecycline, tirofiban, vecuronium, verapamil |
| pH | 2.5-5 |
| Sodium content | Negligible |
| Storage | Store below 25°C in original packaging |
| Excipients | Contains sulfites (may cause allergic reactions). |
| Stability after preparation | From a microbiological point of view, should be used immediately; however, prepared infusions may be stored at 2-8°C and infused (at room temperature) within 24 hours. |

## Monitoring

| Measure | Frequency | Rationale |
|---|---|---|
| Blood pressure | Continuously | • Response to therapy.<br>• If a disproportionate rise in diastolic pressure (i.e. a marked decrease in pulse pressure) is observed, the infusion rate should be decreased and the patients observed carefully for further evidence of predominant vasoconstriction activity, unless such an effect is desired. |
| ECG/Heart rate | | • ↑Pulse.<br>• Rhythm disturbance. |
| Urine output | Hourly | • Response to therapy.<br>• ↓Urine output in absence of ↓BP may signal need for dose reduction, especially when infusion rate is high. |
| Infusion site | | • Possible necrosis on extravasation; see Additional information below for management. |

(continued)

## Monitoring (*continued*)

| Measure | Frequency | Rationale |
|---|---|---|
| Extremities | | • Patients with peripheral vascular disease should be closely monitored for any changes in colour or temperature of the skin of the extremities. Benefits of continued dopamine infusion should be weighed against the risk of possible necrosis. Ischaemic changes may be reversed by ↓rate or discontinuation. Phentolamine may reverse the ischaemia (see the Phentolamine monograph). |
| Renal function and serum Na and K | Periodically | • Monitor particularly during high dose regimens (>20 microgram/kg/minute) as decreased renal blood flow can occur. |

## Additional information

| | |
|---|---|
| Common and serious undesirable effects | *Infusion-related:* Local: Extravasation – necrosis and sloughing of the surrounding tissue. Ischaemia can be reversed by infiltration of the affected area with phentolamine (see the Phentolamine monograph).<br>*Other:* ↑Pulse, anginal pain, ectopic beats, palpitation, dyspnoea, ↓BP, vasoconstriction, headache, nausea and vomiting. |
| Pharmacokinetics | Serum half-life <2 minutes; duration of action <10 minutes. |
| Significant interactions | • Risk of hypertensive crisis with the following:<br>MAOIs, moclobemide, rasagiline, selegiline. |
| Action in case of overdose | ↑BP and vasoconstriction respond rapidly to ↓rate or discontinuation. |
| Counselling | Headache, nausea, dyspnoea may occur; report pain at infusion site. |

| | |
|---|---|
| Risk rating: **AMBER** | Score = 5<br>Moderate-risk product: Risk-reduction strategies are recommended. |

This assessment is based on the full range of preparation and administration options described in the monograph. These may not all be applicable in some clinical situations.

## Bibliography

SPC Dopamine 40mg/ml sterile concentrate, Hospira UK Ltd (accessed 29 April 2009).

**Table D8** Dopamine rate of infusion using dopamine 400 mg in a 250-mL infusion bag, i.e. 1.6 mg/mL (1600 micrograms/mL)

| Weight in kg | Infusion rate (micrograms/kg/minute) | | | | | | |
|---|---|---|---|---|---|---|---|
| | 1 | 2.5 | 5 | 7.5 | 10 | 15 | 20 |
| | Rate of infusion (mL/hour) | | | | | | |
| 40 | 1.5 | 3.8 | 7.5 | 11.3 | 15.0 | 22.5 | 30.0 |
| 45 | 1.7 | 4.2 | 8.4 | 12.7 | 16.9 | 25.3 | 33.8 |
| 50 | 1.9 | 4.7 | 9.4 | 14.1 | 18.8 | 28.1 | 37.5 |
| 55 | 2.1 | 5.2 | 10.3 | 15.5 | 20.6 | 30.9 | 41.3 |
| 60 | 2.3 | 5.6 | 11.3 | 16.9 | 22.5 | 33.8 | 45.0 |
| 65 | 2.4 | 6.1 | 12.2 | 18.3 | 24.4 | 36.6 | 48.8 |
| 70 | 2.6 | 6.6 | 13.1 | 19.7 | 26.3 | 39.4 | 52.5 |
| 75 | 2.8 | 7.0 | 14.1 | 21.1 | 28.1 | 42.2 | 56.3 |
| 80 | 3.0 | 7.5 | 15.0 | 22.5 | 30.0 | 45.0 | 60.0 |
| 85 | 3.2 | 8.0 | 15.9 | 23.9 | 31.9 | 47.8 | 63.8 |
| 90 | 3.4 | 8.4 | 16.9 | 25.3 | 33.8 | 50.6 | 67.5 |
| 95 | 3.6 | 8.9 | 17.8 | 26.7 | 35.6 | 53.4 | 71.3 |
| 100 | 3.8 | 9.4 | 18.8 | 28.1 | 37.5 | 56.3 | 75.0 |
| 110 | 4.1 | 10.3 | 20.6 | 30.9 | 41.3 | 61.9 | 82.5 |
| 120 | 4.5 | 11.3 | 22.5 | 33.8 | 45.0 | 67.5 | 90.0 |
| 130 | 4.9 | 12.2 | 24.4 | 36.6 | 48.8 | 73.1 | 97.5 |
| 140 | 5.3 | 13.1 | 26.3 | 39.4 | 52.5 | 78.8 | 105.0 |

**Table D9** Dopamine rate of infusion using dopamine 800 mg in a 250-mL infusion bag, i.e. 3.2 mg/mL (3200 micrograms/mL)

| Weight in kg | Infusion rate (micrograms/kg/minute) | | | | | | |
| | 1 | 2.5 | 5 | 7.5 | 10 | 15 | 20 |
|---|---|---|---|---|---|---|---|
| | Rate of infusion (mL/hour) | | | | | | |
| 40 | 0.8 | 1.9 | 3.8 | 5.6 | 7.5 | 11.3 | 15.0 |
| 45 | 0.8 | 2.1 | 4.2 | 6.3 | 8.4 | 12.7 | 16.9 |
| 50 | 0.9 | 2.3 | 4.7 | 7.0 | 9.4 | 14.1 | 18.8 |
| 55 | 1.0 | 2.6 | 5.2 | 7.7 | 10.3 | 15.5 | 20.6 |
| 60 | 1.1 | 2.8 | 5.6 | 8.4 | 11.3 | 16.9 | 22.5 |
| 65 | 1.2 | 3.0 | 6.1 | 9.1 | 12.2 | 18.3 | 24.4 |
| 70 | 1.3 | 3.3 | 6.6 | 9.8 | 13.1 | 19.7 | 26.3 |
| 75 | 1.4 | 3.5 | 7.0 | 10.5 | 14.1 | 21.1 | 28.1 |
| 80 | 1.5 | 3.8 | 7.5 | 11.3 | 15.0 | 22.5 | 30.0 |
| 85 | 1.6 | 4.0 | 8.0 | 12.0 | 15.9 | 23.9 | 31.9 |
| 90 | 1.7 | 4.2 | 8.4 | 12.7 | 16.9 | 25.3 | 33.8 |
| 95 | 1.8 | 4.5 | 8.9 | 13.4 | 17.8 | 26.7 | 35.6 |
| 100 | 1.9 | 4.7 | 9.4 | 14.1 | 18.8 | 28.1 | 37.5 |
| 110 | 2.1 | 5.2 | 10.3 | 15.5 | 20.6 | 30.9 | 41.3 |
| 120 | 2.3 | 5.6 | 11.3 | 16.9 | 22.5 | 33.8 | 45.0 |
| 130 | 2.4 | 6.1 | 12.2 | 18.3 | 24.4 | 36.6 | 48.8 |
| 140 | 2.6 | 6.6 | 13.1 | 19.7 | 26.3 | 39.4 | 52.5 |

**Table D10**  Dopamine rate of infusion (central line administration only) using dopamine 200 mg made up to 50 mL in a 50-mL syringe pump, i.e. 4 mg/mL (4000 micrograms/mL)

| Weight in kg | Infusion rate (micrograms/kg/minute) | | | | | | |
| --- | --- | --- | --- | --- | --- | --- | --- |
| | 1 | 2.5 | 5 | 7.5 | 10 | 15 | 20 |
| | Rate of infusion (mL/hour) | | | | | | |
| 40 | 0.6 | 1.5 | 3.0 | 4.5 | 6.0 | 9.0 | 12.0 |
| 45 | 0.7 | 1.7 | 3.4 | 5.1 | 6.8 | 10.1 | 13.5 |
| 50 | 0.8 | 1.9 | 3.8 | 5.6 | 7.5 | 11.3 | 15.0 |
| 55 | 0.8 | 2.1 | 4.1 | 6.2 | 8.3 | 12.4 | 16.5 |
| 60 | 0.9 | 2.3 | 4.5 | 6.8 | 9.0 | 13.5 | 18.0 |
| 65 | 1.0 | 2.4 | 4.9 | 7.3 | 9.8 | 14.6 | 19.5 |
| 70 | 1.1 | 2.6 | 5.3 | 7.9 | 10.5 | 15.8 | 21.0 |
| 75 | 1.1 | 2.8 | 5.6 | 8.4 | 11.3 | 16.9 | 22.5 |
| 80 | 1.2 | 3.0 | 6.0 | 9.0 | 12.0 | 18.0 | 24.0 |
| 85 | 1.3 | 3.2 | 6.4 | 9.6 | 12.8 | 19.1 | 25.5 |
| 90 | 1.4 | 3.4 | 6.8 | 10.1 | 13.5 | 20.3 | 27.0 |
| 95 | 1.4 | 3.6 | 7.1 | 10.7 | 14.3 | 21.4 | 28.5 |
| 100 | 1.5 | 3.8 | 7.5 | 11.3 | 15.0 | 22.5 | 30.0 |
| 110 | 1.7 | 4.1 | 8.3 | 12.4 | 16.5 | 24.8 | 33.0 |
| 120 | 1.8 | 4.5 | 9.0 | 13.5 | 18.0 | 27.0 | 36.0 |
| 130 | 2.0 | 4.9 | 9.8 | 14.6 | 19.5 | 29.3 | 39.0 |
| 140 | 2.1 | 5.3 | 10.5 | 15.8 | 21.0 | 31.5 | 42.0 |

# Dopexamine hydrochloride

**10 mg/ml solution in 5-mL ampoules**

* Dopexamine is a mildly inotropic sympathomimetic agent. It stimulates $beta_2$-adrenoceptors and peripheral dopamine receptors; it inhibits neuronal uptake of noradrenaline.
* It is used for afterload reduction in treatment of exacerbations of chronic heart failure, or to provide short-term haemodynamic support in heart failure associated with cardiac surgery.
* It has also been used (unlicensed) in critically ill patients to ↑splanchnic blood flow with the aim of preventing renal and GI dysfunction.

## Pre-treatment checks

* An inadequate circulating blood volume should be restored prior to and during treatment with dopexamine.
* Do not use in phaeochromocytoma, thrombocytopenia, left ventricular outlet obstruction such as hypertrophic obstructive cardiomyopathy or aortic stenosis.
* Caution in MI or recent angina, ↓K, hyperglycaemia, ↓BP; restrict sodium and fluid load during administration.

*Biochemical and other tests (not all are necessary in an emergency situation)*

Blood glucose                         Electrolytes: serum K
Bodyweight                            Platelets

## Dose

**Standard dose:** initiate at 500 nanograms/kg/minute by IV infusion into a central or large peripheral vein. This can be increased to 1 microgram/kg/minute and further increased up to 6 micrograms/kg/minute in increments of 0.5–1 microgram/kg/minute at intervals of not less than 15 minutes.

* Discontinue treatment gradually.
* Therapy beyond 48 hours has not been fully evaluated.

## Continuous intravenous infusion

The concentration used is dependent on the patient's dosage and fluid requirements.
The final concentration must be no greater than 1 mg/mL via a large peripheral vein, or 4 mg/mL via a central line.

*Preparation of a 0.8 mg/mL (800 micrograms/mL) solution*

1. Withdraw 20 mL from a 250-mL bag of NaCl 0.9%, Gluc 5% or Hartmann's and discard.
2. Withdraw 200 mg (20 mL) of the dopexamine concentrate into a syringe.
3. Add the dopexamine concentrate to the prepared infusion bag and mix well. This gives a solution containing 800 micrograms/mL.
4. The solution should be clear and colourless to very pale pink. Inspect visually for particulate matter or discoloration prior to administration and discard if present.

*Administration*

1. Give by IV infusion via a volumetric infusion device into a large vein at an initial rate of 500 nanograms/kg/minute.
2. Adjust dose according to clinical response.
3. Prepare a fresh infusion bag every 24 hours.

## Continuous intravenous infusion via a syringe pump

For administration via a central line only.

*Preparation of a 4 mg/mL (4000 micrograms/mL) solution*

1. Withdraw 200 mg (20 mL) of the dopexamine concentrate and make up to 50 mL in a syringe pump with NaCl 0.9%, Gluc 5% or Hartmann's.
2. Cap the syringe and mix well to give a solution containing 4 mg/mL (4000 micrograms/mL).
3. The solution should be clear and colourless to very pale pink. Inspect visually for particulate matter or discoloration prior to administration and discard if present.

*Administration*

1. Give by IV infusion via a syringe pump into a central line at an initial rate of 500 nanograms/kg/minute.
2. Adjust dose according to clinical response.
3. Prepare a fresh syringe every 24 hours.

**Calculation of infusion rate:**

$$\text{Infusion rate (mL/hour)} = \frac{\text{Weight (kg)} \times \text{required rate (micrograms/minute)} \times 60}{\text{Concentration of prepared infusion (micrograms/mL)}}$$

See Tables D11 and D12 below for dosage charts detailing pre-calculated infusion rates for each bodyweight using 800 micrograms/mL and 4 mg/mL (4000 micrograms/mL) solutions.

## Technical information

| | |
|---|---|
| Incompatible with | Sodium bicarbonate and other alkaline solutions.<br>Contact with metal parts in infusion apparatus should be minimised. |
| Compatible with | **Flush**: NaCl 0.9%<br>**Solutions**: NaCl 0.9%, Gluc 5%, Gluc NaCl, Hartmann's<br>**Y-site**: No information |
| pH | 3.7–5.7 |
| Sodium content | Negligible |
| Storage | Store below 25°C in original packaging. |
| Stability after preparation | From a microbiological point of view, should be used immediately; however, prepared infusions may be stored at 2–8°C and infused (at room temperature) within 24 hours. |

## Monitoring

| Measure | Frequency | Rationale |
|---|---|---|
| Heart rate/ECG | Continuously | • ↑ or ↓ pulse.<br>• Rhythm disturbances may occur. |

*(continued)*

## Monitoring (continued)

| Measure | Frequency | Rationale |
| --- | --- | --- |
| Blood pressure | Hourly | • ↑Systolic and MAP BP with doses >2 micrograms/kg/minute. |
| Urine output | | • Response to therapy. |
| Cardiac output (where possible) | | • Response to therapy. |
| Serum K | Daily | • May cause ↓K. |
| Blood glucose | | • May cause hyperglycaemia. |

## Additional information

| | |
| --- | --- |
| Common and serious undesirable effects | *Common:* Tachyarrhythmias, ↑ or ↓pulse, worsening heart failure leading to asystole and cardiac arrest, angina, myocardial infarction, cardiac enzyme changes and non-specific ECG changes have occurred, nausea and vomiting, tremor, headache, sweating, dyspnoea, reversible thrombocytopenia. |
| Pharmacokinetics | Serum half-life is 6-7 minutes; up to 11 minutes in heart failure. |
| Significant interactions | • Risk of hypertensive crisis with the following: MAOIs, moclobemide, rasagiline.<br>• Dopexamine may ↑levels or effect of the following drugs (or ↑side-effects): adrenaline (epinephrine), noradrenaline (norepinephrine). |
| Action in case of overdose | Effects are short lived and typically require supportive measures only. |
| Counselling | Nausea, vomiting, chest pain may occur. |

| Risk rating: **AMBER** | Score = 5<br>Moderate-risk product: Risk-reduction strategies are recommended. |
| --- | --- |

This assessment is based on the full range of preparation and administration options described in the monograph. These may not all be applicable in some clinical situations.

## Bibliography

SPC Dopacard, Cephalon Limited (accessed 4 May 2009).

**Table D11** Dopexamine rate of infusion using dopexamine 200 mg in a 250-mL infusion bag, i.e. 800 micrograms/mL

| Weight (kg) | Infusion rate (micrograms/kg/minute) | | | | | | | | | | |
|---|---|---|---|---|---|---|---|---|---|---|---|
| | 0.5 | 1.0 | 1.5 | 2.0 | 2.5 | 3.0 | 3.5 | 4.0 | 4.5 | 5.0 | 6.0 |
| | Rate of infusion (mL/hour) | | | | | | | | | | |
| 40 | 1.5 | 3.0 | 4.5 | 6.0 | 7.5 | 9.0 | 10.5 | 12.0 | 13.5 | 15.0 | 18.0 |
| 45 | 1.7 | 3.4 | 5.1 | 6.8 | 8.4 | 10.1 | 11.8 | 13.5 | 15.2 | 16.9 | 20.3 |
| 50 | 1.9 | 3.8 | 5.6 | 7.5 | 9.4 | 11.3 | 13.1 | 15.0 | 16.9 | 18.8 | 22.5 |
| 55 | 2.1 | 4.1 | 6.2 | 8.3 | 10.3 | 12.4 | 14.4 | 16.5 | 18.6 | 20.6 | 24.8 |
| 60 | 2.3 | 4.5 | 6.8 | 9.0 | 11.3 | 13.5 | 15.8 | 18.0 | 20.3 | 22.5 | 27.0 |
| 65 | 2.4 | 4.9 | 7.3 | 9.8 | 12.2 | 14.6 | 17.1 | 19.5 | 21.9 | 24.4 | 29.3 |
| 70 | 2.6 | 5.3 | 7.9 | 10.5 | 13.1 | 15.8 | 18.4 | 21.0 | 23.6 | 26.3 | 31.5 |
| 75 | 2.8 | 5.6 | 8.4 | 11.3 | 14.1 | 16.9 | 19.7 | 22.5 | 25.3 | 28.1 | 33.8 |
| 80 | 3.0 | 6.0 | 9.0 | 12.0 | 15.0 | 18.0 | 21.0 | 24.0 | 27.0 | 30.0 | 36.0 |
| 85 | 3.2 | 6.4 | 9.6 | 12.8 | 15.9 | 19.1 | 22.3 | 25.5 | 28.7 | 31.9 | 38.3 |
| 90 | 3.4 | 6.8 | 10.1 | 13.5 | 16.9 | 20.3 | 23.6 | 27.0 | 30.4 | 33.8 | 40.5 |
| 95 | 3.6 | 7.1 | 10.7 | 14.3 | 17.8 | 21.4 | 24.9 | 28.5 | 32.1 | 35.6 | 42.8 |
| 100 | 3.8 | 7.5 | 11.3 | 15.0 | 18.8 | 22.5 | 26.3 | 30.0 | 33.8 | 37.5 | 45.0 |
| 110 | 4.1 | 8.3 | 12.4 | 16.5 | 20.6 | 24.8 | 28.9 | 33.0 | 37.1 | 41.3 | 49.5 |
| 120 | 4.5 | 9.0 | 13.5 | 18.0 | 22.5 | 27.0 | 31.5 | 36.0 | 40.5 | 45.0 | 54.0 |
| 130 | 4.9 | 9.8 | 14.6 | 19.5 | 24.4 | 29.3 | 34.1 | 39.0 | 43.9 | 48.8 | 58.5 |
| 140 | 5.3 | 10.5 | 15.8 | 21.0 | 26.3 | 31.5 | 36.8 | 42.0 | 47.3 | 52.5 | 63.0 |

**Table D12** Dopexamine rate of infusion (central line administration only) using dopexamine 200 mg made up to 50 mL in a 50-mL syringe pump, i.e. 4 mg/mL (4000 micrograms/mL)

| Weight (kg) | Infusion rate (micrograms/kg/minute) | | | | | | | | | | |
|---|---|---|---|---|---|---|---|---|---|---|---|
| | 0.5 | 1.0 | 1.5 | 2.0 | 2.5 | 3.0 | 3.5 | 4.0 | 4.5 | 5.0 | 6.0 |
| | Rate of infusion (mL/hour) | | | | | | | | | | |
| 40 | 0.3 | 0.6 | 0.9 | 1.2 | 1.5 | 1.8 | 2.1 | 2.4 | 2.7 | 3.0 | 3.6 |
| 45 | 0.3 | 0.7 | 1.0 | 1.4 | 1.7 | 2.0 | 2.4 | 2.7 | 3.0 | 3.4 | 4.1 |
| 50 | 0.4 | 0.8 | 1.1 | 1.5 | 1.9 | 2.3 | 2.6 | 3.0 | 3.4 | 3.8 | 4.5 |
| 55 | 0.4 | 0.8 | 1.2 | 1.7 | 2.1 | 2.5 | 2.9 | 3.3 | 3.7 | 4.1 | 5.0 |
| 60 | 0.5 | 0.9 | 1.4 | 1.8 | 2.3 | 2.7 | 3.2 | 3.6 | 4.1 | 4.5 | 5.4 |
| 65 | 0.5 | 1.0 | 1.5 | 2.0 | 2.4 | 2.9 | 3.4 | 3.9 | 4.4 | 4.9 | 5.9 |
| 70 | 0.5 | 1.1 | 1.6 | 2.1 | 2.6 | 3.2 | 3.7 | 4.2 | 4.7 | 5.3 | 6.3 |
| 75 | 0.6 | 1.1 | 1.7 | 2.3 | 2.8 | 3.4 | 3.9 | 4.5 | 5.1 | 5.6 | 6.8 |
| 80 | 0.6 | 1.2 | 1.8 | 2.4 | 3.0 | 3.6 | 4.2 | 4.8 | 5.4 | 6.0 | 7.2 |
| 85 | 0.6 | 1.3 | 1.9 | 2.6 | 3.2 | 3.8 | 4.5 | 5.1 | 5.7 | 6.4 | 7.7 |
| 90 | 0.7 | 1.4 | 2.0 | 2.7 | 3.4 | 4.1 | 4.7 | 5.4 | 6.1 | 6.8 | 8.1 |
| 95 | 0.7 | 1.4 | 2.1 | 2.9 | 3.6 | 4.3 | 5.0 | 5.7 | 6.4 | 7.1 | 8.6 |
| 100 | 0.8 | 1.5 | 2.3 | 3.0 | 3.8 | 4.5 | 5.3 | 6.0 | 6.8 | 7.5 | 9.0 |
| 110 | 0.8 | 1.7 | 2.5 | 3.3 | 4.1 | 5.0 | 5.8 | 6.6 | 7.4 | 8.3 | 9.9 |
| 120 | 0.9 | 1.8 | 2.7 | 3.6 | 4.5 | 5.4 | 6.3 | 7.2 | 8.1 | 9.0 | 10.8 |
| 130 | 1.0 | 2.0 | 2.9 | 3.9 | 4.9 | 5.9 | 6.8 | 7.8 | 8.8 | 9.8 | 11.7 |
| 140 | 1.1 | 2.1 | 3.2 | 4.2 | 5.3 | 6.3 | 7.4 | 8.4 | 9.5 | 10.5 | 12.6 |

# Doripenem

**500-mg dry powder vials**

- Doripenem is a synthetic carbapenem beta-lactam antibiotic related to other carbapenems (e.g. ertapenem, imipenem, meropenem). It is more stable to renal dehydropeptidase I than imipenem, meaning that it does not need to be combined with cilastatin to be effective.
- It is used to treat nosocomial pneumonia (including ventilator-associated pneumonia), complicated intra-abdominal infections and complicated urinary tract infections.

## Pre-treatment checks

- Do not give if there is known hypersensitivity to any carbapenem antibacterial agent or previous immediate hypersensitivity reaction to penicillins or cephalosporins.

*Biochemical and other tests*

Renal function: U, Cr, CrCl (or eGFR)

## Dose

Doripenem must not be given by inhalation as this has resulted in pneumonitis.

**Standard dose**: 500 mg every 8 hours.
**Dose in renal impairment**: adjusted according to creatinine clearance:
- CrCl >50 mL/minute: dose as in normal renal function.
- CrCl 30–50 mL/minute: 250 mg every 8 hours.
- CrCl <30 mL/minute: 250 mg every 12 hours.

## Intermittent intravenous infusion

*Preparation and administration*

1. Add 10 mL WFI or NaCl 0.9% to each 500-mg vial and shake to form a suspension.
2. Withdraw the contents of the vial and add to 100 mL NaCl 0.9%.
3. Mix until completely dissolved.
4. The solution should be clear and colourless to slightly yellow. Inspect visually for particulate matter or discoloration prior to administration and discard if present.
5. Give by IV infusion over 1 hour (in the case of severe infections including nosocomial pneumonia this may be increased to 4 hours, which allows the serum concentration to be maintained above the MIC for a longer period of time).

*Preparation of a 250-mg dose*

The manufacturer recommends following steps 1–4 above and removing and discarding 55 mL of the prepared solution from the infusion bag. Give the remainder by IV infusion over 1 hour.

## Technical information

| | |
|---|---|
| Incompatible with | Amphotericin, diazepam, propofol. |
| Compatible with | **Flush**: NaCl 0.9%<br>**Solutions**: NaCl 0.9%, less stable in Gluc 5% (see Stability below)<br>**Y-site**: Aciclovir, amikacin, aminophylline, bumetanide, calcium gluconate, ciprofloxacin, dexamethasone sodium phosphate, digoxin, dobutamine, dopamine, esmolol, fentanyl, fluconazole, furosemide, gentamicin, granisetron, hydrocortisone sodium succinate, labetalol, linezolid, magnesium sulfate, methylprednisolone sodium succinate, metoclopramide, metronidazole, midazolam, noradrenaline (norepinephrine), ondansetron, pantoprazole, potassium chloride, ranitidine, tigecycline, tobramycin, vancomycin |
| pH[1] | 4.5-5.5 |
| Sodium content | Nil |
| Storage | Store below 25°C in original packaging. |
| Displacement value | Negligible |
| Stability after preparation | Infusions prepared in Gluc 5% should be used immediately and infused over 1 hour (insufficiently stable for 4-hour infusion).<br>From a microbiological point of view, infusions prepared in NaCl 0.9% should be used immediately; however, they may be stored at 2-8°C and infused (at room temperature) within 24 hours. |

## Monitoring

| Measure | Frequency | Rationale |
|---|---|---|
| Renal function | Periodically | • Monitor U, Cr and CrCl particularly in patients with moderate to severe impairment.<br>• Changes in function may require a dose adjustment. |
| Development of seizures | Throughout treatment | • Although rare, seizures do sometimes occur, most likely in elderly patients and those with pre-existing CNS disorders (e.g. brain lesions or history of seizures) and/or renal impairment. |
| Development of diarrhoea | Throughout and up to 2 months after treatment | • Development of severe, persistent diarrhoea may be suggestive of *Clostridium difficile*-associated diarrhoea and colitis (pseudomembranous colitis). Discontinue drug and treat. Do not use drugs that inhibit peristalsis. |

## Additional information

| | |
|---|---|
| Common and serious undesirable effects | *Immediate:* Anaphylaxis has occurred rarely.<br>*Infusion-related:* Local: Phlebitis.<br>*Other:* Oral and vaginal candidiasis, headache, nausea, diarrhoea, †hepatic enzymes, pruritus, rash, *C. difficile* colitis. |

*(continued)*

| **Additional information** (*continued*) | |
|---|---|
| Pharmacokinetics | Elimination half-life is about 1 hour. |
| Significant interactions | No significant interactions. |
| Action in case of overdose | *Antidote:* No known antidote but haemodialysis may be effective. Stop administration and give supportive therapy as appropriate. |

Risk rating: **GREEN**   Score = 2
Lower-risk product: Risk-reduction strategies should be considered.

This assessment is based on the full range of preparation and administration options described in the monograph. These may not all be applicable in some clinical situations.

## Reference

1. Communication with manufacturer, 24 April 2009.

## Bibliography

SPC Doribax 500 mg powder for solution for infusion (accessed 13 April 2009).

# Doxapram hydrochloride

### 2 mg/mL solution in 500-mL infusion bag
### 20 mg/mL solution in 5-mL ampoules

* Doxapram hydrochloride is a central and respiratory stimulant with a brief duration of action. It acts by stimulating peripheral chemoreceptors and central respiratory centres. Despite ↑respiratory rate and volume, arterial $O_2$ is rarely improved because doxapram ↑work of breathing (i.e. ↑$O_2$ consumption = ↑$CO_2$ production).
* Doxapram antagonises the respiratory depressant effects of opioids without interfering with their analgesic properties.
* It is used for postoperative respiratory depression to stimulate ventilation and ↓pulmonary complications.
* It has been used in the treatment of ventilatory failure in patients with COPD, but has been largely superseded by ventilatory support. However, if ventilatory support is contraindicated in patients with hypercapnic respiratory failure who are becoming drowsy or comatose, doxapram may revive patients so that they can cooperate and clear secretions.

## Pre-treatment checks

- Respiratory stimulants can be harmful in respiratory failure as they also stimulate non-respiratory muscles. They must only be given under expert supervision in hospital combined with physiotherapy.
- Do not use in severe hypertension, status asthmaticus, coronary artery disease, thyrotoxicosis, epilepsy, recent head injury or physical obstruction of the respiratory tract.
- Give with caution in hypertension (avoid if severe), impaired cardiac reserve, hepatic impairment (doxapram is primarily metabolised by the liver).
- Use in pregnancy only if compelling reasons.
- Protect the airway because of the risk of vomiting and aspiration.
- Give with oxygen in severe irreversible airways obstruction or severely decreased lung compliance (because of ↑workload of breathing).
- Give with a beta$_2$-agonist in bronchoconstriction.
- Delay doxapram use for at least 10 minutes following discontinuation of anaesthetics known to sensitise the myocardium to catecholamines, e.g. halothane, because of possible ↑adrenaline release.

*Biochemical and other tests*

ABGs and pH                                   Bodyweight
Blood pressure and pulse                      LFTs

## Dose

> Doxapram has a narrow margin of safety so the minimum effective dosage should be used.

**Postoperative respiratory depression:**
- 1–1.5 mg/kg bodyweight by IV injection. Repeat at 1-hour intervals if necessary.
- May also be given by IV infusion at an initial rate of 2–3 mg/minute adjusted according to patient response.

**Respiratory failure**: 1.5–4 mg/minute by IV infusion depending on condition and response of the patient. Table D13 shows a dosage regimen that has been shown to result in the rapid achievement of a steady-state plasma concentration of doxapram.

**Table D13**  A doxapram dosing regimen

| Time from start of infusion (minutes) | Rate (mg/minute) | Using 2 mg/mL infusion solution: | |
| --- | --- | --- | --- |
| | | Rate (mL/minute) | Rate (mL/hour) |
| 0-15 | 4.0 | 2 | 120 |
| 15-30 | 3.0 | 1.5 | 90 |
| 30-60 | 2.0 | 1 | 60 |
| 60 onwards | 1.5 | 0.75 | 45 |

## Intravenous injection

*Preparation and administration*

1. Using the 20 mg/mL preparation, withdraw the required dose.
2. The solution should be clear and colourless. Inspect visually for particulate matter or discoloration prior to administration and discard if present.
3. Give by IV injection over 30 seconds.

## Continuous intravenous infusion

*Preparation and administration*

1. Use the pre-prepared IV infusion containing doxapram 2 mg/mL in Gluc 5%.
2. Give by IV infusion up to a maximum rate of 4 mg/minute (i.e. 2 mL/minute, 120 mL/hour).

## Technical information

| | |
|---|---|
| Incompatible with | Sodium bicarbonate.<br>Aminophylline, cefotaxime, cefuroxime, clindamycin phosphate, dexamethasone sodium phosphate, diazepam, digoxin, dobutamine, folic acid, furosemide, hydrocortisone sodium succinate, methylprednisolone sodium succinate, Pabrinex. |
| Compatible with | **Flush**: NaCl 0.9%<br>**Solutions**: NaCl 0.9%, Gluc 5%, Gluc-NaCl (Y-site)<br>**Y-site**: Adrenaline (epinephrine), amikacin, ampicillin, bumetanide, calcium gluconate, ceftazidime, chlorpromazine, dopamine, erythromycin lactobionate, fentanyl, gentamicin, metoclopramide, metronidazole, ranitidine, terbutaline, tobramycin, vancomycin |
| pH | 3.5-5 |
| Sodium content | Nil |
| Storage | *Ampoules:* Store below 25°C in original packaging. Do not refrigerate.<br>*Infusion:* Store below 25°C. |

## Monitoring

| Measure | Frequency | Rationale |
|---|---|---|
| Arterial blood gases and pH | Every 30 minutes during treatment | • To enable dosage adjustment. |
| Respiratory function | | • The effect of doxapram may be shorter than the effects of any respiratory depressant drugs.<br>• Respiratory depression may recur after dosing with doxapram: the patient should be closely monitored until fully alert for 30-60 minutes.<br>• Doxapram may temporarily mask the residual effects of curare-type muscle relaxant drugs. |
| Blood pressure and pulse | | • Stop treatment if sudden ↓BP develops.<br>• ↑BP and ↑pulse are early signs of toxicity. |
| Deep tendon reflexes | | • ↑Deep tendon reflexes are an early sign of toxicity. |

## Additional information

| | |
|---|---|
| Common and serious undesirable effects | *Injection/infusion-related:* None.<br>*Other:* Pyrexia, sweating, flushing, headache, dizziness, hyperactivity, confusion, hallucinations, perineal warmth, muscle fasciculation, dyspnoea, cough, ↑BP, arrhythmias, ↑ or ↓pulse, extrasystoles, chest pain, chest tightness, nausea, vomiting, salivation, desire to defecate, convulsions, bronchospasm, laryngospasm. |
| Pharmacokinetics | Rapidly distributed into tissues after IV injection. Onset of respiratory stimulation usually occurs in 20-40 seconds; peak effect is achieved in 1-2 minutes. Duration of effect following a single dose varies from 5-12 minutes. |
| Significant interactions | The following may ↑doxapram levels or effect (or ↑side-effects):<br>linezolid (theoretical risk of ↑BP), MAOIs (risk of ↑BP), sympathomimetics (risk of ↑BP), theophylline (↑CNS stimulation, e.g. agitation, muscle twitching).<br>Doxapram may ↓levels or effect of muscle relaxants (may mask residual effects). |
| Action in case of overdose | *Symptoms to watch for:* ↑BP, ↑pulse, arrhythmias, ↑deep tendon reflexes, dyspnoea, clonic and generalised seizures.<br>*Antidote:* No known antidote.<br>Stop administration and give supportive therapy as appropriate. |

| Risk rating: **AMBER** | Score = 4<br>Moderate-risk product: Risk-reduction strategies are recommended. |
|---|---|

This assessment is based on the full range of preparation and administration options described in the monograph. These may not all be applicable in some clinical situations.

## Bibliography

SPC Dopram infusion: doxapram hydrochloride 2 mg/ml solution for infusion (received by e-mail 16 February 2009).

SPC Dopram injection (received by e-mail 16 February 2009).

# Enfuvirtide

### 90 mg/mL dry powder vials with solvent (WFI)

* Enfuvirtide is an HIV fusion inhibitor that interferes with entry of HIV into cells.
* It is used with other antiretrovirals in the management of HIV infection.

## Pre-treatment checks

* Use with caution in hepatic impairment.

## Dose

**Standard dose:** 90 mg twice daily.

## Subcutaneous injection

*Preparation and administration*

Vials contain 108 mg of enfuvirtide providing 90 mg/mL after reconstitution.

1. Withdraw 1.1 mL of the diluent (WFI) and add to the powder vial.
2. Gently tap the vial with a fingertip until the powder begins to dissolve. The vial **must not** be shaken or turned upside down as this will cause excessive foaming.
3. After the powder begins to dissolve it may be set aside to allow complete dissolution; this may take up to 45 minutes. Gently rolling the vial between the hands may reduce this time.
4. The resulting solution contains 90 mg/mL enfuvirtide. It should be clear and bubble-free. Inspect visually for visible particles or cloudiness and discard if present.
5. Withdraw the required dose from the vial and give by SC injection into the upper arm, anterior thigh or abdomen (avoiding the navel).

* Each injection should be given at a site different from the preceding injection.
* Injections should not be made into areas where the skin shows signs of a previous injection site reaction or near anatomical areas where large nerve tracts lie close to the skin, e.g. near the elbow, knee, groin, inferior or medial section of the buttocks.
* Also avoid injecting directly over blood vessels, into skin abnormalities, moles, scars (including surgical scars), bruises, tattoos or burn sites.

## Technical information

| | |
|---|---|
| Incompatible with | Not relevant |
| Compatible with | Not relevant |
| pH | 9.0 |
| Sodium content | Negligible |
| Storage | Store below 25°C in original packaging. |

*(continued)*

## Technical information (continued)

| | |
|---|---|
| Displacement value | Nil |
| Stability after reconstitution | From a microbiological point of view, should be used immediately; however, reconstituted solutions may be stored at 2-8°C and injected (at room temperature) within 24 hours. |

## Monitoring

| Measure | Frequency | Rationale |
|---|---|---|
| Signs of a systemic hypersensitivity reaction | Throughout treatment | • Treatment must be stopped immediately and not restarted if this occurs.<br>• Signs include: rash, fever, nausea, vomiting, chills, rigors, low BP, respiratory distress, glomerulonephritis, and ↑liver enzymes. |
| Signs of Immune Reactivation Syndrome | | • Inflammatory symptoms are more likely to occur in the first few weeks or months after initiation of therapy and should be evaluated, with treatment instituted as appropriate.<br>• Complications that may occur include cytomegalovirus retinitis, mycobacterial infections, and *Pneumocystis carinii* pneumonia. |
| Viral load and CD4 cell count | | • To monitor efficacy of the combined treatment. |

## Additional information

| | |
|---|---|
| Common and serious undesirable effects | *Immediate:* Hypersensitivity reactions (may also be delayed).<br>*Injection-related:* Local injection site reactions - pain, erythema, induration, nodules and cysts, pruritus, ecchymosis.<br>*Other:* Pancreatitis, GORD, anorexia, weight loss; hypertriglyceridaemia; peripheral neuropathy, asthenia, tremor, anxiety, nightmares, irritability, impaired concentration, vertigo; pneumonia, sinusitis, influenza-like illness; diabetes mellitus; haematuria; renal calculi, lymphadenopathy; myalgia; conjunctivitis; dry skin, acne, skin papilloma. |
| Pharmacokinetics | Elimination half-life is 3.8 hours. |
| Significant interactions | None reported. |
| Action in case of overdose | No specific antidote. Stop administration and give supportive therapy as appropriate. |
| Counselling | Patients should be advised to seek medical advice if they experience joint aches and pain, joint stiffness or difficulty in movement (possible signs of osteonecrosis). Also to seek immediate medical advice if there are signs of hypersensitivity. |

| Risk rating: **AMBER** | Score = 3<br>Moderate-risk product: Risk-reduction strategies are recommended. |

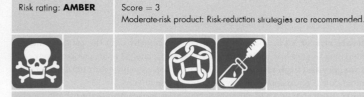

This assessment is based on the full range of preparation and administration options described in the monograph. These may not all be applicable in some clinical situations.

## Bibliography

SPC Fuzeon (accessed 16 March 2009).

# Enoxaparin sodium

**100 mg/mL solution in 20-mg, 40-mg, 60-mg, 80-mg, 100-mg pre-filled syringes and 3-mL vials**
**150 mg/mL solution in 120-mg, 150-mg pre-filled syringes**

* Enoxaparin sodium is low-molecular-weight heparin.
* It is used in the treatment of STEMI and also in the acute coronary syndromes: unstable angina and NSTEMI.
* It is used in the treatment of VTE, i.e. pulmonary embolism and deep vein thrombosis.
* It is used for prophylaxis of VTE in surgical and medical patients and to prevent thrombus formation in extracorporeal circulation during haemodialysis.
* Not all products are licensed for all indications.
* Enoxaparin sodium 1 mg ≅ 100 units of anti-Factor Xa activity.

## Pre-treatment checks

* Avoid in acute bacterial endocarditis, major bleeding or high risk of uncontrolled haemorrhage including recent haemorrhagic stroke.
* In treatment dosage it is contraindicated in patients undergoing locoregional anaesthesia in elective surgical procedures.
* Placement or removal of a spinal/epidural catheter should be delayed for 10–12 hours after administration of prophylactic doses, whereas patients receiving higher doses (1.5 mg/kg once daily) require a 24 hours delay. Subsequent enoxaparin doses should be given no sooner than 4 hours after catheter removal.
* Caution with other drugs affecting haemostasis, such as aspirin or clopidogrel.
* Use with extreme caution in patients with a history of HIT.
* Patients with severe renal or hepatic impairment may need a reduced dose (or at least closer monitoring of ADRs).

*Biochemical and other tests (not all are necessary in an emergency situation)*

| | |
|---|---|
| Bodyweight (for certain indications) | LFTs |
| Electrolytes: serum K | Platelet count |
| INR | Renal function: U, Cr, CrCl (or eGFR) |

## Dose

*Prophylaxis*

**Low to moderate risk of VTE:** 20 mg by SC injection once daily until the patient is mobile. In patients undergoing surgery, the initial dose is given approximately 2 hours preoperatively.

**Orthopaedic surgery and high risk of VTE:** 40 mg by SC injection once daily until the patient is mobile. The initial dose is given approximately 12 hours preoperatively.

**Medical patients (high risk of VTE):** 40 mg by SC injection once daily until the patient is mobile for a maximum of 14 days.

**Prevention of extracorporeal thrombus formation during haemodialysis**: 1 mg/kg introduced into the arterial line at the start of dialysis session. A second dose of 0.5–1 mg/kg may be given after 4 hours if fibrin rings are found. For patients at a high risk of haemorrhage the dose should be reduced to 0.5 mg/kg for double vascular access or 0.75 mg/kg for single vascular access.

*Treatment*

**Treatment of VTE:** 1.5 mg/kg by SC injection once daily for at least 5 days and until INR is >2.

**Treatment of ACS:** 1 mg/kg by SC injection every 12 hours, for a minimum of 2 days until clinically stable.

**Treatment of acute STEMI:** 30 mg by IV injection plus 1 mg/kg by SC injection. This is followed by 1 mg/kg by SC injection every 12 hours (maximum 100 mg for the first two SC doses only) for 8 days or until hospital discharge, whichever comes first. **For patients ≥75 years of age**, omit the IV dose and give 0.75 mg/kg by SC injection every 12 hours (maximum 75 mg for the first two SC doses only).

**Use in acute STEMI with a fibrinolytic:** as above but give enoxaparin between 15 minutes before and 30 minutes after the start of fibrinolytic therapy.

**Use in acute STEMI with PCI:** if the last SC dose of enoxaparin was given <8 hours before balloon inflation, no additional dosing is needed. If the last SC dose was given >8 hours before balloon inflation, give 0.3 mg/kg enoxaparin by IV injection.

**Dose in renal impairment:** dose is adjusted depending on indication and CrCl. See Table E1.

**Table E1**  Enoxaparin dosing in renal impairment

| Standard dose | Creatinine clearance <30 mL/minute |
|---|---|
| 1 mg/kg twice daily | 1 mg/kg once daily |
| 1.5 mg/kg once daily | 1 mg/kg once daily |
| 40 mg once daily | 20 mg once daily |
| 20 mg once daily | 20 mg once daily |
| 30 mg IV injection plus a 1 mg/kg SC injection followed by 1 mg/kg SC twice daily | 30 mg IV injection plus a 1 mg/kg SC injection followed by 1 mg/kg SC once daily |
| *Patients ≥75 years of age (for acute STEMI indication only)* | |
| 0.75 mg/kg SC twice daily without initial IV dose | 1 mg/kg SC once daily without initial IV dose |

## Subcutaneous injection

*Preparation and administration*

1. Select the correct pre-filled syringe. Pre-filled syringes are ready for immediate use: do not expel the air bubble.
   If using multidose vials, withdraw the required dose using a needle suitable for SC administration.
2. The patient should be seated or lying down.
3. Pinch up a skin fold on the abdominal wall between the thumb and forefinger and hold throughout the injection.
4. Give by deep SC injection into the thick part of the skin fold at right angles to the skin. Do not rub the injection site after administration. Alternate doses between the right and left sides.

## Intravenous injection (acute STEMI only)

*Preparation and administration*

1. Withdraw the required dose from a multidose vial, or select an appropriately sized pre-filled syringe and expel the air bubble and excess enoxaparin.
2. The solution should be clear and colourless to pale yellow. Inspect visually for particulate matter or discoloration prior to administration and discard if present.
3. Flush the line with NaCl 0.9% or Gluc 5%.
4. Give by IV injection over 5 seconds and then flush with NaCl 0.9% or Gluc 5%.

## Arterial line injection (haemodialysis circuits)

*Preparation and administration*

1. Withdraw the required dose from a multidose vial, or select an appropriately sized pre-filled syringe and expel the air bubble and excess enoxaparin.
2. The solution should be clear and colourless to pale yellow. Inspect visually for particulate matter or discoloration prior to administration and discard if present.
3. Give over 5 seconds via a port into the arterial limb of the haemodialysis circuit.

| Technical information | |
|---|---|
| Incompatible with | No information |
| Compatible with | **Flush**: NaCl 0.9%, Gluc 5%<br>**Solutions**: NaCl 0.9%, Gluc 5%<br>**Y-site**: No information |
| pH | 5.5-7.5 |
| Sodium content | Negligible |
| Excipients | Vials contain benzyl alcohol. |
| Storage | Store below 25°C in original packaging but do not refrigerate.<br>*In use*: Vial contents should be used within 28 days of first use. |

## Monitoring

| Measure | Frequency | Rationale |
|---|---|---|
| INR | Daily | • If used for the treatment of VTE. |
| Platelets | Regularly from day 5 to day 21 | • Thrombocytopenia can occur from days 5 to 21 of therapy.<br>• A 50%↓ in platelets is indicative of HIT and therapy should be switched to a non-heparin-derived agent.<br>• The manufacturer does not recommend a specific frequency of monitoring, but one suggested regimen is to test on days 5, 10 and 15. |
| Serum K | After 7 days | • Heparins ↓secretion of aldosterone and may cause ↑K.<br>• K should be monitored in all patients with risk factors, particularly those receiving enoxaparin for more than 7 days.<br>• Risk factors include: diabetes mellitus, chronic renal failure, pre-existing metabolic acidosis, ↑plasma K or if taking potassium-sparing drugs. |
| Evidence of bleeding | Throughout treatment | • There is higher risk of bleeding with prophylactic enoxaparin doses if body weight is low: in women <45 kg and in men <57 kg. |
| Anti-Xa activity | If indicated | • Not required routinely but may be considered in patients at ↑risk of bleeding or who are actively bleeding. |

## Additional information

| | |
|---|---|
| Common and serious undesirable effects | *Immediate:* Anaphylaxis has been reported rarely.<br>*Injection/infusion-related:* Local: Pain, haematoma and mild local irritation may follow the SC injection of enoxaparin.<br>*Other:* Risk of bleeding with organic lesions, invasive procedures, asymptomatic thrombocytopenia during the first days of therapy, clinically significant ↑K in patients with diabetes or chronic renal failure. |
| Pharmacokinetics | Rapidly absorbed after SC injection with an elimination half-life of 4-5 hours.<br>Elimination is prolonged in renal impairment. |
| Significant interactions | • The following may ↑risk of bleeding with enoxaparin: aspirin, diclofenac IV (avoid combination), ketorolac (avoid combination).<br>• Glyceryl trinitrate infusion may ↓enoxaparin levels or effect. |
| Action in case of overdose | *Symptoms to watch for:* Bleeding.<br>*Antidote:* Protamine sulfate may be used to ↓bleeding risk if clinically required. See the Protamine sulfate monograph. |
| Counselling | Instruction in injection technique, safe disposal of sharps and use within 28 days if using multiple dose vial (if appropriate).<br>Report any bleeding or bruising and any injection site effects. |

| Risk rating: **GREEN** | Score = 1<br>Lower-risk product. Risk-reduction strategies should be considered. |

This assessment is based on the full range of preparation and administration options described in the monograph. These may not all be applicable in some clinical situations.

## Bibliography

SPC Clexane pre-filled syringes and multi-dose vial (accessed 2 June 2009).

# Enoximone

### 5 mg/mL solution in 20-mL ampoules

* Enoximone is a phosphodiesterase type 3 inhibitor with positive inotropic and vasodilator activity.
* It is now used parenterally only for short-term management of heart failure unresponsive to other treatments.

## Pre-treatment checks

* Use with caution in heart failure associated with hypertrophic cardiomyopathy, stenotic or obstructive valvular disease or other outlet obstruction.
* The injection solution is strongly alkaline and must be diluted with an equal volume of NaCl 0.9% or WFI before use.

*Biochemical and other tests (not all are necessary in an emergency situation)*

| Bodyweight | Platelet count |
| LFTs | Renal function: U, Cr, CrCl (or eGFR) |

## Dose

* **Standard dose by IV injection:** initially 0.5–1 mg/kg by slow IV injection, then 500 micrograms/kg every 30 minutes until satisfactory response or total of 3 mg/kg given. For maintenance, the initial dose of up to 3 mg/kg may be repeated every 3–6 hours as required.
* **Standard dose by IV infusion:** initially 90 micrograms/kg/minute by IV infusion over 10–30 minutes, followed by intermittent or continuous infusion of 5–20 micrograms/kg/minute. Total dose over 24 hours should not usually exceed 24 mg/kg.
* **Dose in renal and hepatic impairment:** doses should be reduced and ideally levels should be monitored during continuous infusions.

## Intravenous injection

Enoximone is incompatible with Gluc 5%.
See Special handling and Spillage below.

*Preparation and administration*

1. Withdraw the required dose and dilute with an equal volume of NaCl 0.9% or WFI to give a solution containing 2.5 mg/mL.
2. The solution should be clear and yellow in colour. Inspect visually for particulate matter or discoloration prior to administration and discard if present.
3. Give by slow IV injection at a maximum rate of 12.5 mg/minute (5 mL/minute of the diluted injection solution).

## Continuous intravenous infusion via a syringe pump

Enoximone is incompatible with Gluc 5%.
See *Special handling* and *Spillage* below.

*To prepare a 2.5 mg/mL (2500 micrograms/mL) solution*

1. Withdraw 100 mg (20 mL) of injection and make up to 40 mL in a syringe with NaCl 0.9%.
2. Cap the syringe and mix well to produce a solution containing 2.5 mg/mL (2500 micrograms/mL).
3. The solution should be clear and yellow in colour. Inspect visually for particulate matter or discoloration prior to administration and discard if present.

*Administration*

1. Give by IV infusion via a syringe pump as described under Dose above.
2. Adjust the dose according to clinical response.
3. Prepare a fresh syringe every 24 hours.

**Calculation of infusion rate:**

$$\text{Infusion rate (mL/hour)} = \frac{\text{Weight in kg} \times \text{required rate (micrograms/minute)} \times 60}{\text{Concentration of prepared infusion (micrograms/mL)}}$$

See Table E2 below for a dosage chart detailing pre-calculated infusion rates for each bodyweight using a 2.5 mg/mL (2500 micrograms/mL) solution.

## Technical information

| | |
|---|---|
| Incompatible with | Enoximone is incompatible with Gluc 5%. Crystal formation can occur if glass syringes or containers are used. |
| Compatible with | **Flush**: NaCl 0.9% <br> **Solutions**: NaCl 0.9%, WFI <br> **Y-site**: No information |
| pH | About 12 |
| Sodium content | Negligible |
| Excipients | Contains ethanol (may interact with metronidazole, possible religious objections). Contains propylene glycol (adverse effects seen in ↓renal function, may interact with disulfiram and metronidazole). |
| Storage | Store below 25°C in original packaging. Do not refrigerate or freeze (crystals may form). |
| Special handling | Extremely caustic. |
| Spillage | Protective clothing required. |

*(continued)*

## Technical information (continued)

| | |
|---|---|
| Stability after preparation | From a microbiological point of view, should be used immediately; however, prepared infusions may be stored at room temperature and infused within 24 hours. Do not refrigerate as crystals may form. |

## Monitoring

| Measure | Frequency | Rationale |
|---|---|---|
| Clinical improvement | Throughout treatment | • Monitor the signs and symptoms of congestive heart failure. |
| Ventricular arrhythmias | Continuously | • Enoximone may ↑ventricular response rate in patients with uncontrolled atrial flutter/fibrillation.<br>• Stop infusion if arrhythmias occur. |
| Blood pressure and heart rate | Continuously during loading | • May ↓BP through vasodilatation. |
| Signs of extravasation | Hourly | • Stop immediately if apparent – the solution is caustic. |
| Platelet count | Daily | • Thrombocytopenia has been reported. |
| Liver enzyme values | Periodically | • Deranged values reported; may require a dose adjustment. |

## Additional information

| | |
|---|---|
| Common and serious undesirable effects | *Common:* ↓BP, insomnia, headache, thrombocytopenia, ↑transaminases and bilirubin. |
| Pharmacokinetics | The plasma elimination half-life varies widely from 1 to 4 hours in healthy subjects and about 3 to 8 hours in patients with heart failure. |
| Significant interactions | • Enoximone should not be used with anagrelide.<br>• Injectable preparation contains ethanol: may interact with disulfiram and metronidazole. |
| Action in case of overdose | *Symptoms to watch for:* ↓BP.<br>Reduce dose or stop administration and give supportive therapy as appropriate. |

| | |
|---|---|
| Risk rating: **AMBER** | Score = 5<br>Moderate-risk product: Risk-reduction strategies are recommended. |

This assessment is based on the full range of preparation and administration options described in the monograph. These may not all be applicable in some clinical situations.

## Bibliography

SPC Perfan from INCA-Pharm GmbH, last revised June 2008.

**Table E2** Enoximone rate of infusion using enoximone 100 mg (20 mL) made up to 40 mL in a syringe pump, i.e. 2.5 mg/mL (2500 micrograms/mL)

| Weight in kg | Infusion rate (micrograms/kg/minute) | | | | |
| | Loading dose: 90 (10–30 minutes only) | 5 | 10 | 15 | 20 |
| | Rate of infusion (mL/hour) | | | | |
|---|---|---|---|---|---|
| 40 | 86.4 | 4.8 | 9.6 | 14.4 | 19.2 |
| 45 | 97.2 | 5.4 | 10.8 | 16.2 | 21.6 |
| 50 | 108.0 | 6.0 | 12.0 | 18.0 | 24.0 |
| 55 | 118.8 | 6.6 | 13.2 | 19.8 | 26.4 |
| 60 | 129.6 | 7.2 | 14.4 | 21.6 | 28.8 |
| 65 | 140.4 | 7.8 | 15.6 | 23.4 | 31.2 |
| 70 | 151.2 | 8.4 | 16.8 | 25.2 | 33.6 |
| 75 | 162.0 | 9.0 | 18.0 | 27.0 | 36.0 |
| 80 | 172.8 | 9.6 | 19.2 | 28.8 | 38.4 |
| 85 | 183.6 | 10.2 | 20.4 | 30.6 | 40.8 |
| 90 | 194.4 | 10.8 | 21.6 | 32.4 | 43.2 |
| 95 | 205.2 | 11.4 | 22.8 | 34.2 | 45.6 |
| 100 | 216.0 | 12.0 | 24.0 | 36.0 | 48.0 |
| 110 | 237.6 | 13.2 | 26.4 | 39.6 | 52.8 |
| 120 | 259.2 | 14.4 | 28.8 | 43.2 | 57.6 |
| 130 | 280.8 | 15.6 | 31.2 | 46.8 | 62.4 |
| 140 | 302.4 | 16.8 | 33.6 | 50.4 | 67.2 |

# Ephedrine hydrochloride

**3 mg/mL solution in 10-mL ampoules; 30 mg/mL solution in 1-mL ampoules**

* Ephedrine hydrochloride is a sympathomimetic with direct and indirect effects on adrenergic receptors. It is less potent than adrenaline (epinephrine) but has a more prolonged action. It ↑BP by both peripheral vasoconstriction and by ↑cardiac output. It is less likely than adrenaline to ↑pulse.
* It is given parenterally to combat ↓BP during spinal or epidural anaesthesia; the risk of ↓BP with spinal or epidural block is greater than with other forms of nerve block. It is ineffective in ↓BP due to shock, circulatory collapse or haemorrhage.

## Pre-treatment checks

* Caution in hyperthyroidism, diabetes mellitus, ischaemic heart disease, hypertension, susceptibility to angle-closure glaucoma, elderly patients, pregnancy.
* May cause acute urine retention in prostatic hypertrophy.

*Biochemical and other tests (not all are necessary in an emergency situation)*

Blood pressure
TFTs

## Dose

**Reversal of hypotension from spinal or epidural anaesthesia**: 3–6 mg (max. 9 mg) given by slow IV injection of a solution containing 3 mg/mL. This is repeated every 3–4 minutes according to response up to a maximum of 30 mg.

## Intravenous injection

*Preparation and administration*

Note: the total maximum dose of 30 mg is given gradually in increments of 3–6 mg.

1. Withdraw the required dose. If using the 30 mg/mL product, dilute to 3 mg/mL with NaCl 0.9%.
2. The solution should be clear and colourless. Inspect visually for particulate matter or discoloration prior to administration and discard if present.
3. Give by IV injection over 3–4 minutes in increments of 3–6 mg (1–2 mL of the dilute 3 mg/mL injection).

## Technical information

| Incompatible with | No information |
|---|---|
| Compatible with | **Flush**: NaCl 0.9%<br>**Solutions**: NaCl 0.9%<br>**Y-site**: No information |
| pH | 4.5–7.0 |
| Sodium content | Nil |
| Storage | Store below 25°C in original packaging. |
| Stability after preparation | Use prepared dilutions immediately. |

## Monitoring

| Measure | Frequency | Rationale |
| --- | --- | --- |
| Blood pressure | Throughout therapy | • BP should be elevated to slightly less than the patient's normal BP.<br>• In previously normotensive patients, systolic BP should be maintained at 80-100 mmHg.<br>• In previously hypertensive patients, the systolic BP should be maintained at 30-40 mmHg below their usual BP.<br>• When used during labour, only a sufficient dosage should be administered to maintain the BP at ≤130/80 mmHg. |
| Heart rate, ECG and urine output | | • To check for therapeutic/toxic effect. |

## Additional information

| | |
| --- | --- |
| Common and serious undesirable effects | Nausea, vomiting, anorexia; ↑pulse (sometimes ↓pulse), arrhythmias, anginal pain, vasoconstriction with ↑BP, vasodilation with ↓BP, dizziness and flushing; dyspnoea; headache, anxiety, restlessness, confusion, psychoses, insomnia, tremor; difficulty in micturition, urine retention; sweating, ↑salivation; ↑blood glucose concentration. |
| Pharmacokinetics | Elimination half-life is 3-6 hours. If urine pH is low elimination is closer to 3 hours. |
| Significant interactions | • Ephedrine may ↑levels or effect of the following drugs (or ↑side-effects): rasagiline (avoid combination), MAOIs (risk of hypertensive crisis, avoid combination and use within 2 weeks of withdrawal), moclobemide (risk of hypertensive crisis, avoid combination, and use within 2 weeks of withdrawal).<br>• Ephedrine may ↓levels or effect of adrenergic neurone blockers (↓hypotensive effect). |
| Action in case of overdose | No specific antidote. Stop administration and give supportive therapy as appropriate. |

| Risk rating: **AMBER** | Score = 3<br>Moderate-risk product: Risk-reduction strategies are recommended. |
| --- | --- |

This assessment is based on the full range of preparation and administration options described in the monograph. These may not all be applicable in some clinical situations.

## Bibliography

SPC Ephedrine hydrochloride injection 3 mg/mL Aurum, September 2005 version.

# Epoprostenol (PGI$_2$, PGX, prostacyclin)

**0.5-mg and 1.5-mg dry powder vials with 50 mL glycine buffer solvent and filter**

> Epoprostenol must not be confused with its analogue iloprost (both names are sometimes erroneously used interchangeably).

- Epoprostenol is a prostaglandin that causes vasodilatation and has platelet de-aggregant properties.
- It is used to prevent platelet aggregation in extracorporeal circuits, e.g. in renal dialysis particularly where use of heparin is contraindicated because of ↑risk of bleeding or for other reasons.
- It is also indicated for the treatment of primary pulmonary hypertension (PPH) in NYHA Class III and Class IV patients who do not respond adequately to conventional therapy. It was originally introduced into the management of end-stage PPH to sustain patients long enough for them to have heart–lung transplantation; however, long-term therapy may also have a role as an alternative to transplantation.
- Epoprostenol has many unlicensed uses including peripheral vascular disease, e.g. severe Raynaud syndrome.
- Many centres have their own protocols for dosing and handling epoprostenol and these should be followed where available.
- Doses are expressed in terms of the base:
  Epoprostenol 1 nanogram ≅ 1.06 nanograms epoprostenol sodium.

## Pre-treatment checks

- Avoid in severe left ventricular dysfunction.
- Caution in concomitant anticoagulant therapy or drugs that ↑risk of bleeding (monitoring is required when given with heparin).
- Other cautions include: haemorrhagic diathesis; dose titration for PPH should be in hospital (risk of pulmonary oedema); and pregnancy.
- Caution also in elderly patients (dose choice should reflect the greater frequency of ↓hepatic, renal or cardiac function and of concomitant disease or other drug therapy in this cohort).

*Biochemical and other tests (not all are necessary in an emergency situation)*

| | |
|---|---|
| Blood glucose level in diabetic patients | FBC including platelets |
| Blood pressure | Heart rate |
| Bodyweight | Renal function: U, Cr |

## Dose

**Renal dialysis**: 4 nanograms/kg/minute by IV infusion prior to dialysis, then during dialysis give 4 nanograms/kg/minute as a continuous infusion into the arterial inlet of the dialyser. Stop the infusion at the end of dialysis.

**Primary pulmonary hypertension:** see product literature for details.

**Severe Raynaud's syndrome (unlicensed):** doses vary – consult your local protocol.

**Calculation of infusion rate (see also Table E3 below):**

$$\text{Infusion rate (mL/hour)} = \frac{\text{Dose (nanograms/kg/minute)} \times \text{bodyweight} \times 60}{\text{Concentration of prepared infusion (micrograms/mL)}}$$

## Continuous intravenous infusion (other than for PPH)

*Preparation of a 2000 nanograms/mL solution*

1. Reconstitute each 0.5-mg vial with approximately 10 mL of the provided solvent and shake gently until the powder has dissolved.
2. Withdraw the entire contents of the drug vial and inject into the residue of the 50-mL solvent vial.
3. Mix well to produce a concentrated solution containing 10 000 nanograms/mL.
4. Withdraw 50 mL from a 250 mL NaCl 0.9% infusion bag and discard.
5. Withdraw 50 mL epoprostenol solution from the vial.
6. Attach the filter provided to the syringe and using firm but not excessive pressure transfer the concentrated solution into the prepared infusion bag of NaCl 0.9% (it takes about 70 seconds to filter 50 mL). Discard the filter unit.
7. Mix well to produce a solution containing 2000 nanograms/mL.
8. The solution should be clear and colourless. Inspect visually for particulate matter or discoloration prior to administration and discard if present.

*Administration*

Give by IV infusion using a volumetric infusion device or syringe pump at the specified rate (see Table E3).

**Fluid restriction:** the concentrated solution may be given undiluted.

**Table E3**   Epoprostenol rate of infusion using a 2000 nanograms/mL solution

| | Infusion rate (nanograms/kg/minute) | | | | |
|---|---|---|---|---|---|
| | **1** | **2** | **3** | **4** | **5** |
| **Weight in kg** | **Rate of infusion(mL/hour)** | | | | |
| 30 | 0.9 | 1.8 | 2.7 | 3.6 | 4.5 |
| 40 | 1.2 | 2.4 | 3.6 | 4.8 | 6.0 |
| 50 | 1.5 | 3.0 | 4.5 | 6.0 | 7.5 |
| 60 | 1.8 | 3.6 | 5.4 | 7.2 | 9.0 |
| 70 | 2.1 | 4.2 | 6.3 | 8.4 | 10.5 |
| 80 | 2.4 | 4.8 | 7.2 | 9.6 | 12.0 |
| 90 | 2.7 | 5.4 | 8.1 | 10.8 | 13.5 |
| 100 | 3.0 | 6.0 | 9.0 | 12.0 | 15.0 |

## Continuous intravenous infusion for PPH

See product literature.

## Technical information

| Incompatible with | No information but do not mix with any other drug. |
|---|---|
| Compatible with | **Flush**: NaCl 0.9%<br>**Solutions**: manufacturers diluent, NaCl 0.9%<br>**Y-site**: No information but likely to be unstable |
| pH | 10.2–10.8 |
| Sodium content | 2.4 mmol/50 mL (in reconstituted vial) |
| Storage | Store below 25°C in original packaging. Do not freeze. |
| Displacement value | Negligible |
| Stability after preparation | Prepared infusions must be infused at room temperature within 12 hours. For PPH the infusion must be completed within 24 hours held in a cold pouch at 2–8°C (which should be changed as necessary throughout the day) |

## Monitoring

| Measure | Frequency | Rationale |
|---|---|---|
| Blood pressure and heart rate | Frequently through administration – at least every 30 minutes | • ↓BP and ↓or ↑heart rate may occur.<br>• If excessive ↓BP occurs during administration, the dose should be reduced or the infusion discontinued.<br>• The recommended doses should be exceeded only with careful monitoring of BP.<br>• ↓BP may be profound in overdose and may result in loss of consciousness. |
| Signs of clotting in the dialysis circuit | Frequently through administration | • Epoprostenol is not a conventional anticoagulant. Although successfully used instead of heparin in renal dialysis, in a small proportion of dialyses clotting has developed, which requires termination of dialysis. |
| Platelets | Periodically | • ↓Platelet count may occur. |
| Blood glucose | Periodically in diabetic patients | • ↑Serum glucose levels have been reported. |
| ECG | If indicated | • This has been suggested in patients with coronary artery disease. |

## Additional information

| Common and serious undesirable effects | *Immediate:* ↓BP, ↑pulse, arrhythmia, nausea, vomiting.<br>*Injection/infusion-related:* Local: Reddening and pain at the infusion site. Extravasation causes tissue damage.<br>*Other:* Sepsis, septicaemia (mostly related to delivery system), ↓platelet count, anxiety, nervousness, headache, facial flushing (seen even in anaesthetised patients), abdominal colic/discomfort, jaw pain. |
|---|---|
| Pharmacokinetics | Elimination half-life is 3–5 minutes. The cardiovascular effects during infusion disappear within 30 minutes of the end of administration. |

(continued)

| **Additional information** (*continued*) | |
|---|---|
| Significant interactions | • The following may ↑epoprostenol levels or effect (or ↑side-effects): other anticoagulants or antiplatelet agents, other vasodilators.<br>• Epoprostenol may reduce the thrombolytic efficacy of tissue plasminogen activator (t-PA). |
| Action in case of overdose | Reduce the dose or discontinue the infusion and initiate appropriate supportive measures as necessary, e.g. plasma volume expansion. |

| Risk rating: **RED** | Score = 7<br>High-risk product: Risk-reduction strategies are required to minimise these risks. |
|---|---|

This assessment is based on the full range of preparation and administration options described in the monograph. These may not all be applicable in some clinical situations.

## Bibliography

SPC Flolan 0.5 mg injection (accessed 31 March 2010).
SPC Flolan 1.5 mg injection (accessed 31 March 2010).

# Eptifibatide

### 2 mg/mL solution in 10-mL vials; 0.75 mg/mL solution in 100-mL vials

• Eptifibatide is an antiplatelet drug that reversibly inhibits binding of fibrinogen, von Willebrand factor, and other adhesive molecules to the glycoprotein IIb/IIIa receptor of platelets.
• It is used, usually in combination with aspirin and heparin, in the management of unstable angina and in patients undergoing coronary angioplasty and coronary artery stenting.

## Pre-treatment checks

• Avoid in abnormal bleeding within 30 days, major surgery or severe trauma within 6 weeks, stroke within last 30 days or any history of haemorrhagic stroke, intracranial disease (aneurysm, neoplasm or arteriovenous malformation), severe ↑BP, haemorrhagic diathesis, ↑PT or INR, thrombocytopenia, significant hepatic impairment; breast feeding.
• Caution in renal impairment.
• The number of vascular punctures and IM injections should be minimised during the treatment.
• IV access should only be obtained at compressible sites of the body.
• All vascular puncture sites should be documented and closely monitored (caution if there is puncture of a non-compressible vessel within 24 hours).
• The use of urinary catheters, nasotracheal intubation and nasogastric tubes should be critically considered before commencing therapy.

*Biochemical and other tests (not all are necessary in an emergency situation)*

| | |
|---|---|
| ACT | FBC (including platelets, Hb and haematocrit) |
| APTT | LFTs |
| Blood pressure | Prothrombin time |
| Bodyweight | Renal function: U, Cr, CrCl (or eGFR) |

## Dose

**Unstable angina or non-Q-wave MI**: 180 micrograms/kg by IV injection as soon as possible after diagnosis, followed by 2 micrograms/kg/minute by IV infusion for up to 72 hours, until initiation of CABG surgery, or until discharge from the hospital (whichever occurs first).

* **If PCI is performed during eptifibatide therapy**, continue the infusion for 20–24 hours post PCI for an overall maximum duration of therapy of 96 hours.
* **If emergency or urgent cardiac surgery is required** during the infusion, terminate the eptifibatide immediately.
* **If the patient requires semi-elective surgery**, stop the infusion at an appropriate time to allow time for platelet function to return towards normal.

**Concomitant therapy with unfractionated heparin in unstable angina or non-Q-wave MI:**
* Patients ≥70 kg: 5000 units by IV injection, followed by 1000 units/hour by IV infusion.
* Patients <70 kg, 60 units/kg by IV injection, followed by 12 units/kg/hour by IV infusion.

**Dose in renal impairment**: adjusted according to creatinine clearance,
* CrCl 30–50 mL/minute: IV injection dose as in normal renal function, IV infusion dose 1 microgram/kg/minute for the duration of therapy.
* CrCl <30 mL/minute: do not use.

**Dose in hepatic impairment:** contraindicated in clinically significant hepatic impairment.

## Intravenous injection

*Preparation and administration*

1. Using the 2 mg/mL strength, withdraw the required dose.
2. The solution should be clear and colourless. Inspect visually for particulate matter or discoloration prior to administration and discard if present.
3. Give by IV injection over 1–2 minutes.

## Continuous intravenous infusion

*Preparation and administration*

1. The 0.75 mg/mL strength is pre-prepared for use.
2. The solution should be clear and colourless. Inspect visually for particulate matter or discoloration prior to administration and discard if present.
3. Spike the vial with a vented infusion set, taking care to centre the spike within the circle on the stopper top.
4. Give by IV infusion at the required rate via a volumetric infusion device.

| Technical information | |
|---|---|
| Incompatible with | Furosemide |
| Compatible with | **Flush**: NaCl 0.9%<br>**Solutions**: NaCl 0.9%, Gluc 5%, (both including added KCl)<br>**Y-site**: Alteplase, atropine sulfate, bivalirudin, dobutamine, glyceryl trinitrate, lidocaine, micafungin, midazolam, morphine sulfate, verapamil |

*(continued)*

## Technical information (*continued*)

| | |
|---|---|
| pH | 5.3 |
| Sodium content | Negligible |
| Storage | Store at 2-8°C in original packaging. Protect from light.<br>Vial contents are single use only - discard any unused portion. |
| Stability after preparation | Use prepared infusions immediately. |

## Monitoring

| Measure | Frequency | Rationale |
|---|---|---|
| Platelets | Within 6 hours of administration and at least daily (more frequently if signs of bleeding) | • If platelets fall to <100 000/mm$^3$ discontinue eptifibatide and unfractionated heparin.<br>• Monitor and treat as appropriate - consider platelet transfusions on an individual basis.<br>• Further platelet counts may be required to rule out pseudo thrombocytopenia. |
| Hb and haematocrit | | • To check for any adverse events or bleeding.<br>• Monitor for fall in Hb of >3 g/dL. |
| APTT in UA/NQMI | Every 30 minutes | • Target is to maintain a value between 50 and 70 seconds.<br>• APTT >70 seconds has ↑risk of bleeding. |
| ACT if PCI to be performed | | • The target is to maintain a value between 300 and 350 seconds.<br>• Stop heparin if the ACT >300 seconds; do not administer until the ACT falls below 300 seconds. |
| Blood pressure | Frequently | • ↓BP may occur. |

## Additional information

| | |
|---|---|
| Common and serious undesirable effects | *Injection-related:* Local: Phlebitis.<br>*Other:* Shock, ↓BP, cardiac arrest, ventricular fibrillation, ventricular tachycardia, congestive heart failure, AV block, atrial fibrillation. |
| Pharmacokinetics | Elimination half-life is 1.1-2.5 hours. Antiplatelet effects persist for about 4 hours after stopping an infusion. |
| Significant interactions | Antiplatelet drugs may ↑eptifibatide levels or effect (or ↑side-effects): possibly not significant. |
| Action in case of overdose | *Symptoms to watch for:* Thrombocytopenia or uncontrolled bleeding.<br>*Antidote:* No specific antidote. Platelet transfusion could be considered; however, activity is rapidly halted by discontinuation of infusion. |

| Risk rating: **AMBER** | Score = 4<br>Moderate-risk product. Risk-reduction strategies are recommended. | |
|---|---|---|

  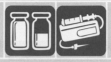

This assessment is based on the full range of preparation and administration options described in the monograph. These may not all be applicable in some clinical situations.

## Bibliography

SPC Integrilin 2 mg solution for injection, 0.75 mg solution for infusion (accessed 30 March 2010).

# Ergocalciferol (calciferol, vitamin D₂)

**300 000 units/mL oily solution in 1-mL and 2-mL ampoules**
* The term vitamin D is used for a range of closely related sterol compounds including alfacalcidol, calcitriol, colecalciferol and ergocalciferol. Vitamin D compounds possess the property of preventing or curing rickets.
* Ergocalciferol injection is indicated in patients with gastrointestinal, liver or biliary disease associated with malabsorption of vitamin D, resulting in hypophosphataemia, rickets, and osteomalacia.
* Ergocalciferol 1 mg is considered to be equivalent to 40 000 units of vitamin D; however, dose comparisons between the different vitamin D compounds are imperfect and may not truly reflect relative vitamin D activity.

## Pre-treatment checks

* Do not give to patients with ↑Ca, including ↑Ca of malignancy.
* Avoid use in hypoparathyroidism.
* Because of the effect on serum Ca, give to patients with renal stones only when benefits outweigh risks.
* For treatment to be effective, patients should be receiving an adequate daily intake of calcium (dietary or prescribed). Phosphate supplements may also be prescribed if appropriate.

*Biochemical and other tests*

Electrolytes: serum Ca, $PO_4$
Liver function: Alk Phos
Renal function: U, Cr, CrCl (or eGFR) (risk of ↑Ca in renal impairment)

## Dose

There are reports of ergocalciferol injections being given daily, weekly, monthly, every 2 months or even annually. However, as the duration of action of ergocalciferol injection is approximately 2 months, one option is to give 300 000 units and review Ca and $PO_4$ levels at 8 weeks. The dose can then be repeated if necessary.
Doses should not normally exceed 40 000 units/day for adults.

## Intramuscular injection

*Preparation and administration*

1. Withdraw the required dose.
2. Give by IM injection.

### Technical information

| | |
|---|---|
| Incompatible with | Not relevant |
| Compatible with | Not relevant |
| pH | Not relevant |
| Sodium content | None |
| Storage | Store below 25°C in original packaging. |

### Monitoring

| Measure | Frequency | Rationale |
|---|---|---|
| Serum Ca and PO$_4$ | See Rationale | • The manufacturer recommends initially monitoring weekly until dose and plasma Ca and PO$_4$ are stable, then monthly; and also whenever nausea or vomiting occurs. In practice many centres check 8 weeks after a single dose.<br>• ↑Ca and ↑PO$_4$ can occur during treatment with pharmacological doses of compounds having vitamin D activity.<br>• Plasma PO$_4$ concentrations should be controlled to reduce the risk of ectopic calcification. |
| Alkaline phosphatase | Monthly | • A fall in serum Alk Phos levels often precedes the appearance of ↑Ca. |
| Ophthalmological examination | Periodically | • To check for ectopic calcification. |
| Signs/symptoms of toxicity | | • E.g. persistent constipation or diarrhoea, constant headache, loss of appetite, mental changes. |

### Additional information

| | |
|---|---|
| Common and serious undesirable effects | ↑Ca (persistent constipation or diarrhoea, constant headache, vertigo, loss of appetite, polyuria, thirst, sweating), rash. |
| Pharmacokinetics | There is a lag of 10–24 hours between administration of ergocalciferol and initiation of its action in the body. Maximum effects occur about 4 weeks after administration and the duration of action can be ≥2 months. Ergocalciferol is hydroxylated in the liver and further metabolism occurs in the kidney. |
| Significant interactions | No significant interactions. |

*(continued)*

| Additional information (continued) | |
|---|---|
| Action in case of overdose | Stop treatment if ↑Ca develops. However, effects can persist for more than 2 months after ergocalciferol treatment ceases. In severe ↑Ca give supportive therapy as appropriate. |
| Counselling | Advise to report symptoms of ↑Ca: persistent constipation or diarrhoea, constant headache, vertigo, loss of appetite, polyuria, thirst, sweating. |

| Risk rating: **GREEN** | Score = 0 Lower-risk product: Risk-reduction strategies should be considered. |
|---|---|

| | | | | | | | |
|---|---|---|---|---|---|---|---|

This assessment is based on the full range of preparation and administration options described in the monograph. These may not all be applicable in some clinical situations.

## Bibliography

SPC Ergocalciferol Injection BP 300,000U and 600,000U SPC, UCB Pharma Ltd (accessed 26 January 2009).

# Ertapenem

### 1-g dry powder vials

- Ertapenem sodium is a carbapenem beta-lactam antibacterial.
- It is used in the treatment of susceptible infections including intra-abdominal infections, acute gynaecological infections, urinary tract infections, skin and skin structure infections (including diabetic foot infections), community-acquired pneumonia and prophylactically in colorectal surgery.
- Doses are expressed in terms of base:
  Ertapenem 1 g ≅ 1.04 g ertapenem sodium.

### Pre-treatment checks

- Do not give if there is known hypersensitivity to any carbapenem antibacterial agent or previous immediate hypersensitivity reaction to penicillins or cephalosporins.

*Biochemical tests*

FBC
LFTs
Renal function: U, Cr, CrCl (or eGFR)

## Dose

**Standard dose:** 1 g by IV infusion daily.

**Surgical prophylaxis:** 1 g by IV infusion within 1 hour before the start of surgery. Check local policies.

**Dose in renal impairment**: adjusted according to creatinine clearance:[1]

* CrCl 10–30 mL/minute: 500 mg–1 g daily.
* CrCl <10 mL/minute: 500 mg daily or 1 g three times a week.

## Intermittent intravenous infusion

*Preparation and administration*

Ertapenem is incompatible with Gluc 5%, Gluc-NaCl, Hartmann's, Ringer's.

1. Reconstitute each 1-g vial with 10 mL WFI or NaCl 0.9% to produce a 100 mg/mL solution. Shake well.
2. Withdraw the required dose and add to 50 mL NaCl 0.9% (final concentration must be no more than 20 mg/mL).
3. The solution should be clear and colourless. Inspect visually for particulate matter or discoloration prior to administration and discard if present.
4. Give by IV infusion over 30 minutes.

## Technical information

| | |
|---|---|
| Incompatible with | Ertapenem is incompatible with Gluc 5%, Gluc-NaCl, Hartmann's, Ringer's.<br>Anidulafungin, mannitol, sodium bicarbonate. |
| Compatible with | **Flush**: NaCl 0.9%<br>**Solutions**: WFI, NaCl 0.9% (including added KCl)<br>**Y-site**: Dextran 40, dextran 70 |
| pH | 7.5 |
| Sodium content | 6 mmol/1-g vial |
| Storage | Store below 25°C in original packaging. |
| Displacement value | Negligible |
| Stability after preparation | From a microbiological point of view, should be used immediately; however:<br>• Prepared infusions may be stored at 2–8°C and infused (at room temperature) within 24 hours.<br>• Vials reconstituted for IM injection should be used within 1 hour. |

## Monitoring

| Measure | Frequency | Rationale |
|---------|-----------|-----------|
| U&Es | Periodically | • ↑U and ↑Cr occur occasionally.<br>• If CrCl falls below 30 mL/minute a review of dosing will be required. |
| LFTs | | • ↑ALT, ↑AST, ↑Alk Phos occur frequently. Bilirubin may also rise. |
| FBC | | • Platelet count rises frequently. Other changes in red and white cell parameters may occur but are uncommon. |
| Development of seizures | Throughout treatment | • Although rare, seizures do sometimes occur, most likely in elderly patients and those with pre-existing CNS disorders (e.g. brain lesions or history of seizures) and/or renal impairment. |
| Signs of supra-infection or superinfection | | • May result in the overgrowth of non-susceptible organisms – appropriate therapy should be commenced; treatment may need to be interrupted. |
| Development of diarrhoea | Throughout and up to 2 months after treatment | • Development of severe, persistent diarrhoea may be suggestive of *Clostridium difficile*-associated diarrhoea and colitis (pseudomembranous colitis). Discontinue drug and treat. Do not use drugs that inhibit peristalsis. |

## Additional information

| | |
|---|---|
| Common and serious undesirable effects | *Immediate:* Allergy has rarely been reported.<br>*Injection/infusion-related:* Local: Infusion site reactions, phlebitis/thrombophlebitis.<br>*Other:* Headache, diarrhoea, nausea, vomiting, rash, pruritus. |
| Pharmacokinetics | Elimination half-life is 4 hours. |
| Significant interactions | No significant interactions. |
| Action in case of overdose | *Antidote:* No known antidote but may be removed to some extent by haemodialysis. Stop administration and give supportive therapy as appropriate. |

| | |
|---|---|
| Risk rating: **AMBER** | Score = 3<br>Moderate-risk product: Risk-reduction strategies are recommended. |

 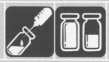

This assessment is based on the full range of preparation and administration options described in the monograph. These may not all be applicable in some clinical situations.

## Reference

1. Ashley C, Currie A, eds. *The Renal Drug Handbook*, 3rd edn. Oxford: Radcliffe Medical Press, 2009.

## Bibliography

SPC INVANZ 1 g powder for concentrate for solution for infusion (accessed 17 March 2009).

# Erythromycin lactobionate

**1-g dry powder vials**

- Erythromycin is a macrolide antibacterial with a broad spectrum of activity.
- It may be used in the treatment of a wide range of infections caused by susceptible organisms including: *Bacillus anthracis, Listeria monocytogenes, Clostridium* spp., *Neisseria meningitidis, Neisseria gonorrhoeae* and *Legionella* spp.
- It is given by IV infusion where high blood levels are required or when the oral route is compromised. Erythromycin was formerly given by IM injection, but such injections are painful and result in unpredictable levels.
- Erythromycin also stimulates gut motility apparently by acting as a motilin receptor agonist. It is sometimes used for its prokinetic action in patients with ↓GI motility, particularly in critically ill patients.
- Doses are expressed in terms of the base:
  Erythromycin 1 g ≅ 1.49 g erythromycin lactobionate.

## Pre-treatment checks

- Erythromycin lactobionate **must not** be given by direct IV injection (risk of fatal ventricular arrhythmias).
- Contraindicated in patients with known hypersensitivity to macrolide antibiotics.
- Avoid in acute porphyria.
- Caution if predisposition to QT interval prolongation (including electrolyte disturbances, concomitant use of drugs that prolong QT interval).

*Biochemical and other tests (not all are necessary in an emergency situation)*

| | |
|---|---|
| Bodyweight in certain indications | LFTs |
| ECG | Renal function: U, Cr, CrCl (or eGFR) |

## Dose

**Intermittent IV infusion:** 250–500 mg every 6 hours for mild to moderate infections.
**Continuous IV infusion:** 25–50 mg/kg per day (up to a maximum of 4 g/day in severe infections).
**Prokinetic dose (unlicensed):** 250 mg four times daily has been used.[1]
**Dose in renal impairment:** CrCl <10 mL/minute: maximum 2 g daily.[2]

## Intermittent intravenous infusion

*Preparation and administration*

Erythromycin lactobionate is incompatible with Gluc 5% (unless buffered, see below), Gluc-NaCl, Hartmann's and Ringer's.

1. Reconstitute each vial with 20 mL WFI and shake vigorously to produce a solution containing 50 mg/mL.
2. Withdraw the required dose and add to a minimum of 100 mL NaCl 0.9% to give a solution containing 1–5 mg/mL. Mix well.
3. The solution should be clear and colourless to very pale yellow. Inspect visually for particulate matter or discoloration prior to administration and discard if present.
4. Give by IV infusion over 60 minutes. Give more slowly in patients with risk factors or previous history of arrhythmias.

## Continuous intravenous infusion

*Preparation and administration*

1. Reconstitute each 1-g vial with 20 mL WFI and shake vigorously to produce a solution containing 50 mg/mL.
2. Withdraw the required dose and add to a suitable volume of NaCl 0.9% to give a final concentration of about 1 mg/mL. Mix well. Concentrations up to 5 mg/mL have been used but may ↑venous irritation.
3. The solution should be clear and colourless to very pale yellow. Inspect visually for particulate matter or discoloration prior to administration and discard if present.
4. Give by IV infusion. Prepare a fresh infusion bag at least every 24 hours if required.

| Technical information | |
|---|---|
| Incompatible with | Erythromycin lactobionate is incompatible with Gluc 5% (unless buffered, see below), Gluc-NaCl, Hartmann's, and Ringer's.<br>Ceftazidime, chloramphenicol sodium succinate, flucloxacillin, furosemide, heparin sodium, linezolid, metoclopramide, Pabrinex. |
| Compatible with | **Flush**: NaCl 0.9%<br>**Solutions**: WFI, NaCl 0.9% (including added KCl), buffered Gluc 5% (add 5 mL sodium bicarbonate 8.4% to each 1000 mL Gluc 5% and mix well)<br>**Y-site**: Aciclovir, aminophylline, ampicillin, benzylpenicillin, esmolol, foscarnet, fusidate sodium, hydrocortisone sodium succinate, labetalol, magnesium sulfate, midazolam, ranitidine, verapamil |
| pH | 6.5–7.5 (reconstituted) |
| Sodium content | Nil |
| Storage | Store below 25°C in original packaging. |
| Displacement value | Negligible |
| Stability after preparation | From a microbiological point of view, should be used immediately; however:<br>• Reconstituted vials may be stored at 2–8°C for 24 hours.<br>• Prepared infusions may be stored at 2–8°C and infused (at room temperature) within 24 hours. |

## Monitoring

| Measure | Frequency | Rationale |
|---|---|---|
| Physical signs of infection | Daily | • Monitor patient response (e.g. FBC, normalisation of observations) for signs of infection resolution – consider review to oral erythromycin as appropriate. |
| LFTs | Weekly | • Monitor in patients with pre-existing hepatic impairment or history of jaundice.<br>• Can cause idiosyncratic hepatotoxicity. |
| Renal function | | • Monitor in patients with worsening renal function as dose reduction may be necessary. |
| ECG | Ongoing | • Use with caution and monitor in patients at risk of prolonged QT interval or ventricular tachycardia. |
| Blood pressure | | • Rapid infusion rates can cause ↓BP. |
| Injection-site reaction | | • Thrombophlebitis can occur. |
| Signs of supra-infection or superinfection | Throughout treatment | • May result in the overgrowth of non-susceptible organisms – appropriate therapy should be commenced; treatment may need to be interrupted. |
| Development of diarrhoea | Throughout and up to 2 months after treatment | • Development of severe, persistent diarrhoea may be suggestive of *Clostridium difficile*-associated diarrhoea and colitis (pseudomembranous colitis). Discontinue drug and treat. Do not use drugs that inhibit peristalsis. |

## Additional information

| | |
|---|---|
| Common and serious undesirable effects | *Infusion-related:*<br>• Too rapid administration: ↓BP, ↑QT interval, ventricular arrhythmias (some fatal).<br>• Local: Venous irritation, thrombophlebitis (↓infusion rate if necessary).<br><br>*Other:* Nausea, vomiting, abdominal discomfort, diarrhoea (antibiotic-associated colitis has been reported), hearing loss (reversible, usually associated with doses >4 g per day), urticaria, rashes, cholestatic jaundice, pancreatitis, cardiac effects (including chest pain and arrhythmias), Stevens-Johnson syndrome and toxic epidermal necrolysis. |
| Pharmacokinetics | Elimination half-life in normal renal function is about 2 hours. In severe impairment it may be 4-7 hours. |

*(continued)*

## Additional information (continued)

| | |
|---|---|
| Significant interactions | • Sirolimus may ↑erythromycin levels or effect (or ↑side-effects).<br>• Cilostazol may ↓erythromycin levels or effect (avoid combination).<br>• Erythromycin may ↑risk of arrhythmias with the following drugs: amiodarone (avoid combination), amisulpride (avoid combination), atomoxetine, droperidol (avoid combination), ivabradine (avoid combination), moxifloxacin (avoid combination), pentamidine isetionate, pimozide (avoid combination), sertindole (avoid combination), sulpiride, zuclopenthixol (avoid combination).<br>• Erythromycin may ↑levels or effect of the following drugs (or ↑side-effects):<br>artemether/lumefantrine (avoid combination), carbamazepine, ciclosporin, cilostazol (avoid combination), clozapine (possible ↑risk of convulsions), colchicine, coumarins (monitor INR), disopyramide, eletriptan (avoid combination), ergotamine (avoid combination), methysergide (avoid combination), midazolam, mizolastine (avoid combination), reboxetine (avoid combination), rifabutin (↑risk of uveitis, ↓rifabutin dose), simvastatin (↑risk of myopathy, avoid combination), sirolimus, tacrolimus, theophylline (monitor levels), verapamil, vinblastine (avoid combination). |
| Action in case of overdose | *Symptoms to watch for:* Severe nausea, vomiting and diarrhoea.<br>Stop administration and give supportive therapy as appropriate. |
| Counselling | Inform the patient of any alterations to their medication while they are being treated with erythromycin, e.g. withholding statins or theophylline. |

| | |
|---|---|
| Risk rating: **AMBER** | Score = 4<br>Moderate-risk product: Risk-reduction strategies are recommended. |

This assessment is based on the full range of preparation and administration options described in the monograph. These may not all be applicable in some clinical situations.

## References

1. Reignier J *et al.* Erythromycin and early enteral nutrition in mechanically ventilated patients. *Crit Care Med.* 2002; 30(6): 1386–1387.
2. Ashley C, Currie A, eds. *The Renal Drug Handbook*, 3rd edn. Oxford: Radcliffe Medical Press, 2009.

## Bibliography

SPC Erythromycin lactobionate for intravenous infusion 1 g, Hospira UK Ltd (accessed 28 September 2009).
SPC Erythrocin IV lactobionate injection (accessed 28 September 2009).

# Erythropoietins (epoetins, recombinant human erythropoietins)

- Erythropoietin is a glycosylated protein hormone and a hematopoietic growth factor secreted primarily by the kidneys, which regulates erythropoiesis.
- Epoetins (recombinant human erythropoietins) are used to treat symptomatic anaemia associated with erythropoietin deficiency in chronic renal failure, to ↑yield of autologous blood in normal individuals and to shorten the period of symptomatic anaemia in patients receiving cytotoxic chemotherapy.
- There are five forms currently marketed in the UK: epoetin alfa, epoetin beta, epoetin zeta, darbepoetin alfa and methoxy polyethylene glycol-epoetin beta (pegzerepoetin alfa).
- The scope of this monograph is to describe the monitoring requirements that are required for them. Individual dosing regimens vary widely and standard literature sources should be used to check these.

## MHRA/CHM advice (December 2007, July 2008)

Overcorrection of Hb concentration in patients with chronic kidney disease (CKD) may ↑risk of death and serious cardiovascular events, and in patients with cancer may ↑risk of death and thrombosis and related complications:

- Patients should not be treated with erythropoietins (within the licensed indications) in CKD or cancer unless symptoms of anaemia are present.
- Hb concentration should be maintained within the range 10–12 g/dL (Hb >12 g/dL should be avoided).
- The aim of treatment is to relieve symptoms of anaemia, and in patients with CKD to avoid the need for blood transfusion; the Hb concentration should not be increased beyond that which provides adequate control of symptoms.
- Erythropoietins licensed for treatment for symptomatic anaemia associated with cancer are licensed **only** for patients who are receiving chemotherapy. The decision to treat should be based on assessment of benefits and risks and in some cases blood transfusion may be a preferred option.

## Pre-treatment checks

- Contraindicated in poorly controlled ↑BP, in patients with advanced head and neck cancer receiving radiation therapy, and in breast feeding.
- Caution advised in hepatic impairment, sickle-cell anaemia, epilepsy and pregnancy.
- The needle cover of some formulations of pre-filled syringes may contain dry natural rubber (latex derivative), which may cause allergic reactions.

*Biochemical and other tests (not all are necessary in an emergency situation)*

Blood pressure
Bodyweight

FBC (any deficiency in iron status should be identified and corrected before treatment in order to ensure effective erythropoiesis)
LFTs

## Dose

Consult specific product literature for individual drugs.

## Technical information

| | |
|---|---|
| Excipients | Consult individual product literature: some products contain L-phenylalanine and benzyl alcohol. |
| Storage | Store at 2-8°C in original packaging. Do not freeze.<br>*In use:* For most products, pre-filled syringes may be stored at 25°C for up to 3 days to enable ambulatory use. Consult individual product literature. |

## Monitoring

| Measure | Frequency | Rationale |
|---|---|---|
| Haemoglobin | Every 1-2 weeks until stable following commencement of treatment or any adjustments in dose or route, then as often as clinically indicated | • Target range of 10-12 g/dL (6.2-7.5 mmol/L).<br>• Sustained Hb levels >12 g/dL should be avoided, as should a rise in Hb of > 2 g/dL over a 4-week period.<br>• Treatment should be suspended if the Hb level exceeds 13 g/dL (8.1 mmol/L), and reinstated at approximately 75% of the previous dose once the Hb level has fallen to ≤12 g/dL (7.5 mmol/L).<br>• Patient tolerability may dictate the Hb dose range, and the ideal target should be decided on an individual basis. |
| Serum ferritin | | • Sufficient iron is required for effective erythropoiesis, and supplementation may be necessary if a deficiency is detected.<br>• If an inadequate response to therapy is seen, further investigations into deficiencies of folic acid and/or vitamin B$_{12}$ should also be made. |
| Platelets | Every 2-4 weeks during first 8 weeks of treatment, then as often as clinically indicated | • ↑Risk of thromboembolic events possible due to ↑platelets and thrombocythaemia<br>• May be required to diagnose PRCA (see Reticulocyte count below). |
| Red blood cell count | | • Polycythaemia may occur. |
| White blood cell count | As indicated | • May be required to diagnose PRCA (see Reticulocyte count below). |
| Packed cell volume | Every 3 months | • Excessive ↑PCV can cause cardiovascular complications. |
| Reticulocyte count in patients treated with epoetin alfa | Every 2-4 weeks during first 8 weeks of treatment, then as often as clinically indicated | • Indicative of response.<br>• If reticulocyte index (i.e. reticulocyte count corrected for anaemia) is low (<0.5%, <20 000/mm$^3$) while platelet and white blood cell counts are normal, anti-erythropoietin antibodies should be determined and a bone marrow examination should be considered to diagnose PRCA. If suspected, treatment with epoetin therapy should be discontinued immediately. |

*(continued)*

## Monitoring (continued)

| Measure | Frequency | Rationale |
|---------|-----------|-----------|
| Blood pressure | Ongoing during treatment, more frequently during initiation | • Can cause ↑BP and hypertensive crisis may occur.<br>• Consider commencing/increasing antihypertensive therapy, and reducing or temporarily withholding therapy if ↑BP occurs. |
| Serum K | | • ↑K reported. |
| Tumour size (if applicable) | Ongoing during treatment | • Theoretical potential for ↑tumour growth if erythropoietin receptors are present on the tumour surface. |

## Additional information

| | |
|---|---|
| Common and serious undesirable effects | *Injection-related:*<br>• Too rapid administration: Flu-like symptoms (minimised by slower IV administration).<br>• Local: Injection-site pain.<br><br>*Other:* Pyrexia, GI disturbances, headache, ↑BP, thrombosis of vascular access, arthralgia, myalgia, porphyria, peripheral oedema, PE, thrombocythaemia. Rarely, allergic reactions (dyspnoea, skin rash, urticaria), convulsions, tumour progression, neutralising anti-erythropoietin antibody-mediated PRCA, cardiovascular and thromboembolic events, including angina, thrombosis, stroke, congestive heart failure, dysrhythmias, myocardial infraction, cardiac arrest. |
| Significant drug interactions | • Erythropoietins may ↓levels or effect of the following drugs:<br>ACE inhibitors and angiotensin-II receptor antagonists (↓hypotensive effect, ↑risk of ↑K), heparin (dialysis patients may need ↑dose owing to the likely ↑PCV). |
| Overdose | If clinically indicated, phlebotomy may be performed, and general supportive measures should be provided. |
| Counselling | Reinforce the need for maintaining treatment with antihypertensive medicines. Patients should be advised to report any side-effects, especially symptoms of thrombotic events such as chest pain, lower leg pain, headache etc. |

| Risk rating: **GREEN** | Score = 1<br>Lower-risk product: Risk-reduction strategies should be considered. |
|---|---|

This assessment is based on the full range of preparation and administration options described in the monograph. These may not all be applicable in some clinical situations.

## Bibliography

SPC Eprex 2000, 4000 and 10000 IU/ml solution for injection in pre-filled syringe (accessed 1 October 2009).

SPC Eprex 40,000 IU/ml solution for injection in pre-filled syringe (accessed 1 October 2009).

SPC Binocrit solution for injection in a pre-filled syringe (accessed 1 October 2009).

SPC Aranesp SureClick (accessed 1 October 2009).

SPC Aranesp (accessed 1 October 2009).

SPC Mircera solution for injection in pre-filled syringe (accessed 1 October 2009).

SPC Neorecormon multidose powder and solvent for solution for injection (accessed 1 October 2009).

SPC NeoRecormon powder and solvent for solution for injection in cartridge (accessed 1 October 2009).

SPC Neorecormon solution for injection in pre-filled syringe (accessed 1 October 2009).

SPC Retacrit solution for injection in pre-filled syringe (accessed 1 October 2009).

# Esmolol hydrochloride

**10 mg/mL solution in 10-mL vials and 250-mL infusion bags**

- Esmolol hydrochloride is a cardioselective beta-adrenoceptor blocker with a very short duration of action.
- It is given IV for rapid control of ventricular rate in patients with AF or atrial flutter in perioperative, postoperative or other circumstances where short-term control of ventricular rate is required. Esmolol is also indicated in perioperative ↑BP.

## Pre-treatment checks

- Use with caution in patients with a history of wheezing or asthma and peripheral circulatory conditions.
- Treatment should be avoided in sick sinus syndrome, heart block greater than first degree, cardiogenic shock and overt heart failure, and hypersensitivity to the substance.

*Biochemical and other tests (not all are necessary in an emergency situation)*

Blood pressure
Bodyweight

Heart rate
Renal function: U, Cr, CrCl (or eGFR)

## Dose

**Supraventricular tachyarrhythmias:** 50–200 micrograms/kg/minute. Dose must be individualised by titration as described in Table E4, in which each step consists of a loading dose followed by a maintenance dose. As the desired end point is approached, omit the loading dose and increase the interval between titration steps from 5 to 10 minutes.

**Table E4**  Esmolol loading and maintenance dose regimens

|  | **Loading dose** | **Maintenance dose** |
|---|---|---|
| Initially | 500 micrograms/kg over 1 minute | 50 micrograms/kg/minute for 4 minutes |
| If adequate response | Maintain infusion rate of 50 micrograms/kg/minute | |
| Inadequate response | 500 micrograms/kg over 1 minute | 100 micrograms/kg/minute for 4 minutes |
| If adequate response | Maintain infusion rate of 100 micrograms/kg/minute | |
| Inadequate response | 500 micrograms/kg over 1 minute | 150 micrograms/kg/minute for 4 minutes |
| If adequate response | Maintain infusion rate of 150 micrograms/kg/minute | |
| Inadequate response | 500 micrograms/kg over 1 minute | 200 micrograms/kg/minute for 4 minutes |
| If adequate response | Maintain infusion rate of 200 micrograms/kg/minute for up to 48 hours | |

When transferring a patient to another antiarrhythmic drug, e.g. verapamil or digoxin, the infusion rate of esmolol hydrochloride is reduced by 50% 30 minutes after starting the alternative drug, and may be stopped 1 hour after the second dose of that drug if it is effective.

**Loading dose calculation:**
* 500 micrograms/kg = bodyweight (kg) divided by 20 = dose in mL of esmolol 10 mg/mL.

For example, for a 70-kg individual, dose = 70/20 = 3.5 mL esmolol 10 mg/mL.

**Maintenance dose calculation:**
* 50 micrograms/kg/minute = bodyweight (kg) × 60/200 = dose in mL of esmolol 10 mg/mL/hour.
* 100 micrograms/kg/minute = bodyweight (kg) × 60/100 = dose in mL of esmolol 10 mg/mL/hour.
* 150 micrograms/kg/minute = bodyweight (kg) × 60/66 = dose in mL of esmolol 10 mg/mL/hour.
* 200 micrograms/kg/minute = bodyweight (kg) × 60/50 = dose in mL of esmolol 10 mg/mL/hour.
* 250 micrograms/kg/minute = bodyweight (kg) × 60/40 = dose in mL of esmolol 10 mg/mL/hour.
* 300 micrograms/kg/minute = bodyweight (kg) × 60/33 = dose in mL of esmolol 10 mg/mL/hour.

**Control of perioperative hypertension and/or tachycardia:**
* **During anaesthesia:** a loading dose of 80 mg (8 mL) by IV injection over 15–30 seconds followed by 150 micrograms/kg/minute by IV infusion, increased as necessary up to 300 micrograms/kg/minute (see dose calculation above).
* **On waking from anaesthesia:** 500 micrograms/kg/minute for 4 minutes; followed by 300 micrograms/kg/minute by IV infusion as required. Alternatively if time for titration is available, dose as for supraventricular tachyarrhythmias as above.

## Intravenous injection (for loading doses)

*Preparation and administration*

1. Withdraw the required dose (see above for calculation).
2. The solution should be clear and colourless to light yellow. Inspect visually for particulate matter or discoloration prior to administration and discard if present.
3. Give by IV injection at the rate specified above for the particular indication.

## Intravenous infusion (for maintenance doses)

*Preparation and administration*

1. Esmolol hydrochloride is available as pre-prepared infusion solution containing 10 mg/mL in a 250-mL infusion bag.
2. The solution should be clear and colourless to light yellow. Inspect visually for particulate matter or discoloration prior to administration and discard if present.
3. Give by IV infusion via a volumetric infusion device at rate appropriate to dosing regimen (see above for calculation).

## Technical information

| | |
|---|---|
| Incompatible with | Amphotericin, diazepam, furosemide, pantoprazole, sodium bicarbonate. |
| Compatible with | **Flush:** NaCl 0.9%<br>**Solutions:** NaCl 0.9%, Gluc 5%, Gluc-NaCl, Hartmann's (all with added KCl)<br>**Y-site:** Amikacin, aminophylline, ampicillin, atracurium, benzylpenicillin, ceftazidime, chloramphenicol sodium succinate, cisatracurium, clindamycin, co-trimoxazole, dopamine, erythromycin, fentanyl, gentamicin, glyceryl trinitrate, hydrocortisone sodium succinate, labetalol, linezolid, magnesium sulfate, metronidazole, micafungin, midazolam, phenytoin, propofol, ranitidine, remifentanil, tobramycin, vancomycin, vecuronium bromide |
| pH | 4.5-5.5 |
| Sodium content | 30 mmol in each 250 mL infusion bag. |
| Storage | Store below 25°C in original packaging. Do not refrigerate or freeze. |

## Monitoring

| Measure | Frequency | Rationale |
|---|---|---|
| Blood pressure | Continuously | • ↓BP is the most frequent side-effect. |
| ECG, heart rate | | • Response to therapy.<br>• Reduce or stop infusion if pulse <50-55 beats/minute |
| Infusion site | Every 30 minutes | • Risk of extravasation injury. |
| Respiratory function | During initiation in patients with respiratory history | • Bronchospasm is possible. |

## Additional information

| | |
|---|---|
| Common and serious undesirable effects | *Injection/infusion-related:* Local: Venous irritation, thrombophlebitis, local skin necrosis.<br>*Other:* ↓BP, ↓pulse, nausea, dizziness, bronchospasm. |
| Pharmacokinetics | Elimination half-life is approximately 9 minutes. |

*(continued)*

| **Additional information** (*continued*) | |
|---|---|
| Significant interactions | • The following may ↑esmolol levels or effect (or ↑side-effects): adrenaline (risk of severe ↑BP and ↓pulse), alpha-blockers (severe ↓BP), amiodarone (risk of ↓pulse and AV block), anti-arrhythmics (risk of myocardial depression), clonidine (↑risk of withdrawal ↑BP), diltiazem (risk of ↓pulse and AV block), dobutamine (risk of severe ↑BP and ↓pulse), flecainide (risk of myocardial depression and ↓pulse), moxisylyte (severe ↓BP), nifedipine (severe ↓BP and heart failure), noradrenaline (risk of severe ↑BP and ↓pulse), verapamil (risk of asystole and severe ↓BP). |
| Action in case of overdose | *Symptoms to watch for:* ↓BP, ↓pulse, EMD, loss of consciousness. Stop administration (esmolol has a 9-minute elimination half-life) and give supportive therapy as appropriate. |
| Counselling | Report nausea, respiratory difficulties and pain at infusion site. |

| Risk rating: **AMBER** | Score = 5<br>Moderate-risk product: Risk-reduction strategies are recommended. |
|---|---|

This assessment is based on the full range of preparation and administration options described in the monograph. These may not all be applicable in some clinical situations.

## Bibliography

SPC Brevibloc injection (accessed 26 January 2009).

# Esomeprazole

### 40-mg dry powder vials

- Esomeprazole sodium is a proton pump inhibitor (PPI), being the *S*-isomer of omeprazole.
- It is used to prevent re-bleeding following therapeutic endoscopy for acute bleeding gastric or duodenal ulcers.
- It may also be used IV when the oral route is temporarily unavailable, to treat conditions where inhibition of gastric acid secretion may be beneficial: treatment and prevention of gastric and duodenal ulcers, gastro-oesophageal reflux disease (GORD) and Zollinger–Ellison syndrome.
- Doses are expressed in terms of esomeprazole:
  Esomeprazole 40 mg ≅ 42.6 mg esomeprazole sodium.

## Pre-treatment checks

* PPIs may mask symptoms of gastric cancer (and delay diagnosis); particular care is required in those whose symptoms change and in those who are middle-aged or older.
* Caution in severe renal impairment (due to lack of experience).

*Biochemical and other tests*

LFTs
Renal function: U, Cr, CrCl (or eGFR)

## Dose

**Prevention of re-bleeding of gastric or duodenal ulcers:** initially 80 mg by IV infusion over 30 minutes, followed by 8 mg/hour by continuous IV infusion for 72 hours.
**GORD:** 40 mg daily.
**Symptomatic reflux disease without oesophagitis, treatment of NSAID-associated gastric ulcer, prevention of NSAID-associated gastric or duodenal ulcer:** 20 mg daily.
**Dose in hepatic impairment:** severe impairment (Child–Pugh Class C) maximum 20 mg daily.

## Intravenous injection

*Preparation and administration*

1. Reconstitute each vial with 5 mL NaCl 0.9% to give a solution containing 40 mg/5 mL.
2. Withdraw the required dose.
3. The solution should be clear and colourless to very slightly yellow. Inspect visually for particulate matter or discoloration prior to administration and discard if present.
4. Give by IV injection over at least 3 minutes.

## Intermittent intravenous infusion

*Preparation and administration*

1. Reconstitute each vial with 5 mL NaCl 0.9% to give a solution containing 40 mg/5 mL.
2. Withdraw the required dose and add to 50–100 mL NaCl 0.9%.
3. The solution should be clear and colourless to very slightly yellow. Inspect visually for particulate matter or discoloration prior to administration and discard if present.
4. Give by IV infusion over 10–30 minutes (30 minutes for 80-mg dose).

## Continuous intravenous infusion

*Preparation and administration*

1. Reconstitute each vial with 5 mL NaCl 0.9%.
2. Add 80 mg to 100 mL NaCl 0.9% or other compatible infusion fluid (but see Stability below).
3. The solution should be clear and colourless to very slightly yellow. Inspect visually for particulate matter or discoloration prior to administration and discard if present.
4. Give by IV infusion over 10 hours (8 mg/hour).

| Technical information | |
|---|---|
| Incompatible with | No information |
| Compatible with | **Flush**: NaCl 0.9%<br>**Solutions**: NaCl 0.9%, Hartmann's, Gluc 5% (limited stability, see below)<br>**Y-site**: No information |
| pH | 9-11 |
| Sodium content | Negligible |

*(continued)*

## Technical information (*continued*)

| | |
|---|---|
| Storage | Store below 30°C in original packaging. |
| Displacement value | Negligible |
| Stability after preparation | From a microbiological point of view, should be used immediately; however, reconstituted vials and prepared infusions may be stored at room temperature and used within 12 hours of preparation (6 hours if Gluc 5% is used). |

## Monitoring

| Measure | Frequency | Rationale |
|---|---|---|
| Renal function | Periodically | • Acute interstitial nephritis has been reported with PPIs.<br>• ↓Na has been reported with PPIs. |
| LFTs | | • Altered LFTs and hepatitis have been reported. |
| Vitamin $B_{12}$ | | • Malabsorption of cyanocobalamin (vitamin $B_{12}$) has been reported due to long duration (>3 years) of acid suppressant therapy. |
| Signs of infection | Throughout treatment | • Use of antisecretory drugs may ↑risk of infection, e.g. community acquired pneumonia, salmonella, campylobacter and *Clostridium difficile*-associated disease. |

## Additional information

| | |
|---|---|
| Common and serious undesirable effects | *Immediate:* Hypersensitivity reactions including anaphylaxis and bronchospasm have been reported very rarely.<br>*Injection/infusion-related:* Local: Administration site reactions, particularly with prolonged infusion.<br>*Other:* Nausea, vomiting, abdominal pain, flatulence, diarrhoea, constipation, headache, dry mouth, peripheral oedema, dizziness, sleep disturbances, fatigue, paraesthesia, arthralgia, myalgia, rash, and pruritus. |
| Pharmacokinetics | Elimination half-life is 1–1.4 hours (IV). |
| Significant interactions | • Tipranavir may ↓esomeprazole levels or effect.<br>• Esomeprazole may ↑levels or effect of the following drugs (or ↑side-effects): coumarins (monitor INR); phenytoin (monitor levels).<br>• Esomeprazole may ↓levels or effect of the following drugs: atazanavir (avoid combination); clopidogrel (avoid combination).<br>• Esomeprazole may affect the following tests:<br>Antisecretory drug therapy may cause a false-negative urea breath test. May give false positive tetrahydrocannabinol (THC) urine screening test results. |
| Action in case of overdose | Stop administration and give supportive therapy as appropriate. Esomeprazole is extensively plasma protein bound and is therefore not readily dialysable. |

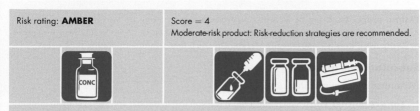

Risk rating: **AMBER**

Score = 4
Moderate-risk product: Risk-reduction strategies are recommended.

This assessment is based on the full range of preparation and administration options described in the monograph. These may not all be applicable in some clinical situations.

## Bibliography

SPC Nexium IV (accessed 28 September 2009).

# Etanercept

**25-mg dry powder vials with solvent; 25-mg and 50-mg pre-filled syringes; 50-mg pre-filled pens**

* Etanercept is a cytokine modulator; it must only be used under specialist supervision.
* It is licensed for use in the treatment of rheumatoid arthritis, psoriatic arthritis, ankylosing spondylitis and plaque psoriasis.
* In the UK, if treatment is for any rheumatological condition other than those listed above, the patient should be entered on the British Society of Rheumatology's Biologics Register.[1]
* Etanercept has been assessed by NICE and in the UK should be used in accordance with the appropriate guidance.

## Pre-treatment checks

* Do not give if the patient has any active infections including chronic or localised infections; record results on a patient alert card. There is a risk of false-negative tuberculin skin test results in patients who are severely ill or immunocompromised.
* Monitor patients for hepatitis B virus: reactivation of hepatitis B has occurred in patients who are carriers.
* Caution in congestive heart failure, which may worsen.
* Caution should be exercised when using in patients with demyelinating CNS disorders since there is a risk of exacerbating clinical symptoms.
* Caution in patients with moderate to severe alcoholic hepatitis.

*Biochemical and other tests*

ESR

CRP

U&Es

FBC

LFTs

Disease Activity Score (DAS)

## Dose

**Rheumatoid arthritis, psoriatic arthritis, ankylosing spondylitis**: 25 mg by SC injection twice weekly or 50 mg by SC injection once weekly.

**Plaque psoriasis:** 25 mg by SC injection twice weekly or 50 mg by SC injection once weekly. Alternatively, 50 mg may be given twice weekly for a maximum of 12 weeks followed, if required, by 25 mg twice weekly or 50 mg once weekly. The usual total treatment duration is 24 weeks.

## Subcutaneous injection

*Preparation and administration*

1. **For dry powder vials:** Slowly add 1 mL WFI (supplied) to the vial and swirl gently to minimise foaming until all the powder has completely dissolved. The solution then contains 25 mg/mL. If the powder has not all dissolved within 10 minutes then discard the vial.
2. **For all presentations:** Either withdraw the required dose or select the appropriate pre-filled syringe. (If using the MYCLIC pre-filled pen, follow detailed instructions in the package insert.)
3. The solution should be clear and colourless to pale yellow. Inspect visually to make sure there are no lumps, flakes or particles.
4. Allow the injection to reach room temperature (approximately 15–30 minutes). Do not remove the needle cover on pre-filled syringes until room temperature is reached.
5. Give by SC injection into the thigh, abdomen, or upper arm. Rotate injection sites for subsequent injections.

## Technical information

| | |
|---|---|
| Incompatible with | Not relevant |
| Compatible with | Not relevant |
| pH | Not relevant |
| Sodium content | Negligible |
| Excipients | Pre-prepared solutions contain L-arginine (may cause hypersensitivity reactions). |
| Storage | Store at 2–8°C in original packaging. Do not freeze. All presentations are single use only. |
| Displacement value | Negligible |
| Stability after preparation | From a microbiological point of view, should be used immediately; however, reconstituted vials may be stored at 2–8°C for a maximum of 6 hours. |

## Monitoring

| Measure | Frequency | Rationale |
|---|---|---|
| Injection-site reactions | Post injection | • Reactions including bleeding, bruising, erythema, itching, pain, and swelling have been commonly reported. They usually occurred in the first month of treatment. |
| Infections | During and after treatment | • Serious infections including tuberculosis may occur. |
| LFTs | Periodically during and after treatment | • Hepatitis B infections have been reported from 3 weeks to 20 months after treatment with etanercept was initiated. |

*(continued)*

## Monitoring (continued)

| Measure | Frequency | Rationale |
|---------|-----------|-----------|
| FBC | Periodically | • Blood dyscrasias may occur (rarely). |
| Clinical improvement, e.g. DAS | | • Stop treatment if no adequate response after 6 months (NICE guidelines). |
| Skin examination | | • ↑Risk of non-melanoma skin cancer, particularly in patients with psoriasis. |

## Additional information

| | |
|---|---|
| Common and serious undesirable effects | *Injection-related:* Local: Injection-site reactions including bleeding, bruising, erythema, itching, pain, swelling. <br> *Other:* Infections (including upper respiratory tract infections, bronchitis, cystitis, skin infections), pruritus. |
| Pharmacokinetics | Elimination half-life is 70 hours (range 7–300 hours). |
| Significant interactions | • The following may ↑etanercept levels or effect (or ↑side-effects): abatacept (↑incidence of serious ADRs), anakinra (↑risk of infection), sulfasalazine (significant ↓WCC). |
| Action in case of overdose | There is no known antidote. |
| Counselling | Report signs or symptoms of infection, especially tuberculosis infection during or after treatment with etanercept, e.g. persistent cough, wasting/weight loss, low-grade fever. <br> Report symptoms of blood disorders, e.g. fever, sore throat, bruising or bleeding and seek medical help if these occur. <br> Patients should be given an Alert Card. <br> Patients should avoid live vaccines. |

| | |
|---|---|
| Risk rating: **GREEN** | Score = 1 <br> Lower-risk product: Risk-reduction strategies should be considered. |

This assessment is based on the full range of preparation and administration options described in the monograph. These may not all be applicable in some clinical situations.

## Reference

1. BSR (2010). *British Society for Rheumatology Biologics Register* (BSRBR). London: British Society for Rheumatology www.medicine.manchester.ac.uk/epidemiology/research/arc/inflammatorymus-culoskeletal/pharmacoepidemiology/bsrbr/ (accessed 18 January 2010).

**Bibliography**

SPC Enbrel 25 mg powder and solvent for solution for injection (accessed 18 January 2010).
SPC Enbrel 25mg solution for injection in pre-filled syringe accessed (accessed 18 January 2010).
SPC Enbrel 50 mg solution for injection in pre-filled pen accessed (accessed 18 January 2010).
SPC Enbrel 50mg solution for injection in pre-filled syringe accessed (accessed 18 January 2010).

# Ethanolamine oleate (monoethanolamine oleate)

**5% solution in 2-mL and 5-mL ampoules**

* Ethanolamine oleate is a sclerosing agent that, when injected into a vein, irritates the endothelium, resulting in thrombus formation and occlusion of the vein. Fibrous tissue develops to permanently obliterate the occluded vessel.
* It is used in the local treatment of small uncomplicated varicose veins in the lower extremities.
* It has also been used as a sclerosing agent in oesophageal varices (unlicensed indication).

## Pre-treatment checks

* Do not give in local or systemic infection, marked arterial or cardiac disease or severe renal impairment.
* Contraindicated if the patient is unable to walk; in acute phlebitis, obese legs, superficial thrombophlebitis and deep vein thrombosis in the region of the varicose veins.
* Do not use if there is a history of uncontrolled metabolic disorders, e.g. diabetes mellitus.
* Do not use if the patient is taking oral contraceptives.

*Biochemical and other tests*

Body temperature
FBC
Renal function: U, Cr, CrCl (or eGFR)

## Dose

**Sclerosis of varicose veins:** a total dose of 2–5 mL is slowly injected directly into the empty isolated sections of varicose vein in divided doses between three or four sites. Dose can be repeated at weekly intervals to achieve required clinical result.

**Sclerosis of oesophageal varices (unlicensed indication):** a dose of 1.5–5 mL is injected per varix, up to a maximum of 20 mL per treatment session. Treatment may be given in the initial management of bleeding varices, then repeated at intervals (usually after 1 week, 6 weeks, 3 months and 6 months as indicated) until all varices are occluded.

## Local injection into vein

*Preparation and administration*

1. Withdraw the required volume.
2. Slowly inject the prepared volume of solution into affected section(s) of varicose vein, or into oesophageal varix/varices, taking care not to leak solution into surrounding tissue (extravasation may cause necrosis of tissues, and there is a risk of sloughing and ulceration).

## Technical information

| | |
|---|---|
| Incompatible with | Not relevant |
| Compatible with | Not relevant |
| pH | 8-9 |
| Sodium content | Nil |
| Excipients | Contains benzyl alcohol (must not be used in neonates). |
| Storage | Store below 25°C in original packaging. |

## Monitoring

| Measure | Frequency | Rationale |
|---|---|---|
| Observation of injection site | During injection and in immediate post-injection period | • Extravasation may cause tissue damage, and potentially necrosis. |
| Patient response | | • Allergic reactions can occur - monitor for clinical signs (e.g. dyspnoea, anaphylaxis, nausea and vomiting). |
| Endoscopy (for oesophageal varices) | Every 3-6 months or as indicated. | • Monitor for recurrent bleeding, effective obliteration, and development of new varices or tissue ulceration/necrosis. |
| Renal function | Regular intervals throughout treatment | • Acute nephrotoxicity reported in overdose - monitor trends in renal function from baseline. |

## Additional information

| | |
|---|---|
| Common and serious undesirable effects | *Immediate:* Allergic reactions and anaphylaxis have been reported following use of sclerosing agents.<br>*Injection-related:* Local: Extravasation can cause sloughing, ulceration, necrosis.<br>*Other:* Burning and cramping sensations, urticaria. |
| Pharmacokinetics | Systemic absorption is not expected, as ethanolamine oleate is a locally acting agent. |
| Significant interactions | None known. |
| Action in case of overdose | Acute nephrotoxicity has been reported in two patients given a total volume of 15-20 mL.[1] Stop further administration and give supportive therapy as appropriate. |
| Counselling | Report injection site reactions, in order to detect tissue damage at earliest possible opportunity. |

| Risk rating: **GREEN** | Score = 2<br>Lower-risk product: Risk-reduction strategies should be considered. |
|---|---|

This assessment is based on the full range of preparation and administration options described in the monograph. These may not all be applicable in some clinical situations.

## Reference

1. Maling TJB, Cretney MJ. Ethanolamine oleate and acute renal failure. *N Z Med J.* 1975; 82: 269–270.

## Bibliography

SPC Ethanolamine Oleate Injection BP, UCB Pharma Ltd (accessed 28 September 2009).

# Exenatide

**5 micrograms/dose and 10 micrograms/dose solution in pre-filled pen**

* Exenatide is a synthetic form of exendin-4, a 39-amino-acid peptide isolated from the venom of the Gila monster lizard. It is an incretin mimetic that ↑insulin secretion, ↓glucagon secretion, and slows gastric emptying.
* It is used for the treatment of type 2 diabetes mellitus in combination with metformin and/or a sulfonylurea, in patients who have not achieved adequate glycaemic control with these drugs alone or in combination. It is also licensed for use with glitazones (with or without other oral agents) in the USA.

## Pre-treatment checks

* Do not use in type 1 diabetes mellitus or for the treatment of diabetic ketoacidosis.
* Not licensed in combination with insulin in type 2 diabetes.
* Do not use in severe renal impairment (CrCl or eGFR <30 mL/minute).
* Avoid in severe gastrointestinal disease (including gastroparesis) because of GI side-effects.
* Avoid in pregnancy and breast feeding – insulin is a safe alternative.
* Consider reducing the dose of sulfonylurea when starting therapy.
* Ensure that the patient reads and understands the user manual.

*Biochemical and other tests*

HbA$_{1c}$
Renal function: U, Cr, CrCl (or eGFR)

## Dose

Initiate at 5 micrograms twice daily by SC injection for at least 1 month, in order to improve tolerability. The dose can then be increased to 10 micrograms twice daily to further improve glycaemic control.

* Give the dose **60 minutes or less before the two main meals of the day** (at least 6 hours apart).
* Exenatide **must not** be injected after a meal.

## Subcutaneous injection

Exenatide must not be injected after a meal.

*Preparation and administration*

1. The solution should be clear and colourless, do not use if cloudy or discoloured or if particles are present.
2. Dial up the dose according to the pen-user manual (see package insert).
3. Give by SC injection into the upper outer thigh, abdomen or upper arm. Remove the needle after use and discard according to local guidelines. Although not specifically recommended by the manufacturer, it would be wise to vary the site of the injection.

## Technical information

| | |
|---|---|
| Incompatible with | Not relevant |
| Compatible with | Not relevant |
| pH | Not relevant |
| Sodium content | Negligible |
| Excipients | Contains metacresol which may cause hypersensitivity reactions. |
| Storage | *Long term:* Store at 2-8°C. Do not freeze. If it has been frozen, do not use. *In use:* Store below 25°C. Do not store the pen with the needle attached. Replace the cap on the pen to protect from light. Each pen contains 60 doses. Discard after 30 days of use even if some medication remains. |

## Monitoring

| Measure | Frequency | Rationale |
|---|---|---|
| Hypersensitivity reactions | At the start of treatment | • May very rarely cause hypersensitivity reactions including anaphylaxis. |
| Renal function | Periodically | • May exacerbate pre-existing renal impairment. |
| Capillary blood glucose | As clinically appropriate | • Has caused hypoglycaemia with concomitant sulfonylurea therapy. |
| HbA$_{1c}$ | Every 3-6 months | • To assess therapeutic response. |

## Additional information

| | |
|---|---|
| Common and serious undesirable effects | *Immediate:* Hypersensitivity reactions (anaphylaxis, rash, pruritus, urticaria, angioedema) occur very rarely (possibly due to metacresol content).<br>*Injection/infusion-related:* Local: Injection-site reactions.<br>*Other:* GI disturbances: nausea (may improve with time), vomiting, diarrhoea, dyspepsia, abdominal pain and distension, gastro-oesophageal reflux disease, ↓appetite; constipation, flatulence, dehydration, taste disturbance. Hypoglycaemia (particularly when given with sulfonylurea). Headache, dizziness, asthenia, drowsiness, jitteriness, ↑sweating. Pancreatitis has rarely been reported (stop immediately if suspected). |
| Pharmacokinetics | Following SC injection exenatide reaches peak plasma concentrations in 2 hours. The mean terminal half-life is 2.4 hours. Clearance is principally renal, and is reduced in renal impairment. |
| Significant interactions | • ↑INR has been reported in patients taking warfarin.<br>• Exenatide slows gastric emptying so may reduce the extent and rate of absorption of some oral medicinal products.<br>• In general, oral antibiotics should be taken one hour before exenatide dose.<br>• Proton pump inhibitors should be taken 1 hour before, or 4 hours after exenatide. |
| Action in case of overdose | *Symptoms to watch for:* Severe nausea, severe vomiting and rapidly declining blood glucose concentrations. Manage symptomatically. |
| Counselling | Use and storage of pens, disposal of pen and needles, discard pens that have been frozen.<br>Timing of dose in relation to food and what to do about missed doses.<br>Warn about the ↑risk of hypoglycaemia at the start of therapy in patients being treated with a sulfonylurea.<br>Warn to report symptoms of pancreatitis i.e. persistent, severe abdominal pain, sometimes accompanied by vomiting.<br>Warn about timing of concomitant antibiotic therapy and other medication if appropriate. |

| Risk rating: **GREEN** | Score = 0<br>Lower-risk product: Risk-reduction strategies should be considered. |
|---|---|

This assessment is based on the full range of preparation and administration options described in the monograph. These may not all be applicable in some clinical situations.

## Bibliography

SPC Byetta 5 micrograms solution for injection, prefilled pen (accessed 15 January 2009).
SPC Byetta 10 micrograms solution for injection, prefilled pen (accessed 15 January 2009).
*MHRA. Drug Safety Update* March 2009; 2(8).

# Fentanyl

### 50 micrograms/mL solution in 2-mL and 10-mL ampoules

* Fentanyl citrate is a potent opioid analgesic chemically related to pethidine.
* It is used parenterally at low doses to provide analgesia during surgery and at higher doses as an analgesic and respiratory depressant during assisted ventilation. It may also be used to provide pain relief in other situations.
* Doses are expressed in terms of the base:
  Fentanyl 100 micrograms $\cong$ 157 micrograms fentanyl citrate.

## Pre-treatment checks

* Avoid in patients with respiratory depression or obstructive airways disease.
* Do not give with monoamine oxidase inhibitors or within 2 weeks of their discontinuation.
* Only give in an environment where the airway can be controlled. Resuscitation equipment should be available.

*Biochemical and other tests (not all are necessary in an emergency situation)*

Bodyweight (use IBW if overweight, to avoid excessive dosing)
Respiratory rate

## Dose

The analgesic/respiratory depressant dose used depends on whether the patient has spontaneous respiration or has assisted ventilation.

**Spontaneous respiration**: initially 50–100 micrograms by IV injection followed by further doses of 50 micrograms if required.

* Maximum initial dose is 200 micrograms on specialist advice only.
* Alternatively, give 50–80 nanograms/kg/minute by IV infusion adjusted according to response.

**Assisted respiration**: initially 300–3500 micrograms followed by further doses of 100–200 micrograms adjusted according to response.

* Alternatively, initially give 1 microgram/kg/minute by IV infusion for 10 minutes followed by 100 nanograms/kg/minute adjusted according to response.
* Higher infusion rates up to 3 micrograms/kg/minute have been used in cardiac surgery.
* Stop infusion about 40 minutes before end of surgery unless it is planned to ventilate postoperatively.

**Premedication**: 50–100 micrograms (1–2 mL) may be given by IM injection 45 minutes before induction of anaesthesia.

## Intravenous injection

*Preparation and administration*

1. Withdraw the required dose.
2. The solution should be clear and colourless. Inspect visually for particulate matter or discoloration prior to administration and discard if present.
3. Give by slow IV injection over 1–2 minutes.
4. Close monitoring of respiratory rate and consciousness recommended.

## Intravenous infusion

*Preparation and administration*

1. Withdraw the required dose and add to a suitable volume of compatible infusion solution.
2. The solution should be clear and colourless. Inspect visually for particulate matter or discoloration prior to administration and discard if present.

*(continued)*

3. Give by IV infusion via a volumetric infusion device or syringe pump at a rate appropriate to the clinical condition of the patient. Adjust dose to clinical response.
4. Close monitoring of respiratory rate and consciousness recommended.

## Intramuscular injection

*Preparation and administration*

1. Withdraw the required dose.
2. The solution should be clear and colourless. Inspect visually for particulate matter or discoloration prior to administration and discard if present.
3. Give by IM injection.
4. Close monitoring of respiratory rate and consciousness is recommended for 30 minutes in patients receiving initial dose, especially elderly patients or those of low bodyweight.

## Technical information

| | |
|---|---|
| Incompatible with | Phenytoin sodium, thiopental. |
| Compatible with | **Flush**: NaCl 0.9%<br>**Solutions**: NaCl 0.9%, Gluc 5% (both with added KCl)<br>**Y-site**: Adrenaline (epinephrine), atracurium, cisatracurium, dexamethasone sodium phosphate, dobutamine, dopamine, esmolol, furosemide, glyceryl trinitrate, hydrocortisone sodium succinate, labetalol, linezolid, lorazepam, metoclopramide, midazolam, propofol, ranitidine, remifentanil |
| pH | 4–7.5 |
| Sodium content | Negligible |
| Storage | Store below 25°C in original packaging. Controlled Drug. |
| Stability after preparation | From a microbiological point of view, should be used immediately; however, prepared infusions may be stored at 2–8°C and infused (at room temperature) within 24 hours. |

## Monitoring

Close monitoring of respiratory rate and consciousness is recommended for 30 minutes in patients receiving initial dose, especially elderly patients or those of low bodyweight.

| Measure | Frequency | Rationale |
|---|---|---|
| Pain or dyspnoea | At regular intervals | • To ensure therapeutic response. |
| Blood pressure, pulse and respiratory rate | | • ↓BP, ↑ or ↓pulse, palpitations and respiratory depression can occur. |
| Sedation | | • May cause sedation (unless being used for sedatory purposes). |
| Monitor for side-effects and toxicity | | • May cause side-effects such as nausea and constipation, which may need treating. |

## Additional information

| | |
|---|---|
| Common and serious undesirable effects | *Common:* Nausea and vomiting, constipation, dry mouth, urticaria, pruritus, biliary spasm, ↑ or ↓pulse, hallucinations, euphoria, drowsiness. *At higher doses:* ↓BP, sedation, respiratory depression, muscle rigidity. |
| Pharmacokinetics | Elimination half-life is 2–14 hours; with prolonged infusions ↑duration of effect of fentanyl. |
| Significant interactions | • The following may ↑fentanyl levels or effect (or ↑side-effects): antihistamines-sedating (↑sedation), MAOIs (avoid combination and for 2 weeks after stopping MAOI), moclobemide, ritonavir.<br>• Fentanyl may ↑levels or effect (or ↑side-effects) of sodium oxybate (avoid combination). |
| Action in case of overdose | *Symptoms to watch for:* ↑Sedation, respiratory depression. *Antidote:* Naloxone (see Naloxone monograph). Stop administration and give supportive therapy as appropriate. |

| Risk rating: **AMBER** | Score = 5<br>Moderate-risk product: Risk-reduction strategies are recommended. |
|---|---|

This assessment is based on the full range of preparation and administration options described in the monograph. These may not all be applicable in some clinical situations.

## Bibliography

SPC Sublimaze (accessed 12 December 2008).

# Filgrastim (G-CSF, r-metHuCSF)

**300 micrograms/mL solution in 1-mL and 1.6-mL vials**
**300 micrograms/0.5 mL and 480 micrograms/0.5 mL solution in 0.5-mL pre-filled syringes**

• Filgrastim is recombinant methionyl human granulocyte-colony stimulating factor (G-CSF), produced using r-DNA technology in *E. coli*. It acts primarily on neutrophil precursors to increase neutrophil levels.
• It is used to treat or prevent neutropenia in patients receiving myelosuppressive cancer chemotherapy (except in chronic myeloid leukaemia and myelodysplastic syndromes), to reduce the duration of neutropenia in patients undergoing bone marrow transplantation and to mobilise peripheral blood progenitor cells in blood stem cell transplantation.
• Doses are expressed in micrograms or units (micrograms are used throughout this monograph): Filgrastim 10 micrograms ≡1 million units.

## Pre-treatment checks

* Prior to commencing treatment for neutropenia, exclude possible causes of transient neutropenia, e.g. viral infections.
* Do not use in severe congenital neutropenia (Kostmann's syndrome) with abnormal cytogenetics.
* Caution in secondary acute myeloid leukaemia, sickle-cell disease; monitor spleen size (risk of rupture); existing osteoporotic bone disease.
* If the patient is receiving cytotoxic chemotherapy, ensure that the first dose of filgrastim is not administered in the first 24 hours following the completion of the cycle of chemotherapy.

*Biochemical and other tests*

Blood pressure
Bodyweight (for certain indications)

FBC including differential white cell and platelet counts
LFTs

## Dose

**Cytotoxic-induced neutropenia:** 5 micrograms/kg once daily by SC injection (preferred route), or by IV infusion. The first dose should be given a minimum of 24 hours after cytotoxic therapy and is usually continued until neutrophil count is within the normal range.

**Myeloablative therapy followed by bone marrow transplantation:** 10 micrograms/kg daily given either by a 30-minute or 24-hour IV infusion, or by a 24-hour SC infusion. The first dose should be given a minimum of 24 hours after cytotoxic therapy and is further titrated according to patient response (see product literature).

**Mobilisation of peripheral blood progenitor cells for autologous infusion:** if filgrastim is being used alone, 10 micrograms/kg daily given by a 24-hour SC infusion or as a single daily SC injection for 5–7 consecutive days until leucopheresis is complete (see product literature).

**Mobilisation of peripheral blood progenitor cells in normal donors for allogeneic infusion:** 10 micrograms/kg daily by SC injection for 4–5 consecutive days (for timing of leucopheresis see product literature).

**Severe chronic neutropenia, congenital:** initially 12 micrograms/kg daily by SC injection as a single dose or divided doses and adjusted according to response. Maintenance dose should be the minimum required to maintain neutrophil count (see product literature).

**Severe chronic neutropenia, idiopathic or cyclic:** initially 5 micrograms/kg daily by SC injection as a single dose or divided doses and adjusted according to response. Maintenance dose should be the minimum required to maintain neutrophil count (see product literature).

**Persistent neutropenia in HIV infection:** initially 1 microgram/kg daily by SC injection titrated up to 4 micrograms/kg daily according to response. Maintenance dose should be the minimum required to maintain neutrophil count (see product literature).

## Subcutaneous injection

*Preparation and administration*

1. Withdraw the required dose from a vial using a needle suitable for SC injection, or select an appropriately sized pre-filled syringe.
2. Give by SC injection. Rotate injection sites for subsequent injections.

## Subcutaneous infusion

*Preparation and administration*

Filgrastim is incompatible with NaCl 0.9%.

1. Withdraw the required dose and add to a suitable volume of Gluc 5%, ensuring that the final concentration is 15 micrograms/mL or more.*

*(continued)*

2. The solution should be clear and colourless. Inspect visually for particulate matter or discoloration prior to administration and discard if present.
3. Give as a continuous SC infusion, preparing a fresh infusion every 24 hours.

*Stability is concentration dependent: if filgrastim concentration is <15 micrograms/mL then human serum albumin must be added to produce a final albumin concentration of 2 mg/mL.

## Intermittent intravenous infusion
*Preparation and administration*

Filgrastim is incompatible with NaCl 0.9%.

1. Withdraw the required dose and add to a suitable volume of Gluc 5%, ensuring that the final concentration is 15 micrograms/mL or more.*
2. The solution should be clear and colourless. Inspect visually for particulate matter or discoloration prior to administration and discard if present.
3. Give by IV infusion over 30 minutes.

*Stability is concentration dependent: if filgrastim concentration is <15 micrograms/mL then human serum albumin must be added to produce a final albumin concentration of 2 mg/mL.

## Continuous intravenous infusion
*Preparation and administration*

Filgrastim is incompatible with NaCl 0.9%.

1. Withdraw the required dose and add to a suitable volume of Gluc 5%, ensuring that the final concentration is 15 micrograms/mL or more.* Mix well.
2. The solution should be clear and colourless. Inspect visually for particulate matter or discoloration prior to administration and discard if present.
3. Give by continuous IV infusion via a volumetric infusion device. Prepare a fresh infusion at least every 24 hours.

*Stability is concentration dependent: if filgrastim concentration is <15 micrograms/mL then human serum albumin must be added to produce a final albumin concentration of 2 mg/mL.

## Technical information

| Incompatible with | Filgrastim is incompatible with NaCl 0.9%.<br>Amphotericin, cefotaxime, ceftriaxone, cefuroxime, clindamycin phosphate, furosemide, gentamicin, heparin sodium, imipenem with cilastatin, methylprednisolone sodium succinate, metronidazole. |
|---|---|
| Compatible with | **Flush**: Gluc 5%<br>**Solutions**: Gluc 5% (concentration dependent)<br>**Y-site**: Aciclovir, amikacin, aminophylline, ampicillin, aztreonam, bumetanide, calcium folinate, calcium gluconate, ceftazidime, co-trimoxazole, dexamethasone sodium phosphate, fluconazole, ganciclovir, granisetron, hydrocortisone sodium succinate, mesna, metoclopramide, ondansetron, potassium chloride, ranitidine, sodium bicarbonate, ticarcillin with clavulanate, tobramycin, vancomycin, zidovudine |

*(continued)*

## Technical information (*continued*)

| | |
|---|---|
| pH | 4 |
| Sodium content | Negligible |
| Storage | Store at 2-8°C (accidental freezing does not adversely affect stability). May be stored at room temperature for up to 24 hours. Vials and pre-filled syringe are for single use only: discard any unused solution. |
| Stability after preparation | From a microbiological point of view, should be used immediately; however, prepared infusions may be stored at 2-8°C and infused (at room temperature) within 24 hours. |

## Monitoring

| Measure | Frequency | Rationale |
|---|---|---|
| Absolute neutrophil count | Initially 2-3 times weekly, reducing in frequency as clinically appropriate | • Monitor ANC to assess patient response and titrate dose if applicable.<br>• In patients with HIV-associated neutropenia, it is recommended that the ANC is measured daily for the first 2-3 days, then at least twice weekly for the first 2 weeks, then weekly or on alternate weeks for the duration of treatment. In an intermittent dosing regimen, it is recommended that the blood sample is taken immediately before a dose is due, in order to measure the ANC nadir. |
| WBC | | • Severe leucocytosis may occur, and treatment should be discontinued if leucocytes are >50 000 cells/mm$^3$ (>50 × 10$^9$/L) after expected nadir; and discontinued or dose reduced if leucocytes are >70 × 10$^9$/L in PBPC mobilisation. |
| Overall FBC | | • Especially if receiving cytotoxic chemotherapy, the patient may be at higher risk of thrombocytopenia and anaemia.<br>• PBPC donors may develop thrombocytopenia - potentially due to apheresis procedure. Apheresis should not be performed if platelets are <75 000 cells/mm$^3$ (<75 × 10$^9$/L).<br>• Discontinuation of filgrastim should be considered if thrombocytopenia develops in patients with severe chronic neutropenia. |
| Urinalysis | Monthly | • Haematuria and proteinuria have been reported. |
| LFTs | | • ↑Alk Phos and ↑GGT have been reported (reversible and dose dependent). |
| Serum lactate dehydrogenase and uric acid | | • ↑Levels have been reported (reversible and dose-dependent). |

(continued)

## Monitoring (continued)

| Measure | Frequency | Rationale |
|---|---|---|
| Pulmonary observations | Throughout treatment | • Presence of cough, fever and dyspnoea in association with radiological evidence of pulmonary infiltrates and physical deterioration in pulmonary function may be indicative of ARDS - discontinue treatment. |
| Physical examination of spleen size (and ultrasound scan if appropriate) | Periodically, and urgently if patient presents with left upper abdominal pain or shoulder tip pain | • Splenomegaly is a direct effect of filgrastim therapy, but splenic rupture may occur.<br>• Dose reduction may slow or stop progression of enlargement. |
| Blood pressure | Periodically | • May cause ↓BP. |
| Bone density | Consider if treatment >6 months | • Long-term therapy may promote osteoporotic bone disease. |
| Morphological and cytogenetic bone marrow examinations | Regularly every 12 months in long-term therapy for severe congenital neutropenia | • Accurate diagnosis is required before commencing treatment with filgrastim.<br>• Recommended in severe congenital neutropenia owing to risk of myelodysplastic syndromes or leukaemia (discontinue filgrastim immediately if either occurs).<br>• Any changes during treatment should prompt a review of the risks and benefits of continuing treatment. |

## Additional information

| | |
|---|---|
| Common and serious undesirable effects | *Immediate:* Allergic reactions, including anaphylaxis and angioedema, have been reported particularly following IV administration.<br>*Injection-related:* Local: Injection-site pain.<br>*Other:* Headache, musculoskeletal pain, GI disturbances, leucocytosis, thrombocytopenia, ↑Alk Phos, ↑LDH, splenomegaly, transient ↓blood glucose, urticaria, ↓BP. |
| Pharmacokinetics | Elimination half-life is 3.5 hours. |
| Significant interactions | Any drug causing neutropenia may ↓filgrastim levels or effect. |
| Action in case of overdose | Effects not established. Discontinuation of treatment usually results in a 50% decrease in circulating neutrophils within 1-2 days, returning to normal levels in 1-7 days. |
| Counselling | Training in aseptic technique and administration if self-administering.<br>Safe disposal of needles, syringes and unused drug. |

Risk rating: **AMBER**

Score = 5
Moderate-risk product: Risk-reduction strategies are recommended.

This assessment is based on the full range of preparation and administration options described in the monograph. These may not all be applicable in some clinical situations.

## Bibliography

SPC Neupogen (accessed 22 September 2009).

# Flecainide acetate

**10 mg/mL solution in 15-mL ampoules**

* Flecainide is a class 1 (membrane-stabilising) antiarrhythmic agent.
* It is used IV for rapid control of severe symptomatic ventricular arrhythmias such as sustained ventricular tachycardia and severe symptomatic supraventricular arrhythmias.

## Pre-treatment checks

* Contraindicated in the following: heart failure; abnormal left ventricular function; history of myocardial infarction and either asymptomatic ventricular ectopics or asymptomatic non-sustained ventricular tachycardia; long-standing atrial fibrillation where conversion to sinus rhythm is not attempted; haemodynamically significant valvular heart disease. Avoid in sinus node dysfunction, atrial conduction defects, second-degree or greater AV block, bundle branch block or distal block unless pacing rescue is available.
* Caution in patients with a history of cardiac failure, who may become decompensated during the administration (in such patients it is recommended that the initial dose is given over 30 minutes).
* Caution also in patients with pacemakers (especially those who may be pacemaker dependent because the stimulation threshold may rise appreciably), in atrial fibrillation following heart surgery, and in elderly patients (accumulation may occur).
* ECG monitoring and resuscitation facilities must be available.

*Biochemical and other tests (not all are necessary in an emergency situation)*

Bodyweight
ECG
Electrolytes: serum Na, K

LFTs
Renal function: U, Cr

## Dose

**Initial dose:** 2 mg/kg (maximum 150 mg) given by IV injection over at least 10 minutes, or as a small-volume infusion in Gluc 5% over 10–30 minutes. This may be followed by IV infusion if appropriate.

**Intravenous infusion:** 1.5 mg/kg/hour for the first hour, followed by 100–250 micrograms/kg/hour for a maximum of 24 hours.

* The cumulative dose in the first 24 hours should not exceed 600 mg.
* Oral therapy should be started as soon as possible, the first oral dose being given as the infusion is stopped.

**Dose in renal impairment**: if CrCl <35 mL/minute, reduce each of the above doses by half.
**Dose in hepatic impairment**: avoid (or reduce dose) in severe liver disease.

## Initial dose

1. Withdraw the required dose. Use undiluted or dilute with 20–100 mL Gluc 5%.
2. The solution should be clear and colourless. Inspect visually for particulate matter or discoloration prior to administration and discard if present.
3. Give by IV injection over a minimum of 10 minutes or by small-volume infusion over 10–30 minutes.

## Continuous intravenous infusion

1. Withdraw the required dose and add to a suitable volume of Gluc 5%. Mix well.
2. The solution should be clear and colourless. Inspect visually for particulate matter or discoloration prior to administration and discard if present.
3. Give by IV infusion as specified above for a maximum of 24 hours.

## Technical information

| | |
|---|---|
| Incompatible with | Limited stability in sodium-containing infusion fluids: dose must be diluted to 500 mL if using NaCl 0.9% or Hartmann's to avoid precipitation. |
| Compatible with | **Flush**: Gluc 5% <br> **Solutions**: Gluc 5% <br> **Y-site**: No information |
| pH | 6.7–7.1 |
| Sodium content | Negligible |
| Storage | Store below 30°C in original packaging. Do not freeze. |
| Stability after preparation | There is little information on stability after preparation, therefore it would be prudent to use the infusion immediately after preparation. |

## Monitoring

| Measure | Frequency | Rationale |
|---|---|---|
| ECG | Continuously | • Response to therapy. <br> • Flecainide may cause arrhythmia. |
| Plasma flecainide level monitoring (where the assay is available) | Suggested after 12 hours | • Target trough level is 200–1000 nanograms/mL. <br> • Toxicity is frequent with trough serum levels >1000 nanograms/mL. <br> • Recommended in patients receiving infusion at the upper end of the dose range and for those with significant renal or hepatic impairment. |

## Additional information

| | |
|---|---|
| Common and serious undesirable effects | Dizziness, visual disturbances, headache and nausea. |
| Pharmacokinetics | Elimination half-life is 7-20 hours. |
| Significant interactions | • The following may ↑flecainide levels or effect (or ↑side-effects): amiodarone (halve flecainide doses), artemether/lumefantrine (avoid combination), quinine, verapamil.<br>• ↑Risk of arrhythmias with the following drugs:<br>clozapine, dolasetron (avoid combination), tricyclic antidepressants, fosamprenavir (avoid combination), indinavir (avoid combination), lopinavir (avoid combination), mizolastine (avoid combination), ritonavir (avoid combination), tolterodine.<br>• Flecainide may ↑levels or effect (or ↑side-effects) of beta-blockers (↑risk of bradycardia). |
| Action in case of overdose | Life threatening - no specific antidote; there is no known way of rapidly removing flecainide from the body. Stop administration and give supportive therapy as appropriate. |

| Risk rating: **AMBER** | Score = 5<br>Moderate-risk product: Risk-reduction strategies are recommended. |
|---|---|

This assessment is based on the full range of preparation and administration options described in the monograph. These may not all be applicable in some clinical situations.

## Bibliography

SPC Tambocor injection (accessed 1 October 2009).

# Flucloxacillin (floxacillin)

### 250-mg, 500-mg, 1-g dry powder vials

* Flucloxacillin sodium is a penicillin with a mode of action similar to that of benzylpenicillin, but it is resistant to staphylococcal penicillinase.
* It is particularly useful in infections caused by staphylococci resistant to benzylpenicillin. These include bone and joint infections, endocarditis and soft-tissue infections.
* Dose are expressed in terms of flucloxacillin:
  Flucloxacillin 1 g ≡ 1.09 g flucloxacillin sodium.

## Pre-treatment checks

* Do not give if there is known hypersensitivity to penicillin.
* Avoid in patients with a history of hepatic dysfunction associated with flucloxacillin.
* Flucloxacillin is considered unsafe in porphyria (associated with acute attacks).

*Biochemical and other tests (not all are necessary in an emergency situation)*

Bodyweight in certain indications
FBC

LFTs
Renal function: U, Cr, CrCl (or eGFR)

## Dose

> If used in combination with an aminoglycoside (e.g. amikacin, gentamicin, tobramycin), preferably administer at a different site. If this is not possible then flush the line with a compatible solution between drugs.

**Standard dose:** 250 mg–2 g by IM or IV injection or IV infusion every 6 hours.
**Osteomyelitis:** 2 g by IV injection or infusion every 6–8 hours.
**Endocarditis:** bodyweight ≤85 kg: 2 g by IV injection or infusion every 6 hours; bodyweight >85 kg: 2 g every 4 hours.
**Surgical prophylaxis:** 1–2 g at induction by IV injection or infusion followed by (for high risk procedures), up to four further doses of 500 mg orally or parenterally every 6 hours. Check local policies.
**Intrapleural injection:** 250 mg once daily.
**Intra-articular injection:** 250–500 mg once daily.
**Nebulised:** 125–250 mg every 6 hours.
**Dose in renal impairment:** adjusted according to creatinine clearance:[1]
* CrCl >10 mL/minute: dose as in normal renal function.
* CrCl <10 mL/minute: dose as in normal renal function (maximum total daily dose 4 g).

**Dose in hepatic impairment:** use with caution (risk of cholestatic jaundice and hepatitis).

## Intravenous injection

*Preparation and administration*

> See Special handling below.
> If used in combination with an aminoglycoside (e.g. amikacin, gentamicin, tobramycin), preferably administer at a different site. If this is not possible then flush the line with a compatible solution between drugs.

1. Dissolve each 250 mg in 5 mL WFI (i.e. use 10 mL for a 500-mg vial, 20 mL for 1-g vial).
2. Withdraw the required dose.
3. The solution should be clear and colourless. Inspect visually for particulate matter or discoloration prior to administration and discard if present.
4. Give by IV injection over 3–4 minutes.

## Intermittent intravenous infusion

*Preparation and administration*

> See Special handling below.
> If used in combination with an aminoglycoside (e.g. amikacin, gentamicin, tobramycin), preferably administer at a different site. If this is not possible then flush the line with a compatible solution between drugs.

1. Reconstitute each 250-mg vial with 5 mL WFI (use 10 mL for each 500-mg vial, 20 mL for each 1-g vial).
2. Withdraw the required dose and add to a suitable volume of compatible infusion fluid (usually 100 mL NaCl 0.9%).
3. The solution should be clear and colourless. Inspect visually for particulate matter or discoloration prior to administration and discard if present.
4. Give by IV infusion over 30–60 minutes.

## Intramuscular injection (maximum dose 500 mg)

*Preparation and administration*

See Special handling below.

1. Reconstitute each 250-mg vial with 1.5 mL WFI (use 2 mL for each 500-mg vial).
2. Withdraw the required dose.
3. Give by IM injection into a large muscle such as the gluteus or the lateral aspect of the thigh. Rotate injection sites for subsequent injections.

## Other routes

See Special handling below.

- **Intrapleural injection:** dissolve 250 mg in 5–10 mL WFI.
- **Intra-articular injection:** dissolve 250–500 mg in up to 5 mL of WFI. If pain occurs, 0.5% lidocaine may be used for reconstitution (see the Lidocaine monograph for cautions and monitoring)
- **Nebulised:** dissolve 250 mg in 3 mL of WFI.

| Technical information | |
|---|---|
| Incompatible with | Sodium bicarbonate.<br>Amikacin, amiodarone, benzylpenicillin, calcium gluconate, ciprofloxacin, clarithromycin, diazepam, dobutamine, erythromycin lactobionate, gentamicin, metoclopramide, midazolam, ofloxacin, tobramycin, verapamil. |
| Compatible with | **Flush**: NaCl 0.9%<br>**Solutions**: NaCl 0.9%, Gluc 5%, Gluc-NaCl, Hartmann's (all with added KCl), WFI<br>**Y-site**: Adrenaline (epinephrine), aminophylline, ampicillin, bumetanide, ceftazidime, cefuroxime, dexamethasone sodium phosphate, digoxin, hydrocortisone sodium succinate, isosorbide dinitrate, metronidazole, ranitidine, sodium fusidate |
| pH | 5-7 |
| Sodium content | 2.3 mmol per 1-g vial |
| Storage | Store below 25°C in original packaging. |
| Displacement value | 0.2 mL/250 mg |
| Special handling | Avoid skin contact as may cause sensitisation. |

*(continued)*

## Technical information (*continued*)

| | |
|---|---|
| Stability after preparation | From a microbiological point of view, should be used immediately; however:<br>• Reconstituted vials may be stored at 2-8°C for 24 hours.<br>• Prepared infusions may be stored at 2-8°C and infused (at room temperature) within 24 hours. |

## Monitoring

| Measure | Frequency | Rationale |
|---|---|---|
| LFTs | Intermittently if on long-term/high-dose treatment and if otherwise indicated | • Changes in LFTs may occur; reversible on discontinuation of treatment.<br>• Hepatitis and cholestatic jaundice can occur up to 2 months post treatment; the effects can last several months and are not related to either dose or route of administration.<br>• Older patients and those receiving more than 2 weeks' treatment at higher risk. |
| Renal function | | • Reduction of dose or extension of dosing interval is required if CrCl <10 mL/minute. |
| FBC | | • Agranulocytosis has been associated rarely with flucloxacillin. Neutropenia and thrombocytopenia can also occur but are reversible when treatment is stopped.<br>• Neutropenia is reported with high doses of beta-lactams with an incidence of from 5% to 15% in patients treated for more than 10 days. |

## Additional information

| | |
|---|---|
| Common and serious undesirable effects | *Immediate:* Anaphylaxis and other hypersensitivity reactions have been reported.<br>*Injection/infusion-related:* Phlebitis following IV infusion.<br>*Other:* Urticaria, fever, joint pains, rashes, angioedema, anaphylaxis, serum sickness-like reaction, nausea, vomiting and diarrhoea (pseudomembranous reported rarely). Patients treated for syphilis or neurosyphilis may develop a Jarisch-Herxheimer reaction (occurs 2-12 hours after initiation of therapy - headache, fever, chills, sweating, sore throat, myalgia, arthralgia, malaise, ↑pulse and ↑BP followed by a ↓BP. Usually subsides within 12-24 hours. Corticosteroids may ↓incidence and severity). |
| Pharmacokinetics | Half-life is approximately 1 hour. |
| Significant interactions | No significant interactions. |
| Action in case of overdose | *Symptoms to watch for:* Large doses have been associated with seizures.<br>*Antidote:* None; stop administration and give supportive therapy as appropriate. |
| Counselling | Women taking the combined contraceptive pill should be should be advised to take additional precautions during and for 7 days after the course. |

| Risk rating: **GREEN** | Score = 2<br>Lower-risk product: Risk-reduction strategies should be considered. |
|---|---|

This assessment is based on the full range of preparation and administration options described in the monograph. These may not all be applicable in some clinical situations.

## Reference

1. Ashley C, Currie A, eds. *The Renal Drug Handbook*, 3rd edn. Oxford: Radcliffe Medical Press, 2009.

## Bibliography

SPC Flucloxacillin 500 mg powder for solution for injection or infusion, Wockhardt (accessed 28 September 2009).

# Fluconazole

**2 mg/mL solution in 50-mL, 100-mL, 200-mL infusion bags; 25-mL, 100-mL infusion vials**

* Fluconazole is a triazole antifungal drug that in sensitive fungi selectively inhibits cytochrome P450-dependent enzymes resulting in impairment of ergosterol synthesis, an essential component of fungal cell membranes.
* It is used IV to treat systemic fungal infections including candidiasis, coccidioidomycosis and cryptococcosis.

## Pre-treatment checks

Do not use in acute porphyria.

*Biochemical and other tests (not all are necessary in an emergency situation)*

| | |
|---|---|
| Electrolytes: serum K | Renal function: U, Cr, CrCl (or eGFR) |
| FBC | Consider baseline ECG (caution in susceptibility |
| LFTs | to QT interval prolongation) |

## Dose

**Invasive candidal infections (including candidaemia and disseminated candidiasis) and cryptococcal infections (including meningitis):** 400 mg by IV infusion on first day then 200–400 mg daily; unlicensed doses of 800–1000 mg daily have been used in severe infections with treatment continued according to response (at least 8 weeks for cryptococcal meningitis).

**Prevention of relapse of cryptococcal meningitis in AIDS patients after completion of primary therapy:** 100–200 mg daily by IV infusion (or orally).

**Prevention of fungal infections in immunocompromised patients:** 50–400 mg daily by IV infusion (or orally), adjusted according to risk: 400 mg daily if there is high risk of systemic infections, e.g. following bone-marrow transplantation. Commence treatment before the anticipated onset of neutropenia and continue for 7 days after the neutrophil count has reached the desirable range.

**Dosing in renal impairment (in patients who will receive multiple doses):** the normal dose is given according to indication on day 1, then the dose is adjusted according to creatinine clearance, i.e.

* CrCl >50 mL/minute – dose as in normal renal function.
* CrCl 11–50 mL/minute (no dialysis) – 50% of normal dose.
* Patients receiving regular dialysis – one normal dose after every dialysis session.

## Intermittent intravenous infusion

*Preparation and administration*

1. The solution should be clear and colourless. Inspect visually for particulate matter or discoloration prior to administration and discard if present.
2. Give by IV infusion at a rate of 5–10 mL/minute (300–600 mL/hour). In the USA, a maximum infusion rate of 100 mL/hour is recommended.

## Technical information

| | |
|---|---|
| Incompatible with | Amphotericin, ampicillin, calcium gluconate, cefotaxime, ceftazidime, ceftriaxone, cefuroxime, chloramphenicol sodium succinate, clindamycin phosphate, co-trimoxazole, diazepam, digoxin, furosemide, imipenem with cilastatin, pantoprazole. |
| Compatible with | **Flush**: NaCl 0.9%<br>**Solutions**: NaCl 0.9%, Gluc 5%, Hartmann's, Ringer's (all including added KCl)<br>**Y-site**: Aciclovir, amikacin, aminophylline, aztreonam, benzylpenicillin, ciprofloxacin, cisatracurium, dexamethasone sodium phosphate, dobutamine, dopamine, foscarnet, ganciclovir, gentamicin, glyceryl trinitrate, linezolid, meropenem, metronidazole, midazolam, ondansetron, phenytoin sodium, piperacillin with tazobactam, propofol, ranitidine, remifentanil, ticarcillin with clavulanate, tigecycline, tobramycin, vancomycin, vasopressin (synthetic), vecuronium bromide |
| pH | 4–8 in NaCl 0.9% |
| Sodium content | 15 mmol/100 mL |
| Storage | Store below 25°C in original packaging. Do not freeze.<br>Infusions are single use only - discard any unused portion. |

## Monitoring

| Measure | Frequency | Rationale |
|---|---|---|
| LFTs | Periodically and if liver toxicity is suspected | • Transient rises (1.5-3 × ULN) in AST, ALT, Alk Phos, GGT and bilirubin occur occasionally, returning to normal during or after treatment.<br>• Rare, but reversible, hepatic abnormalities occur. If serious hepatic injury is suspected fluconazole should be discontinued: >8 × ULN, ↑ALT and ↑AST are indicative of this. |

*(continued)*

## Monitoring (*continued*)

| Measure | Frequency | Rationale |
|---|---|---|
| U&Es | Periodically | • If renal function changes a dose reduction may be required.<br>• Occasional ↑Cr and ↑U occur.<br>• ↓K has been reported – supplementation may be necessary. |
| FBC | | • Eosinophilia, leucopenia, neutropenia, thrombocytopenia and anaemia have occasionally been reported. |
| Symptoms of exfoliative skin reactions, e.g. Stevens-Johnson syndrome and toxic epidermal necrolysis | Throughout treatment | • If a rash develops attributable to fluconazole: discontinue for a patient with a superficial fungal infection; for a patient with invasive/systemic fungal infections, monitor closely and discontinue if bullous lesions or erythema multiforme develop. |
| ECG anomalies | If indicated | • Use with caution in patients with pro-arrhythmic conditions.<br>• Torsade de pointes and QT prolongation have occurred (rarely). |

## Additional information

| | |
|---|---|
| Common and serious undesirable effects | *Immediate:* Anaphylaxis (including angioedema) has rarely been reported.<br>*Other:* Headache, rash, abdominal pain, diarrhoea, nausea, hepatotoxicity (more common in HIV patients).<br>*Rarely:* Dizziness, seizures, taste perversion, exfoliative skin disorders, blood dyscrasias, hypercholesterolaemia, hypertriglyceridaemia, ↓K, QT prolongation, torsade de pointes. |
| Pharmacokinetics | Elimination half-life is 30 hours. |
| Significant interactions | • Rifampicin may ↓fluconazole levels or effect (↑fluconazole dose if necessary).<br>• Fluconazole may ↑levels or effect of the following drugs (or ↑side-effects): bosentan (avoid combination), ciclosporin (monitor levels closely), coumarin anticoagulants (may ↑INR), ergotamine (avoid combination), methysergide (avoid combination), midazolam, nevirapine, pimozide (avoid combination), phenytoin (monitor levels), reboxetine (avoid combination), rifabutin (↑risk of uveitis), sertindole (avoid combination), sulphonylureas (risk of hypoglycaemia), tacrolimus (monitor levels closely), theophylline (monitor levels) |
| Action in case of overdose | No known antidote but a 3-hour haemodialysis session should decrease plasma level by half. Stop administration and give supportive therapy as appropriate. |

| Risk rating: **GREEN** | Score = 1<br>Lower-risk product: Risk-reduction strategies should be considered. |
|---|---|

This assessment is based on the full range of preparation and administration options described in the monograph. These may not all be applicable in some clinical situations.

## Bibliography

SPC Diflucan capsules 50 mg and 200 mg, powder for oral suspension 50 mg/5 mL and 200 mg/5 mL, intravenous infusion 2 mg/mL (accessed 17 March 2009).
SPC Fluconazole 2 mg/mL intravenous infusion, Hospira UK Ltd (accessed 17 March 2009).

# Flucytosine

### 2.5 g/250 mL (10 mg/mL) solution in infusion bottles

- Flucytosine is a fluorinated pyrimidine antifungal.
- It is used in the treatment of systemic fungal infections. Because there is a high incidence of primary resistance amongst target organisms, it is usually used synergistically with amphotericin or fluconazole in the treatment of severe systemic candidiasis and cryptococcal meningitis.

### Pre-treatment checks

*Biochemical and other tests (not all are necessary in an emergency situation)*

FBC
LFTs
Renal function: U, Cr, CrCl (or eGFR)

Cultures for sensitivity testing should ideally be taken before treatment and repeated at regular intervals during therapy; however it is not necessary to delay treatment until these test results are known.

### Dose

**Standard dose**: 50 mg/kg four times a day by IV infusion, usually for no more than 7 days.
**Patients harbouring extremely sensitive organisms**: 25–37.5 mg/kg by IV infusion four times a day may be sufficient.
**Cryptococcal meningitis (with amphotericin)**: 25 mg/kg daily four times a day by IV infusion for at least 4 months.
**Dose in renal impairment:** adjusted according to creatinine clearance:

- CrCl >20–40 mL/minute: 50 mg/kg every 12 hours.
- CrCl 10–20 mL/minute: 50 mg/kg every 24 hours.
- CrCl <10 mL/minute: an initial single dose of 50 mg/kg with subsequent doses adjusted according to the serum concentration of the drug (see Monitoring below).

### Intermittent intravenous infusion

*Preparation and administration*

1. The infusion is pre-prepared for use. It should be clear and colourless. Inspect visually for particulate matter or discoloration prior to administration and discard if present.
2. Give the required dose by IV infusion over 20–40 minutes.

## Technical information

| | |
|---|---|
| Incompatible with | Do not mix with other drugs during infusion. |
| Compatible with | **Flush**: NaCl 0.9%<br>**Solutions**: NaCl 0.9%, Gluc 5%, Gluc-NaCl<br>**Y-site**: No information |
| pH | 7.4 |
| Sodium content | 34.5 mmol/250-mL bottle |
| Storage | Store at 18–25°C in original packaging.<br>Precipitation may occur below 18°C. Decomposition, with the formation of fluorouracil, may occur with prolonged storage above 25°C. |

## Monitoring

| Measure | Frequency | Rationale |
|---|---|---|
| Flucytosine serum concentration | Two to three times a week in renal impairment. Periodically in prolonged therapy | • Samples should be taken shortly before an infusion is due to commence (trough level).<br>• Concentration for optimum response is 25–50 mg/L (200–400 micromol/L) and should not be allowed to exceed 80 mg/L (620 micromol/L). |
| Renal function | At least weekly | • Frequency of testing may be higher in renal impairment.<br>• Na content of infusion is high so this needs close monitoring in patients with renal impairment, cardiac failure or electrolyte disturbances.<br>• Dose adjustment may be necessary if renal function changes. |
| FBC | | • Moderate hypoplasia of bone marrow can occur with leucopenia, thrombocytopenia, agranulocytosis and aplastic anaemia reported.<br>• ↑Risk of bone marrow toxicity with prolonged, high serum concentrations.<br>• Bone marrow toxicity can be irreversible and may lead to death in immunosuppressed patients. |
| LFTs | | • ↑Alk Phos, ↑AST, ↑ALT and ↑bilirubin are usually dose dependent.<br>• Hepatitis and hepatic necrosis have been reported. |
| Microorganism cultures | At regular intervals throughout treatment | • To ensure efficacy. |

## Additional information

| | |
|---|---|
| Common and serious undesirable effects | Nausea, vomiting, diarrhoea and skin rashes may occur and are usually transient. |
| Pharmacokinetics | Elimination half-life is 3–6 hours in normal renal function. |

*(continued)*

| **Additional information** (*continued*) | |
|---|---|
| Significant interactions | • The following may ↑flucytosine levels or effect (or ↑side-effects): cytarabine (monitor FBC more frequently); drugs that impair renal function, e.g. amphotericin may ↓flucytosine elimination and ↑toxicity (monitor flucytosine levels and renal function more frequently).<br>• Cytarabine may oppose the antifungal effects, or ↓flucytosine (monitor levels) or effect. |
| Action in case of overdose | Stop administration and give supportive therapy as appropriate. Haemodialysis produces a rapid fall in the serum concentration. |

| Risk rating: **AMBER** | Score = 3<br>Moderate-risk product: Risk-reduction strategies are recommended. |
|---|---|

This assessment is based on the full range of preparation and administration options described in the monograph. These may not all be applicable in some clinical situations.

## Bibliography

SPC Ancotil 2.5 g/250 mL solution for infusion (accessed 17 March 2009).

# Flumazenil

**100 microgram/mL solution in 5-mL ampoules**

* Flumazenil is a benzodiazepine antagonist that acts competitively at CNS benzodiazepine receptors.
* It is used in anaesthesia and intensive care for complete or partial reversal of sedation caused by benzodiazepines.
* It may also be used to diagnose or treat benzodiazepine toxicity in certain circumstances.

## Pre-treatment checks

* Avoid in patients with a known hypersensitivity to benzodiazepines.
* Flumazenil is not recommended for use in epileptic patients who have been receiving benzodiazepine treatment for a prolonged time.
* Use cautiously in alcoholic patients to avoid precipitation of alcohol withdrawal seizures.
* Do not give to patients who have been given a benzodiazepine for control of a potentially life-threatening situation.
* Caution is required in cases of mixed intoxication with benzodiazepines and tricyclic antidepressants where there are symptoms of severe intoxication with tricyclics, e.g. cardiovascular symptoms (the toxicity of the antidepressants can be masked by the protective benzodiazepine effects).

*Biochemical and other tests (not all are necessary in an emergency situation)*

LFTs
Respiratory rate
Sedation levels

## Dose

**By IV injection**: 200 micrograms over 15 seconds, then 100 micrograms at 60-second intervals if required.
* The usual dose range is 300–600 micrograms.
* The maximum total dose is 1 mg (or 2 mg in intensive care settings).
* If there is no response question the diagnosis.

**By IV infusion**: if drowsiness recurs, give 100–400 micrograms/hour (adjust rate according to response).

**Dose in hepatic impairment**: flumazenil is mainly metabolised in the liver; careful titration is recommended in patients with impaired hepatic function.

## Intravenous injection

*Preparation and administration*

1. Withdraw the required dose.
2. The solution should be clear and colourless. Inspect visually for particulate matter or discoloration prior to administration and discard if present.
3. Give by IV injection over 15 seconds. Injection into a freely running IV infusion line can reduce pain at the injection site.

## Continuous intravenous infusion

*Preparation and administration*

1. Withdraw the required dose and add to a suitable volume of Gluc 5% or NaCl 0.9%. Mix well.
2. The solution should be clear and colourless. Inspect visually for particulate matter or discoloration prior to administration and discard if present.
3. Give by IV infusion at a rate of 100–400 micrograms/hour (adjusted according to response).

| Technical information | |
|---|---|
| Incompatible with | No information |
| Compatible with | **Flush**: NaCl 0.9%<br>**Solutions**: Gluc 5%, NaCl 0.9%<br>**Y-site**: Aminophylline, dobutamine, dopamine, ranitidine |
| pH | 3.5-4.5 |
| Sodium content | Negligible |
| Storage | Store below 25°C in original packaging. |
| Stability after preparation | From a microbiological point of view, should be used immediately; however, prepared infusions may be stored at 2-8°C and infused (at room temperature) within 24 hours. |

## Monitoring

| Measure | Frequency | Rationale |
|---|---|---|
| Respiratory rate | Throughout treatment | • To ensure that respiratory rate returns to normal.<br>• Closely observe until all possible central effects of benzodiazepines have subsided. |
| Re-sedation | | • To check further doses are not required. |
| Seizures | On presentation | • The reversal of benzodiazepine effects may be associated with onset of seizures.<br>• Most likely to occur in patients who have been receiving benzodiazepines for long-term sedation or in patients who have taken an overdose of benzodiazepines and other psychotropic drugs (especially tricyclic antidepressants). |

## Additional information

| | |
|---|---|
| Common and serious undesirable effects | Nausea and vomiting (occasionally).<br>If patients are awakened rapidly they may become agitated, anxious or fearful.<br>Transient ↑BP and pulse may occur on awakening in intensive care patients. |
| Pharmacokinetics | Elimination half-life is 40–80 minutes. |
| Significant interactions | None known. |
| Action in case of overdose | There is no antidote. Treatment should be symptomatic, however no symptoms observed even when doses of 100 mg administered IV. |
| Counselling | Advise patient not to undertake any activities requiring complete mental alertness.<br>Do not drive or operate machinery until there are no residual sedative effects of benzodiazepines.<br>Avoid alcohol or non-prescription drugs for 24 hours after administration of flumazenil or until there are no residual sedative effects of benzodiazepines. |

| Risk rating: **AMBER** | Score = 3<br>Moderate-risk product: Risk-reduction strategies are recommended. |
|---|---|

This assessment is based on the full range of preparation and administration options described in the monograph. These may not all be applicable in some clinical situations.

## Bibliography

SPC Anexate (accessed 28 January 2008).

# Flupentixol decanoate (flupenthixol decanoate)

**20 mg/mL oily solution in 1-mL and 2-mL ampoules; 1-mL and 2-mL syringes; 10-mL vials**
**100 mg/mL oily solution in 0.5-mL and 1-mL ampoules; 5-mL vials**
**200 mg/mL oily solution in 1-mL ampoules**

* Flupentixol decanoate is a thioxanthene antipsychotic presented as a long-acting depot injection.
* It is used in the treatment of schizophrenia and other psychoses.
* Doses are expressed in terms of flupentixol decanoate.

## Pre-treatment checks

* Avoid in patients in comatose states, including alcohol, barbiturate, or opiate poisoning.
* Not recommended for excitable or agitated patients.
* Concomitant treatment with other antipsychotics should be avoided.
* Caution in epilepsy, Parkinson disease, liver disease, renal failure, cardiac disease, depression, myasthenia gravis, prostatic hypertrophy, narrow-angle glaucoma, hypothyroidism, hyperthyroidism, phaeochromocytoma, severe respiratory disease or if there are risk factors for stroke.

*Biochemical and other tests*

| | |
|---|---|
| Blood pressure | LFTs |
| Bodyweight | Renal function: U, Cr, CrCl (or eGFR) |
| ECG | TFTs |
| FBC | |

## Dose

**Test dose:** 20 mg to assess tolerability. Reduce test dose to 5 or 10 mg if patient is elderly.
**Maintenance dose**: commence at least one week after test dose, usual dose range 50 mg every 4 weeks up to 300 mg every 2 weeks. Some patients may require up to 400 mg weekly.

## Intramuscular injection

*Preparation and administration*

1. Withdraw the required dose. The maximum volume to be administered at one site is 2 mL. Volumes >2 mL should be distributed between two injection sites.
2. Give by deep IM injection into the upper outer buttock or lateral thigh. Aspirate before injection to avoid inadvertent intravascular injection. Rotate injection sites for subsequent injections.

| Technical information | |
|---|---|
| Incompatible with | Do not mix with other drugs in the same syringe. |
| Compatible with | Flupentixol decanoate products made by the same manufacturer may be mixed in the same syringe. |

*(continued)*

## Technical information (continued)

| | |
|---|---|
| pH | Not relevant - oily injection |
| Sodium content | Nil |
| Storage | Store below 25°C in original packaging. |

## Monitoring

| Measure | Frequency | Rationale |
|---|---|---|
| Therapeutic improvement | Periodically | • To ensure that treatment is effective. |
| EPSEs | During dose adjustment and every 3 months | • Causes extrapyramidal symptoms, e.g. dystonias. |
| Renal function | At least annually | • As part of regular health check. |
| LFTs | | |
| Blood pressure | | |
| Blood glucose | | |
| Lipids (including cholesterol, HDL, LDL and triglycerides) | | |
| Weight and obesity | | • As part of regular health check.<br>• May cause weight gain<br>• Obesity measured by waist:hip ratio or waist circumference. |
| ECG | Annually | • Can ↑QT interval. |
| Prolactin | See rationale | • If symptoms of hyperprolactinaemia develop. |

## Additional information

| | |
|---|---|
| Common and serious undesirable effects | *Injection-related:* Occasionally erythema, swelling or nodules have been reported.<br>*Other:* EPSEs, blurring of vision, ↑pulse, urinary incontinence and frequency. Dose-related postural ↓BP may occur, particularly in elderly patients. Weight gain. |
| Pharmacokinetics | Elimination half-life is 8 days (single dose); 17 days (multiple doses). |

(continued)

## Additional information (*continued*)

| | |
|---|---|
| Significant interactions | • The following may ↑flupentixol levels or effect (or ↑side-effects): anaesthetics-general (↑hypotensive effect), artemether with lumefantrine, clozapine (↑risk of agranulocytosis), myelosuppressive drugs, ritonavir, sibutramine.<br>• Flupentixol may ↑risk of ventricular arrhythmias with the following drugs: antiarrhythmics, antidepressants-tricyclic, atomoxetine, methadone.<br>• Flupentixol may ↓effect of the following drugs (lowers convulsive threshold): barbiturates, carbamazepine, ethosuximide, oxcarbazepine, phenytoin, primidone, valproate. |
| Action in case of overdose | Treat EPSE with anticholinergic antiparkinsonian drugs.<br>If agitation or convulsions occur treat with benzodiazepines.<br>If the patient is in shock treatment with metaraminol or noradrenaline may be appropriate.<br>Adrenaline must not be given (may further ↓BP). |
| Counselling | Advise patients not to drink alcohol, especially at beginning of treatment.<br>May impair alertness so do not drive or operate machinery until susceptibility is known. |

| Risk rating: **GREEN** | Score = 2<br>Lower-risk product: Risk-reduction strategies should be considered. |
|---|---|

This assessment is based on the full range of preparation and administration options described in the monograph. These may not all be applicable in some clinical situations.

### Bibliography

SPC Depixol (accessed 15 October 2007).

NICE (2009). *Clinical Guideline 82: Core interventions in the treatment and management of schizophrenia in primary and secondary care (update)*. London: National Institute for Health and Clinical Excellence. http://guidance.nice.org.uk/CG82 (accessed 1 October 2009).

# Folic acid

### 15 mg/mL solution in 1-mL ampoules

• Folic acid is a member of the vitamin B group.
• It is used to treat folate-deficient megaloblastic anaemias, usually due to poor nutrition, pregnancy, or antiepileptic drugs.
• It is used to prevent folate deficiency in renal dialysis patients or chronic haemolytic states.

- The parenteral route should only be considered when oral administration is not feasible, or when malabsorption is suspected (although most patients with malabsorption states can absorb adequate amounts of oral folic acid).
- Folic acid injection is an unlicensed product in the UK.

## Pre-treatment checks

Do not give alone for pernicious anaemia and other vitamin $B_{12}$ deficiency states (may precipitate subacute combined degeneration of the spinal cord).

*Biochemical and other tests*

FBC
Red cell folate levels
Vitamin $B_{12}$ levels

## Dose

- **Folate-deficient megaloblastic anaemia**: usually 5 mg daily for 4 months (or until term in pregnant women); doses of up to 15 mg daily may be required in malabsorption states Maintenance dosing of 5 mg every 1–7 days may be required.
- **Prevention of methotrexate-induced side-effects in rheumatic disease** (unlicensed indication): 5 mg once weekly, on a separate day to methotrexate treatment.
- **Prophylaxis in chronic haemolytic states/folate deficiency of dialysis**: 5 mg every 1–7 days depending on clinical condition.

## Intramuscular injection (unlicensed)

*Preparation and administration*

1. Withdraw the required dose.
2. Give by deep IM injection.

## Intravenous injection (unlicensed)

*Preparation and administration*

- Withdraw the required dose.
- The solution should be clear and yellow. Inspect visually for particulate matter or discoloration prior to administration and discard if present.
- Give by IV injection over 3–5 minutes. Dilute with NaCl 0.9% in the syringe if necessary.

## Subcutaneous injection (unlicensed)

*Preparation and administration*

1. Withdraw the required dose.
2. Give by SC injection.

| Technical information | |
|---|---|
| Incompatible with | No information |
| Compatible with | **Flush**: NaCl 0.9%<br>**Solutions**: NaCl 0.9%<br>**Y site**: No information |
| pH | 8–11 |

*(continued)*

## Technical information (continued)

| | |
|---|---|
| Sodium content | Negligible |
| Storage | Store below 25°C in original packaging. |

## Monitoring

| Measure | Frequency | Rationale |
|---|---|---|
| Neurological function | Ongoing through treatment | • Monitor for improvement in folate-deficient peripheral neuropathy if clinically applicable. |
| Mean cell volume | Once weekly during acute phase of treatment | • Response to treatment can be judged by cell size reducing to normal range. |
| Haemoglobin | | • Monitor level of haemoglobin to assess response to treatment. |
| WCC | Once weekly during acute phase of treatment if baseline abnormal | • Production may be affected in megaloblastic anaemia, neutrophils may be hypersegmented. |
| Platelets | | • Production may be affected in megaloblastic anaemia, resulting in thrombocytopenia. |
| Red cell folate levels | Every 1-2 weeks | • Close physiological indicator of folate stores (do not use serum folate, as subject to changes in dietary intake therefore not accurate predictor of overall stores). |
| Physical assessment of patient | Ongoing | • Assess patient symptoms to assess relief of typical anaemic presentation (tiredness, pallor, fainting, exertional dyspnoea, etc.).<br>• More specific symptoms of folate deficiency: glossitis, angular stomatitis, diarrhoea, altered bowel habit, mild jaundice, neuropathy. |

## Additional information

| | |
|---|---|
| Common and serious undesirable effects | *Immediate:* Bronchospasm, anaphylactoid reaction (both very rare).<br>*Other:* Hypersensitivity (erythema, rash, itching), altered sleep patterns, irritability, confusion, lack of concentration, ↓serum vitamin $B_{12}$ levels. |
| Pharmacokinetics | Elimination half-life is difficult to distinguish owing to hepatic storage, wide inter-subject variability. |
| Significant interactions | None significant. |
| Action in case of overdose | Unlikely to require interventional treatment in the event of overdose. |
| Counselling | Patients with a dietary folic acid deficiency require appropriate nutritional advice to support their pharmaceutical supplementation. |

| Risk rating: **GREEN** | Score = 1 Lower-risk product: Risk-reduction strategies should be considered. |
|---|---|

This assessment is based on the full range of preparation and administration options described in the monograph. These may not all be applicable in some clinical situations.

# Fondaparinux sodium

**5 mg/mL solution in pre-filled syringes: 1.5 mg/0.3 mL and 2.5 mg/0.5 mL**
**12.5 mg/mL solution in pre-filled syringes: 5 mg/0.4 mL, 7.5 mg/0.6 mL and 10 mg/0.8 mL**

* Fondaparinux sodium is a synthetic pentasaccharide that acts as a selective inhibitor of Factor Xa.
* It is used in the treatment of STEMI and also in the acute coronary syndromes (ACS): unstable angina and NSTEMI.
* It is used in the treatment of VTE, i.e. pulmonary embolism and deep vein thrombosis.
* It is used for prophylaxis of VTE in surgical and medical patients.
* Routine coagulation tests such as PT and APTT are **not** useful for monitoring.

## Pre-treatment checks

* Avoid in active bleeding; bacterial endocarditis.
* Do not give if CrCl <20 mL/minute in the UK (in the USA the cut off is CrCl <30 mL/minute).
* Caution in patients who have developed HIT.
* Use with caution in patients with bodyweight <50 kg as at ↑risk of bleeding (elimination ↓with weight). In the USA it is contraindicated in such patients undergoing hip-fracture, hip-replacement, knee-replacement, or abdominal surgery due to ↑incidence of major bleeding.
* Caution also in any bleeding disorders, active GI ulcer disease; recent intracranial haemorrhage; brain, spinal, or ophthalmic surgery; spinal or epidural anaesthesia (risk of spinal haematoma – avoid if using treatment doses); risk of catheter thrombus during PCI; elderly patients; concomitant use of drugs that ↑risk of bleeding, hepatic impairment, pregnancy and breast feeding.
* Not licensed in the UK for adults <17 years of age.

*Biochemical and other tests (not all are necessary in an emergency situation)*

| | |
|---|---|
| Blood pressure | LFTs |
| Bodyweight | Renal function: U, Cr, CrCl (or eGFR) |
| FBC (including platelets) | |

## Dose

*Prophylaxis*

**General or orthopaedic surgery with high risk of VTE:** 2.5 mg by SC injection 6 hours after surgery then 2.5 mg once daily until the patient is mobile for at least 5–9 days.

**Medical patients (high risk of VTE):** 2.5 mg by SC injection once daily until the patient is mobile.

*Treatment*

**Treatment of VTE:** give by SC injection once daily based on bodyweight as indicated in Table F1. Treat for at least 5 days and until INR >2.

**Table F1**  Treatment doses of fondaparinux for VTE

| Bodyweight (kg) | Syringe to use |
| --- | --- |
| <50 | 5 mg (0.4 mL) |
| 50-100 | 7.5 mg (0.6 mL) |
| >100 kg | 10 mg (0.8 mL) |

**Treatment of ACS:** 2.5 mg by SC injection once daily for up to 8 days or until hospital discharge, whichever comes first.

Unfractionated heparin should be used in patients undergoing PCI and fondaparinux reinstituted as specified in local protocols.

**Treatment of acute STEMI:** 2.5 mg by IV injection or infusion on first day, thereafter 2.5 mg by SC injection once daily for up to 8 days or until hospital discharge, whichever comes first.

**Dose in renal impairment:** adjusted according to creatinine clearance and indication,

**Prophylaxis of VTE:**

* CrCl 20–50 mL/minute: 1.5 mg once daily.
* CrCl <20 mL/minute: do not use.

**Treatment of VTE:**

* CrCl 30–50 mL/minute: in patients > 100 kg after initial 10 mg dose, reduce to 7.5 mg daily.
* CrCl <30 mL/minute: do not use.

**Treatment of ACS and STEMI:**

* CrCl >20 mL/minute: dose as in normal renal function.
* CrCl <20 mL/minute: do not use.

**Dose in hepatic impairment:** caution in severe hepatic impairment (↑risk of bleeding).

## Subcutaneous injection

*Preparation and administration*

1. Select the correct pre-filled syringe. Pre-filled syringes are ready for immediate use; do not expel the air bubble.
2. The patient should be seated or lying down.
3. Pinch up a skin fold on the abdominal wall between the thumb and forefinger and hold throughout the injection.
4. Give by deep SC injection (push the plunger of the syringe the full length of the syringe barrel) into the thick part of the skin fold at right angles to the skin. Do not rub the injection site after administration. Alternate doses between the right and left sides.
5. Once the plunger is released, the needle automatically withdraws from the skin and retracts into the security sleeve.

## Intravenous injection (first dose in STEMI only)

*Preparation and administration*

1. Select a 2.5-mg pre-filled syringe.
2. The solution should be clear and colourless to slightly yellow. Inspect visually for particulate matter or discoloration prior to administration and discard if present.
3. Give by IV injection via an existing IV line.
4. Flush with NaCl 0.9% after injection to ensure that the entire dose is administered.
5. Once the plunger is released, the needle automatically retracts into the security sleeve.

## Intravenous infusion (alternative route for first dose in STEMI only)

*Preparation and administration*

1. Select a 2.5-mg pre-filled syringe and add the contents to 50 mL NaCl 0.9%.
2. The solution should be clear and colourless to slightly yellow. Inspect visually for particulate matter or discoloration prior to administration and discard if present.
3. Give by IV infusion over 1–2 minutes.
4. Once the plunger is released, the needle automatically retracts into the security sleeve.

## Technical information

| | |
|---|---|
| Incompatible with | No information |
| Compatible with | **Flush**: NaCl 0.9%<br>**Solutions**: NaCl 0.9%<br>**Y-site**: No information |
| pH | 5–8 |
| Sodium content | Negligible |
| Storage | Store below 25°C in original packaging. Do not freeze. |
| Stability after preparation | From a microbiological point of view prepared infusions should be used immediately, however known to be stable at room temperature for up to 24 hours. |

## Monitoring

| Measure | Frequency | Rationale |
|---|---|---|
| Blood pressure | At least daily | • ↓BP may indicate bleeding is occurring somewhere. |
| Renal function | Periodically | • Changes in renal function may require a dose adjustment or cessation of therapy if CrCl drops below 20 mL/minute (30 mL/minute in USA). |
| FBC including platelets | | • Monitor for signs of thrombocytopenia.<br>• ↓Hb and haematocrit may indicate bleeding. |
| Signs and symptoms of bleeding | | • Check stools for faecal occult blood to indicate whether bleeding is occurring in GI tract.<br>• Other symptoms include epistaxis, haematoma. |

## Additional information

| | |
|---|---|
| Common and serious undesirable effects | *Immediate:* Allergic reactions have been reported rarely.<br>*Other:* ↑Risk of bleeding, nausea, vomiting, rash, pruritus, ↑LFTs, oedema. |
| Pharmacokinetics | Rapidly absorbed SC with 100% bioavailability.<br>Elimination half-life is 17-21 hours but is prolonged in patients with renal impairment, in elderly patients, and in those with bodyweight <50 kg. |
| Significant interactions | No significant interactions. |
| Action in case of overdose | *Symptoms to watch for:* Bleeding.<br>*Antidote:* No known antidote but seek haematology advice. If overdose is associated with bleeding complications, stop treatment then search for the primary cause. Initiation of appropriate therapy such as surgical haemostasis, blood replacements, fresh plasma transfusion, plasmapheresis should be considered. |

| Risk rating: **GREEN** | Score = 1<br>Lower-risk product: Risk-reduction strategies should be considered. |
|---|---|

This assessment is based on the full range of preparation and administration options described in the monograph. These may not all be applicable in some clinical situations.

## Bibliography

SPC Arixtra 1.5 mg/0.3 mL solution for injection, pre-filled syringe (accessed 21 August 2009).
SPC Arixtra 2.5mg/0.5 mL solution for injection, pre-filled syringe (accessed 21 August 2009).
SPC Arixtra 5 mg, 7.5 mg, 10 mg solution for injection, pre-filled syringe (accessed 21 August 2009).

# Foscarnet sodium

### 24 mg/mL solution in 250-mL and 500-mL infusion bottles

* Foscarnet sodium is a non-nucleoside analogue with activity against herpes viruses.
* It is used for the treatment of CMV retinitis in AIDS patients and for aciclovir-resistant muco-cutaneous HSV infections in immunocompromised patients.

## Pre-treatment checks

* Caution in patients with neurological or cardiac abnormalities because of electrolyte disturbances.
* Ensure adequate hydration to establish diuresis by giving 500 mL–1 L of NaCl 0.9% or Gluc 5% concurrently with each infusion.

*Biochemical tests*

Electrolytes: serum Ca, K, Mg, PO$_4$

FBC

LFTs

Renal function: U, Cr, CrCl (or eGFR)

## Dose

**CMV retinitis:**

* Induction: 60 mg/kg every 8 hours for 2–3 weeks.
* Maintenance: 60 mg/kg daily (increased to 90–120 mg/kg if tolerated and/or in progressive retinitis). If retinitis continues to progress on the maintenance dose, then repeat the induction regimen.

**Mucocutaneous herpes simplex infection**: 40 mg/kg every 8 hours for 2–3 weeks or until lesions heal. (No maintenance schedule has been determined for this indication.)

**Dose in renal impairment**: in the UK the manufacturer recommends dosage adjustment according to creatinine clearance expressed as mL/kg/minute. (Calculate the CrCl or eGFR in the normal way and divide the result by the patient's ideal bodyweight.) The dose is then reduced according to the calculated creatinine clearance and the indication, see Table F2.

NB: a different dosing schedule is used in the USA.

**Table F2** Foscarnet dosing in renal impairment

| CrCl (mL/kg/minute) | CMV: induction (mg/kg every 8 hours) | CMV: maintenance (mg/kg daily) | HSV dosing (mg/kg every 8 hours) |
|---|---|---|---|
| >1.6 | 60 | 60 | 40 |
| >1.4-1.6 | 55 | 55 | 37 |
| >1.2-1.4 | 49 | 49 | 33 |
| >1.0-1.2 | 42 | 42 | 28 |
| >0.8-1.0 | 35 | 35 | 24 |
| >0.6-0.8 | 28 | 28 | 19 |
| 0.4-0.6 | 21 | 21 | 14 |
| <0.4 | Not recommended | Not recommended | Not recommended |

## Intermittent intravenous infusion

*Preparation and administration*

* See Special handling below.
* Foscarnet sodium is incompatible with Hartmann's, Ringer's and other solutions or preparations containing calcium.
* Foscarnet sodium must not be given by rapid IV infusion or injection.
* The 24 mg/mL solution may be given without dilution via a central vein.
* If a peripheral vein is used, the solution must be diluted to give a solution containing 12 mg/mL before administration.

1. Calculate the required total dose. To minimise the risk of overdosage, any drug in excess of the patient's calculated dose should be removed from the infusion bottle and discarded prior to administration.
2. If the infusion is to be given via a peripheral vein, dilute the dose with an equal quantity of NaCl 0.9% before administration. Alternatively, some centres piggyback 1 L NaCl 0.9% to run concurrently with the foscarnet dose.
3. The solution should be clear and colourless. Inspect visually for particulate matter or discoloration prior to administration and discard if present.
4. Give by IV infusion using a controlled infusion device. Give up to 60 mg/kg over a minimum of 60 minutes; for higher doses the infusion time should be increased proportionately.

## Technical information

| | |
|---|---|
| Incompatible with | Foscarnet sodium is incompatible with Hartmann's, Ringer's and other solutions or preparations containing calcium. Aciclovir, amphotericin, co-trimoxazole, diazepam, digoxin, dobutamine, ganciclovir, midazolam, pentamidine isetionate, vancomycin. |
| Compatible with | **Flush**: NaCl 0.9%<br>**Solutions**: NaCl 0.9% (including added KCl), Gluc 5%<br>**Y-site**: Amikacin, aminophylline, ampicillin, aztreonam, benzylpenicillin, ceftazidime, ceftriaxone, cefuroxime, chloramphenicol sodium succinate, clindamycin phosphate, dexamethasone sodium phosphate, dopamine, erythromycin lactobionate, fluconazole, furosemide, gentamicin, hydrocortisone sodium succinate, imipenem with cilastatin, metoclopramide, metronidazole, phenytoin, ranitidine, ticarcillin with clavulanate, tobramycin |
| pH | 7.4 |
| Sodium content | 60 mmol/250 mL (also contains phosphate 19.8 mmol/250 mL) |
| Storage | Store below 30°C but do not refrigerate.<br>Precipitation may occur if refrigerated which may be brought into solution again by keeping the bottle at room temperature and repeatedly shaking.<br>Bottles are single use only - discard any unused portion. |
| Special handling | Contact with the skin or eye may cause local irritation and a burning sensation. Rinse the affected area with water. |
| Stability after reconstitution | From a microbiological point of view, should be used immediately; however, prepared dilutions may be stored at 2-8°C and infused (at room temperature) within 24 hours. |

## Monitoring

| Measure | Frequency | Rationale |
|---|---|---|
| CrCl (or eGFR) | Every second day during induction; once weekly during maintenance | • Foscarnet is nephrotoxic and changes in renal function may require a dose adjustment.<br>• Renal toxicity can be reduced by adequate hydration of the patient. |

*(continued)*

## Monitoring (continued)

| Measure | Frequency | Rationale |
|---------|-----------|-----------|
| Serum Ca, Mg, K and PO$_4$ concentrations | Every second day during induction; once weekly during maintenance | • Foscarnet may chelate bivalent metal ions therefore there may be an acute decrease of ionised serum Ca and Mg, which may not be reflected in total serum concentrations.<br>• Patients must report signs of ↓Ca, e.g. perioral tingling, numbness in the extremities, paraesthesias. If these occur, stop the infusion and review before recommencing.<br>• Changes in electrolytes are reversible and a lower infusion rate, e.g. 1 mg/kg/minute may lessen the effects. |
| LFTs | Periodically | • ↑ALT, ↑AST and ↑GGT may occur. |
| FBC | | • ↓Haemoglobin concentration, leucopenia, granulocytopenia, thrombocytopenia have been reported. |
| Ophthalmological examination | Every 4-6 weeks (more frequently if indicated) | • To detect the progression or recurrence of CMV retinitis. |

## Additional information

| | |
|---|---|
| Common and serious undesirable effects | *Infusion-related:* Thrombophlebitis if given undiluted by peripheral vein.<br>*Other:* Nausea, vomiting, diarrhoea (occasionally constipation), dyspepsia, abdominal pain, anorexia; changes in BP and ECG; headache, fatigue, mood disturbances (including psychosis), asthenia, paraesthesia, convulsions (in up to 10% of patients), tremor, dizziness, and other neurological disorders; rash; genital irritation and ulceration. |
| Pharmacokinetics | Elimination half-life is 3-6 hours. |
| Significant interactions | • Foscarnet may ↑nephrotoxicity of the following drugs (monitor CrCl): aminoglycosides, amphotericin, ciclosporin.<br>• Foscarnet may cause ↓Ca with pentamidine isetionate (monitor serum Ca). |
| Action in case of overdose | No known antidote but haemodialysis may be effective.<br>Stop administration and give supportive therapy as appropriate. |
| Counselling | Patients should pay extra attention to personal hygiene after micturition to lessen the potential of local irritation (foscarnet may be excreted in high concentrations in the urine and can lead to genital irritation or even ulceration). |

| | |
|---|---|
| Risk rating: **AMBER** | Score = 5<br>Moderate-risk product: Risk-reduction strategies are recommended. |

This assessment is based on the full range of preparation and administration options described in the monograph. These may not all be applicable in some clinical situations.

**Bibliography**

SPC Foscavir (accessed 18 March 2009).

# Fosphenytoin sodium

**75 mg/mL solution in 10-mL vials ≡ 50 mg/mL phenytoin sodium ≡ 50 mg PE/mL**

* Fosphenytoin is a pro-drug of phenytoin. Phenytoin sodium is a hydantoin antiepileptic agent believed to act by preventing the spread of seizure activity, rather than raising seizure threshold.
* Fosphenytoin sodium is used in the management of status epilepticus, as a substitute for phenytoin when parenteral therapy is indicated, and for prophylactic control of seizures in neurosurgery or following serious head injury.

Fosphenytoin sodium doses are expressed in terms of phenytoin sodium equivalents (PE):

All labelling and all prescriptions must specify doses as phenytoin sodium equivalents (PE) to avoid confusion:

* Fosphenytoin sodium 1.5 mg ≡1 mg PE (phenytoin sodium equivalent).
* Fosphenytoin 1 mmol is metabolised to 1 mmol phenytoin.

### UK CSM advice (May 2000)

IV infusion of fosphenytoin has been associated with severe cardiovascular reactions including asystole, ventricular fibrillation, and cardiac arrest. ↓BP, ↓pulse and heart block have also been reported. The CSM advises:

* Monitor heart rate, BP and respiratory function for duration of infusion.
* Observe the patient for at least 30 minutes after the end of the infusion.
* If ↓BP occurs, reduce the infusion rate or discontinue administration.
* A lower loading dose and/or infusion rate may be required in elderly patients and in those with renal or hepatic impairment.

## Pre-treatment checks

* Ensure that resuscitation facilities are available.
* Avoid in acute porphyria.
* Caution in ↓BP, ↓pulse, heart failure, previous myocardial infarction, sinoatrial block, second- and third-degree heart block and Stokes–Adams syndrome.

*Biochemical and other tests (not all are necessary in an emergency situation)*

| | |
|---|---|
| Blood pressure | FBC |
| Bodyweight | LFTs including albumin |
| ECG | Pregnancy test |

## Dose

For existing epilepsy patients switched from oral phenytoin maintenance to parenteral fosphenytoin:
* Capsules (containing phenytoin sodium) 100 mg ≡ 100 mg PE fosphenytoin IV.
* Suspension (containing phenytoin base) 90 mg ≅ 100 mg PE fosphenytoin IV.

Phenytoin exhibits non-linear pharmacokinetics (minor dose changes can have a significant effect on phenytoin levels) – always monitor levels closely when the route is changed.

**Status epilepticus:** 20 mg (PE)/kg by IV infusion then 4–5 mg (PE)/kg daily in 1–2 divided doses by IV infusion or IM injection. Adjust dosage according to phenytoin levels and change to oral phenytoin as soon as possible.

**Seizure prophylaxis or treatment during neurosurgery or following head injury:** 10–15 mg (PE)/kg by IV infusion or IM injection, then 4–5 mg (PE)/kg daily in 1–2 divided doses by IV infusion or IM injection. Adjust dosage according to phenytoin levels and change to oral phenytoin as soon as possible.

**Temporary replacement of oral phenytoin:** see dosage statement above.

**Dose in elderly patients and in renal and hepatic impairment:** the manufacturer recommends a 10–25% reduction in dose or infusion rate be considered (except initial dose for status epilepticus). No reference is made to the degree of renal or hepatic impairment requiring such reductions; be guided by clinical response and plasma concentrations.

## Intravenous infusion

*Preparation and administration*

1. Withdraw the required dose and add to a suitable volume of NaCl 0.9% or Gluc 5% to give a solution containing 1.5–25 mg (PE)/mL. Use 25 mg (PE)/mL for status epilepticus.
2. The solution should be clear and colourless to faintly yellow. Inspect visually for particulate matter or discoloration prior to administration and discard if present.
3. Give by IV infusion using a rate controlled infusion device at a maximum rate of 150 mg (PE)/minute:
   * Rate for status epilepticus loading dose: 100–150 mg (PE)/minute.
   * Rate for all other indications and further doses 50–100 mg (PE)/minute.

## Intramuscular injection

This route is not suitable for status epilepticus.

*Preparation and administration*

1. Withdraw the required dose.
2. Give by deep IM injection.

## Technical information

| | |
|---|---|
| Incompatible with | Drotrecogin alfa (activated), midazolam. |
| Compatible with | **Flush**: NaCl 0.9%<br>**Solutions**: NaCl 0.9%, Gluc 5% (both with added KCl)<br>**Y-site**: Lorazepam, mannitol, phenobarbital sodium |
| pH | 8.6-9.0 |

(continued)

## Technical information (continued)

| | |
|---|---|
| Sodium content | 3.7 mmol/10-mL vial |
| Storage | Store between 2 and 8°C in original packaging. |
| Stability after preparation | Use prepared infusions immediately. |

## Monitoring

| Measure | Frequency | Rationale |
|---|---|---|
| ECG and blood pressure | During IV administration | • There is a risk of serious arrhythmias and ↓BP. |
| Infusion solution and rate of infusion | During administration | • Discard if precipitate present or becomes discoloured. <br>• Over rapid administration can lead to serious adverse effects. |
| Seizures | Continuously | • For therapeutic effect. |
| Blood glucose | Frequently | • May ↑blood glucose concentration. <br>• Adjust dosage of insulin or oral antidiabetic drugs if required. |
| Phenytoin serum levels | At steady state to ensure in therapeutic window (after 5-7 half-lives). If dosage adjustments are required. If toxicity or a drug interaction is suspected | • Phenytoin levels are measured for fosphenytoin therapy. <br>• Therapeutic total plasma-phenytoin level for optimum response: 10-20 mg/L (40-80 micromoles/L) or unbound plasma-phenytoin levels: 1-2 mg/L (4-8 micromoles/L). <br>• Care should be taken if dosage is to be adjusted when levels are in the upper range as a small increase in dosage may produce a large increase in serum concentration. |
| LFTs including albumin | Periodically | • Albumin levels should also be measured to indicate if protein binding is affected. If albumin is low, free phenytoin levels will be high even if total plasma-phenytoin levels are in range. <br>• Liver dysfunction sometimes occurs. |
| FBC | | • Thrombocytopenia, leucopenia, granulocytopenia, agranulocytosis, pancytopenia and aplastic anaemia have all been reported. |
| Pregnancy test | If pregnancy suspected | • May cause blood clotting abnormalities and congenital malformations in the neonate. |

## Additional information

| | |
|---|---|
| Common and serious undesirable effects | *Injection/infusion-related:*<br>• Too rapid administration: Arrhythmias, ↓pulse, heart block, vasodilation, ↓BP, cardiovascular collapse, asystole, impaired respiratory function and respiratory arrest. Transient itching, burning, warmth or tingling in the groin (lessened by ↓infusion rate).<br>• Local: Injection-site reaction or pain. Inadvertent SC, intra-arterial or perivascular injection may cause severe local tissue damage due to the high pH.<br>*Other:* Nausea, vomiting, constipation, anorexia, insomnia, transient nervousness, tremor, paraesthesia, dizziness, headache, peripheral neuropathy, dyskinesia, rash, megaloblastic anaemia, leucopenia, thrombocytopenia, aplastic anaemia, hepatotoxicity, lymphadenopathy, polyarteritis nodosa, lupus erythematosus, Stevens-Johnson syndrome, toxic epidermal necrolysis, pneumonitis, interstitial nephritis. |
| Pharmacokinetics | Elimination half-life fosphenytoin is 15 minutes - converted to phenytoin. Elimination half-life of phenytoin is usually 10-15 hours; may take many weeks to reach steady state. The half-life may increase if the metabolism pathway becomes saturated - risk of toxicity. |
| Significant interactions | • The following may ↑phenytoin levels or effect (or ↑side-effects): amiodarone, azapropazone (avoid combination), chloramphenicol (monitor), cimetidine, co-trimoxazole, diltiazem, disulfiram (monitor levels), esomeprazole, ethosuximide, fluconazole-multiple dosing (monitor levels), fluoxetine, fluvoxamine, indinavir, isoniazid, metronidazole-systemic, miconazole, NSAIDs-systemic, sulphinpyrazone, topiramate, trimethoprim, voriconazole (monitor levels).<br>• The following may ↓phenytoin levels or effect: antipsychotics (↓seizure threshold), mefloquine, pyrimethamine, rifabutin, rifampicin, theophylline, SSRIs (↓seizure threshold), St John's wort, tricyclic antidepressants (↓seizure threshold).<br>• Fosphenytoin may ↑levels or effect (or ↑side-effects) of coumarins.<br>• Fosphenytoin may ↓levels or effect of the following drugs: aripiprazole, ciclosporin, corticosteroids, coumarins, diltiazem, eplerenone (avoid combination), ethosuximide, imatinib (avoid combination), indinavir, itraconazole (avoid combination), ketoconazole, lapatinib (avoid combination), mianserin, nifedipine, oestrogens (↓contraceptive effect), posaconazole, progestogens (↓contraceptive effect), telithromycin (avoid combination), theophylline, topiramate, tricyclic antidepressants, voriconazole (↑dose needed). |
| Action in case of overdose | *Symptoms:* ↑ or ↓pulse, asystole, respiratory or circulatory depression, cardiac arrest, syncope, ↓Ca, metabolic acidosis and death.<br>*Antidote:* No known antidote but haemodialysis may be used, as about 10% of phenytoin is not protein bound.<br>Stop administration and give supportive therapy as appropriate. Phenytoin plasma levels should be checked as soon as possible. |
| Counselling | Women who have been relying on the combined contraceptive pill should be advised to take additional precautions. |

| Risk rating: **AMBER** | Score = 5<br>Moderate-risk product: Risk-reduction strategies are recommended. |
|---|---|

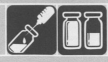

This assessment is based on the full range of preparation and administration options described in the monograph. These may not all be applicable in some clinical situations.

## Bibliography

SPC Pro-Epanutin concentrate for infusion/solution for injection (accessed 10 October 2008).

# Furosemide (frusemide)

### 10 mg/mL solution in 2-mL, 5-mL and 25-mL ampoules or vials

- Furosemide is a loop diuretic with a rapid action.
- It is indicated for use when prompt and effective diuresis is required.
- The IV formulation is appropriate for use in emergencies or when the oral route is unavailable or ineffective: indications include cardiac, pulmonary, hepatic and renal oedema.

## Pre-treatment checks

- Do not use in hypovolaemia, dehydration, severe ↓K, severe ↓Na; comatose or precomatose states associated with liver cirrhosis; renal failure due to nephrotoxic or hepatotoxic drugs, anuria.
- Caution in ↓BP; prostatic enlargement; impaired micturition; gout; diabetes; hepatorenal syndrome; hepatic impairment; renal impairment.
- Fluid balance and electrolytes should be carefully controlled and, in particular, in patients with shock, measures should be taken to correct BP and circulating blood volume before commencing treatment.

*Biochemical and other tests (not all are necessary in an emergency situation)*

| | |
|---|---|
| Blood glucose | LFTs |
| Blood pressure | Renal function: U, Cr, CrCl (or eGFR) |
| Electrolytes: serum Na, K, Mg | |

## Dose

**Standard initial dose**: 20–50 mg. If larger doses are required, they should be given increasing by 20-mg increments and not given more often than every 2 hours.

**Oliguria in acute or chronic renal failure** (GFR <20 mL/minute but >5 mL/minute): the following doses have been used:

1. Initially 250 mg infused over 1 hour.
2. If urine output is insufficient within the next hour, this dose may be followed by 500 mg infused over about 2 hours.

3. If a satisfactory urine output has still not been achieved within 1 hour of the end of the second infusion, then a third dose of 1 g may be infused over about 4 hours.
4. If the response is satisfactory, the effective dose (up to 1 g) may then be repeated every 24 hours.

The recommended maximum daily dose is 1500 mg.

## Intravenous infusion (preferred route for doses >50 mg)

*Preparation and administration*

1. Withdraw the required dose. Depending on hydration status, either give undiluted using a syringe pump or add to a convenient volume of NaCl 0.9%.
2. The solution should be clear and colourless or almost colourless. Inspect visually for particulate matter or discoloration prior to administration and discard if present.
3. Give by IV infusion at a rate no greater than 4 mg/minute, i.e. a dose of 100 mg must be infused over at least 25 minutes. In severe renal impairment the rate may be reduced to 2.5 mg/minute to reduce the likelihood of ototoxicity.

## Intravenous injection (may be suitable for doses ≤50 mg)

*Preparation and administration*

1. Withdraw the required dose.
2. The solution should be clear and colourless or almost colourless. Inspect visually for particulate matter or discoloration prior to administration and discard if present.
3. Give by IV injection over 3–5 minutes. Note: rapid injection may cause tinnitus and deafness.

## Intramuscular injection

*Preparation and administration*

> Restrict to exceptional cases (and only for doses ≤50 mg) where neither the oral nor IV routes are available. IM use is not suitable for the treatment of acute conditions such as pulmonary oedema.

1. Withdraw the required dose.
2. Give by IM injection.

| Technical information | |
|---|---|
| Incompatible with | Furosemide is incompatible with Gluc solutions.<br>Adrenaline (epinephrine), amikacin, amiodarone, ciprofloxacin, cisatracurium, clarithromycin, diazepam, dobutamine, dopamine, doxapram, drotrecogin alfa (activated), erythromycin lactobionate, esmolol, fluconazole, gentamicin, hydralazine, hydrocortisone sodium succinate, labetalol, metoclopramide, midazolam, noradrenaline (norepinephrine), ondansetron, pantoprazole, tobramycin, vasopressin, vecuronium. |
| Compatible with | **Flush**: NaCl 0.9%<br>**Solutions**: NaCl 0.9% (with added KCl)<br>**Y-site**: Aminophylline, aztreonam, benzylpenicillin, calcium gluconate, ceftazidime, cefuroxime, dexamethasone sodium phosphate, digoxin, glyceryl trinitrate, granisetron, isosorbide dinitrate, linezolid, meropenem, micafungin, piperacillin with tazobactam, ranitidine, remifentanil, sodium bicarbonate |
| pH | 8-9.3 |

*(continued)*

## Technical information (continued)

| | |
|---|---|
| Sodium content | Negligible |
| Storage | Store below 25°C in original packaging. |
| Stability after preparation | Use prepared infusions immediately and complete infusion within 24 hours. |

## Monitoring

| Measure | Frequency | Rationale |
|---|---|---|
| Urinary output and relief of symptoms | Throughout treatment | • Response to therapy. |
| Fluid balance, serum electrolytes, and bicarbonate | Periodically | • Fluid balance should be carefully controlled. Electrolyte disturbances and metabolic alkalosis may occur. Replace if necessary. Disturbances may require temporary discontinuation of therapy.<br>• ↓K may precipitate coma (use potassium-sparing diuretic to prevent this).<br>• Increased risk of ↓Mg in alcoholic cirrhosis. |
| Renal function | | • Changes in renal function may require a different dose or rate of infusion.<br>• A marked ↑blood urea or the development of oliguria or anuria indicates severe progression of renal disease and treatment should be stopped. |
| Blood pressure | | • Potential for ↓BP and circulatory collapse resulting from rapid mobilisation of oedema fluid. |
| Blood glucose | | • Reduced serum potassium may blunt response to insulin in patients with diabetes mellitus. |

## Additional information

| | |
|---|---|
| Common and serious undesirable effects | *Immediate:* Anaphylaxis and other hypersensitivity reactions have been reported.<br>*Injection/infusion-related:* Too rapid administration: Tinnitus and deafness.<br>*Other:* ↓Ca, ↓K, ↓Na, ↑uric acid levels, ↑blood glucose, ↓BP, dehydration, blood dyscrasias. |
| Pharmacokinetics | Elimination half-life is about 2 hours; prolonged in patients with renal and hepatic impairment. |
| Significant interactions | • Furosemide may ↑risk of ototoxicity with the following drugs: aminoglycosides, polymyxins, vancomycin.<br>• ↓K due to furosemide may ↑risk of cardiotoxicity with the following drugs: amisulpride, atomoxetine, cardiac glycosides, disopyramide, flecainide, pimozide, sertindole, sotalol.<br>• Furosemide may cause ↓BP with the following drugs: ACE inhibitors, alpha-blockers, ATII receptor antagonists.<br>• Furosemide may ↑levels (or ↑side-effects) of lithium (avoid combination or monitor levels).<br>• Furosemide may ↓effect of lidocaine (↓K antagonises action). |

*(continued)*

## Additional information (*continued*)

| | |
|---|---|
| Action in case of overdose | Treat with fluid replacement and electrolytes as necessary. |
| Counselling | Advise the patient to report muscle pains/cramps and hearing disturbance. |

| | |
|---|---|
| Risk rating: **AMBER** | Score = 4<br>Moderate-risk product: Risk-reduction strategies are recommended. |

This assessment is based on the full range of preparation and administration options described in the monograph. These may not all be applicable in some clinical situations.

## Bibliography

SPC Furosemide Injection BP, Hameln (accessed 14 September 2009).

SPC Furosemide Injection BP 10 mg/ml, 2 mL, 5 mL and 25 mL, Goldshield (accessed 14 September 2009).

SPC Furosemide Injection BP Minijet 10 mg/ml solution for injection, International Medication Systems (accessed 14 September 2009).

SPC Lasix injection 20 mg/2 mL (accessed 14 September 2009).

# Ganciclovir

**500-mg dry powder vials**
* Ganciclovir sodium is a synthetic nucleoside analogue of guanine.
* It is used for the treatment and suppression of life-threatening or sight-threatening CMV infections in immunocompromised patients.
* Doses are expressed in terms of the base:
  Ganciclovir 500 mg $\cong$ 545 mg ganciclovir sodium.

## Pre-treatment checks

* Do not give if there is known hypersensitivity to ganciclovir, valganciclovir, aciclovir or valaciclovir.
* Ensure that the patient is adequately hydrated (excretion depends on adequate renal function).

*Biochemical and other tests*

Bodyweight
FBC (do not initiate if the absolute neutrophil count is <500 cells/mm$^3$ ($0.5 \times 10^9$/L), or platelet count <25 000/mm$^3$ ($25 \times 10^9$/L), or haemoglobin <8 g/dL)
Ophthalmological examination
Renal function: U, Cr, CrCl (or eGFR)

## Dose

> Ganciclovir sodium must not be given by IV injection as excessive plasma levels result in ↑toxicity. It must not be given by IM or SC injection because the high pH causes tissue irritation.

*CMV infection*

**Induction**: 5 mg/kg every 12 hours for 14–21 days.
**Maintenance**: 6 mg/kg once daily 5 days per week, or 5 mg/kg once daily 7 days per week (used for immunocompromised patients at risk of relapse of CMV retinitis). If retinitis continues to progress on the maintenance dose then repeat the induction regimen.

*Prevention of CMV disease*

**Induction**: 5 mg/kg infused every 12 hours for 7–14 days.
**Maintenance**: 6 mg/kg once daily 5 days per week, or 5 mg/kg once daily 7 days per week.

**Dose in renal impairment:** adjusted according to creatinine clearance.
* CrCl >70 mL/minute: dose as in normal renal function.
* CrCl 50–69 mL/minute: 2.5 mg/kg every 12 hours (induction); 2.5 mg/kg every 24 hours (maintenance).
* CrCl 25–49 mL/minute: 2.5 mg/kg every 24 hours (induction); 1.25 mg/kg every 24 hours (maintenance).
* CrCl 10–24 mL/minute: 1.25 mg/kg every 24 hours (induction); 0.625 mg/kg every 24 hours (maintenance).
* CrCl <10 mL/minute: 1.25 mg/kg shortly after haemodialysis (induction); 0.625 mg/kg shortly after haemodialysis (maintenance). NB: In the USA a maximum of 3 doses per week is recommended.

## Intermittent intravenous infusion

Give via a large peripheral or central vein.
See Special handling below.

*Preparation and administration*

1. Add 10 mL WFI to the vial and shake to dissolve. This gives a concentration of 50 mg/mL.
2. Withdraw the required dose and transfer to 50–250 mL of compatible infusion fluid (usually 100 mL NaCl 0.9% is used). The final concentration must not exceed 10 mg/mL.
3. The solution should be clear and colourless. Inspect visually for particulate matter or discoloration prior to administration and discard if present.
4. Give by IV infusion at a constant rate over 60 minutes via a large peripheral or central vein (↑blood flow is essential to ensure rapid dilution and distribution). A controlled-infusion device is recommended for more concentrated solutions.

## Technical information

| | |
|---|---|
| Incompatible with | WFI containing parabens.<br>Aztreonam, foscarnet, ondansetron, piperacillin with tazobactam. |
| Compatible with | **Flush**: NaCl 0.9%<br>**Solutions**: NaCl 0.9%, Gluc 5%, Hartmann's Ringer's<br>**Y-site**: Cisatracurium, fluconazole, granisetron, linezolid, propofol, remifentanil |
| pH | 11 |
| Sodium content | 2 mmol/500-mg vial |
| Storage | Store below 30°C in original packaging. |
| Displacement value | Negligible |
| Special handling | Ganciclovir is considered a potential teratogen and carcinogen in humans.<br>The use of latex gloves and protective eyewear is recommended.<br>Avoid inhalation or direct contact of the dry powder or reconstituted solution with skin or mucous membranes. If contact occurs, wash thoroughly with soap and water; rinse the eyes thoroughly with sterile water (or plain water if sterile water is unavailable). |
| Stability after preparation | From a microbiological point of view, should be used immediately, however:<br>• Reconstituted vials may be stored at room temperature for up to 12 hours.<br>• Prepared infusions may be stored at 2–8°C and infused (at room temperature) within 24 hours. |

## Monitoring

| Measure | Frequency | Rationale |
|---------|-----------|-----------|
| FBC (including platelets) | Alternate days during induction; at least weekly thereafter | • If severe leucopenia, neutropenia, anaemia, thrombocytopenia or pancytopenia occurs, treatment with haematopoietic growth factors and/or dose interruption should be considered.<br>• Monitor FBC daily if there is a history of leucopenia, if neutrophil count is <1000 cells/mm³ (1 × 10⁹/L), and in haemodialysis.<br>• If neutropenia and/or thrombocytopenia occur, dosage adjustment and/or interruption of therapy may be necessary. |
| Renal function | At least fortnightly | • Serum Cr may become raised, necessitating a dose adjustment. |
| Ophthalmological examination | At least every 6 weeks | • To detect the possibility of progression and/or recurrence of cytomegalovirus retinitis.<br>• These examinations should continue after cessation of treatment. |

## Additional information

| | |
|---|---|
| Common and serious undesirable effects | *Immediate:* Anaphylaxis has rarely been reported.<br>*Injection/infusion-related:* Local: Injection-site reactions.<br>*Other:* Sepsis, anaemia, blood dyscrasias, anorexia, depression, insomnia, convulsions, taste disturbance, eye disorders, dyspnoea, diarrhoea, nausea, vomiting, altered LFTs, dermatitis, night sweats, pruritus, myalgia, muscle cramps, renal impairment, fatigue, pyrexia, chest pain. |
| Pharmacokinetics | Elimination half-life is 2.5–5 hours in normal renal function; up to 29 hours in renal impairment. |
| Significant interactions | • The following may ↑ganciclovir levels or effect (or ↑side-effects): imipenem with cilastatin (↑risk of convulsions); zidovudine (profound myelosuppression – avoid combination). |
| Action in case of overdose | No known antidote but rehydration and haemodialysis may be effective. Stop administration and give supportive therapy as appropriate. |
| Counselling | Potentially teratogenic and may cause temporary or permanent inhibition of spermatogenesis. Women of child-bearing potential must use effective contraception during treatment, and men must use barrier contraception during and for at least 90 days after treatment (unless certain that the female partner is not at risk of pregnancy). |

| | |
|---|---|
| Risk rating: **AMBER** | Score = 5<br>Moderate-risk product: Risk-reduction strategies are recommended. |

  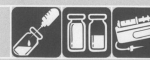

This assessment is based on the full range of preparation and administration options described in the monograph. These may not all be applicable in some clinical situations.

**Bibliography**

SPC Cymevene powder for infusion (accessed 11 March 2008).

# Gelatin

**3%, 3.5% and 4% solutions (with varying amounts of electrolytes) in 500-mL or 1000-mL infusion containers**

* Gelatin preparations are colloidal plasma substitutes. They contain large molecules that do not readily leave the intravascular space where they exert osmotic pressure to maintain circulatory volume. Compared with crystalloids, smaller volumes are required to produce the same expansion of blood volume.
* They are used in the initial short-term management of hypovolaemic shock caused by conditions such as burns, septicaemia, haemorrhage, acute trauma or surgery. Blood products should be given as soon as available if appropriate.
* Use of gelatin-containing infusion fluids may ↑risk of bleeding owing to dilution of clotting factors.
* Table G1 shows the gelatin and electrolyte content of the commercially available products.

**Table G1**  Gelatin and electrolyte content of some gelatin-containing infusion fluids

| Product | Gelofusine | Geloplasma | Haemaccel | Isoplex | Volplex |
|---|---|---|---|---|---|
| Volume | 500 mL | 500 mL | 500 mL | 500 mL | 500 mL |
| Gelatin (%)[a] | 4 | 3 | 3.5 | 4 | 4 |
| Sodium (mmol) | 77 | 75 | 72.5 | 72.5 | 77 |
| Potassium (mmol) | - | 2.5 | 2.55 | 2 | - |
| Magnesium (mmol) | - | 0.75 | - | 0.45 | - |
| Calcium (mmol) | - | - | 3.125 | - | - |
| Chloride (mmol) | 60 | 50 | 72.5 | 52.5 | 62.5 |
| Lactate (mmol) | - | 15 | - | 12.5 | - |

[a]As either succinylated gelatin (Gelofusine, Geloplasma, Isoplex, Volplex) or polygeline (Haemaccel)

## Pre-treatment checks

* Preparations containing lactate are contraindicated in patients with liver disease.
* Extreme caution should be used in those patients likely to develop circulatory overload such as in congestive cardiac failure, renal failure and pulmonary oedema.
* Caution should also be used in those patients at risk of liver disease and bleeding disorders.

- Patients with known allergic disorders (e.g. asthma) may be more likely to suffer an allergic reaction.
- Dehydration should be corrected prior to or during treatment.

*Biochemical and other tests (not all are necessary in an emergency situation)*

Electrolytes: serum Na, K
FBC
Urinary output

## Dose

**Hypovolaemic shock:** initial volumes of 500–1000 mL may be required. The volume given and rate of infusion will depend on the condition of the patient. In severe acute blood loss may be given rapidly (500 mL in 5–10 minutes).

## Intravenous infusion

*Preparation and administration*

Preparations containing Ca are not compatible with citrated blood.

1. If the infusion is to be given rapidly, warm container to no more than 37°C if possible.
2. The infusion is pre-prepared for use. It should be clear and pale yellow or straw coloured. Inspect visually for particulate matter or discoloration prior to administration and discard if present.
3. Give by IV infusion at the required rate; pressure may be applied to the container to hasten administration.
4. Discard any unused portion. Do not reconnect partially used infusion containers.

## Technical information

| Incompatible with | Preparations containing Ca are not compatible with citrated blood. |
|---|---|
| Compatible with | Non-Ca-containing preparations may be given through the same giving set as blood. |
| pH | 3.8-7.6 |
| Electrolyte content | See Table G1. |
| Storage | Do not store above 25°C. Do not freeze or refrigerate. |

## Monitoring

| Measure | Frequency | Rationale |
|---|---|---|
| Serum Na and K concentration | During treatment | • Close monitoring is required at all times as the patient's condition is likely to be unstable. <br>• All aspects of fluid and volume replacement need to be taken into account. <br>• Dehydration should be corrected prior to or during treatment and adequate amounts of fluid provided daily. |

*(continued)*

## Monitoring (continued)

| Measure | Frequency | Rationale |
|---------|-----------|-----------|
| FBC and coagulation screen | During treatment | • Adequate haematocrit should be maintained and not allowed to fall below 25-30%, observe for early signs of bleeding complications.<br>• Dilutional effects upon coagulation should be avoided.<br>• Coagulation factor deficiencies should be corrected. |
| Signs of anaphylaxis | | • Severe anaphylaxis has occurred. |
| CVP (and signs of circulatory overload) | | • Monitoring of CVP during the initial period of infusion will aid the detection of fluid overload. |
| Urine output | | • Monitor for oliguria or renal failure.<br>• ↓Urine output secondary to shock is not a contraindication unless there is no improvement after the initial dose is administered. |

## Additional information

| | |
|---|---|
| Common and serious undesirable effects | *Immediate:* Anaphylaxis and other hypersensitivity reactions (e.g. wheezing, dyspnoea, rashes, urticaria) have been reported.<br>*Other:* Tremor, ↑pulse, ↑ or ↓BP, hypoxia, chills, pyrexia and transient ↑bleeding time. |
| Pharmacokinetics | Elimination half-lives: succinylated (modified fluid/liquid gelatin), 4 hours; Polygeline (gelatin derivative), 5-8 hours. |
| Significant interactions | None significant in the emergency situation. |
| Action in case of overdose | *Symptoms to watch for:* Circulatory overload and electrolyte imbalance. Stop administration and give supportive therapy as appropriate. |

| Risk rating: **GREEN** | Score = 2<br>Lower-risk product: Risk-reduction strategies should be considered. |
|---|---|

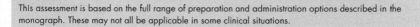

This assessment is based on the full range of preparation and administration options described in the monograph. These may not all be applicable in some clinical situations.

## Bibliography

SPC Volplex 4% solution for infusion (accessed 7 May 2010).
SPC Isoplex 4% solution for infusion (accessed 14 September 2009).

# Gentamicin

**40 mg/mL solution in 1-mL or 2-mL ampoules or vials; 10 mg/mL solution in 2-mL vials**

* Gentamicin sulfate is classed as an aminoglycoside antibiotic and is a mixture of antibiotic substances produced by the growth of *Micromonospora purpurea.*
* It is active against many Gram-negative aerobic bacteria and against some species of staphylococci.
* It has a narrow therapeutic range, with its two most serious adverse reactions – ototoxicity and nephrotoxicity – being dose related.
* Dose is calculated on the basis of renal function (as it is almost completely renally excreted) and body weight. However, gentamicin is not lipophilic, so dose should be based on ideal bodyweight (IBW) rather than actual bodyweight (ABW). Some authorities recommend using a 'dosing weight' calculated by adding IBW to 40% of the difference between ABW and IBW. Whichever method is employed it is important to check these criteria to avoid overdosing, e.g. in short, obese individuals with impaired renal function.
* Traditionally gentamicin has been given every 8 or 12 hours, but many hospitals have now adopted once-daily dosing regimens, with diverse methods of dosing, monitoring and subsequent dose adjustment. Seek out your local policy.
* Doses are expressed in terms of gentamicin base.

## Pre-treatment checks

* Do not give in myasthenia gravis.
* Ensure good hydration status (dehydration ↑risk of toxicity).

*Biochemical and other tests*

Baseline check of auditory and vestibular function
Bodyweight (and possibly height if patient over-weight)
FBC
Renal function: U, Cr, CrCl (or eGFR)

## Dose

> To avoid excessive dosing, doses for all regimens should be calculated on the basis of ideal bodyweight (IBW) in obese patients.

*Multiple daily dosing regimen*

**Standard dose**: give by IV injection or infusion every 6–8 hours to provide a total daily dose of 3–5 mg/kg.

**Endocarditis**: 1 mg/kg every 8 hours (in combination with other antibacterials).

**Dose in renal impairment**: adjusted according to creatinine clearance:[1]

* CrCl >70 mL/minute: 80 mg* every 8 hours and monitor levels.
* CrCl >30–70 mL/minute: 80 mg* every 12 hours and monitor levels.
* CrCl 10–30 mL/minute: 80 mg* every 24 hours and monitor levels.
* CrCl <10 mL/minute: 80 mg* every 48 hours and monitor levels.

*If bodyweight <60 kg, use 60 mg.

*Once-daily dosing regimen*

**Standard dose**: 5–7 mg/kg by IV infusion every 24 hours (or according to local guidelines). It is suggested that the dose be rounded to the nearest 20 mg to facilitate measurement.

**Dose in renal impairment**: adjusted according to creatinine clearance:[2]

* CrCl 30–70 mL/minute: 3–5 mg/kg IBW every 24 hours and monitor levels.
* CrCl 10–30 mL/minute: 2–3 mg/kg IBW every 24 hours and monitor levels.
* CrCl 5–10 mL/minute: 2 mg/kg IBW every 48–72 hours and monitor levels.

## Intermittent intravenous infusion

*Preparation and administration*

If used in combination with a penicillin or cephalosporin, preferably administer at a different site. If this is not possible then flush the line thoroughly with a compatible solution between drugs.

1. Withdraw the required dose and add to a suitable volume of compatible infusion fluid (usually 100 mL NaCl 0.9%).
2. The solution should be clear and colourless to very pale yellow. Inspect visually for particulate matter or discoloration prior to administration and discard if present.
3. Give by IV infusion over 30–60 minutes.

## Intramuscular injection

*Preparation and administration*

1. Withdraw the required dose.
2. Give by IM injection into a large muscle such as the gluteus or the lateral aspect of the thigh. Volumes >4 mL should be distributed between two or more injection sites.

## Intravenous injection

*Preparation and administration*

Direct IV injection should not be used for once-daily dosing regimen: ↑risk of neuromuscular blockade.
If used in combination with a penicillin or cephalosporin, preferably administer at a different site. If this is not possible then flush the line thoroughly with a compatible solution between drugs.

1. Withdraw the required dose.
2. The solution should be clear and colourless to pale yellow. Inspect visually for particulate matter or discoloration prior to administration and discard if present.
3. Give by IV injection over a minimum of 3–5 minutes.

## Technical information

| | |
|---|---|
| Incompatible with | Amoxicillin, amphotericin, ampicillin, cefotaxime, cefradine, ceftazidime, ceftriaxone, cefuroxime, clindamycin phosphate, drotrecogin alfa (activated), flucloxacillin, furosemide, heparin sodium, propofol, sodium bicarbonate, sodium fusidate. |
| Compatible with | **Flush**: NaCl 0.9%<br>**Solutions**: NaCl 0.9%, Gluc 5%, Gluc-NaCl<br>**Y-Site**: Aciclovir, atracurium, ciprofloxacin, cisatracurium, clarithromycin, esmolol, fluconazole, foscarnet, granisetron, labetalol, levofloxacin, linezolid, magnesium sulfate, midazolam, ondansetron, remifentanil, tigecycline, vecuronium bromide |

*(continued)*

## Technical information (continued)

| | |
|---|---|
| pH | 3-5.5 |
| Sodium content | Negligible |
| Excipients | Some products contain sulfites (may cause hypersensitivity reactions). |
| Storage | Store below 25°C in original packaging. Do not freeze or refrigerate. Vials are intended for single use only - discard any unused solution. |
| Stability after preparation | From a microbiological point of view, should be used immediately; however, prepared infusions may be stored at 2-8°C and infused (at room temperature) within 24 hours. |

## Monitoring

| Measure | Frequency | Rationale |
|---|---|---|
| Temperature | Minimum daily | • For clinical signs of fever declining. |
| Vestibular and auditory function | Daily | • Ototoxicity is a potential effect of overexposure to gentamicin. <br>• Check there is no deterioration of balance or hearing - if there is, this may be indicative of toxic levels. |
| Gentamicin serum concentration. For meaningful interpretation of results the laboratory request form must state <br>• the time the previous dose was given <br>• the time the blood sample was taken | See right hand column for details of first measurement, then twice weekly in normal renal function; more frequently if renal function is impaired | For a multiple daily dosing regimen the first measurements should be made around the third dose. <br>• A trough level is taken just before this dose and should be <2 mg/L (<1 mg/L in endocarditis). <br>• A peak level is taken 1 hour after the dose has been given and should be 5-10 mg/L (3-5 mg/L in endocarditis). <br>• Toxicity is usually observed at concentrations >12 mg/L. <br>For a once-daily dosing regimen the first measurement should be made before the second dose. <br>• A trough level is taken just before this dose and should be plotted on whichever nomogram is used by local guidelines. An assessment then needs to be made whether it is safe to continue with the current dose or if an adjustment is required (preferably before giving the next dose). <br>• Peak levels are not monitored in once-daily regimens. |
| U&Es | Twice weekly in normal renal function; more frequently if renal function is impaired | • Gentamicin is nephrotoxic. <br>• ↑Cr may indicated toxicity and require a reduction in dose. <br>• ↓K has been reported (rarely). |

(continued)

## Monitoring (continued)

| Measure | Frequency | Rationale |
|---------|-----------|-----------|
| FBC | Periodically | • WCC: for signs of the infection resolving.<br>• Blood dyscrasias have been reported rarely. |
| Serum Ca and Mg | Occasionally if therapy is prolonged | • ↓Mg and ↓Ca have been reported (rarely). |

## Additional information

| | |
|---|---|
| Common and serious undesirable effects | Vestibular and auditory damage, nephrotoxicity. |
| Pharmacokinetics | Elimination half-life is 2 hours (may be more than doubled depending on degree of renal impairment). |
| Significant interactions | • Gentamicin may ↑risk of nephrotoxicity with the following drugs: ciclosporin, platinum compounds, tacrolimus.<br>• Gentamicin may ↑levels or effect of the following drugs (or ↑side-effects): diuretics-loop (↑risk of ototoxicity), muscle relaxants-non depolarising, suxamethonium.<br>• Gentamicin may ↓levels or effect of the following drugs: neostigmine, pyridostigmine. |
| Action in case of overdose | *Antidote:* No known antidote but haemodialysis may be effective.<br>Stop administration and give supportive therapy as appropriate. |

| Risk rating: **AMBER** | Score = 3<br>Moderate-risk product: Risk-reduction strategies are recommended. |
|---|---|

This assessment is based on the full range of preparation and administration options described in the monograph. These may not all be applicable in some clinical situations.

## References

1. SPC Gentamicin Paediatric 20 mg/2 mL Solution for Injection, Sanofi-Aventis (accessed 19 March 2009).
2. Ashley C, Currie A, eds. *The Renal Drug Handbook*, 3rd edn. Oxford: Radcliffe Medical Press, 2009.

## Bibliography

SPC Cidomycin Adult Injectable 80 mg/2 mL (accessed 19 March 2009).

# Glatiramer acetate

**20 mg/mL solution in 1-mL pre-filled syringe**

* Glatiramer is a peptide (a random polymer of L-alanine, L-glutamic acid, L-lysine, and L-tyrosine) that has some structural resemblance to myelin basic protein.
* It is used to ↓frequency of relapses in the management of relapsing-remitting multiple sclerosis.
* Doses are expressed as glatiramer acetate:
  Glatiramer acetate 20 mg ≅ 18 mg glatiramer base.

## Pre-treatment checks

* Do not give if hypersensitive to mannitol or glatiramer.
* Caution in patients with pre-existing cardiac disorders.

*Biochemical tests*

Renal function: U, Cr

## Dose

**Standard dose:** 20 mg daily by SC injection.

## Subcutaneous injection

*Preparation and administration*

1. Remove the syringe from the refrigerator and allow to warm to room temperature for 20 minutes before use.
2. Give by SC injection into the abdomen, arm, hip or thigh. Injection-site rotation should be planned for subsequent injections so that any one area is not injected more than once a week.

| Technical information | |
|---|---|
| Incompatible with | Not relevant |
| Compatible with | Not relevant |
| pH | Not relevant |
| Sodium content | Nil |
| Storage | Store at 2–8°C in original packaging.<br>*In use:* Pre-filled syringes may be stored at room temperature (15-25°C) for up to 1 month. |

| Monitoring | | |
|---|---|---|
| **Measure** | **Frequency** | **Rationale** |
| Injection-site reactions or hypersensitivity | For 30 minutes after first injection | • To ensure safety with future injections; the majority of these symptoms are short-lived and resolve quickly. |

*(continued)*

## Monitoring (continued)

| Measure | Frequency | Rationale |
|---------|-----------|-----------|
| Neurological examination | 3-monthly | • To assess stabilisation/improvement on therapy, i.e. any disability, relapses and their general condition. |
| Renal function | | • Only applicable to patients with pre-existing renal impairment. While there is no evidence of glomerular deposition of immune complexes in patients, the possibility cannot be excluded. |

## Additional information

| | |
|---|---|
| Common and serious undesirable effects | *Immediate:* Anaphylaxis and other hypersensitivity reactions have been reported: flushing, chest pain, palpitation, ↑pulse and dyspnoea may occur within minutes of injection. Most reactions are short-lived and resolve quickly. *Injection-related:* Local: injection-site reactions: erythema, pain, pruritus, oedema, inflammation (more common in patients being treated with corticosteroids). *Other:* Nausea, constipation, diarrhoea, syncope, anxiety, asthenia, depression, dizziness, headache, tremor, sweating, oedema, lymphadenopathy, hypertonia, back pain, arthralgia, influenza-like symptoms, rash. |
| Pharmacokinetics | No information available. |
| Significant interactions | No significant interactions. |
| Action in case of overdose | *Antidote:* No known antidote; stop administration and give supportive therapy as appropriate. |
| Counselling | Injection technique as in the patient information leaflet. Sites for self-injection include the abdomen, arms, hips and thighs. A planned rotation of sites within an area should be followed so that any one area is not injected more than once each week. Give guidance on how to safely dispose of the syringe in line with any local policy. |

**Risk rating: GREEN**    Score = 1
Lower-risk product: Risk-reduction strategies should be considered.

This assessment is based on the full range of preparation and administration options described in the monograph. These may not all be applicable in some clinical situations.

## Bibliography

SPC Copaxone 20 mg/mL, solution for injection, pre-filled syringe (accessed 23 February 2010).

# Glucagon

**1-mg dry powder vials with pre-filled syringes containing 1.1 mL WFI**

- Glucagon is an endogenous polypeptide hormone produced by the alpha cells of the pancreatic islets of Langerhans. Its release mobilises glucose by activating hepatic glycogenolysis.
- It is used in the treatment of severe hypoglycaemia when the patient cannot take glucose by mouth and the use of IV glucose is not feasible.
- Glucagon may be used to relax specific areas of the GI tract for diagnostic purposes because it has a relaxant effect on smooth muscle.
- It is also used (unlicensed) in beta-blocker overdose to bypass blocked beta-receptors in severe ↓BP, heart failure or cardiogenic shock because it has chronotropic and inotropic effects that are independent of a response to catecholamine
- Although structurally identical to endogenous human glucagon, commercially available glucagon is prepared using recombinant DNA technology.
- Glucagon 1 mg ≡1 unit glucagon.

## Pre-treatment checks

- Avoid use in phaeochromocytoma.
- Use with caution in glucagonoma and insulinoma.
- Use with caution if using for diagnostic purposes in patients with diabetes mellitus or in elderly patients with known cardiac disease.
- The hyperglycaemic action of glucagon is dependent on the presence of liver glycogen. It is unlikely to be effective in starvation, adrenal insufficiency, chronic hypoglycaemia or alcohol-induced hypoglycaemia.

*Biochemical and other tests (not all are necessary in an emergency situation)*

Blood glucose
Blood pressure and pulse
Electrolytes: serum K, Ca

## Dose

**Hypoglycaemia:** 1 mg by SC or IM injection. The patient will normally respond within 10 minutes. When the patient has responded to the treatment, give oral carbohydrate to restore the liver glycogen and prevent further hypoglycaemia. If the patient does not respond within 10 minutes, give IV glucose.

**Diagnostic aid in GI examinations to inhibit motility:** usual dose for relaxation of the stomach, duodenal bulb, duodenum and small bowel is 0.2–0.5 mg by IV injection or 1 mg by IM injection; the usual dose to relax the colon is 0.5–0.75 mg by IV injection or 1–2 mg by IM injection.

- Onset of action after IV injection occurs within 1 minute and the duration of effect is 5–20 minutes.
- Onset of action after IM injection occurs after 5–15 minutes and lasts approximately 10–40 minutes.

**Beta-blocker overdose (unlicensed):**

It is essential to consult a poisons information service, e.g. Toxbase at www.toxbase.org (password or registration required) for full details of the management of beta-blocker toxicity.

5–10 mg by slow IV injection over 10 minutes (to reduce the likelihood of vomiting); followed by an infusion of 1–5 mg/hour (50 micrograms/kg/hour) titrated to clinical response.[1]

## Intramuscular injection

*Preparation and administration*

1. Inject the WFI provided (1.1 mL) into the vial. Shake gently until completely dissolved to give a solution containing 1 mg/mL (1 unit/mL).
2. The solution should be clear and colourless. If the solution shows signs of fibril formation (↑viscosity) or insoluble matter it should be discarded.
3. Withdraw the required dose
4. Give by IM injection.

## Subcutaneous injection

*Preparation and administration*

1. Inject the WFI provided (1.1 mL) into the vial. Shake gently until completely dissolved to give a solution containing 1 mg/mL (1 unit/mL).
2. The solution should be clear and colourless. If the solution shows signs of fibril formation (↑viscosity) or insoluble matter it should be discarded.
3. Withdraw the required dose.
4. Give by SC injection.

## Intravenous injection

*Preparation and administration*

1. Inject the WFI provided (1.1 mL) into the vial. Shake gently until completely dissolved to give a solution containing 1 mg/mL (1 unit/mL).
2. Withdraw the required dose.
3. The solution should be clear and colourless. If the solution shows signs of fibril formation (↑viscosity) or insoluble matter it should be discarded.
4. Give by IV injection. Give doses >1 mg slowly over 10 minutes to ↓likelihood of nausea and vomiting.

## Intravenous infusion (unlicensed)

NB: The solvent provided no longer contains preservative and is safe to use for the reconstitution of large doses.

*Preparation and administration*

1. Inject the WFI provided (1.1 mL) into the vial. Shake gently until completely dissolved to give a solution containing 1 mg/mL (1 unit/mL).
2. Withdraw the required dose and add to a suitable volume of Gluc 5%.
3. The solution should be clear and colourless. If the solution shows signs of fibril formation (↑viscosity) or insoluble matter it should be discarded.
4. Give by IV infusion via a volumetric infusion device. Adjust rate to clinical response.

| Technical information | |
|---|---|
| Incompatible with | No information |
| Compatible with | **Flush**: Gluc 5%, NaCl 0.9%<br>**Solutions**: Gluc 5%<br>**Y-site**: No information |
| pH | 2.5–3.5 |

*(continued)*

## Technical information (*continued*)

| | |
|---|---|
| Sodium content | Negligible |
| Storage | *Long term:* Store at 2–8° C. Do not freeze.<br>*For emergency use:* May be stored below 25°C in original packaging for up to 18 months (provided this is within the expiry date). |
| Displacement value | Negligible |
| Stability after preparation | Use prepared infusions immediately. |

## Monitoring

| Measure | Frequency | Rationale |
|---|---|---|
| Monitor nausea and vomiting | Regularly during infusion | • Nausea and vomiting are common side-effects particularly at doses use for beta-blocker overdose.<br>• Some centres pre-treat with a suitable antiemetic. If necessary, protect the airway.<br>• Replace fluids and electrolytes as necessary. |
| Blood glucose | | • Hyperglycaemia (and sometimes hypoglycaemia) is a known side-effect. |
| Serum potassium | | • ↓K is a known side-effect. Treat with oral or IV KCl as necessary. |
| Serum calcium | | • ↓Ca is a known side-effect but is often transient in nature. |
| Blood pressure and pulse | | • ↓BP and both ↓and ↑pulse have been reported. |

## Additional information

| | |
|---|---|
| Common and serious undesirable effects | *Immediate:* ↓BP and anaphylactic shock are rare.<br>*Other:* In management of beta-blocker overdose side-effects include nausea, vomiting, hyperglycaemia (sometimes hypoglycaemia, ↓K and ↓Ca). Hypersensitivity reactions including rash are rare. |
| Pharmacokinetics | Glucagon is cleared rapidly by the liver in 3–6 minutes. |
| Significant interactions | • The following may ↓glucagon levels or effect:<br>  insulin, indometacin (may even produce hypoglycaemia). |
| Action in case of overdose | Adverse effects of overdose have not been reported. Give supportive therapy as appropriate. |
| Counselling | Learn to recognise symptoms of low blood sugar.<br>Read the leaflet that comes with your injection so that you know how to use it. A family member or friend should be taught how to use glucagon before an emergency occurs.<br>After the dose, you should lie down on your right side in case you feel sick. When you wake up and are able to swallow, eat carbohydrate to stop low blood sugar recurring. |

| Risk rating: **AMBER** | Score = 4<br>Moderate-risk product: Risk-reduction strategies are recommended. |
|---|---|

This assessment is based on the full range of preparation and administration options described in the monograph. These may not all be applicable in some clinical situations.

## Reference

1. Toxbase at www.toxbase.org (accessed 2 May 2010).

## Bibliography

SPC GlucaGen Hypokit 1 mg (accessed 2 May 2010).

# Glucose (dextrose monohydrate)

**5%, 10%, 20%, 25% and 50% solution in ampoules and infusion bags of various volumes**
**50% solution in 50-mL pre-filled syringes**

* Glucose is a monosaccharide which, when dissolved in water, is used as an electrolyte-free crystalloid intravenous fluid that disperses through the intra- and extracellular fluid as water. It is sometimes referred to as dextrose (see also Appendix 1) but should always be prescribed as glucose in the UK.
* It is given by IV infusion to treat fluid depletion and maintain hydration. However, sole use of electrolyte-free glucose-containing infusion fluids causes electrolyte depletion. Glucose is also used as an energy source in combination with other nutrients in parenteral nutrition.
* Glucose is given by IV injection or infusion in the treatment of hypoglycaemia; it is also given by IV infusion to maintain blood glucose levels in patients receiving insulin infusions.
* It is given alongside insulin in the treatment of severe ↑K, so that hypoglycaemia is avoided (see the Insulins monograph).
* Gluc 5% may be used as a vehicle or diluent for the administration of compatible parenteral drugs. It may also be given (unlicensed) by SC infusion (hypodermoclysis).
* The concentration of glucose solutions for IV use in the UK (and in this monograph) are expressed in terms of the percentage w/v of anhydrous glucose. In the USA and some other countries, concentrations are expressed in terms of the percentage w/v of glucose monohydrate.

## Pre-treatment checks

* Hypertonic glucose solutions are contraindicated in patients with anuria, intraspinal or intracranial haemorrhage, ischaemic stroke and hyperglycaemic coma and in patients with delirium tremens.
* Caution in patients with diabetes mellitus and impaired glucose tolerance, severe under-nutrition, thiamine deficiency, ↓$PO_4$, haemodilution, sepsis, trauma, shock, metabolic acidosis or severe dehydration.

- Gluc 5% solutions are used mainly to treat fluid depletion but should be given alone only when there is no significant loss of electrolytes (prolonged administration of glucose solutions without electrolytes can lead to ↓Na and other electrolyte disturbances).

*Biochemical and other tests (not all are necessary in an emergency situation)*

Blood glucose
Electrolytes: serum Na
Fluid balance

## Dose

Glucose 5% is approximately isotonic with plasma and may be given via peripheral vein. Solutions >5% are hypertonic (see osmolarity below) and where possible should be given via a central line, although some sources suggest that 10% solutions may be given via a large peripheral vein for short periods provided the infusion site is changed at least daily.
In emergency situations it may be necessary to administer hypertonic solutions peripherally.

**Treatment or prevention of fluid depletion:** dose is dependent upon the age, weight, biochemistry and clinical condition of the patient. Normal fluid requirements are generally about 40 mL/kg/24 hours. Glucose solutions are usually used in combination with electrolyte-containing solutions so that electrolyte depletion is avoided. The use of colloid solutions should be considered where plasma expansion is required due to ↑losses.

**Treatment of severe hypoglycaemia:** 50 mL Gluc 20% (preferred)[1] or 20–50 mL Gluc 50% by slow IV injection into a large vein; the dose may be repeated as necessary according to the patient's response. Gluc 50% is available in a pre-filled syringe but is very viscous, making it difficult to administer.

Lower concentrations are equally effective, and carry less risk of venous irritation, but larger volumes are required, e.g. up to 250 mL Gluc 5%, or 100 mL Gluc 10%, titrated to patient response.

- Once the patient has regained consciousness oral carbohydrate is given to prevent relapse.
- Hypoglycaemia caused by insulin or oral hypoglycaemic agents requires close monitoring as the duration of action of these agents may be prolonged; further glucose administration may be required.

## Intravenous infusion

*Preparation and administration*

1. The infusion is pre-prepared for use. It should be clear and colourless. Inspect visually for particulate matter or discoloration prior to administration and discard if present.
2. Give by IV infusion at the required rate; give hypertonic solutions via a central venous catheter (see information above).
3. Discard any unused portion. Do not reconnect partially used infusion containers.

## Intravenous injection (emergency treatment of hypoglycaemia)

*Preparation and administration*

1. Withdraw the required dose from an IV infusion bag or (if using 50% glucose) assemble a pre-filled syringe in accordance with the manufacturer's instructions.
2. The solution should be clear and colourless. Inspect visually for particulate matter or discoloration prior to administration and discard if present.
3. Give by slow IV injection over 1–2 minutes.
4. Give oral carbohydrate once the patient has regained consciousness.

## Technical information

| | |
|---|---|
| Incompatible with | The following drugs are incompatible with glucose solutions (however this list may not be exhaustive, check individual drug monographs): alteplase, amoxicillin, caspofungin, co-amoxiclav, dantrolene, daptomycin, enoximone, ertapenem, erythromycin lactobionate, furosemide, hydralazine, isoniazid, itraconazole, phenytoin sodium, urokinase. |
| Compatible with | **Flush**: Not relevant <br> **Y-site**: See individual drug monographs |
| pH | 3.5–6.5 |
| Sodium content | Nil |
| Osmolarity (plasma osmolality = 280–300 mOsmol/L)[2] | Gluc 5% $\cong$ 278 mOsmol/L <br> Gluc 10% $\cong$ 555 mOsmol/L <br> Gluc 20% $\cong$ 1110 mOsmol/L <br> Gluc 50% $\cong$ 2775 mOsmol/L |
| Storage | Store below 25°C. |

## Monitoring

| Measure | Frequency | Rationale |
|---|---|---|
| Confusion and loss of consciousness | During and after treatment | • Symptomatic of hyperglycaemia or hyperosmolar syndrome. |
| Blood/urine glucose | | • Hyperglycaemia can occur. <br> • Prolonged use in parenteral nutrition may affect insulin production. |
| Fluid balance, U&Es, acid-base balance | | • Fluid and electrolyte disturbances can occur. |

## Additional information

| | |
|---|---|
| Common and serious undesirable effects | *Immediate:* Anaphylactoid reactions have been reported rarely in patients with asthma and diabetes mellitus. <br> *Injection/infusion-related:* <br> • Too rapid administration: Hyperglycaemia and glycosuria. <br> • Local: Pain, irritation, inflammation, thrombophlebitis. Extravasation may cause tissue damage. <br> *Other:* Water intoxication (with excessive use of dilute solutions); dehydration (with hypertonic solutions if blood glucose is not controlled), ↓Na, ↓K, ↓Mg, ↓$PO_4$; precipitation of Wernicke's encephalopathy in thiamine-deficient patients; glucose metabolism generates ↑$CO_2$ which may be important in respiratory failure. |
| Pharmacokinetics | Not applicable. |
| Significant interactions | No significant interactions. |

(continued)

| **Additional information** (*continued*) | |
|---|---|
| Action in case of overdose | *Symptoms to watch for:* Hyperglycaemia and glycosuria. This can lead to dehydration, hyperosmolar coma and death.<br>*Antidote:* Stop administration and give supportive therapy as appropriate; insulin may be administered. |

| Risk rating: **GREEN** | Score = 1<br>Lower-risk product: Risk-reduction strategies should be considered. |
|---|---|

This assessment is based on the full range of preparation and administration options described in the monograph. These may not all be applicable in some clinical situations.

### References

1. *Safe and Effective Use of Insulin in Hospitalised Patients*.www.diabetes.nhs.uk (accessed 15 May 2010).
2. Longmore M *et al.*, eds. *Oxford Handbook of Clinical Medicine*, 6th edn. Oxford: Oxford University Press, 2004.

### Bibliography

SPC Glucose Injection BP Minijet, International Medication Systems (accessed 5 May 2010).
SPC Glucose infusions 5%, 10%, 20%, 50%, Baxter (accessed 05 May 2010).

# Glyceryl trinitrate (GTN, nitroglycerin, nitroglycerol)

**1 mg/mL solution in 5-mL and 10-mL ampoules and 25-mL and 50-mL vials**
**5 mg/mL solution in 5-mL and 10-mL ampoules; 10 mg/mL solution in 10-mL ampoules**

* Glyceryl trinitrate relaxes smooth vascular muscle, reducing cardiac filling pressure and volume (pre-load), and lowering myocardial oxygen demand.
* It is used in unresponsive congestive heart failure, acute left-sided heart failure, acute MI, refractory unstable angina pectoris and coronary insufficiency including Prinzmetal's angina.
* It is also used in induction of controlled hypotension for surgery and in the control of hypertensive episodes and/or myocardial ischaemia during and after cardiac surgery.

### Pre-treatment checks

* Do not give in hypersensitivity to nitrates, severe anaemia, ↑intracranial pressure due to head trauma or cerebral haemorrhage, uncorrected hypovolaemia and hypotensive shock, arterial hypoxaemia and angina caused by hypertrophic obstructive cardiomyopathy, constrictive pericarditis, pericardial tamponade or toxic pulmonary oedema.
* Caution in severe renal/hepatic impairment, hypothyroidism, malnutrition, or hypothermia.

*Biochemical and other tests (not all are necessary in an emergency situation)*

Electrolytes: serum Na, K

Renal function: U, Cr, CrCl (or eGFR)

## Dose

Initiate at the following doses then titrate against individual clinical response (usual range 10–200 micrograms/minute):

**Congestive heart failure**: initially 10 micrograms/minute.

**Refractory unstable angina pectoris**: initially 10–15 micrograms/minute increasing in increments of 5–10 micrograms approximately every 30 minutes either until angina is relieved, headache limits further dose increase or mean arterial pressure falls by >20 mmHg.

**Surgery**: initially 5–25 micrograms/minute (or according to local protocol), titrating gradually to desired systolic arterial pressure.

## Continuous intravenous infusion via syringe pump

*Preparation and administration*

Avoid use of PVC infusion containers, administration sets and in-line filters if possible. Significant losses (>40%) occur by adsorption or absorption, requiring higher infusion rates to be employed. This effect is not significant with rigid plastics, e.g. polyethylene or polypropylene syringes and administration sets. Administration using a syringe pump is the most effective way of giving glyceryl trinitrate by infusion.

1. Withdraw 50 mL of the 1 mg/mL strength into a syringe suitable for use with a syringe pump. Alternatively, withdraw 10 mL of the 5 mg/mL strength and make up to 50 mL with NaCl 0.9%. Cap the syringe and mix well to give a solution containing 1 mg/mL.
2. The solution should be clear and colourless to slightly yellow. Inspect visually for particulate matter or discoloration prior to administration and discard if present.
3. Give by IV infusion using a syringe pump. For most indications the starting infusion rate is 10 micrograms/minute (0.6 mL/hour). Adjust the dose to clinical response as indicated above.

| Technical information | |
|---|---|
| Incompatible with | Avoid use of PVC infusion containers, administration sets and in-line filters if possible. Rigid plastics, e.g. polyethylene or polypropylene administration sets and syringes, should be used if available.<br>Alteplase, hydralazine, pantoprazole, phenytoin |
| Compatible with | **Flush**: NaCl 0.9%<br>**Solutions**: NaCl 0.9%, Gluc 5%<br>**Y-site**: Adrenaline (epinephrine), atracurium, cisatracurium, dobutamine, dopamine, esmolol, fentanyl, furosemide, labetalol, linezolid, micafungin, midazolam, noradrenaline (norepinephrine), propofol, ranitidine, remifentanil, vecuronium |
| pH | 3–6.5 |
| Sodium content | Nil |

*(continued)*

## Technical information (continued)

| | |
|---|---|
| Excipients | Hospira, Nitrocine and Goldshield products contain propylene glycol (risk of lactic acidosis if used for more than three successive days; adverse effects seen in ↓renal function; may interact with disulfiram and metronidazole).<br>Hospira and Goldshield products contain ethanol (possible intoxication if used for prolonged periods, may interact with metronidazole; possible religious objections). |
| Storage | Store below 25°C in original packaging.<br>All ampoules/vials are single use only - discard any unused portion. |
| Stability after preparation | From a microbiological point of view, should be used immediately; however, prepared infusions may be stored at 2-8°C and infused (at room temperature) within 24 hours provided use of PVC containers is avoided. |

## Monitoring

| Measure | Frequency | Rationale |
|---|---|---|
| Blood pressure | Continuous | • ↓BP may occur. |
| Heart rate | | • ↑Pulse may occur (↓pulse very rarely). |
| Angina pain and symptoms | | • Response to therapy.<br>• Relative haemodynamic and antianginal tolerance may develop during prolonged infusions; titrate dose accordingly. |
| Pulmonary capillary wedge pressure, cardiac output and precordial ECG depending on the clinical picture | | |
| Ethanol intoxication | As necessary (ethanol-containing products only) | • Very high infusion rates (e.g. 2 mg/minute) with the ethanol-containing products may lead to intoxication. |
| Serum osmolarity | Daily during high-dose therapy (propylene glycol-containing products only) | • Infusion of solutions with propylene glycol can lead to hyperosmolality. |

## Additional information

| | |
|---|---|
| Common and serious undesirable effects | *Immediate:* Anaphylaxis and other hypersensitivity reactions have been reported.<br>*Injection/infusion-related:* Too rapid administration: Headache, dizziness, flushing, ↑pulse.<br>*Other:* Nausea, sweating, restlessness, retrosternal discomfort, paradoxical ↓pulse (all reversible on ↓infusion rate or discontinuing treatment) |
| Pharmacokinetics | Elimination half-life is 1-4 minutes. |

(continued)

| **Additional information** (*continued*) | |
|---|---|
| Significant interactions | • The following may ↑glyceryl trinitrate levels or effect (or ↑side-effects): other hypotensive drugs, phosphodiesterase type-5 inhibitors (sildenafil is contraindicated).<br>• Glyceryl trinitrate may ↑levels or effect (or ↑side-effects) of opioid analgesics.<br>• Glyceryl trinitrate may ↓levels or effect of heparin.<br>• Hospira and Goldshield products contain ethanol: may interact with disulfiram and metronidazole. |
| Action in case of overdose | Symptoms are rapidly reversed by discontinuing treatment; give supportive therapy as appropriate. |
| Counselling | Advise of risk of headache, and symptoms of ↓BP. |

| Risk rating: **AMBER** | Score = 5<br>Moderate-risk product: Risk-reduction strategies are recommended |
|---|---|

This assessment is based on the full range of preparation and administration options described in the monograph. These may not all be applicable in some clinical situations.

## Bibliography

SPC Glyceryl trinitrate 1 mg/mL solution for infusion, Hameln Pharmaceuticals Ltd (accessed 21 April 2009).

SPC Glyceryl trinitrate 5 mg/mL sterile concentrate, Hospira UK Ltd (accessed 21 April 2009).

# Glycopyrronium bromide (glycopyrrolate)

### 200 micrograms/mL solution in 1-mL and 3-mL ampoules

* Glycopyrronium bromide is an antimuscarinic agent with largely peripheral actions. It has anti-spasmodic actions on smooth muscle and reduces salivary and bronchial secretions. It depresses the vagus and thereby increases the heart rate.
* It is used preoperatively to reduce secretions; to treat symptomatic sinus bradycardia induced by drugs; to prevent muscarinic effects on the heart (e.g. ↓pulse) during surgery; and in combination with neostigmine during reversal of effect of non-depolarising muscle relaxants.
* Glycopyrronium bromide may also be given (unlicensed) by SC infusion in palliative care to reduce excessive respiratory secretions and relieve bowel colic.

## Pre-treatment checks

- Use with caution in patients with coronary artery disease, congestive heart failure, cardiac arrhythmias, myasthenia gravis, hypertension and thyrotoxicosis.
- Care should also be taken in pyrexial patients due to the inhibition of sweating.

*Biochemical and other tests*

Blood pressure
Bodyweight

## Dose

**Premedication:** 200–400 micrograms *or* 4–5 micrograms/kg (maximum 400 micrograms) by IM or IV injection.

**Intraoperative use:** 200–400 micrograms *or* 4–5 micrograms/kg (maximum 400 micrograms) by IV injection, repeated if necessary.

**Control of muscarinic side-effects of neostigmine in reversal of non-depolarising neuromuscular block:** 200 micrograms per 1 mg of neostigmine *or* 10–15 micrograms/kg per 50 micrograms of neostigmine by IV injection. The two drugs can be mixed in the same syringe which provides greater cardiovascular stability.

## Intravenous injection

*Preparation and administration*

1. Withdraw the required dose.
2. The solution should be clear and colourless. Inspect visually for particulate matter or discoloration prior to administration and discard if present.
3. Give by slow IV injection over 1 minute.

## Intramuscular injection

*Preparation and administration*

1. Withdraw the required dose.
2. Give by IM injection.

| Technical information | |
|---|---|
| Incompatible with | Diazepam, methylprednisolone sodium succinate, thiopental sodium. |
| Compatible with | **Flush**: NaCl 0.9%<br>**Solutions**: Gluc 5%, NaCl 0.9%, Gluc-NaCl, Ringer's<br>**Y-site**: Neostigmine (in-syringe compatible), propofol |
| pH | 2–3 |
| Sodium content | Negligible |
| Storage | Store below 25°C in original packaging. |

| Monitoring | | |
|---|---|---|
| **Measure** | **Frequency** | **Rationale** |
| Clinical improvement | Periodically | • To that ensure treatment is effective. |
| Signs and symptoms of cholinergic toxicity | | • To observe for side-effects. |

## Additional information

| | |
|---|---|
| Common and serious undesirable effects | Dry mouth, difficulty in micturition, dilatation of the pupils with loss of accommodation, ↑pulse, palpitations, inhibition of sweating. |
| Pharmacokinetics | Elimination half-life is 0.55–1.25 hours (but not well studied). |
| Significant interactions | No significant interactions. |
| Action in case of overdose | *Symptoms to watch for:* Peripheral antimuscarinic effects.<br>*Antidote:* Stop administration and give supportive therapy as appropriate. Neostigmine may be used to reverse antimuscarinic effects. |

| Risk rating: **GREEN** | Score = 1<br>Lower-risk product: Risk-reduction strategies should be considered. |
|---|---|

This assessment is based on the full range of preparation and administration options described in the monograph. These may not all be applicable in some clinical situations.

## Bibliography

SPC Glycopyrronium bromide (accessed 18 December 2008).

# Goserelin

### 3.6-mg or 10.8-mg implant with sterile applicator

- Goserelin acetate is a synthetic analogue of gonadorelin (gonadotrophin-releasing hormone).
- It is used for the suppression of testosterone in the treatment of prostate cancer, and for the treatment breast cancer in pre- and perimenopausal women.
- It is used in the treatment of endometriosis and uterine fibroids. It may also be given before surgery for endometrial ablation and as an adjunct to ovulation induction with gonadotrophins for infertility.
- Doses are expressed in terms of goserelin base.

### Pre-treatment checks

Caution in diabetes and osteoporosis (or those at risk, i.e. chronic alcohol and/or tobacco use, strong family history of osteoporosis, or chronic use of drugs that can reduce bone mass such as anticonvulsants or corticosteroids).

*Biochemical and other tests*

Blood pressure
Bone mineral density: consider if treatment is to be prolonged

Pregnancy test (for assisted reproduction)
Testosterone level (in prostate cancer)

## Dose

**Prostate cancer:** 3.6 mg by SC injection every 28 days or 10.8 mg every 12 weeks. An antiandrogen agent may be given for 3 days before until 3 weeks after commencement to ↓risk of disease flare, e.g. cyproterone acetate 100 mg three times daily.

**Breast cancer**: 3.6 mg by SC injection every 28 days.

**Endometriosis:** 3.6 mg by SC injection every 28 days for a maximum 6 months (do not repeat). Supplementary combined HRT may reduce bone mineral density loss and vasomotor symptoms.

**Endometrial thinning before intrauterine surgery**: 3.6 mg (may be repeated after 28 days if the uterus is large or to allow flexible surgical timing).

**Before surgery in women who have anaemia due to uterine fibroids**: 3.6 mg every 28 days (with supplementary iron) for a maximum duration 3 months.

**Assisted reproduction:** 3.6 mg is administered to down-regulate the pituitary gland. Serum estradiol levels should decline to levels similar to those in the early follicular phase in 7–21 days. Gonadotrophin is then administered following the protocol of the individual clinic.

## Subcutaneous injection

*Preparation and administration*

1. A local anaesthetic may be given prior to implantation.
2. Give by SC injection into the anterior abdominal wall.

### Technical information

| Incompatible with | Not relevant |
|---|---|
| Compatible with | Not relevant |
| pH | Not relevant |
| Sodium content | Nil |
| Storage | Store below 25°C. Use immediately after opening the pouch. |

### Monitoring

| Measure | Frequency | Rationale |
|---|---|---|
| Blood glucose in diabetic patients | Regularly | • ↑Blood glucose levels can occur (↓glucose tolerance). |
| Blood pressure | Periodically | • ↓BP or ↑BP can occur (rarely) and may require medical intervention or withdrawal of treatment. |
| Serum testosterone in men | If indicated | • Consider if the anticipated clinical or biochemical response in prostate cancer has been achieved. |
| Serum prostate-specific antigen (PSA) in men | | • ↓PSA may indicate the duration of progression-free status; however, it may occur independently of tumour response and cannot be solely relied upon. |

*(continued)*

## Monitoring (continued)

| Measure | Frequency | Rationale |
|---|---|---|
| Monitor for signs of OHSS in women | During treatment | • When combined with gonadotrophins there is a higher risk of OHSS than with gonadotrophins alone.<br>• The stimulation cycle should be monitored carefully to identify patients at risk of developing OHSS and hCG should be withheld if necessary.<br>• Symptoms include abdominal pain, feeling of abdominal tension, ↑abdominal girth, occurrence of ovarian cysts, nausea, vomiting, massive enlargement of the ovaries, dyspnoea, diarrhoea, oliguria, haemoconcentration, hypercoagulability. |

## Additional information

| | |
|---|---|
| Common and serious undesirable effects | *Immediate:* Anaphylaxis and other hypersensitivity reactions are rare. In the event that the implant needs to be removed, it may be located by ultrasound.<br>*Injection-related:* Local: Mild bruising at injection site.<br>*Other:* ↓BMD, hot flushes, sweating, ↓libido, breast tenderness (infrequently).<br>*In women:* Headaches, mood changes, depression, vaginal dryness, change in breast size. Some women experience vaginal bleeding of variable duration and intensity (usually in the first month). |
| Pharmacokinetics | Elimination half-life in men is 4.2 hours; in women 2.3 hours. Formulations are long-acting, however. |
| Significant interactions | No significant interactions. |
| Action in case of overdose | No clinically relevant adverse effects have been seen. There is no specific treatment and should be managed symptomatically. |
| Counselling | Discuss the nature of product, treatment course and likely side-effects. Fertile women should use non-hormonal barrier methods of contraception during the entire treatment period. |

| Risk rating: **GREEN** | Score = 1<br>Lower-risk product: Risk-reduction strategies should be considered. |
|---|---|

This assessment is based on the full range of preparation and administration options described in the monograph. These may not all be applicable in some clinical situations.

## Bibliography

SPC Zoladex 3.6 mg implant (accessed 23 March 2009).
SPC Zoladex LA 10.8 mg (accessed 23 March 2009).

# Granisetron

**1 mg/mL solution in 1-mL and 3-mL ampoules**

* Granisetron hydrochloride is a 5-HT$_3$ antagonist with antiemetic activity.
* It is used to treat nausea and vomiting associated with cytotoxic chemotherapy and radiotherapy, and also to prevent and treat PONV.
* Co-administration of dexamethasone or methylprednisolone may ↑efficacy of granisetron.
* Doses are expressed in terms of the base:
  Granisetron 1 mg ≡1.12 mg granisetron hydrochloride.

## Pre-treatment checks

Patients with signs of subacute intestinal obstruction should be monitored following administration as granisetron may ↓lower bowel mobility.

## Dose

**Prevention of nausea and vomiting induced by cytotoxic chemotherapy**: 1–3 mg by IV injection or infusion not less than 30 minutes prior to start of chemotherapy. Most patients only require a single dose but up to two additional doses of 3 mg may be given in a 24-hour period (not less than 10 minutes apart).

**Treatment of nausea and vomiting induced by cytotoxic chemotherapy:** 3 mg by IV injection or infusion. Up to two additional doses of 3 mg may be administered in a 24-hour period. These additional doses must be given at least 10 minutes apart.

**Prevention of PONV**: 1 mg by IV injection before induction of anaesthesia.

**Treatment of PONV**: 1 mg by IV injection; maximum 2 mg in 24 hours.

## Intravenous injection

*Preparation and administration*

1. Withdraw the required dose and dilute each 1 mg (1 mL) to 5 mL with NaCl 0.9% in the syringe.
2. The solution should be clear and colourless. Inspect visually for particulate matter or discoloration prior to administration and discard if present.
3. Give by IV injection over a minimum of 30 seconds.

## Intravenous infusion

*Preparation and administration*

1. Withdraw the required dose and add to 50 mL of compatible infusion fluid (usually NaCl 0.9%).
2. The solution should be clear and colourless. Inspect visually for particulate matter or discoloration prior to administration and discard if present.
3. Give by IV infusion over 5 minutes.

## Technical information

| | |
|---|---|
| Incompatible with | Amphotericin |
| Compatible with | **Flush**: NaCl 0.9%<br>**Solutions**: NaCl 0.9%, Gluc 5%<br>**Y-site**: Aciclovir, amikacin, aminophylline, ampicillin, aztreonam, bumetanide, calcium gluconate, cefotaxime, ceftazidime, ceftriaxone, cefuroxime, ciprofloxacin, clindamycin phosphate, co-trimoxazole, dexamethasone sodium phosphate, dobutamine, dopamine, fluconazole, furosemide, ganciclovir, gentamicin, hydrocortisone sodium succinate, imipenem with cilastatin, linezolid, magnesium sulfate, methylprednisolone sodium succinate, metoclopramide, metronidazole, piperacillin with tazobactam, propofol, ranitidine, ticarcillin with clavulanate, tobramycin, vancomycin |
| pH | 4-7 |
| Sodium content | Negligible |
| Storage | Store below 25°C in original packaging. Do not freeze. |
| Stability after preparation | From a microbiological point of view, should be used immediately; however, prepared infusions may be stored at 2-8°C and infused (at room temperature) within 24 hours. |

## Monitoring

| Measure | Frequency | Rationale |
|---|---|---|
| Clinical improvement | Periodically | To ensure efficacy. |

## Additional information

| | |
|---|---|
| Common and serious undesirable effects | *Immediate:* Hypersensitivity reactions (including anaphylaxis) have very rarely been reported.<br>*Other:* Constipation, headache, rash. Rarely: rash, dystonias, dyskinesias. |
| Pharmacokinetics | Elimination half-life is approximately 9 hours but there is a wide variation. |
| Significant interactions | None reported. |
| Action in case of overdose | Stop administration and give supportive therapy as appropriate. |

| | |
|---|---|
| Risk rating: **GREEN** | Score = 1<br>Lower-risk product: Risk-reduction strategies should be considered. |

This assessment is based on the full range of preparation and administration options described in the monograph. These may not all be applicable in some clinical situations.

## Bibliography

SPCs Kytril 1 mg and 3 mg (accessed 5 September 2009).

# Guanethidine monosulfate

**10 mg/mL solution in 1-mL ampoules**
* Guanethidine monosulfate is a peripheral sympathetic blocking drug that is thought to lower BP by depleting and inhibiting reformation of noradrenaline at nerve endings.
* It has been used in hypertensive crises, but its use has largely been superseded. It is now restricted to situations where alternative treatments are not effective.

## Pre-treatment checks

* Do not use in patients with phaeochromocytoma or on MAOI drugs, in cardiac failure not associated with ↑BP, and where renal function is compromised (CrCl <41 mL/minute).
* Treatment with guanethidine should be stopped 2 or 3 days prior to surgery.

*Biochemical and other tests (not all are necessary in an emergency situation)*

Renal function: U, Cr, CrCl (or eGFR)

## Dose

**Standard dose**: 10–20 mg by IM injection; repeat after 3 hours if necessary (longer in renal impairment to avoid accumulation).
**Dose in renal impairment:** extend dosing interval in moderate renal impairment; avoid use in severe renal impairment.

## Intramuscular injection

*Preparation and administration*

1. Withdraw the required dose.
2. Give by IM injection.

| Technical information | |
|---|---|
| Incompatible with | Not relevant |
| Compatible with | Not relevant |
| pH | 4.7-5.7 |
| Sodium content | Negligible |
| Storage | Store below 30°C in original packaging. Do not freeze. |

## Monitoring

| Measure | Frequency | Rationale |
| --- | --- | --- |
| Blood pressure | Every 30 minutes | Response to therapy. Maximal response should be achieved within 1-2 hours.<br>Be aware of risk of orthostatic ↓BP. |
| Serum creatinine | Daily | Stop therapy if CrCl falls below 41 mL/minute. |
| Electrolytes and urine output | Periodically | Heart failure is a potential complication of prolonged treatment. |
| Pyrexia | On presentation | If fever develops, the dose should be reduced. |

## Additional information

| | |
| --- | --- |
| Common and serious undesirable effects | *Common:* Postural ↓BP, sinus ↓pulse, dizziness, tiredness, paraesthesia, headache, syncope, fluid retention.<br>*Rare:* Myalgia, muscle tremor. |
| Pharmacokinetics | Biological effects are maintained for 4-6 hours. Terminal serum elimination half-life is around 5 days and elimination is prolonged in renal impairment.<br>An injection of 10-20 mg will usually cause a fall in BP within 30 minutes. The effect reaches a maximum in 1-2 hours and is maintained for 4-6 hours. |
| Significant interactions | • The following may ↑guanethidine levels or effect (or ↑side-effects): MAOIs, beta-blockers, phenothiazine or tricyclic antidepressant drugs.<br>• Guanethidine may ↑levels or effect (or ↑side-effects) of sympathomimetics. |
| Action in case of overdose | *Symptoms to watch for:* Postural ↓BP, syncope and sinus ↓pulse.<br>*Antidote:* None known. Keep the patient lying down and consider administration of fluid and electrolytes. |
| Counselling | Report dizziness and fainting. |

| Risk rating: **GREEN** | Score = 1<br>Lower-risk product. Risk-reduction strategies should be considered. |
| --- | --- |

This assessment is based on the full range of preparation and administration options described in the monograph. These may not all be applicable in some clinical situations.

## Bibliography

SPC Ismelin ampoules 10 mg/mL (accessed 6 September 2009).

# Haloperidol

**5 mg/mL solution in 1-mL ampoules**

This preparation must not be confused with the depot preparation.

* Haloperidol is a butyrophenone antipsychotic with a wide range of actions. It is a dopamine inhibitor and has antiemetic activity.
* It is used parenterally in the short-term management of acutely disturbed patients suffering from schizophrenia or other psychoses, mania, hypomania and other mental or behavioural problems. Oral treatment should succeed parenteral administration as soon as is practicable.
* Haloperidol may also be given (unlicensed) by SC infusion in palliative care to treat nausea and vomiting and also restlessness and confusion.

## Pre-treatment checks

* Avoid in comatose states, CNS depression, Parkinson disease, lesions of basal ganglia, clinically significant cardiac disorders, QTc interval prolongation, history of ventricular arrhythmias or torsade de pointes, ↓pulse or second- or third-degree heart block.
* Do not give with other QT prolonging drugs or to patients with uncorrected ↓K.
* Caution in patients with liver disease, renal failure, phaeochromocytoma, epilepsy, and conditions predisposing to epilepsy (e.g. alcohol withdrawal and brain damage) or convulsions.
* Use with great caution in patients with disturbed thyroid function.
* When using for rapid tranquillisation, an antimuscarinic medication such as procyclidine or benzatropine should be available to treat any dystonia or EPSE.

*Biochemical and other tests (not all are necessary in an emergency situation)*

ECG
Electrolytes: serum K, Ca, Mg
LFTs

Renal function: U, Cr, CrCl (or eGFR)
TFTs

## Dose

Bioavailability from the oral route is about 60% of that from the IM route, and adjustment of dose may be required.

**Control of acutely agitated patients with moderate symptoms**: 2–10 mg by IM injection. Depending on response subsequent doses may be given every 4–6 hours, up to a maximum of 18 mg/day.

## Intramuscular injection

*Preparation and administration*

1. Withdraw the required dose.
2. Give by IM injection.

## Technical information

| Incompatible with | Do not mix with other drugs in the same syringe. |
|---|---|
| Compatible with | Do not mix with other drugs in the same syringe. |
| pH | 2.7-4.7 |
| Sodium content | Nil |
| Storage | Store below 25°C in original packaging. |

## Monitoring

| Measure | Frequency | Rationale |
|---|---|---|
| Clinical effectiveness | Post administration | • To ensure that treatment is effective. |
| Respiratory rate | Monitor every 15 minutes for 2 hours after the injection | • Can cause respiratory depression.<br>• Closer monitoring is required when haloperidol is being used for rapid tranquillisation. |
| Blood pressure | Post injection | • ↓BP occurs rarely, but if a patient is predisposed (e.g. an elderly patient) or if the drug is being used for rapid tranquillisation then closer monitoring is required. |
| ECG | Periodically and baseline (if possible) | • Torsade de pointes and QT prolongation, including sudden death, have been reported especially when haloperidol is given IV or at doses higher than recommended.<br>• ↓Dose if QT is prolonged and discontinue if QTc exceeds 500 milliseconds. |
| Temperature | Periodically after injection | • Very rarely may cause neuroleptic malignant syndrome. |
| Motor side-effects | | • May cause EPSE. |
| LFTs | 6-monthly | • If treatment is long term. |

## Additional information

| Common and serious undesirable effects | *Injection-related:* Local: Injection-site reactions.<br>*Other:*<br>• Common: EPSE (consider giving an antimuscarinic such as procyclidine or benzatropine), confusional states, epileptic fits, depression, sedation, agitation, drowsiness, insomnia, headache, vertigo.<br>• Rare: neuroleptic malignant syndrome, QT prolongation, ventricular arrhythmias, sudden death. |
|---|---|
| Pharmacokinetics | Elimination half-life is 21 hours (range: 10-38 hours). |

*(continued)*

## Additional information (*continued*)

| | |
|---|---|
| Significant interactions | • The following may ↑haloperidol levels or effect (or ↑side-effects): antiarrhythmics, CNS depressants, buspirone, fluoxetine, quinidine.<br>• The following may ↓haloperidol levels or effect: enzyme-inducing drugs such as carbamazepine, phenobarbital and rifampicin. |
| Action in case of overdose | *Antidote:* None specific. A patent airway should be established and maintained. In view of isolated reports of arrhythmia, ECG monitoring is strongly advised.<br>↓BP and circulatory collapse should be treated by plasma volume expansion and other appropriate measures. Adrenaline should not be used. Monitor body temperature and adequate fluid intake should be maintained.<br>In cases of severe EPSE, appropriate antimuscarinic medication should be administered, e.g. procyclidine. |

| | |
|---|---|
| Risk rating: **GREEN** | Score = 1<br>Lower-risk product: Risk-reduction strategies should be considered. |

This assessment is based on the full range of preparation and administration options described in the monograph. These may not all be applicable in some clinical situations.

### Bibliography

SPC Haldol (accessed 3 October 2007).

# Haloperidol decanoate

**50 mg/mL and 100 mg/mL oily solution in 1-mL ampoules**

This preparation is a depot preparation and must not be confused with haloperidol injection for rapid tranquillisation.

* Haloperidol decanoate is a butyrophenone antipsychotic presented as a long-acting depot injection.
* It is used in the treatment of schizophrenia and other psychoses.
* Doses are expressed in terms of the base:
  Haloperidol 100 mg ≅ 141 mg haloperidol decanoate.

### Pre-treatment checks

* Do not administer to patients in comatose states, including alcohol, barbiturate or opiate poisoning or patients with Parkinson's disease.

- Caution if suffering from epilepsy, liver disease, renal failure, cardiac disease, depression, myasthenia gravis, prostatic hypertrophy, narrow-angle glaucoma, hypothyroidism, hyperthyroidism, phaeochromocytoma, severe respiratory disease or if there are risk factors for stroke.
- Concomitant treatment with other antipsychotics should be avoided.

*Biochemical and other tests*

| | |
|---|---|
| Blood pressure | LFTs |
| Bodyweight | TFTs |
| ECG | U&Es |
| FBC | |

## Dose

**Test dose**: 50 mg to assess tolerability. Reduce dose to 12.5–25 mg for elderly patients.

**Maintenance dose**: repeat dose every 4 weeks, increasing if necessary by 50-mg increments to 300 mg every 4 weeks. Some patients may require higher doses. If fortnightly administration is preferred doses should be halved.

## Intramuscular injection

*Preparation and administration*

1. Before use warm the ampoule in the hands to aid withdrawal of the contents.
2. Withdraw the required dose. Maximum volume to be administered at one site is 2 mL. Volumes >2 mL should be distributed between two injection sites.
3. Give by deep IM injection into the gluteal region. Aspirate before injection to avoid inadvertent intravascular injection. Rotate injection sites for subsequent injections.

## Technical information

| | |
|---|---|
| Incompatible with | Do not mix with other drugs in the same syringe. |
| Compatible with | Do not mix with other drugs in the same syringe. |
| pH | Not relevant - oily injection |
| Sodium content | Nil |
| Excipients | Contains benzyl alcohol.<br>Contains sesame oil (may cause hypersensitivity reactions). |
| Storage | Store below 25°C in original packaging. Do not refrigerate or freeze. |

## Monitoring

| Measure | Frequency | Rationale |
|---|---|---|
| Therapeutic improvement | Periodically | • To that ensure treatment is effective |
| EPSEs | During dose adjustment and every 3 months | • Causes extrapyramidal symptoms, e.g. dystonias. |

*(continued)*

## Monitoring (continued)

| Measure | Frequency | Rationale |
|---------|-----------|-----------|
| U&Es | At least annually | • Electrolyte imbalance ↑risk of QT interval prolongation. |
| ECG | | • Can ↑QTc interval. The dose should be reduced if QTc is prolonged and stopped if QTc> 500 milliseconds. |
| Bodyweight | | • May cause weight gain.<br>• As part of regular health check, measure waist hip ratio or waist circumference. |
| Blood pressure, blood glucose, LFTs | | • As part of regular health check. |
| Lipid profile | | • As part of regular health check. Include cholesterol, HDL, LDL and triglycerides. |
| Prolactin | | • If symptoms of hyperprolactinaemia develop. |

## Additional information

| | |
|---|---|
| Common and serious undesirable effects | *Injection-related:* Local: Injection-site reactions.<br>*Other:* EPSE (consider giving an antimuscarinic such as procyclidine or benzatropine), confusional states, epileptic fits, depression, sedation, agitation, drowsiness, insomnia, headache, vertigo. Rarely: neuroleptic malignant syndrome, QT prolongation, ventricular arrhythmias, sudden death. |
| Pharmacokinetics | Elimination half-life is 18-21 days. |
| Significant interactions | • The following may ↑haloperidol levels or effect (or ↑side-effects): antiarrhythmics, CNS depressants, buspirone, fluoxetine, quinidine.<br>• The following may ↓haloperidol levels or effect: enzyme-inducing drugs such as carbamazepine, phenobarbital and rifampicin. |
| Action in case of overdose | Give supportive therapy as appropriate. Adrenaline must not be given (may further ↓BP). |
| Counselling | Advise patients not to drink alcohol especially at beginning of treatment. May impair alertness so do not drive or operate machinery until susceptibility is known. |

| Risk rating: **GREEN** | Score = 2<br>Lower-risk product: Risk-reduction strategies should be considered. |
|---|---|

This assessment is based on the full range of preparation and administration options described in the monograph. These may not all be applicable in some clinical situations.

## Bibliography

SPC Haldol (accessed 3 October 2007).

NICE (2009) *Clinical Guideline 82: Core interventions in the treatment and management of schizophrenia in primary and secondary care (update)*. London: National Institute for Health and Clinical Excellence. http://guidance.nice.org.uk/CG82 (accessed 1 October 2009).

# Hartmann's solution (sodium lactate compound, Ringer-lactate)

### 500-mL and 1-L infusion bags

- Hartmann's solution is a crystalloid intravenous fluid that behaves like NaCl 0.9% but more closely mimics extracellular fluid.
- Each 1000 mL contains: sodium chloride 6 g, sodium lactate 3.2 g, potassium chloride 400 mg, calcium chloride 270 mg.
- It is used to replenish extracellular fluid in place of NaCl 0.9% to ↓risk of hyperchloraemic acidosis, particularly where fluid replacement is required over a prolonged period.
- Table H1 shows the electrolyte content of different volumes of the solution.

**Table H1**  Electrolyte content of Hartmann's solution

| Volume | 500 mL | 1000 mL |
|---|---|---|
| Sodium (mmol) | 65.5 | 131 |
| Potassium (mmol) | 2.5 | 5 |
| Calcium (mmol) | 1 | 2 |
| Bicarbonate, as lactate (mmol) | 14.5 | 29 |
| Chloride (mmol) | 55.5 | 111 |

## Pre-treatment checks

- Use with caution in patients with ↑BP, heart failure, and peripheral or pulmonary oedema, renal impairment, and liver cirrhosis, pre-eclampsia, toxaemia of pregnancy or other conditions associated with Na retention.
- Caution in patients receiving corticosteroids and in geriatric or postoperative patients.
- Bicarbonate-forming compounds should **not** generally be given in respiratory alkalosis or any condition where lactate levels are elevated.
- Lactate solutions should **not** be used in severe acidosis requiring immediate repletion of plasma bicarbonate as the production of bicarbonate from lactate is delayed for 1–2 hours after administration. They should **not** be used to treat lactic acidosis.

*Biochemical and other tests (not all are necessary in an emergency situation)*

Blood pH

Electrolytes: serum Na, K, Ca

## Dose

**Treatment or prevention of fluid depletion:** dose is dependent upon the age, weight, biochemistry and clinical condition of the patient. Normal fluid requirements are generally about 40 mL/kg/ 24 hours. The use of colloid solutions should be considered where plasma expansion is required owing to ↑losses.

## Intravenous infusion

*Preparation and administration*

1. The infusion is pre-prepared for use. It should be clear and colourless. Inspect visually for particulate matter or discoloration prior to administration and discard if present.
2. Give by IV infusion at the required rate.
3. Discard any unused portion. Do not reconnect partially used infusion containers.

| Technical information | |
|---|---|
| Incompatible with | The following drugs are incompatible with Hartmann's solution (however, this list may not be exhaustive: check individual drug monographs): amiodarone, amoxicillin, amphotericin, ampicillin, ceftriaxone, clodronate sodium, co-amoxiclav, co-fluampicil, dantrolene, diazepam, enoximone, ertapenem, erythromycin lactobionate, filgrastim, foscarnet, ibandronate, imipenem with cilastatin, itraconazole, metronidazole, mycophenolate, pamidronate disodium, parecoxib, phenytoin sodium, piperacillin with tazobactam, quinupristin with dalfopristin, zoledronic acid. |
| Compatible with | **Flush**: Not relevant<br>**Y-site**: See individual drug monographs |
| pH | 5-7 |
| Electrolyte content | See Table H1. |
| Storage | Store below 25°C. |

| Monitoring | | |
|---|---|---|
| **Measure** | **Frequency** | **Rationale** |
| Plasma electrolytes | Regularly throughout treatment | • Too rapid correction of Na can lead to severe neurological adverse effects.<br>• Excessive IV administration may result in ↓K. |
| Acid-base balance | | • Lactate-induced metabolic acidosis can occur with excessive administration of lactate-containing compounds.<br>• Na is associated with chloride and bicarbonate in the regulation of acid-base balance. |

*(continued)*

## Monitoring (continued)

| Measure | Frequency | Rationale |
|---------|-----------|-----------|
| Fluid balance/ accumulation | Regularly throughout treatment | • Retention of excess Na can lead to the accumulation of extracellular fluid and may result in pulmonary and peripheral oedema and their consequent effects. |

## Additional information

| | |
|---|---|
| Common and serious undesirable effects | *Immediate:* Anaphylaxis and other hypersensitivity reactions have been reported, e.g. urticaria, skin rash, erythema, pruritus, facial oedema, laryngeal oedema.<br>*Infusion-related:* Local: Phlebitis, thrombophlebitis.<br>*Other:* Electrolyte disturbances, metabolic acidosis, panic attacks. |
| Pharmacokinetics | Not applicable. |
| Significant interactions | No significant interactions. |
| Action in case of overdose | Stop administration and give supportive therapy as appropriate. |

| Risk rating: **GREEN** | Score = 0<br>Lower-risk product: Risk-reduction strategies should be considered. |
|---|---|

| | | | | | | | |
|---|---|---|---|---|---|---|---|
| | | | | | | | |

This assessment is based on the full range of preparation and administration options described in the monograph. These may not all be applicable in some clinical situations.

## Bibliography

SPC. 2010, Compound Sodium Lactate Intravenous Infusion BP (Hartman's) at http://www.baxter-healthcare.co.uk (accessed 3 May 2010).

# Heparin

**1000 units/mL solution in 1-mL, 5-mL and 20-mL ampoules or vials**
**5000 units/mL solution in 1-mL and 5-mL ampoules or vials**
**25 000 units/mL in 0.2-mL and 1-mL ampoules or vials**
**1 unit/mL solution in NaCl 0.9% 500-mL infusion bag**
**Flush: 10 units/mL solution in 5-mL ampoules; 100 units/mL solution in 2-mL ampoules**

Heparin calcium has also been used for the prophylaxis and treatment of VTE in similar doses to heparin sodium.

* Heparin sodium is an anticoagulant agent derived from animal mucosa.
* It may be given by continuous IV infusion in the treatment of VTE, i.e. PE and DVT, STEMI and also in the acute coronary syndromes: unstable angina and NSTEMI, particularly where ↓renal function precludes the use of some LMWHs.
* It is used for prophylaxis of VTE in surgical and medical patients and to prevent thrombus formation in extracorporeal circulation during haemodialysis.
* It may be used to maintain patency of central intravenous lines.
* Not all products are licensed for all indications.

## Pre-treatment checks

* Do not use in patients who are haemorrhaging.
* Use extreme care in those at serious risk of haemorrhage, e.g. in cases of haemorrhagic blood disorders, thrombocytopenia, peptic ulcer disease, cerebrovascular disorders, bacterial endocarditis, severe ↑BP, oesophageal varices, or after recent surgery where haemorrhage remains a risk.
* Caution in hepatic and renal impairment, and in elderly patients.

*Biochemical and other tests*

Electrolytes: serum K                                Renal function: U, Cr, CrCl (or eGFR)
Platelet count                                       Treatment dose only: APTT or APTT ratio

## Dose

*Prophylaxis*

**General or orthopaedic surgery with high risk of VTE:** 5000 units by SC injection 2 hours preoperatively and then every 8–12 hours until the patient is mobile.
**VTE prophylaxis in other patients:** 5000 units SC every 8–12 hours.

*Treatment*

**Standard dose using heparin by IV infusion:** 5000 units by IV injection (for major PE give 10 000 units) followed by 18 units/kg/hour* by IV infusion adjusting to APTT or APTT ratio.
* Omit the loading dose if initial APTT ratio is 1.5–2.5.
* If initial APTT ratio is > 2.5 review the need to start therapy.

*Many hospitals use an initial rate of 1000 units/hour for all patients, then check APTT or APTT ratio after 2–6 hours and adjust rate accordingly. Table H2 is an example of a dose adjustment protocol – check local policy.

**Table H2** An example of a dose adjustment protocol for heparin infusion using 50 000 units in a 50-mL syringe pump, i.e. 1000 units/mL.

Goal of therapy: therapeutic APTT of 50–70 seconds (for control 26–36 seconds); APTT ratio ≅ 1.6–2.2

| APTT (seconds) Control 26–36 seconds | APTT ratio | Further IV dose (units) | Stop infusion (minutes) | Rate change (mL/hour) | Repeat APTT (hours) |
|---|---|---|---|---|---|
| <40 | <1.3 | 3000 | 0 | +0.1 mL/hour | 6 hours |
| 40-49 | 1.3-1.5 | 0 | 0 | +0.1 mL/hour | 6 hours |
| 50-70 (target) | 1.6-2.2 | 0 | 0 | 0 (no change) | 12-24 hours |
| 71-85 | 2.3-2.7 | 0 | 0 | −0.1 mL/hour | 12-24 hours |
| 86-100 | 2.8-3.2 | 0 | 30 minutes | −0.1 mL/hour | 6 hours |
| 101-150 | 3.3-4.8 | 0 | 60 minutes | −0.2 mL/hour | 6 hours |
| 151-200 | 4.9-6.5 | 0 | 60 minutes | −0.3 mL/hour | 6 hours |
| >200 | >6.5[a] | 0 | 180 minutes | −0.4 mL/hour | 3 hours |

[a]Seek medical advice and consider reversal with protamine sulfate if at risk of bleeding or oozing blood from drain sites or puncture sites (see the Protamine sulfate monograph).

*Flushes and locks*

As there are risks of repeated exposure to heparin and the risk of dosing errors, the use of heparin solutions for flushing or locking peripheral cannulas is not recommended.[1]

Choice of solution concentration and volume for central line lock varies according to the IV device used and local policies.

**Dose in hepatic impairment:** reduce dose in severe liver disease.

## Continuous intravenous infusion via a syringe pump

*Preparation and administration*

Make sure you have selected the correct strength of heparin injection.

1. Withdraw 50 mL of pre-prepared solution containing 1000 units/mL into a suitable syringe.*
2. The solution should be clear and colourless to pale straw in colour. Inspect visually for particulate matter or discoloration prior to administration and discard if present.
3. Give by IV infusion using a syringe pump. Adjust dose to clinical response.

*Alternatively, if a pre-prepared solution containing 1000 units/mL is not available, then withdraw 50 000 units (ensure you have selected the correct strength of injection) and make up to 50 mL with NaCl 0.9% in a syringe pump. This gives a solution containing 1000 units/mL. Diluted solutions must always be inverted at least 6 times during mixing to ensure thorough distribution of drug.

## Subcutaneous injection

*Preparation and administration*

Make sure you have selected the correct strength of heparin injection.

1. Withdraw the required dose.
2. The patient should be seated or lying down.
3. Pinch up a skin fold on the abdominal wall between the thumb and forefinger and hold throughout the injection.
4. Give by deep SC injection into the thick part of the skin fold at right angles to the skin. Do not rub the injection site after administration. Alternate doses between the right and left sides.

## Intravenous injection

*Preparation and administration*

Make sure you have selected the correct strength of heparin injection.

1. Withdraw the required dose.
2. The solution should be clear and colourless to pale straw in colour. Inspect visually for particulate matter or discoloration prior to administration.
3. Give by IV injection over 3–5 minutes.

| Technical information | |
|---|---|
| Incompatible with | Alteplase, amiodarone, ciprofloxacin, cisatracurium, clarithromycin, diazepam, dobutamine, drotrecogin alfa (activated), gentamicin, labetalol, methylprednisolone sodium succinate, phenytoin sodium, tobramycin, vancomycin. |
| Compatible with | **Flush**: NaCl 0.9%<br>**Solutions**: NaCl 0.9%<br>**Y-site**: Furosemide, linezolid, metoclopramide |
| pH | 5–7.5 |
| Sodium content | Negligible |
| Excipients | Some preparations contain benzyl alcohol. |
| Storage | Store below 25°C in original packaging.<br>*In use*: Vial contents should be used within 28 days of first use. |
| Stability after preparation | From a microbiological point of view, should be used immediately; however, prepared infusions may be stored at 2–8°C and infused (at room temperature) within 24 hours. |

## Monitoring

| Measure | Frequency | Rationale |
|---------|-----------|-----------|
| APTT ratio | At least daily - see dosing above | • Therapeutic (anticoagulation) dosing must be monitored for titration to target anticoagulation range.<br>• Monitoring is not required for prophylactic therapy. |
| Injection/infusion site | Daily | • Tissue necrosis is a rare adverse effect. |
| Platelet count | Alternate days, commencing 3-5 days after start of dosing, until day 14 | • Risk of heparin-induced thrombocytopenia.<br>• Stop immediately if this occurs. Caution as consequent platelet aggregation and thrombosis may exacerbate the condition being treated.<br>• Patients exposed to heparin within the previous 100 days may be sensitised - on re-exposure check platelet count within 24 hours. |
| Serum potassium | After 7 days | • Heparin inhibits the secretion of aldosterone and so may cause ↑K.<br>• K should be monitored in all patients with risk factors, particularly those receiving heparin for >7 days. |
| Bone mineral density | After extended therapy, e.g. >3 months | • Consider anti-osteoporosis measures. |

## Additional information

| | |
|---|---|
| Common and serious undesirable effects | *Immediate*: Anaphylaxis and other hypersensitivity reactions have been reported<br>*Injection/infusion-related*: Local: Rarely local irritation and skin necrosis<br>*Other*: ↑Risk of bleeding, thrombocytopenia, clinically significant ↑K in patients with diabetes or chronic renal failure, reversible ↑liver transaminase. |
| Pharmacokinetics | Serum half-life is between 1 and 6 hours (average 1.5). |
| Significant interactions | • The following may ↑risk of bleeding with heparin: aspirin, diclofenac IV (avoid combination), ketorolac (avoid combination).<br>• Glyceryl trinitrate infusion may ↓heparin levels or effect. |
| Action in case of overdose | *Symptoms to watch for*: Bleeding.<br>*Antidote*: Protamine sulfate may be used to ↓bleeding risk if clinically required. See the Protamine sulfate monograph |
| Counselling | Report bleeding or skin reactions. |

| | | |
|---|---|---|
| Risk rating: **AMBER** | Score = 4<br>Moderate-risk product: Risk-reduction strategies are recommended. | |

This assessment is based on the full range of preparation and administration options described in the monograph. These may not all be applicable in some clinical situations.

## References

1. NPSA (2008) NPSA/2008/RRR002: *Risks with Intravenous Heparin Flush Solutions*. London: National
   Patient Safety Agency. www.nrls.npsa.nhs.uk/resources/type/alerts/?entryid45=59892&p=3
   (accessed 5 February 2010).

## Bibliography

SPC Heparin (Mucous) Injection BP, Leo Laboratories Ltd. (accessed 12 May 2009).

SPC Heparin sodium 1,000 IU/mL solution for injection or concentrate for solution for infusion
(with preservative), Wockhardt UK Ltd (accessed 12 February 2009).

SPC Heparin sodium 10 IU/mL IV flush solution, Leo Laboratories Ltd (accessed 12 February 2009).

SPC Heparin calcium 25,000 IU/mL solution for injection or concentrate for solution for infusion,
Wockhardt UK Ltd (accessed 12 February 2009).

# Hyaluronidase

**1500-unit dry powder ampoules**

- Hyaluronidase is an enzyme that makes body tissue more permeable to injected fluids.
- It may be used to enhance the absorption of SC fluids, local anaesthetics and SC or IM injections
  and to promote the resorption of excess fluids and blood in the tissues.

## Pre-treatment checks

- Do not use to reduce the swelling of bites or stings, or for anaesthetic procedures in unexplained
  premature labour.
- Ensure that the site selected for administration is healthy, clean, non-oedematous and convenient
  for the patient's comfort.

## Dose

Hyaluronidase must not be used with IV injections.

**With SC infusions (hypodermoclysis):** 1500 units by SC injection or injected into the tubing of
the infusion site. This is sufficient for administration of 500–1000 mL of most fluids. (NB: in the USA
the usual dose is 150 units/1000 mL of fluid.)

**With SC or IM injections:** 1500 units dissolved directly in solution to be injected (check
compatibility).

**Extravasation:** where dispersal rather than localisation is indicated, 1500 units infiltrated into
affected area (as soon as possible after extravasation is noticed).

**Haematoma:** 1500 units infiltrated into the affected area.

## With subcutaneous infusions

Care should be taken to control the speed and total volume of fluid administered and to avoid
over-hydration, especially in renal impairment.

*Preparation and administration*

1. Dissolve 1500 units in 1 mL WFI or NaCl 0.9%.
2. Give by SC injection into the site before the infusion is set up. Alternatively, it may be injected into the tubing of the infusion set (about 2 cm back from the needle) at the start of the infusion.

## With subcutaneous or intramuscular injections

*Preparation and administration*

1. Dissolve 1500 units directly in the solution to be injected (check compatibility).
2. Give immediately by SC or IM injection as appropriate.

## Extravasation or haematoma

*Preparation and administration*

1. Dissolve 1500 units in 1 mL of WFI or NaCl 0.9%.
2. Infiltrate into the affected area.

## Technical information

| | |
|---|---|
| Incompatible with | Benzodiazepines, furosemide, heparin sodium, phenytoin. |
| Compatible with | **Flush**: Not relevant<br>**Solutions**: NaCl 0.9%, Gluc 5%, Gluc-NaCl (all with added KCl up to 34 mmol/L)<br>In syringe: No information<br>**Y-site**: Not relevant |
| pH | 4.5–7.5 |
| Sodium content | Negligible |
| Storage | Store below 25°C in original packaging. |

## Monitoring

| Measure | Frequency | Rationale |
|---|---|---|
| Infusion site | When the bag is changed or more frequently for solutions other than NaCl 0.9% | • The site should be moved if pain is experienced at the infusion site, if the site becomes inflamed, white or hard, or if blood is observed in the giving set. |

## Additional information

| | |
|---|---|
| Common and serious undesirable effects | *Immediate:* Anaphylaxis has been reported rarely.<br>*Injection/infusion-related:* Local: Irritation, infection, bleeding, bruising (all rare).<br>*Other:* Oedema. |
| Pharmacokinetics | Not applicable. |
| Significant interactions | None reported. |
| Action in case of overdose | No cases of overdose appear to have been reported. |

| Risk rating: **GREEN** | Score = 1 Lower-risk product: Risk-reduction strategies should be considered. |

This assessment is based on the full range of preparation and administration options described in the monograph. These may not all be applicable in some clinical situations.

## Bibliography

SPC Hyalase (accessed 12 December 2008).

---

# Hydralazine hydrochloride

**20-mg dry powder ampoules**

1. Hydralazine is a vasodilator acting mainly on the arterioles to lower peripheral resistance and ↓arterial BP.
2. The injection is used in management of hypertension with renal complications and hypertensive emergencies particularly those associated with pre-eclampsia and toxaemia of pregnancy.

## Pre-treatment checks

- Avoid in patients with idiopathic systemic lupus erythematosus, severe ↑pulse, high output heart failure, myocardial insufficiency due to mechanical obstruction, cor pulmonale, dissecting aortic aneurysm; acute porphyria.
- Patients with recent myocardial infarction should not receive hydralazine.
- Patients with suspected or confirmed coronary artery disease should only be given hydralazine under cover of a beta-blocker, which should be commenced a few days before treatment with hydralazine.
- Caution in renal and hepatic impairment.

*Biochemical and other tests (not all are necessary in an emergency situation)*

Blood pressure and pulse
LFTs
Renal function: U, Cr, CrCl (or eGFR)

## Dose

**Hypertensive crisis:** 5–10 mg by IV injection repeated if necessary after 20–30 minutes. Alternatively, give 200–300 micrograms/minute by continuous IV infusion. The rate should be titrated to response and maintenance rate is usually within 50–150 micrograms/minute.
The IM route is unlicensed in the UK, but doses of 10–50 mg have been used in the USA.
**Dose in renal impairment:** if CrCl < 30 mL/minute, the dose or dose interval should be adjusted according to clinical response.

**Dose in hepatic impairment:** the dose or dose interval should be adjusted according to clinical response.

## Intravenous injection

*Preparation and administration*

1. Reconstitute each 20-mg ampoule with 1 mL WFI to give a solution containing 20 mg/mL.
2. Withdraw the required dose and further dilute to 10 mL with NaCl 0.9%.
3. The solution should be clear and colourless. Inspect visually for particulate matter or discoloration prior to administration and discard if present.
4. Give by IV injection over 2–3 minutes.

## Continuous intravenous infusion (large-volume infusion)

*Preparation and administration*

1. Reconstitute each 20-mg ampoule with 1 mL WFI to give a solution containing 20 mg/mL.
2. Withdraw the required dose and add to a suitable volume of NaCl 0.9% (e.g. 20 mg/500 mL gives a solution containing 40 micrograms/mL). Mix well.
3. The solution should be clear and colourless. Inspect visually for particulate matter or discoloration prior to administration and discard if present.
4. Give by IV infusion via a volumetric infusion device at an initial rate of 200–300 micrograms/minute, i.e. 5–7.5 mL/minute (300–450 mL/hour) of a 20 mg/500 mL infusion. Adjust the dose to the clinical response.

## Continuous intravenous infusion via a syringe pump

*Preparation and administration*

1. Reconstitute each 20-mg ampoule with 1 mL WFI to give a solution containing 20 mg/mL.
2. Make 60 mg (3 mL) up to 60 mL in a syringe pump with NaCl 0.9%
3. Cap the syringe and mix well to give a solution containing 1 mg/mL.
4. The solution should be clear and colourless. Inspect visually for particulate matter or discoloration prior to administration and discard if present.
5. Give by IV infusion at an initial rate of 200–300 micrograms/minute, i.e. 0.2–0.3 mL/minute (12–18 mL/hour) of a 1 mg/mL solution. Adjust dose to clinical response.

## Intramuscular injection (unlicensed)

*Preparation and administration*

1. Reconstitute each 20-mg ampoule with 1 mL WFI.
2. Withdraw the required dose.
3. Give immediately by IM injection.

## Technical information

| | |
|---|---|
| Incompatible with | Hydralazine is incompatible with glucose solutions. Aminophylline, ampicillin, furosemide, glyceryl trinitrate. |
| Compatible with | **Flush**: NaCl 0.9% <br> **Solutions**: NaCl 0.9%, Hartmann's, Ringer's (all with added KCl) <br> **Y-site**: Hydrocortisone sodium succinate, verapamil |
| pH | 3.5–4.2 |
| Sodium content | Nil |

*(continued)*

## Technical information (*continued*)

| | |
|---|---|
| Storage | Store below 30°C in original packaging. |
| Displacement value | Negligible |
| Stability after preparation | Use prepared infusions immediately. Contact with metals (e.g. needles) may lead to degradation. |

## Monitoring

| Measure | Frequency | Rationale |
|---|---|---|
| Blood pressure | Continuously until stable then every 15-30 minutes | • Avoid precipitous decreases in arterial BP (critical reduction in cerebral or utero-placental perfusion).<br>• The initial aim is to reduce mean arterial BP by no more than 25% within a few minutes to 1 hour.<br>• A satisfactory response can be defined as a decrease in diastolic BP to 90-100 mmHg. |
| Heart rate | Every 15-30 minutes | • Reflex ↑pulse may occur. |
| Chest pain/ECG changes | After initial dosing | • Angina may be induced. |
| Body temperature and skin reactions | Throughout treatment | • Rash or febrile reactions may signify hypersensitivity reaction and the drug should be withdrawn in such instances. |

## Additional information

| | |
|---|---|
| Common and serious undesirable effects | *Injection/infusion-related:* Local: Pain.<br>*Common:* ↓BP, ↑pulse, palpitation, angina symptoms, flushing, headache, dizziness. Rarely hypersensitivity reactions (e.g. rash, pruritus, urticaria, eosinophilia), development of SLE-like condition after long-term therapy. |
| Pharmacokinetics | Elimination half-life is 2-3 hours but is up to 16 hours in severe renal failure (CrCl <20 mL/minute) and shortened to <1 hour in rapid acetylators. |
| Significant interactions | • The following may ↑hydralazine levels or effect (or ↑side-effects): other antihypertensives, anaesthetics tricyclic antidepressants, major tranquillisers or drugs exerting central depressant actions (including alcohol) - administration shortly before or after diazoxide may give rise to marked ↓BP. |
| Action in case of overdose | *Symptoms to watch for:* ↓BP, ↑pulse, myocardial ischaemia, dysrhythmias and coma.<br>*Antidote:* No known antidote; stop administration and give supportive therapy as appropriate. Use of adrenaline should be avoided. |
| Counselling | Patients should report chest pain and pain at injection site.<br>Warn of symptoms of vasodilatation such as flushing and dizziness. |

| Risk rating: **AMBER** | Score = 5<br>Moderate-risk product. Risk-reduction strategies are recommended. |
| --- | --- |

This assessment is based on the full range of preparation and administration options described in the monograph. These may not all be applicable in some clinical situations.

## Bibliography

SPC Apresoline injection (accessed 24 August 2009).

# Hydrocortisone acetate

**25 mg/mL aqueous suspension in 1-mL ampoules**
* Hydrocortisone acetate is a corticosteroid formulated for local use only.
* It is given by intra-articular or periarticular injection to treat arthritic conditions when few joints are involved.
* It may also be used for the symptomatic treatment of some non-articular inflammatory conditions, e.g. inflamed tendon sheaths and bursas.

## Pre-treatment checks

* Do not inject into unstable joints.
* Do not give in the presence of active infection in or near joints.
* Prior to administration of hydrocortisone acetate a local anaesthetic may be infiltrated into the soft tissue surrounding the joint and/or injected into the joint or mixed in the same syringe (unlicensed).

*Biochemical and other tests*

Early morning stiffness
ESR and CRP

Number of tender or swollen joints
Pain

## Dose

**Standard dose:** 5–50 mg by intra-articular or periarticular injection depending on size of joint.
Do not treat more than three joints in one day. The injection may be repeated at intervals of about 3 weeks.

## Intra-articular or periarticular injection

*Preparation and administration*

1. Withdraw the required dose.
2. Give by the desired route.

## Technical information

| | |
|---|---|
| Incompatible with | Not relevant |
| Compatible with | Not relevant |
| pH | Not relevant |
| Sodium content | Negligible |
| Excipients | Contains benzyl alcohol. |
| Storage | Store at 15-25°C in original packaging. Do not freeze. |

## Monitoring

| Measure | Frequency | Rationale |
|---|---|---|
| Symptoms of septic arthritis | Following intra-articular injection | • Marked ↑pain accompanied by local swelling, further restriction of joint motion, fever, and malaise are suggestive of septic arthritis. |
| Number of tender or swollen joints; pain; early morning stiffness | Periodically | • To check treatment is effective. |
| ESR and CRP | | • To monitor clinical improvement. |

## Additional information

| | |
|---|---|
| Common and serious undesirable effects | *Injection-related:* Intra-articular: Temporary local exacerbation with increased pain and swelling. This normally subsides after a few hours.<br>*Systemic:* Systemic undesirable effects are unlikely but may occur after high or prolonged local dosage: ↑BP, Na and water retention, ↓K, ↓Ca, ↑blood glucose, peptic ulceration and perforation, psychiatric reactions, ↑susceptibility to infection, muscle weakness, tendon rupture, insomnia, ↑intracranial pressure, ↓seizure threshold, impaired healing. For undesirable effects resulting from long-term corticosteroid use refer to the BNF. |
| Pharmacokinetics | Absorption after local injection is very slow and is usually completed 24-48 hours after intra-articular injection. |
| Significant interactions | A small number of local injections are unlikely to have any significant interactions typical of corticosteroids. |
| Action in case of overdose | Overdose is very unlikely, treatment should be symptomatic. |
| Counselling | Patients on long-term corticosteroid treatment should read and carry a Steroid Treatment Card. |

Risk rating: **GREEN**

Score = 2
Lower-risk product: Risk-reduction strategies should be considered.

This assessment is based on the full range of preparation and administration options described in the monograph. These may not all be applicable in some clinical situations.

## Bibliography

SPC Hydrocortistab (accessed 27 June 2009).

# Hydrocortisone sodium phosphate

### 100 mg/mL solution in 1-mL and 5-mL ampoules

- Hydrocortisone sodium phosphate is a corticosteroid with both glucocorticoid and, to a lesser extent, mineralocorticoid activity.
- It is used in the treatment of conditions for which systemic corticosteroid therapy is indicated.
- It is used parenterally when a rapid effect is required in emergencies, e.g. acute adrenocortical insufficiency, and also when the oral route is temporarily unavailable or inappropriate.
- It may also be given by soft-tissue injection for various inflammatory conditions.
- Doses are expressed in terms of the base:
  Hydrocortisone 100 mg $\cong$ 134 mg hydrocortisone sodium phosphate.

### Pre-treatment checks

- Avoid where systemic infection is present (unless specific therapy is given).
- Avoid live virus vaccines in those receiving immunosuppressive doses.
- May activate or exacerbate amoebiasis or strongyloidiasis (exclude before initiating a corticosteroid in those at risk or with suggestive symptoms). Fungal or viral ocular infections may also be exacerbated.
- Caution in patients predisposed to psychiatric reactions, including those who have previously suffered corticosteroid-induced psychosis, or who have a personal or family history of psychiatric disorders.
- Do not use in the treatment of cerebral oedema associated with acute head injury or cerebrovascular accident, as it is unlikely to be of benefit and may even be harmful.

*Biochemical and other tests (not all are necessary in an emergency situation)*

Electrolytes: serum Na, K, Ca

## Dose

**Standard dose:** 100–500 mg by IV injection/infusion or IM injection depending upon the condition being treated. The dose may be repeated 3–4 times in 24 hours as determined by the patient's response.

**Injection into soft tissues:** 100–200 mg daily; may be repeated on 2–3 occasions depending upon the patient's response.

## Intravenous injection

*Preparation and administration*

1. Withdraw the required dose.
2. The solution should be clear and colourless. Inspect visually for particulate matter or discoloration prior to administration and discard if present.
3. Give by IV injection over a minimum of 30–60 seconds.

## Intermittent intravenous infusion

*Preparation and administration*

1. Withdraw the required dose.
2. Add to a convenient volume of compatible infusion fluid.
3. The solution should be clear and colourless. Inspect visually for particulate matter or discoloration prior to administration and discard if present.
4. Give by IV infusion over 20–30 minutes.

## Intramuscular injection

*Preparation and administration*

1. Withdraw the required dose.
2. Give by IM injection.

| Technical information | |
|---|---|
| Incompatible with | No information |
| Compatible with | **Flush**: NaCl 0.9%<br>**Solutions**: NaCl 0.9%, Gluc 5%<br>**Y-site**: No information |
| pH | 7.5–8.5 |
| Sodium content | 0.4 mmol/100 mg |
| Excipients | Contains sulfites (may cause hypersensitivity reactions). |
| Storage | Store below 25°C in original packaging. |
| Stability after preparation | Use prepared infusions immediately. |

## Monitoring

| Measure | Frequency | Rationale |
|---------|-----------|-----------|
| Serum Na, K, Ca | Throughout treatment | • May cause fluid and electrolyte disturbances. |
| Withdrawal symptoms and signs | During withdrawal and after stopping treatment | • During prolonged therapy with corticosteroids, adrenal atrophy develops and can persist for years after stopping. Abrupt withdrawal after a prolonged period can lead to acute adrenal insufficiency, ↓BP or death.<br>• The CSM has recommended that gradual withdrawal of systemic corticosteroids should be considered in patients whose disease is unlikely to relapse. Full details can be found in the BNF. |
| Signs of infection | During treatment | • Prolonged courses ↑susceptibility to infections and severity of infections. Serious infections may reach an advanced stage before being recognised. |
| Signs of chickenpox | | • Unless they have had chickenpox, patients receiving corticosteroids for purposes other than replacement should be regarded as being at risk of severe chickenpox.<br>• Confirmed chickenpox requires urgent treatment; corticosteroids should not be stopped and dosage may need to be increased. |
| Exposure to measles | | • Patients should be advised to take particular care to avoid exposure to measles and to seek immediate medical advice if exposure occurs.<br>• Prophylaxis with IM normal immunoglobulin may be needed. |

## Additional information

| | |
|---|---|
| Common and serious undesirable effects | *Immediate:* Anaphylaxis and other hypersensitivity reactions have been reported.<br>*Injection/infusion-related:* Too rapid administration: Paraesthesia and pain (particularly in the perineal region) that is usually transient.<br>*Short-term use:* Undesirable effects which may result from short-term use (minimise by using the lowest effective dose for the shortest time): ↑BP, Na and water retention, ↓K, ↓Ca, ↑blood glucose, peptic ulceration and perforation, psychiatric reactions, ↑susceptibility to infection, muscle weakness, tendon rupture, insomnia, ↑intracranial pressure, ↓seizure threshold, impaired healing. For undesirable effects resulting from long-term corticosteroid use refer to the BNF. |
| Pharmacokinetics | Elimination half-life is 1–2 hours. |
| Significant interactions | • The following may ↓corticosteroid levels or effect: barbiturates, carbamazepine, phenytoin, primidone, rifabutin, rifampicin.<br>• Corticosteroids may ↑levels or effect of the following drugs (or ↑side-effects): anticoagulants (monitor INR), methotrexate (↑risk of blood dyscrasias). If using IV amphotericin monitor fluid balance and K level closely.<br>• Corticosteroids may ↓effect of vaccines (↓immunological response, ↑risk of infection with live vaccines). |

*(continued)*

| **Additional information** (*continued*) | |
|---|---|
| Action in case of overdose | No known antidote but haemodialysis may be effective.<br>Give supportive therapy as appropriate. Following chronic overdose the possibility of adrenal suppression should be considered. |
| Counselling | Patients on long-term corticosteroid treatment should read and carry a Steroid Treatment Card. |

| Risk rating: **GREEN** | Score = 2<br>Lower-risk product: Risk-reduction strategies should be considered. |
|---|---|

This assessment is based on the full range of preparation and administration options described in the monograph. These may not all be applicable in some clinical situations.

## Bibliography

SPC Efcortesol injection (accessed 9 September 2009).

# Hydrocortisone sodium succinate

**100-mg dry powder vials**

* Hydrocortisone sodium succinate is a corticosteroid with both glucocorticoid and, to a lesser extent, mineralocorticoid activity.
* It is used in the treatment of conditions for which systemic corticosteroid therapy is indicated.
* It is used parenterally when a rapid effect is required in emergencies, e.g. acute adrenocortical insufficiency, and also when the oral route is temporarily unavailable or inappropriate.
* Doses are expressed in terms of the base:
  Hydrocortisone 100 mg $\cong$ 134 mg hydrocortisone sodium succinate.

## Pre-treatment checks

* Avoid where systemic infection is present (unless specific therapy given).
* Avoid live virus vaccines in those receiving immunosuppressive doses.
* May activate or exacerbate amoebiasis or strongyloidiasis (exclude before initiating a corticosteroid in those at risk or with suggestive symptoms). Fungal or viral ocular infections may also be exacerbated.
* Caution in patients predisposed to psychiatric reactions, including those who have previously suffered corticosteroid-induced psychosis, or who have a personal or family history of psychiatric disorders.
* Do not use in the treatment of cerebral oedema associated with acute head injury or cerebrovascular accident, as it is unlikely to be of benefit and may even be harmful.

*Biochemical and other tests (not all are necessary in an emergency situation)*

Electrolytes: serum Na, K, Ca

## Dose

**Standard dose:** 100–500 mg given by IM injection or by IV injection or infusion. The dose depends on the severity of the condition and may be repeated at intervals of 2, 4 or 6 hours as indicated by the patient's response and clinical condition.

### Intravenous injection

*Preparation and administration*

1. Reconstitute each vial with 2 mL WFI to give a solution containing 100 mg/2 mL.
2. Withdraw the required dose.
3. The solution should be clear and colourless. Inspect visually for particulate matter or discoloration prior to administration and discard if present.
4. Give by IV injection over 1–10 minutes.

### Intermittent intravenous infusion

*Preparation and administration*

1. Reconstitute each vial with 2 mL WFI to give a solution containing 100 mg/2 mL.
2. Withdraw the required dose and add to a minimum of 100 mL of compatible infusion fluid.
3. The solution should be clear and colourless. Inspect visually for particulate matter or discoloration prior to administration and discard if present.
4. Give by IV infusion over 20–30 minutes.

**Fluid-restricted patients:** the required dose has been given in 50 mL NaCl 0.9% or Gluc 5% (unlicensed).

### Intramuscular injection

*Preparation and administration*

1. Reconstitute each vial with up to 2 mL WFI then shake to form a solution.
2. Withdraw the required dose
3. Give by IM injection.

## Technical information

| | |
|---|---|
| Incompatible with | Ciprofloxacin, diazepam, midazolam, pantoprazole, phenytoin. |
| Compatible with | **Flush**: NaCl 0.9%<br>**Solutions**: NaCl 0.9%, Gluc 5%, Gluc-NaCl, Hartmann's, Ringer's<br>**Y-site**: Aciclovir, adrenaline (epinephrine), aminophylline, atracurium, aztreonam, benzylpenicillin, calcium gluconate, cisatracurium, digoxin, dopamine, fentanyl, foscarnet, granisetron, hydralazine, linezolid, magnesium sulfate, noradrenaline (norepinephrine), ondansetron, phytomenadione, piperacillin with tazobactam, propofol, remifentanil, sodium bicarbonate, verapamil |
| pH | 7–8 |
| Sodium content | 0.2 mmol/100 mg |
| Storage | Store below 25°C in original packaging. |

*(continued)*

## Technical information (*continued*)

| | |
|---|---|
| Displacement value | Negligible |
| Stability after preparation | From a microbiological point of view, should be used immediately; however, prepared infusions (in NaCl 0.9% or Gluc 5%) may be stored at 2-8°C and infused (at room temperature) within 24 hours. |

## Monitoring

| Measure | Frequency | Rationale |
|---|---|---|
| Serum Na, K, Ca | Throughout treatment | • May cause fluid and electrolyte disturbances. |
| Withdrawal symptoms and signs | During withdrawal and after stopping treatment | • During prolonged therapy with corticosteroids, adrenal atrophy develops and can persist for years after stopping. Abrupt withdrawal after a prolonged period can lead to acute adrenal insufficiency, ↓BP or death.<br>• The CSM has recommended that gradual withdrawal of systemic corticosteroids should be considered in patients whose disease is unlikely to relapse. Full details can be found in the BNF. |
| Signs of infection | During treatment | • Prolonged courses ↑susceptibility to infections and severity of infections. Serious infections may reach an advanced stage before being recognised. |
| Signs of chickenpox | | • Unless they have had chickenpox, patients receiving corticosteroids for purposes other than replacement should be regarded as being at risk of severe chickenpox.<br>• Confirmed chickenpox requires urgent treatment; corticosteroids should not be stopped and dosage may need to be increased. |
| Exposure to measles | | • Patients should be advised to take particular care to avoid exposure to measles and to seek immediate medical advice if exposure occurs.<br>• Prophylaxis with IM normal immunoglobulin may be needed. |

## Additional information

| | |
|---|---|
| Common and serious undesirable effects | *Immediate:* Anaphylaxis and other hypersensitivity reactions have been reported.<br>*Short-term use:* Undesirable effects that may result from short-term use (minimise by using the lowest effective dose for the shortest time): ↑BP, Na and water retention, ↓K, ↓Ca, ↑blood glucose, peptic ulceration and perforation, psychiatric reactions, ↑susceptibility to infection, muscle weakness, tendon rupture, insomnia, ↑intracranial pressure, ↓seizure threshold, impaired healing. For undesirable effects resulting from long-term corticosteroid use refer to the BNF. |
| Pharmacokinetics | Elimination half-life is 1-2 hours. |

*(continued)*

## Additional information (*continued*)

| | |
|---|---|
| Significant interactions | • The following may ↓corticosteroid levels or effect: barbiturates, carbamazepine, phenytoin, primidone, rifabutin, rifampicin.<br>• Corticosteroids may ↑levels or effect of the following drugs (or ↑side-effects): anticoagulants (monitor INR), methotrexate (↑risk of blood dyscrasias). If using IV amphotericin monitor fluid balance and K level closely.<br>• Corticosteroids may ↓effect of vaccines (↓immunological response, ↑risk of infection with live vaccines). |
| Action in case of overdose | No known antidote but haemodialysis may be effective.<br>Give supportive therapy as appropriate. Following chronic overdose the possibility of adrenal suppression should be considered. |
| Counselling | Patients on long-term corticosteroid treatment should read and carry a Steroid Treatment Card. |

| | |
|---|---|
| Risk rating: **AMBER** | Score = 3<br>Moderate-risk product: Risk-reduction strategies are recommended. |

This assessment is based on the full range of preparation and administration options described in the monograph. These may not all be applicable in some clinical situations.

## Bibliography

SPC Solucortef (accessed 9 September 2009).

# Hydroxocobalamin (vitamin B₁₂)

**1 mg/mL solution in 1-mL ampoules**

- Vitamin $B_{12}$, a water soluble vitamin, occurs in the body in various forms including hydroxocobalamin. Deficiency may occur in strict vegetarians, in patients with malabsorption syndromes or metabolic disorders, or in patients following gastrectomy or extensive ileal resection. Deficiency results in megaloblastic anaemias, demyelination and other neurological damage.
- Hydroxocobalamin is used to treat pernicious anaemia, for prophylaxis and treatment of other macrocytic anaemias associated with vitamin $B_{12}$ deficiency and to treat tobacco amblyopia and Leber's optic atrophy.
- Hydroxocobalamin may be used diagnostically as part of the Schilling test to assess absorption of vitamin $B_{12}$ if an absence of intrinsic factor is suspected.
- Hydroxocobalamin may also be used as an emergency treatment for cyanide poisoning (unlicensed indication). The standard hydroxocobalamin preparation is not suitable for this use. Cyanokit, an imported product that contains 2.5 g hydroxocobalamin per vial, is manufactured for this indication.

## Pre-treatment checks

Do not use for the treatment of megaloblastic anaemia of pregnancy unless a definite diagnosis of vitamin $B_{12}$ deficiency has been established.

*Biochemical and other tests (not all are necessary in an emergency situation)*

Electrolytes: serum K (cardiac arrhythmias secondary to ↓K during initial therapy have been reported – correct if necessary).
FBC
Serum folate (to ensure that folate deficiency is not a contributory/causative factor).
A baseline assessment of neurological function is useful to assess impact of treatment in cases of vitamin $B_{12}$ deficiency anaemia with neurological complications.

## Dose

**Pernicious anaemia and other macrocytic anaemias without neurological involvement**: initially 1 mg by IM injection 3 times a week for 2 weeks then 1 mg every 3 months.

**Pernicious anaemia and other macrocytic anaemias with neurological involvement**: initially 1 mg by IM injection on alternate days until there is no further improvement, then 1 mg every 2 months.

**Prophylaxis of macrocytic anaemias associated with vitamin $B_{12}$ deficiency**: 1 mg by IM injection every 2–3 months.

**Tobacco amblyopia and Leber's optic atrophy**: initially 1 mg by IM injection daily for 2 weeks, then 1 mg twice weekly until there is no further improvement, then 1 mg every 1–3 months.

**Schilling test**: involves use of IM hydroxocobalamin as part of the test.

## Intramuscular injection

*Preparation and administration*

1. Withdraw the required dose.
2. Give by IM injection.

| Technical information | |
| --- | --- |
| Incompatible with | Not relevant |
| Compatible with | Not relevant |
| pH | 3.5-5.5 |
| Sodium content | Negligible |
| Storage | Store below 25°C in original packaging. |

| Monitoring | | |
| --- | --- | --- |
| **Measure** | **Frequency** | **Rationale** |
| Serum K | Daily for first 48 hours, then consider 2-3 times weekly during acute phase | • If ↓K occurs, correct potassium levels, consider withdrawing hydroxocobalamin and monitor cardiac function. |

*(continued)*

## Monitoring (continued)

| Measure | Frequency | Rationale |
|---------|-----------|-----------|
| Neurological function | Ongoing through treatment | • Vitamin B$_{12}$ deficiency anaemias with neurological complications require dosing to continue until no further neurological improvement is seen. Inadequate treatment may manifest as a decline in neurological function. |
| Mean cell volume (MCV) | Once weekly during acute phase of treatment | • Vitamin B$_{12}$ anaemia is characterised by macrocytosis, therefore response to treatment can be judged by cell size reducing to normal range. |
| Haemoglobin | | • Monitor level of Hb to assess response to treatment. |
| Reticulocyte and erythrocyte count | | • Generation of new reticulocytes and erythrocytes supports a diagnosis and treatment of vitamin B$_{12}$ deficiency anaemia. |
| WCC and platelets | Once weekly during acute phase of treatment if baseline is abnormal | • Production may be affected in megaloblastic anaemia. |
| Physical assessment of patient | Ongoing | • Assess patient symptoms to assess relief of typical anaemic presentation, in addition to more specific symptoms of vitamin B$_{12}$ deficiency (glossitis, angular stomatitis, diarrhoea, altered bowel habit, mild jaundice, and neuropathy). |

## Additional information

| | |
|---|---|
| Common and serious undesirable effects | *Injection related:* Local: injection-site pain.<br>*Other:* Nausea, headache, dizziness; fever, hypersensitivity reactions including rash and pruritus. |
| Pharmacokinetics | Wide inter-subject variation when given IM due to hepatic storage. 26-31 hours when administered IV. |
| Significant interactions | Vitamin B$_{12}$ assay: Anti-metabolites and most antibiotics may affect vitamin B$_{12}$ assays. |
| Action in case of overdose | Treatment unlikely to be needed in case of overdose. |

| | |
|---|---|
| Risk rating: **GREEN** | Score = 0<br>Lower-risk product: Risk-reduction strategies should be considered. |

This assessment is based on the full range of preparation and administration options described in the monograph. These may not all be applicable in some clinical situations.

## Bibliography

SPC Cobalin-H 1000 mcg/mL (accessed 31 March 2010).
SPC NeoCytamen Injection 1000 mcg/mL (accessed 31 March 2010).

# Hyoscine butylbromide (scopolamine butylbromide)

**20 mg/mL solution in 1-mL ampoules**

This preparation must not be confused with hyoscine *hydrobromide*.

* Hyoscine butylbromide is quaternary ammonium derivative with antimuscarinic activity.
* It is used to relieve smooth-muscle spasm in GI and genitourinary disorders.
* It is licensed for use in radiology for differential diagnosis of obstruction and to reduce spasm and pain in diagnostic procedures where spasm may be a problem.
* Hyoscine butylbromide may also be given (unlicensed) by SC infusion in palliative care to reduce excessive respiratory secretions and relieve bowel colic.
* Doses are expressed as hyoscine butylbromide.

## Pre-treatment checks

* Do not give in myasthenia gravis (but may be used to ↓muscarinic side-effects of anticholinesterases), megacolon, narrow-angle glaucoma, ↑pulse, prostatic enlargement with urinary retention, mechanical stenoses in the region of the GI tract or paralytic ileus.
* Caution in Down's syndrome, in children and in elderly patients, in GORD, diarrhoea, ulcerative colitis, acute MI, ↑BP, conditions characterised by ↑pulse (including hyperthyroidism, cardiac insufficiency, cardiac surgery), pyrexia (may reduce sweating), pregnancy and breast feeding, and in individuals susceptible to angle-closure glaucoma.
* It is considered unsafe in porphyria.

*Biochemical and other tests*

Blood pressure

## Dose

**Acute spasm and spasm in diagnostic procedures:** 20 mg by IM or slow IV injection repeated after 30 minutes if necessary (may be repeated more frequently in endoscopy) up to a maximum of 100 mg daily.

## Intramuscular injection

*Preparation and administration*

1. Withdraw the required dose.
2. Inject into a large muscle such as the gluteus or the lateral aspect of the thigh.

## Intravenous injection

*Preparation and administration*

1. Withdraw the required dose.
2. The solution should be clear and colourless or almost colourless. Inspect visually for particulate matter or discoloration prior to administration and discard if present.
3. Give by IV injection over 3–5 minutes. May be diluted to 10 mL with NaCl 0.9% or Gluc 5% to enable slow administration if necessary.

### Technical information

| | |
|---|---|
| Incompatible with | Dexamethasone sodium phosphate, haloperidol. |
| Compatible with | **Flush**: NaCl 0.9%<br>**Solutions**: NaCl 0.9%, Gluc 5%<br>**Y-site**: No information |
| pH | 3.7–5.5 |
| Sodium content | Negligible |
| Storage | Store below 30°C in original packaging. |

### Monitoring

| Measure | Frequency | Rationale |
|---|---|---|
| Blood pressure | Post dose | • Marked ↓BP has been observed. |

### Additional information

| | |
|---|---|
| Common and serious undesirable effects | *Immediate:* Anaphylaxis and other hypersensitivity reactions have rarely been reported.<br>*Too rapid IV administration:* Marked ↓BP and shock.<br>*Other:* Constipation, transient ↓pulse (followed by ↑pulse, palpitation and arrhythmias), reduced bronchial secretions, urinary urgency and retention, dilatation of the pupils with loss of accommodation, photophobia, dry mouth, flushing and dryness of the skin. Confusion (particularly in elderly patients). |
| Pharmacokinetics | Elimination half-life is 5–8 hours. |
| Significant interactions | • The following may ↑hyoscine butylbromide levels or effect (or ↑side-effects): alcohol, amantadine, antihistamines, disopyramide, tricyclic and MAOI drugs, phenothiazines. |
| Action in case of overdose | Symptoms of overdose respond to parasympathomimetics. For patients with glaucoma, pilocarpine should be given locally. |
| Counselling | Seek urgent ophthalmological advice if a painful red eye develops. |

| Risk rating: **GREEN** | Score = 0<br>Lower-risk product: Risk-reduction strategies should be considered. |
|---|---|

This assessment is based on the full range of preparation and administration options described in the monograph. These may not all be applicable in some clinical situations.

## Bibliography

SPC Buscopan injection (accessed 6 September 2009).

# Hyoscine hydrobromide (scopolamine hydrobromide)

**400 micrograms/mL and 600 micrograms/mL solution in 1-mL ampoules**

This preparation must not be confused with hyoscine *butylbromide*.

- Hyoscine hydrobromide is a tertiary amine with antimuscarinic activity.
- It is used as a preoperative medication to control bronchial, nasal, pharyngeal and salivary secretions. It also helps to prevent bronchospasm and laryngospasm and blocks cardiac vagal inhibiting reflexes during induction of anaesthesia and intubation. It can provide a degree of amnesia, sedation and antiemesis.
- Hyoscine hydrobromide may also be given (unlicensed) by SC injection or infusion in palliative care to reduce excessive respiratory secretions.
- Doses are expressed as hyoscine hydrobromide.

## Pre-treatment checks

- Avoid in narrow-angle glaucoma.
- Caution in cardiovascular disease, gastrointestinal obstruction, paralytic ileus, prostatic enlargement, Down's syndrome, myasthenia gravis, renal or hepatic impairment.

*Biochemical and other tests*

Blood pressure

## Dose

**Premedication**: 200–600 micrograms by SC or IM injection 30–60 minutes before induction of anaesthesia. In acute use the injection may also be administered by IV injection.

**Excessive respiratory secretions** (unlicensed): 400–600 micrograms by SC injection every 4–8 hours, taking care to avoid discomfort caused by dry mouth. Hyoscine hydrobromide may also be given by SC infusion.

## Subcutaneous injection

*Preparation and administration*

1. Withdraw the required dose.
2. Give by SC injection.

## Intramuscular injection

*Preparation and administration*

1. Withdraw the required dose.
2. Give by IM injection.

## Intravenous injection

*Preparation and administration*

1. Withdraw the required dose and dilute to a suitable volume with WFI.
2. The solution should be clear and colourless. Inspect visually for particulate matter or discoloration prior to administration and discard if present.
3. Give by IV injection.

## Technical information

| | |
|---|---|
| Incompatible with | No information |
| Compatible with | **Flush**: NaCl 0.9%<br>**Solutions**: NaCl 0.9%, Gluc 5% (both with added KCl), WFI<br>**Y-site**: Fentanyl, hydrocortisone sodium succinate, propofol |
| pH | 3.5–6.5 |
| Sodium content | Negligible |
| Storage | Store below 25°C in original packaging. |

## Monitoring

| Measure | Frequency | Rationale |
|---|---|---|
| Sedation, decreased salivary/bronchial secretions | Pre-anaesthesia | • To ensure that treatment is effective. |
| Blood pressure | Periodically | • May cause ↓BP if administered with morphine. |
| Pulse | | • Can cause ↑or↓ pulse. |

## Additional information

| | |
|---|---|
| Common and serious undesirable effects | *Common*: Drowsiness, dry mouth, dizziness, blurred vision and difficulty with micturition. |
| Pharmacokinetics | Elimination half-life is 4.8 hours. |

*(continued)*

| **Additional information** (continued) | |
|---|---|
| Significant interactions | • The following may ↑hyoscine hydrobromide levels or effect (or ↑side-effects): alcohol, amantadine, antihistamines, disopyramide, tricyclic and MAOI drugs, phenothiazines.<br>• Hyoscine hydrobromide may ↓effect of sub-lingual nitrates. |
| Action in case of overdose | *Symptoms to watch for:* Dilated pupils, ↑pulse, rapid respiration, hyperpyrexia, restlessness, excitement, delirium and hallucinations.<br>*Antidote:* Stop administration and give supportive therapy as appropriate. Neostigmine and diazepam have been used to control symptoms. |

| Risk rating: **GREEN** | Score = 1<br>Lower-risk product. Risk-reduction strategies should be considered. |
|---|---|

This assessment is based on the full range of preparation and administration options described in the monograph. These may not all be applicable in some clinical situations.

## Bibliography

SPCs Hyoscine hydrobromide 400 and 600 micrograms/mL solution for injection, Wockhardt UK Ltd (accessed 11 June 2008).

# Ibandronic acid

**1 mg/mL solution in 2-mL ampoules and 6-mL vials (Bondronat)**
**1 mg/mL solution in 3-mL pre-filled syringe (Bonviva)**

* Ibandronate is an aminobisphosphonate that is a potent inhibitor of bone resorption.
* Bondronat is indicated for prevention of skeletal events (pathological fractures, bone complications requiring radiotherapy or surgery) in patients with breast cancer and bone metastases and for treatment of tumour-induced ↑Ca with or without metastases.
* Bonviva is indicated for treatment of osteoporosis in postmenopausal women at increased risk of fracture.
* Doses are expressed in terms of the base:
  Ibandronic acid 1 mg ≡ 1.125 mg ibandronic acid monosodium salt, monohydrate.

## Pre-treatment checks

* Do not give to patients already receiving other bisphosphonates.
* Osteonecrosis of the jaw can occur: consider dental examination and preventive dentistry prior to *planned* treatment in patients with risk factors (e.g. cancer, chemotherapy, radiotherapy, corticosteroids, poor oral hygiene). Avoid invasive dental procedures during treatment if possible.
* Give cautiously to patients who have had previous thyroid surgery (increased risk of ↓Ca)
* Contraindicated in pregnancy. Women of child-bearing potential should take contraceptive precautions during *planned* treatment.
* Unless it is being used for ↑Ca, prescribe oral calcium and vitamin D supplements in those at risk of deficiency (e.g. through malabsorption or lack of exposure to sunlight). All patients being treated for osteoporosis should receive supplements.
* Hydrate patient adequately before, during and after infusions (up to 4 L may be given over 24 hours, but over-hydration should be avoided; risk of cardiac failure).

*Biochemical and other tests*

Electrolytes: serum Na, K, Ca, $PO_4$, Mg
Renal function: U, Cr, CrCl (or eGFR)

## Dose

**Prevention of skeletal events in breast cancer and bone metastases (Bondronat):** 6 mg by IV infusion every 3–4 weeks.
**Dose for this indication in renal impairment:** adjusted according to creatinine clearance, see Table I1.

**Table I1** Ibandronic acid dose in renal impairment

| Creatinine clearance (mL/minute) | Dosage (mg) | Minimum duration of infusion | Infusion volume (mL) |
|---|---|---|---|
| ≥50 | 6 mg | 15 minutes | 100 mL |
| 30–49 | 6 mg | 1 hour | 500 mL |
| <30 | 2 mg | 1 hour | 500 mL |

**Treatment of tumour-induced hypercalcaemia (Bondronat):**

The patient must be adequately hydrated using NaCl 0.9% before dosing for ↑Ca.

Dependent on the patient's initial 'corrected' serum Ca; see Table I2. Normalisation of serum Ca is usually seen within 7 days. If normocalcaemia is not achieved within this time, a further dose may be given. The duration of the response varies – treatment can be repeated whenever ↑Ca recurs.

**Table I2** Treatment of tumour-induced hypercalcaemia with ibandronic acid

| Initial serum calcium ('corrected') | | Dose (mg) | Minimum duration of infusion (hours) | Infusion volume (mL) |
|---|---|---|---|---|
| (mmol/L) | (mg/dL) | | | |
| <3.0 | <12.0 | 2 mg | 2 hours | 500 mL |
| ≥3.0 | ≥12.0 | 4 mg | 2 hours | 500 mL |

**Treatment of osteoporosis in postmenopausal women at increased risk of fracture (Bonviva):** 3 mg by IV injection every 3 months. Do not give more often than every 3 months. Do not give for this indication if CrCl <30 mL/minute.

## Intravenous infusion (Bondronat)

*Preparation and administration*

Ibandronic acid is incompatible with Hartmann's and Ringer's (contain Ca).

1. Withdraw the required dose and add to the appropriate volume of NaCl 0.9% or Gluc 5% (dependent on renal function and indication – see information above).
2. The solution should be clear and colourless. Inspect visually for particulate matter or discoloration prior to administration and discard if present.
3. Give by IV infusion over the appropriate period of time (dependent on renal function and indication – see information above).

## Intravenous injection (Bonviva)

*Preparation and administration*

1. Bonviva is supplied as a pre-filled syringe containing 3 mg/3 mL.
2. The solution should be clear and colourless. Inspect visually for particulate matter or discoloration prior to administration and discard if present.
3. Give by IV injection over 15–30 seconds.

## Technical information

| | |
|---|---|
| Incompatible with | Ibandronic acid is incompatible with Hartmann's and Ringer's (contain Ca). |
| Compatible with | **Flush**: NaCl 0.9%<br>**Solutions**: NaCl 0.9%, Gluc 5% (Bondronat). Bonviva should not be mixed with other products.<br>**Y-site**: No information |
| pH | No information |
| Sodium content | Negligible |
| Storage | Store below 30°C in original packaging. |
| Stability after preparation | From a microbiological point of view, should be used immediately; however, prepared infusions may be stored at 2–8°C and infused (at room temperature) within 24 hours. |

## Monitoring

| Measure | Frequency | Rationale |
|---|---|---|
| Hypersensitivity reactions | During and just after treatment | • Pruritus, urticaria, bronchospasm, and angioedema have been reported rarely. |
| Fluid balance | Frequently during therapy for ↑Ca | • Hydration ↑Ca diuresis.<br>• Hydration reduces decline in renal function and decreases formation of calcium renal calculi. |
| U&E, CrCl (or eGFR) | Prior to each dose, periodically post dose | • Enables the infusion to be given at the correct dose and rate.<br>• Decline in renal function has been reported during bisphosphonate therapy.<br>• ↑K, ↓K, ↑Na have been reported. |
| Serum Ca, PO$_4$, Mg | | • Stop treatment if ↓Ca develops.<br>• Serum Ca may determine whether further treatment is required.<br>• PO$_4$ and Ca share common control systems. Disruption to Ca metabolism affects PO$_4$ levels.<br>• ↓Mg occurs commonly during treatment. |

## Additional information

| | |
|---|---|
| Common and serious undesirable effects | *Immediate:* Angioedema and bronchospasm have been reported.<br>*Injection/infusion-related:* Local: Injection-site reactions have been observed. Care should be taken to avoid extravasation or inadvertent intra-arterial administration.<br>*Other:* Renal dysfunction, reversible elevations of parathyroid hormone, lactic acid dehydrogenase, transaminase and alkaline phosphatase, asymptomatic and symptomatic ↓Ca (paraesthesia, tetany), pruritus, urticaria, exfoliative dermatitis, fever and influenza-like symptoms, malaise, rigors, fatigue and flushes (usually resolve spontaneously), jaw osteonecrosis (see above). |

*(continued)*

## Additional information (*continued*)

| | |
|---|---|
| Pharmacokinetics | Ibandronic acid is removed from the circulation via bone absorption (estimated to be 40-50% in postmenopausal women) and the remainder is eliminated unchanged by the kidney.<br>Pharmacological effects are not related to actual plasma concentrations. |
| Significant drug interactions | None |
| Action in case of overdose | *Symptoms to watch for:* Clinically significant ↓Ca (paraesthesia, tetany, ↓BP).<br>*Antidote:* Calcium gluconate infusion.<br>Stop administration and give supportive therapy as appropriate. Monitor serum Ca, PO$_4$, Mg, K. |
| Counselling | Maintain fluid intake during the post-infusion hours.<br>Report any injection-site reactions.<br>Inform of symptoms of ↓Ca (paraesthesia, tetany, muscle cramps, confusion).<br>Advise on the importance of taking calcium and vitamin D supplements as prescribed where these are indicated.<br>Advise patients with risk factors for osteonecrosis of the jaw (see Pre-treatment checks) not to undergo invasive dental procedures during treatment. |

| Risk rating: **AMBER** | Score = 3<br>Moderate-risk product: Risk-reduction strategies are recommended. |
|---|---|

This assessment is based on the full range of preparation and administration options described in the monograph. These may not all be applicable in some clinical situations.

## Bibliography

SPC Bondronat (accessed 11 February 2009).
SPC Bonviva 3 mg/3 mL solution for injection in pre-filled syringe (accessed 11 February 2009).

# Iloprost

**100 micrograms/mL solution in 1-mL ampoules**

Iloprost must not be confused with its analogue epoprostenol (both names are sometimes erroneously used interchangeably).

- Iloprost trometamol is a synthetic analogue of epoprostenol that causes vasodilatation and has platelet de-aggregant properties.
- It is given by IV infusion (as an unlicensed product) to treat peripheral vascular disease and pulmonary hypertension.

- Many centres have their own protocols for dosing and handling iloprost by infusion and these should be followed where available.
- Iloprost trometamol is also given via nebuliser to treat idiopathic or familial pulmonary arterial hypertension, for which a licensed product exists.
- Doses are expressed in terms of the base:
  Iloprost 1 nanogram ≅ 1.3 nanograms iloprost trometamol.

## Pre-treatment checks

- Caution in concomitant anticoagulant therapy or drugs that ↑risk of bleeding.
- Caution in hepatic and renal impairment.

*Biochemical and other tests (not all are necessary in an emergency situation)*

| | |
|---|---|
| Blood pressure | LFTs |
| Bodyweight | Renal function: U, Cr |
| Heart rate | |

## Dose

**Peripheral vascular disease (unlicensed):** 0.5–2 nanograms/kg/minute for 6 hours daily by IV infusion. Up to 4 weeks of treatment may be required.

**Primary pulmonary hypertension (unlicensed):** 1–8 nanograms/kg/minute for 6 hours daily. Alternatively, iloprost may be given via nebuliser (licensed product) at a dose of 2.5–5 micrograms inhaled 6–9 times daily.

**Dose in renal or hepatic impairment:** in liver cirrhosis or in renal impairment requiring dialysis the dose may need to be halved.

**Calculation of infusion rate (see also Table I3):**

$$\text{Infusion rate (mL/hour)} = \frac{\text{Dose (nanograms/kg/minute)} \times \text{bodyweight (kg)} \times 60}{\text{Concentration of infusion (nanograms/mL)}}$$

**Table I3**  Iloprost rate of infusion using a 2000 nanograms/mL solution

| | Infusion rate (nanograms/kg/minute) | | | |
|---|---|---|---|---|
| | **0.5** | **1.0** | **1.5** | **2.0** |
| **Weight (kg)** | **Rate of infusion (mL/hour)** | | | |
| 30 | 0.45 | 0.9 | 1.35 | 1.8 |
| 40 | 0.60 | 1.2 | 1.80 | 2.4 |
| 50 | 0.75 | 1.5 | 2.25 | 3.0 |
| 60 | 0.90 | 1.8 | 2.70 | 3.6 |
| 70 | 1.05 | 2.1 | 3.15 | 4.2 |
| 80 | 1.20 | 2.4 | 3.60 | 4.8 |
| 90 | 1.35 | 2.7 | 4.05 | 5.4 |
| 100 | 1.50 | 3.0 | 4.50 | 6.0 |

## Continuous intravenous infusion via syringe pump

*Preparation of a 2000 nanograms/mL solution*

1. Withdraw 100 micrograms (1 mL) and make up to 50 mL in a syringe pump with NaCl 0.9% or Gluc 5%.
2. Cap the syringe and mix well to give a solution containing 2000 nanograms/mL.
3. The solution should be clear and colourless. Inspect visually for particulate matter or discoloration prior to administration and discard if present.

*Administration*

Give by continuous IV infusion at the required rate. If adverse effects occur stop the infusion and review; may be recommenced after 1 hour at half the previous rate if appropriate.

### Technical information

| Incompatible with | No information, but do not mix with any other drug. |
|---|---|
| Compatible with | **Flush**: NaCl 0.9%, Gluc 5%<br>**Solutions**: NaCl 0.9%, Gluc 5%<br>**Y-site**: No information but likely to be unstable |
| pH | 7.8–8.8 |
| Sodium content | Negligible |
| Excipients | Contains ethanol (may interact with metronidazole, possible religious objections). |
| Storage | Store below 25°C. Do not freeze. Protect from light. |
| Stability after preparation | Use the prepared infusion immediately. |

### Monitoring

| Measure | Frequency | Rationale |
|---|---|---|
| Blood pressure and heart rate | Frequently throughout administration - at least every 30 minutes | • ↓BP and ↓or↑ heart rate may occur.<br>• If excessive ↓BP occurs during administration, the dose should be reduced or the infusion discontinued.<br>• ↓BP may be profound in overdose and may result in loss of consciousness. |
| ECG | If indicated | • This has been suggested in patients with coronary artery disease. |

### Additional information

| Common and serious undesirable effects | *Immediate:* ↓BP, ↑pulse, arrhythmia, nausea, vomiting.<br>*Other:* Sepsis, septicaemia (mostly related to delivery system), ↓platelet count, anxiety, nervousness, headache, facial flushing (seen even in anaesthetised patients), abdominal colic/discomfort, jaw pain. |
|---|---|

*(continued)*

| Additional information | *(continued)* |
|---|---|
| Pharmacokinetics | Elimination half-life is 20–30 minutes. |
| Significant interactions | • The following may ↑iloprost levels or effect (or ↑side-effects): other anticoagulants or antiplatelet agents, antihypertensives and vasodilators.<br>• Injectable preparation contains ethanol: may interact with disulfiram and metronidazole. |
| Action in case of overdose | Reduce the dose or discontinue the infusion and initiate appropriate supportive measures as necessary, e.g. plasma volume expansion. |

| Risk rating: **AMBER** | Score = 4<br>Moderate-risk product: Risk-reduction strategies are recommended. |
|---|---|

This assessment is based on the full range of preparation and administration options described in the monograph. These may not all be applicable in some clinical situations.

## Bibliography

Micromedex Healthcare Series. Iloprost drug evaluation. www.thomsonhc.com (accessed 21 April 2010).

# Imipenem with cilastatin

### 500-mg dry powder vials

* Imipenem is a semisynthetic carbapenem beta-lactam antibacterial that is always given with cilastatin (which inhibits the renal metabolism of imipenem) in a ratio of 1 : 1 by weight.
* It is used for infections caused by susceptible organisms including infections in neutropenic patients, intra-abdominal infections, bone and joint infections, skin and soft-tissue infections, urinary tract infections, biliary tract infections, hospital-acquired pneumonia, and septicaemia.
* It may also be used for surgical infection prophylaxis and as part of a multidrug regimen for the treatment of anthrax.
* Doses are expressed as milligrams of imipenem.

## Pre-treatment checks

* Do not give if there is known hypersensitivity to any carbapenem antibacterial agent or cilastatin, or previous immediate hypersensitivity reaction to penicillins or cephalosporins.
* Caution in CNS disorders (e.g. epilepsy).

*Biochemical and other tests*

FBC

LFTs

Renal function: U, Cr, CrCl (or eGFR)

## Dose

**Mild infections**: 250 mg by IV infusion every 6 hours.

**Moderate infections**: 500 mg by IV infusion every 8 hours.

**Severe, fully susceptible infections**: 500 mg by IV infusion every 6 hours.

**Severe and/or life-threatening infections** due to less sensitive organisms (primarily some strains of *P. aeruginosa*): 1 g by IV infusion every 6–8 hours.

**Surgical prophylaxis**: 1 g by IV infusion at induction repeated after 3 hours, supplemented in high risk (e.g. colorectal) surgery by doses of 500 mg at 8 and 16 hours after induction. Check local policies.

**Dose in renal impairment**: adjusted according to creatinine clearance:

- CrCl 31–70 mL/minute: 500 mg every 6–8 hours.
- CrCl 21–30 mL/minute: 500 mg every 8–12 hours.
- CrCl 6–20 mL/minute: 250 mg (or 3.5 mg/kg, whichever is the lower) every 12 hours or occasionally 500 mg every 12 hours (↑risk of convulsions).
- CrCl 5 mL/minute or less: should only be given if haemodialysis is started within 48 hours; 250 mg (or 3.5 mg/kg, whichever is the lower) should be given after a dialysis session and then every 12 hours.

## Intermittent intravenous infusion

*Preparation and administration*

Imipenem with cilastatin should not be directly mixed with Hartmann's (incompatible with lactate) but may be co-administered via Y-site.

1. Disperse the contents of each 500-mg vial in 10 mL NaCl 0.9% to produce a suspension of the drug.
2. Withdraw the required dose from the vial(s) and add to 100 mL NaCl 0.9%. If necessary use a further 10 mL NaCl 0.9% to effectively 'wash out' the vial (s) and add this to the infusion bag to ensure complete transfer of vial contents.
3. Agitate the bag to ensure complete mixing.
4. The solution should be clear and colourless to yellow. Inspect visually for particulate matter or discoloration prior to administration and discard if present.
5. Give by IV infusion. Give 250–500 mg over 20–30 minutes and 1 g over 40–60 minutes. The infusion rate should be slowed if the patient develops nausea during the infusion.

| Technical information | |
|---|---|
| Incompatible with | Imipenem with cilastatin should not be directly mixed with Hartmann's (incompatible with lactate) but may be co-administered via Y-site. Amiodarone, amphotericin, drotrecogin alfa (activated), fluconazole, lorazepam, midazolam, sodium bicarbonate. |
| Compatible with | **Flush**: NaCl 0.9% <br> **Solutions**: NaCl 0.9%, Gluc 5% <br> **Y-site**: Aciclovir, cisatracurium, foscarnet, gentamicin, granisetron, linezolid, ondansetron, propofol, remifentanil, tigecycline, tobramycin, vasopressin |

*(continued)*

## Technical information (continued)

| | |
|---|---|
| pH | 6.5-7.5 |
| Sodium content | 1.72 mmol/vial |
| Storage | Store below 25°C in original packaging. |
| Displacement value | Negligible |
| Stability after preparation | From a microbiological point of view, should be used immediately; however, prepared infusions may be stored at 2-8°C and infused (at room temperature) within 24 hours. |

## Monitoring

| Measure | Frequency | Rationale |
|---|---|---|
| Renal function | Periodically if on long-term treatment | • Transient ↑Cr and ↑U may occur.<br>• Dosage may need adjusting if renal function changes. |
| LFTs | | • Transient ↑AST, ↑Alk Phos and ↑bilirubin may occur. |
| FBC | | • Various haematological effects occasionally occur. |
| Development of diarrhoea | Throughout treatment | • Development of severe, persistent diarrhoea may be suggestive of Clostridium difficile-associated diarrhoea and colitis (pseudomembranous colitis). Discontinue drug and treat. Do not use drugs that inhibit peristalsis. |
| Development of seizures | | • Most frequently reported in patients with CNS disorders (e.g. history of seizures, brain lesions, recent head trauma) and/or patients with renal impairment.<br>• If focal tremors, myoclonus or seizures occur during therapy, patients should be evaluated neurologically and anticonvulsant therapy should be initiated in patients who are not already receiving such therapy, and the imipenem dose reassessed to determine whether dosage should be decreased or the drug discontinued. |

## Additional information

| | |
|---|---|
| Common and serious undesirable effects | *Immediate:* Anaphylaxis and other hypersensitivity reactions have been reported.<br>*Other:* Nausea, vomiting, diarrhoea, taste disturbances, tooth or tongue discoloration, hearing loss, blood disorders, positive Coombs' test, rash, pruritus, urticaria, Stevens-Johnson syndrome, rarely toxic epidermal necrolysis, exfoliative dermatitis, myoclonic activity, convulsions, confusion, mental disturbances. |
| Pharmacokinetics | Elimination half-life is 1 hour in normal renal function. |

(continued)

| **Additional information** (*continued*) | |
|---|---|
| Significant interactions | • The following may ↑imipenem levels or effect (or ↑side-effects): ganciclovir (↑risk of convulsions), valganciclovir (↑risk of convulsions). |
| Action in case of overdose | No known antidote but haemodialysis may be effective. Stop administration and give supportive therapy as appropriate. |

| Risk rating: **AMBER** | Score = 3 Moderate-risk product: Risk-reduction strategies are recommended. |
|---|---|

 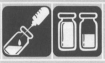

This assessment is based on the full range of preparation and administration options described in the monograph. These may not all be applicable in some clinical situations.

## Bibliography

SPC Primaxin IV injection (accessed 23 March 2009).

# Infliximab

**100-mg dry powder vial**

Infliximab should be used under specialist supervision only.

- Infliximab is a cytokine modulator.
- It is licensed for use in the treatment of rheumatoid arthritis, adult and paediatric Crohn's disease, ulcerative colitis, ankylosing spondylitis, psoriatic arthritis and psoriasis.
- If it is being used for any rheumatologic indication other than rheumatoid arthritis, ankylosing spondylitis or psoriatic arthritis, the patient should be entered on the British Society of Rheumatology's Biologics Register.[1]
- Infliximab has been assessed by NICE and in the UK should be used in accordance with the appropriate guidance.

## Pre-treatment checks

- Screen for tuberculosis, do not give to patients with active tuberculosis or other severe infections.
- Do not give to patients with moderate to severe heart failure.
- Monitor patients for hepatitis B virus, reactivation of hepatitis B has occurred in patients who are carriers.
- Caution should be exercised when using in patients with demyelinating CNS disorders since there is a risk of exacerbating clinical symptoms.
- If the patient has experienced infusion reactions, consider pretreatment with an antihistamine, hydrocortisone and/or paracetamol to prevent mild and transient effects.

*Biochemical and other tests*

| | |
|---|---|
| Bodyweight | LFTs |
| CRP | Skin assessment (if being used for psoriasis) |
| ESR | Tender joint count, swollen joint count (if being |
| FBC | used for psoriatic or rheumatoid arthritis) |

## Dose

**Rheumatoid arthritis**: initially 3 mg/kg by IV infusion, repeated at 2 and 6 weeks after the initial dose and then every 8 weeks thereafter.

**Severe active Crohn's disease**: initially 5 mg/kg by IV infusion, then 5 mg/kg 2 weeks after the initial dose. If the condition has responded, maintenance of *either* 5 mg/kg 6 weeks after initial dose, then 5 mg/kg every 8 weeks *or* a further dose of 5 mg/kg if signs and symptoms recur.

**Fistulating Crohn's disease**: initially 5 mg/kg by IV infusion, repeated at 2 and 6 weeks after the initial dose. If the condition has responded, consult product literature for guidance on further doses.

**Moderate to severe active ulcerative colitis**: initially 5 mg/kg by IV infusion repeated at 2 and 6 weeks after the initial dose, then 5 mg/kg every 8 weeks; discontinue if there is no response 14 weeks after the initial dose.

**Ankylosing spondylitis**: initially 5 mg/kg by IV infusion, repeated at 2 and 6 weeks after the initial dose and then every 6–8 weeks. If there is no response at 6 weeks, no additional treatment with infliximab should be given.

**Psoriatic arthritis**: initially 5 mg/kg by IV infusion, repeated at 2 and 6 weeks after the initial dose, then every 8 weeks thereafter.

**Psoriasis**: initially 5 mg/kg by IV infusion, repeated at 2 and 6 weeks after the initial dose, then every 8 weeks thereafter. If there is no response after 14 weeks, no additional treatment with infliximab should be given.

## Intermittent intravenous infusion

*Preparation and administration*

The infusion should be prepared in a CIVAS unit.

1. Confirm the patient's details on the prepared bag, and that the correct dose has been supplied.
2. The solution should be clear and almost colourless. Inspect visually for particulate matter or discoloration prior to administration and discard if present.
3. Give by IV infusion through a low-protein-binding filter (pore size 1.2 micron or less) over at least 2 hours.

## Technical information

| | |
|---|---|
| Incompatible with | No information |
| Compatible with | **Flush**: NaCl 0.9%<br>**Solutions**: NaCl 0.9%<br>**Y-site**: No information but likely to be unstable |
| pH | 7.2 (reconstituted solution) |
| Sodium content | Negligible |

*(continued)*

## Technical information (*continued*)

| | |
|---|---|
| Storage | Store at 2-8°C in original packaging. |
| Stability after preparation | Be guided by the expiry date/time information provided by the CIVAS unit. From a microbiological point of view, should be used immediately, and prepared infusions should preferably be infused within 3 hours of preparation. However, prepared infusions are known to be stable if stored at 2-8°C and infused (at room temperature) within 24 hours. |

## Monitoring

| Measure | Frequency | Rationale |
|---|---|---|
| Close observation for hypersensitivity reactions | For 1-2 hours post infusion | • Most hypersensitivity reactions are reported during this period.<br>• The risk is greatest in patients receiving their first or second infusion or patients who discontinue other immunosuppressants. |
| Clinical improvement | Periodically | • To check that treatment is effective, e.g. ESR, CRP, DAS. |
| FBC | | • May cause blood dyscrasias. |
| LFTs | | • If jaundice develops and/or $\uparrow$ALT $\geq$ 5 times ULN, stop treatment. |

## Additional information

| | |
|---|---|
| Common and serious undesirable effects | *Immediate* (or with a few hours of administration): Anaphylaxis and other hypersensitivity reactions have been reported.<br>*Infusion-related:* Local: Injection-site reactions.<br>*Other:* Viral infection, serum sickness-like reaction, headache, vertigo, dizziness, flushing, lower and upper respiratory tract infection, abdominal pain, diarrhoea, nausea, dyspepsia, $\uparrow$transaminases, urticaria, rash, pruritus, hyperhidrosis, dry skin, chest pain, fatigue, fever, blood dyscrasias. |
| Pharmacokinetics | Elimination half-life is 8-9.5 days. |
| Significant interactions | • The following may $\uparrow$infliximab levels or effect (or $\uparrow$side-effects): anakinra ($\uparrow$risk of infection), abatacept ($\uparrow$incidence of serious ADRs), live vaccines (avoid combination). |
| Action in case of overdose | No cases reported. Management would be symptomatic. |
| Counselling | Report signs or symptoms of infection, especially a tuberculosis infection during or after treatment with infliximab, e.g. persistent cough, wasting/weight loss, low-grade fever or signs.<br>Report symptoms of blood disorders, e.g. fever, sore throat, bruising or bleeding and seek medical help if these occur.<br>Patients should be given an Alert Card.<br>Patients should avoid live vaccines. |

| Risk rating: **RED** | Score = 6 |
|---|---|
| | High-risk product: Risk-reduction strategies are required to minimise these risks. |

This assessment is based on the full range of preparation and administration options described in the monograph. These may not all be applicable in some clinical situations.

## Reference

1. BSR (2010). *British Society for Rheumatology Biologics Register* (BSRBR). London: British Society for Rheumatology. www.medicine.manchester.ac.uk/epidemiology/research/arc/inflammatorymusculoskeletal/pharmacoepidemiology/bsrbr/ (accessed 18 January 2010).

## Bibliography

SPC Remicade 100mg powder for concentrate for solution for infusion (accessed 18 January 2010).

# Insulins

**Insulin 100 units/mL solution in 10-mL vials**
**3-mL pen cartridges and 3-mL pre-filled pens (see chart below)**
**Restricted use: insulin 500 units/mL solution in 10-mL vials**

- Insulin is a hormone produced by the pancreas that is crucial in the regulation of carbohydrate, protein and fat metabolism. It is secreted when blood glucose levels start to rise; its action is opposed by glucagon; catecholamines, glucocorticoids and growth hormone (the counter-regulatory hormones), and others. Decreased or absent insulin secretion results in the development of diabetes mellitus, although patients with insulin resistance may be markedly hyperinsulinaemic as well as hyperglycaemic.
- The main use of insulin is in the treatment of diabetes mellitus. For maintenance treatment it is given by SC injection (in various regimens) or by continuous SC insulin infusion (CSII).
- Soluble insulin is given by IV infusion in acute illness, e.g. DKA or HHS (formerly known as HONS or HONK), and for maintenance in patients who are temporarily unable to take food by mouth, e.g. perioperatively. The IM route may occasionally be used in the initial treatment of DKA and HHS as a stop-gap measure until IV infusion can be established, as absorption is thought to be slightly faster than via the SC route.
- Insulin is given (unlicensed) by IV infusion in the treatment of moderate to severe ↑K because it increases intracellular uptake of potassium. Glucose is given alongside to counteract hypoglycaemia.
- Rarely insulin containing 500 units/mL may be required for a specific patient. If used it must be kept completely separate from all other insulins, be clearly labelled, and only be administered by staff who have had specific training in its use.[1]
- Insulins were initially produced commercially from animal pancreases (pork and/or beef). Human sequence insulins are now widely available and are produced either by enzymatic modification of porcine insulin (emp), or biosynthetically by recombinant DNA technology using bacteria (crb, prb) or yeast (pyr).

# Prescribing insulin

- Soluble insulin is fairly rapidly absorbed from SC injection sites and insulin has therefore now been produced in many different formulations and types aimed at ↑ or ↓rate of absorption following SC injection. These are grouped according to onset and duration of action (see Table I4 below).
- Insulins should always be prescribed by brand name because release characteristics may vary even between insulins in the same category.
- Insulin doses are expressed in units. Insulin prescriptions should always state the word 'units' in full; the use of abbreviations such as 'U' or 'IU' has caused serious administration errors.[1]
- Insulin should always be measured using insulin syringes designed for the purpose. The use of other syringes has resulted in fatal dosing errors.[1]

## Pre-treatment checks

- Should not be used in hypoglycaemia unless adequate glucose is given alongside.
- JVP, BP and pulse prior to treatment for DKA and HHS, to assess appropriate speed for necessary rehydration.

*Biochemical and other tests (not all are necessary in an emergency situation)*

| | |
|---|---|
| ABG (in DKA) | Bodyweight in certain indications |
| Blood cultures (if infection suspected) | FBC |
| Blood glucose (plus formal laboratory sample as soon as possible in DKA and HHS) | Plasma osmolality (in HHS) |
| | U&Es |
| Blood or urine ketones (in suspected DKA) | |

## Dose

**Diabetic ketoacidosis:** DKA is a medical emergency and its management is complex. Insulin is used in combination with aggressive rehydration, potassium supplementation and many other supportive measures, alongside intensive monitoring.[2]

- Insulin is given by IV infusion via a syringe pump at a fixed rate of 0.1 unit/kg/hour using an insulin infusion containing 1 unit/mL (i.e. 7 mL/hour if weight is 70 kg). If there is a delay in setting up the IV infusion, then a single dose of 0.1 unit/kg may be given by IM injection.
- If the patient is normally maintained on *Lantus* or *Levemir* insulin by SC injection then this should be continued at the usual dose and usual time.
- As soon as the blood glucose falls to 14 mmol/L, give Gluc 10% initially at 125 mL/hour alongside other fluids so that hypoglycaemia is avoided.
- Once ketonaemia has resolved and the patient is biochemically stable and able to eat/drink, insulin by SC injection should be resumed or started. If the patient is unable to eat/drink see NBM management below.

**Hyperosmolar hyperglycaemic state:** HHS management varies from hospital to hospital. Insulin is used in combination with rehydration, potassium and other supportive measures, alongside intensive monitoring.

- Insulin is given as a variable-dose IV infusion (see Table I5 below) adjusted to reduce blood glucose levels by about 3 mmol/hour.
- Patients with HHS may be highly sensitive to insulin. Once the patient is biochemically stable and able to eat/drink, the usual therapy for diabetes treatment should be resumed or started. If the patient is unable to eat/drink, see NBM management below.

**Control of blood glucose in patients who are perioperative or otherwise nil by mouth (NBM):** insulin should be given as a variable-dose infusion (see Table I5) with Gluc 5% or 10% alongside (including KCl unless ↑K) so that hypoglycaemia is avoided.

**Moderate to severe hyperkalaemia (unlicensed):** calcium gluconate is given to stabilise the myocardium (see Calcium gluconate monograph) followed by 5–10 units of soluble insulin with

50 mL Gluc 50% over 5–15 minutes. Effects are seen in 15 minutes and last 4–6 hours.[3] Repeat as necessary or give as a continuous infusion.

**Maintenance regimens for insulin-dependent or insulin-requiring diabetes mellitus:** the regimen chosen depends on the patient's ability to inject, monitor and adjust doses, patient preference and the degree of blood glucose control required. All regimens are given by SC injection with the exception of CSII.

- **Once daily:** usually given as a single daily dose of an intermediate or long-acting insulin. Occasionally a biphasic insulin is used, but the dose must then be given in association with a meal.
- **Twice daily:** usually given as a twice daily dose of an intermediate or biphasic insulin with breakfast and evening meal.
- **Basal-bolus:** an intermediate- or long-acting insulin is given once (or occasionally twice) daily to provide a background or 'basal' level of insulin; doses of a short- or rapid-acting insulin are given with food.
- **Dose adjustment for normal eating (DAFNE):** similar to basal-bolus but patients attend a 5-day course on dose adjustment, and management of sickness.
- **CSII:** given via a programmable external pump containing an insulin reservoir. The pump is set to deliver a basal level of insulin by SC infusion and bolus doses are given using the pump to coincide with food intake.

**Dose in renal impairment:** reduced doses may be required in severe renal impairment.

## Subcutaneous injection

*Preparation and administration*

1. Check that the insulin you have selected is the one specified on the prescription chart.
2. If using an insulin suspension, re-suspend by rolling the vial, cartridge or pen gently between the palms or inverting several times. The insulin suspension should look uniformly milky.
3. Withdraw the required dose using an insulin syringe*, or dial up the correct dose according to the manufacturer's instructions if using an insulin pen.
4. Using an area on the abdomen, outer thigh, upper outer arm or the buttock, pinch up a skin fold between the thumb and forefinger and hold throughout the injection.
5. Give by SC injection into the thick part of the skin fold at right angles to the skin. Leave the needle *in situ* for a few seconds before removal.
6. Do not rub the injection site after administration. Avoid overuse of injection sites as this may impair absorption; rotate sites so that individual sites are not reused within 1 month.

*Some insulins may be mixed in the syringe immediately prior to administration – see individual product literature.

## Continuous intravenous infusion via a syringe pump

This method is used for control of blood glucose.
Only solutions containing 1 unit/mL should be prepared.[1]

*Preparation and administration*

1. Withdraw 49.5 mL NaCl 0.9% into a syringe suitable for use in a syringe pump.
2. Withdraw 50 units (0.5 mL) soluble insulin (e.g. Actrapid, Humulin S) into an insulin syringe and add to the prepared syringe.
3. Cap the syringe and mix well to give a solution containing 1 unit/mL.
4. The solution should be clear and colourless. Inspect visually for particulate matter or discoloration prior to administration and discard if present.

*(continued)*

5.  Give by IV infusion at the required rate.\* Check hydration status, patency of IV access and the pump for malfunction if blood glucose values are higher than expected at any point.
6.  Prepare a fresh syringe at least every 24 hours if required.

\*If the patient is normally maintained on *Lantus* or *Levemir* insulin by SC injection then this should be continued at the usual dose and usual time while the insulin infusion is in progress.[2]

## Intravenous injection or infusion via a syringe pump (unlicensed use for hyperkalaemia only)

> This method is used for the treatment of hyperkalaemia only.
> There are no stability data on insulin added to Gluc 50%; prepared syringes must be used immediately.

*Preparation and administration*

1.  Withdraw 50 mL Gluc 50% into a syringe.
2.  Withdraw the required dose of soluble insulin (e.g. Actrapid, Humulin S) into an insulin syringe and add to the prepared syringe.
3.  Cap the syringe and mix well to disperse the insulin thoroughly. Failure to do this may result in unexpected hypoglycaemia.
4.  The solution should be clear and colourless. Inspect visually for particulate matter or discoloration prior to administration and discard if present.
5.  Give by IV injection or infusion over 5–15 minutes.

## Continuous subcutaneous insulin infusion (CSII)

1.  Prepare following the manufacturer's guidelines.
2.  The cannula should be replaced and repositioned every 3 days.[4]

## Technical information

| | |
|---|---|
| Incompatible with | Insulin is adsorbed on to the surface of infusion containers; this can be decreased by using small-volume containers, e.g. syringe pumps rather than large infusion bags.<br>Drotrecogin alfa (activated), labetalol, micafungin, ranitidine. |
| Compatible with | **Flush**: NaCl 0.9%<br>**Solutions**: NaCl 0.9%, Gluc 5% (including added KCl)<br>**Y-site**: Co-administration of drugs is not recommended because of the risk of inadvertently affecting insulin infusion rate. In DKA insulin may be infused in the same line as infusion fluids provided a Y-connector with a one-way anti-siphon valve is used and a large-bore cannula has been placed.[2] |
| pH | 7-7.8 (but dependent on product) |
| Sodium content | Negligible |
| Excipients | Most insulins contain metacresol (may cause hypersensitivity reactions) - see individual product literature. |
| Storage | Store at 2-8°C in original packaging. Do not freeze.<br>*In use:* May be used and stored at room temperature for up to 28 days (some products are stable for 42 days - see individual product literature).<br>Pens in use should not be stored in the fridge (pens may jam) or with needles attached. Replace the pen cap between injections to protect from light. |

*(continued)*

## Technical information (continued)

| Stability after preparation | Use prepared infusions immediately. |
|---|---|

## Monitoring

| Measure | Frequency | Rationale |
|---|---|---|
| Capillary blood glucose *(during IV infusion)* | Every 60 minutes | • For signs of clinical improvement (in DKA and HHS).<br>• To maintain blood glucose within normal range and avoid hypoglycaemia if the patient is NBM. |
| Capillary blood glucose *(during SC maintenance)* | Pre-meals, at bedtime and if hypoglycaemia is suspected (or as recommended by the patient's clinic) | • To monitor adequacy of insulin regimen and to facilitate dose adjustment.<br>• To ensure that hypoglycaemia is treated appropriately. |
| Blood (or urine) ketones | Every 60 minutes in DKA | • For signs of clinical improvement. |
| U&Es | Every 2 hours in DKA and HHS, daily during IV infusion while NBM | • To assess whether K-containing fluids are required and to avoid ↓K.<br>• To avoid ↓Na and assess state of hydration. |
| Blood bicarbonate, pH | Every 2 hours in DKA – venous samples are adequate[2] | • For signs of clinical improvement. |
| HbA$_{1c}$ | Every 3–6 months | • To assess adequacy of control of diabetes mellitus. |
| Monitoring of diabetic complications | Annually (or more frequently if appropriate) | • To ensure that complications are treated or dealt with, and that the patient is counselled appropriately. |

## Additional information

| Common and serious undesirable effects | *Injection/infusion-related:*<br>• Too rapid administration: Hypoglycaemia.<br>• Local: Pain, itching, swelling or inflammation at SC injection sites that usually reduces with continued use. Injection sites should be rotated. Lipoatrophy or lipohypertrophy from overuse of sites (less common with highly purified insulins).<br><br>*Other:* Hypoglycaemia, ↓K. |
|---|---|
| Pharmacokinetics | Onset of action is instantaneous if given IV irrespective of the formulation used, i.e. an inadvertent IV dose of a long-acting insulin will have immediate effect. Elimination half-life is a few minutes after IV administration.<br>Duration of action is dependent on insulin formulation if give by SC injection. Action may be prolonged in severe renal impairment.<br>In ↑K, effects are seen in 15 minutes and last 4–6 hours.[3] |

(continued)

## Additional information *(continued)*

| | |
|---|---|
| Significant interactions | No significant interactions; however, any medication affecting blood glucose control may necessitate an adjustment in insulin dosage.<br>• The following may ↓blood glucose levels:<br>ethanol, quinine (parenteral).<br>• The following may ↑blood glucose levels:<br>antipsychotics-atypical, beta-agonists (parenteral), combined oral contraceptives, glucocorticoids, protease inhibitors, diuretics-thiazide. |
| Action in case of overdose | *Symptoms to watch for:* Hypoglycaemia: excessive sweating, pallor, palpitations, trembling, feeling cold, impaired vision, irritability, tingling round the lips, inability to concentrate, confusion, personality change, inability to waken.<br>*Antidote:* Rapidly absorbed oral carbohydrate. If unconscious, *glucagon* by IM or SC injection or *glucose* by slow IV injection (see relevant monographs). |
| Counselling | Correct administration of insulin, insulin storage, disposal of sharps, importance of taking doses regularly as prescribed.<br>Training in use of blood glucose, blood ketone or urine glucose monitoring as appropriate.<br>Patients maintained on insulin should always carry glucose (and glucagon if necessary) and should be able to recognise the symptoms of hypoglycaemia.<br>Relatives or carers should be trained to recognise hypoglycaemia and how to treat it appropriately.<br>Contact number for advice for newly diagnosed insulin-treated patients. |

| | |
|---|---|
| Risk rating: **RED** | Score = 6<br>High-risk product: Risk-reduction strategies are required to minimise these risks. |

This assessment is based on the full range of preparation and administration options described in the monograph. These may not all be applicable in some clinical situations.

## References

1. NHS Evidence. *Safe and Effective Use of Insulin in Hospitalised Patients.* www.diabetes.nhs.uk (accessed 15 May 2010).
2. Joint British Diabetes Societies Inpatient Care Group. *The Management of Diabetic Ketoacidosis in Adults.* www.diabetes.nhs.uk (accessed 15 May 2010).
3. CREST(2006). *Guidelines for the Treatment of Hyperkalaemia in Adults.* www.crestni.org.uk/publications/hyperkalaemia-booklet.pdf (accessed 28/04/08).
4. NICE. TA 057 *Continuous Subcutaneous Insulin Infusion for the Treatment of Diabetes Mellitus.* www.nice.org.uk (accessed 15 May 2010).

## Bibliography

SPCs of all products mentioned (accessed 15 May 2010).

**Table 14** Some of the different types and brands of insulin available

| Insulin category | Brand name | Insulin source/type | Licensed routes | Form[a] |
|---|---|---|---|---|
| Rapid-acting human insulin analogues | Apidra | glulisine | SC, IV | C, P, V |
| | Humalog | lispro | SC, CSII, IV, IM | C, P, V |
| | NovoRapid | aspart | SC, CSII, IV | C, P, V |
| Short-acting, also called 'soluble', 'neutral' or 'regular' insulin | Actrapid | human (pyr) soluble | SC, IV | V |
| | Humulin S | human (prb) soluble | SC, IV, IM | C, V |
| | Hypurin Bovine Neutral | beef soluble | SC, IV, IM | C, V |
| | Hypurin Porcine Neutral | pork soluble | SC, IV, IM | C, V |
| | Insuman Rapid | human (crb) soluble | SC, IV | C, P |
| Intermediate- and long-acting | Humulin I | human (prb) isophane | SC | C, P, V |
| | Hypurin Bovine Isophane | beef isophane | SC | C, V |
| | Hypurin Bovine Lente | beef zinc suspension | SC | V |
| | Hypurin Bovine Protamine Zinc | beef protamine zinc | SC | V |
| | Hypurin Porcine Isophane | pork isophane | SC | C, V |
| | Insulatard | human (pyr) isophane | SC | C, P, V |
| | Insuman Basal | human (crb) | SC | C, P, V |
| | Lantus | glargine | SC | C, P, V |
| | Levemir | detemir | SC | C, P |

(continued)

**Table 14** Some of the different types and brands of insulin available *(continued)*

| Insulin category | Brand name | Insulin source/type | Licensed routes | Form[a] |
|---|---|---|---|---|
| Biphasic, also called 'insulin mixtures' | Humalog Mix25 | lispro 25%, lispro protamine 75% | SC | C, P, V |
| | Humalog Mix50 | lispro 50%, lispro protamine 50% | SC | C, P, V |
| | Humulin M3 | human soluble 30%, isophane 70% | SC | C, P, V |
| | Hypurin Porcine 30/70 Mix | pork soluble 30%, isophane 70% | SC | C, V |
| | Insuman Comb 15 | human soluble 15%, isophane 85% | SC | P |
| | Insuman Comb 25 | human soluble 25%, isophane 75% | SC | C, P |
| | Insuman Comb 50 | human soluble 50%, isophane 50% | SC | C, P |
| | Mixtard 30 | human soluble 30%, isophane 70% | SC | C, P, V |
| | NovoMix 30 | aspart 30%, aspart isophane 70% | SC | C, P |

[a]C = cartridges, P = pre-filled pens, V = vials.

**Table 15** An example of a prescription for a variable-dose IV insulin infusion (use local policy if available)

| Capillary glucose (mmol/L) | Insulin infusion (units/hour) |
|---|---|
| 0–4 | 0.5[a] |
| 4.1-7 | 1 |
| 7.1-11 | 2 |
| 11.1-14 | 3 |
| 14.1-17 | 4 |
| 17.1-20 | 5 |
| >20 | 6 (and seek medical input) |

[a]For patients with Type 1 diabetes mellitus, the insulin infusion rate should never be decreased to zero unless Lantus or Levemir insulins are also being given.

# Intralipid

**10% emulsion in 100-mL and 500-mL infusion containers**
**20% emulsion in 100-mL, 250-mL and 500-mL infusion containers**
**30% in 333-mL infusion container**

- Intralipid contains fractionated soya oil in the form of a fat emulsion. It is a rich source of linoleic and linolenic acids, which are essential fatty acids.
- Fat emulsions such as Intralipid are used in combination with other nutrients in parenteral nutrition regimens to provide a high energy intake in a relatively small volume.
- Intralipid may also be used (unlicensed) for 'lipid rescue' to treat severe local anaesthetic toxicity resulting from inadvertent systemic administration of epidural and other preparations.

## Pre-treatment checks

- Do not give to patients with severe egg allergy.
- Use with caution in patients known to be allergic to soya protein, and only after hypersensitivity tests.
- Caution in conditions of impaired lipid metabolism such as renal insufficiency, uncontrolled diabetes mellitus, pancreatitis, certain forms of liver insufficiency, hypothyroidism (if hypertrigly-ceridaemic), metabolic disorders and sepsis.

*Biochemical and other tests (not all are necessary in an emergency situation)*

FBC
LFTs
Lipid profile

Renal function: U, Cr, CrCl (or eGFR)
TFTs

## Dose

**Total parenteral nutrition:** the dose is tailored to the energy requirements and the clinical status of the patient as well as the patient's ability to utilise fat. Energy requirements of individuals must be met if amino acids are to be utilised for tissue maintenance rather than as an energy source. Parenteral feeding should be introduced slowly initially, particularly in those patients at risk of refeeding syndrome, e.g. the chronically malnourished.

**Prevention and correction of essential fatty acid deficiency (EFAD):** when given to prevent or correct essential fatty acid deficiency, 4–8% of non-protein calories should be supplied as Intralipid to provide sufficient amounts of linoleic and linolenic acids.

**Treatment of local anaesthetic induced cardiac arrest that is unresponsive to standard therapy:** data is still extremely limited; there are no standard methods for lipid emulsion therapy. The following regimen has been suggested.[1,2] It should be used only after standard resuscitation methods fail to re-establish sufficient circulatory stability.

The following doses are of Intralipid 20%:

1. 1.5 mL/kg over 1 minute.*
2. Follow immediately with an IV infusion at a rate of 0.25 mL/kg/minute.*
3. Continue chest compressions (lipid must circulate).
4. Repeat 1.5 mL/kg bolus every 3–5 minutes up to 3 mL/kg total dose until circulation is restored.
5. Continue infusion until haemodynamic stability is restored. Increase the rate to 0.5 mL/kg/ minute if BP declines.*
6. A maximum total dose of 8 mL/kg is recommended.

**\*In practice, for a 70-kg adult:**

* Withdraw 50 mL from a 500-mL Intralipid 20% container and give immediately (twice).
* Attach the Intralipid 20% container to a giving set give by IV infusion over the next 15 minutes.
* Repeat the initial bolus up to twice more, if spontaneous circulation has not returned.

### Intravenous infusion

* Intralipid may be given as a separate infusion or (more commonly now) as an 'all-in-one' admixture.
* Parenteral nutrition admixtures must be prepared in a pharmacy aseptic unit and must be compounded for physical stability.
* When separate infusion is preferred, the fat emulsion may be infused into the same central or peripheral vein as carbohydrate/amino acid solutions via a Y-connector close to the infusion site.
* It has been recommended that administration sets used for lipid emulsions be changed within 24 hours of initiating infusion because of the potential for bacterial and fungal contamination.
* On the first day of infusion it is advisable to give a maximum of 5 mL/kg Intralipid 20% or 10 mL/ kg Intralipid 10%. Subsequently the dose is usually increased and, when a larger intake is indicated, the dose may be increased to a maximum of 3 g/kg/day.
* Intralipid 10% 500 mL should be given over a period not less than 3 hours.
* Intralipid 20% 500 mL should be given over a period of not less than 5 hours.
* Intralipid 30%: the rate for the first half-hour should be half the final administration rate. The infusion rate should not exceed 333 mL in 5 hours.

## Technical information

| | |
|---|---|
| Incompatible with | No information but likely to be unstable.<br>Fat emulsions may extract phthalate plasticisers from bags and giving sets and non-phthalate containing equipment should be used wherever possible. |
| Compatible with | **Solutions**: May be added to certain amino acid and carbohydrate solutions.<br>Additives: Vitlipid N Adult, Vitlipid N Infant, Solivito N.<br>**Y-site**: May be infused into the same central or peripheral vein as certain amino acid and carbohydrate solutions. |

*(continued)*

## Technical information (continued)

| | |
|---|---|
| pH | 8 |
| Sodium content | Nil |
| Excipients | Contains egg-yolk phospholipids - avoid in severe egg allergy. |
| Storage | Store below 25°C. Do not freeze.<br>Single use only - discard unused portion. |

## Monitoring

| Measure | Frequency | Rationale |
|---|---|---|
| Fat elimination and triglycerides | Throughout treatment (daily in high-risk patients) | • Patients with conditions involving impaired lipid metabolism are at risk of fat embolism.<br>• Fat embolism has been reported in a few cases when the recommended infusion rate has been exceeded.<br>• Patients given Intralipid for more than one week should also be monitored. |
| Renal function, LFTs, FBC and acid-base balance | Periodically | • In the metabolic and nutritional management of the seriously ill patient, preliminary investigations and continuous monitoring are essential, particularly of electrolyte levels.<br>• Changes in the patient's biochemistry can indicate required changes in formulation to a TPN regimen. |
| Vitamins and trace elements | | • Deficiency can occur, especially in patients receiving long-term parenteral nutrition. |

## Additional information

| | |
|---|---|
| Common and serious undesirable effects | *Immediate:* Anaphylaxis and other hypersensitivity reactions have very rarely been reported. Rarely ↑temperature, chills and nausea/vomiting.<br>*Infusion-related:* Too rapid administration: Prolonged or too rapid infusion of soya oil emulsion or its use in patients with impaired fat metabolism has been associated with the 'fat overload syndrome': hyperlipidaemia, fever, fat infiltration, organ dysfunction and coma.<br>*Other.* Rarely skin rash, urticaria, respiratory symptoms (e.g. tachypnoea, dyspnoea), ↑ or ↓BP, cyanosis, haemolysis, hypercoagulability, reticulocytosis, abdominal pain, headache, tiredness and priapism.<br>↑Transaminases, Alk Phos and bilirubin have been observed in patients receiving parenteral nutrition, with or without Intralipid. If the dosage is reduced, values usually return to normal. Cholestasis has also been reported. |
| Pharmacokinetics | Elimination half-life is approximately 30 minutes. |
| Significant interactions | • Intralipid may ↓levels or effect of the following drugs:<br>coumarin anticoagulants (soybean oil has natural vitamin $K_1$ content).<br>• Intralipid may affect the following tests:<br>some laboratory tests may be affected if blood is taken before fat has adequately cleared; this may take 4-6 hours. |

(continued)

| **Additional information** (*continued*) | |
|---|---|
| Action in case of overdose | *Symptoms to watch for:* Metabolic acidosis has been associated with severe overdosage.<br>All symptoms are usually reversible if the infusion is discontinued. |

Risk rating: **AMBER**     Score = 4
Moderate-risk product: Risk-reduction strategies are recommended.

This assessment is based on the full range of preparation and administration options described in the monograph. These may not all be applicable in some clinical situations.

## References

1. *LipidRescue*. www.lipidrescue.org (accessed 11 May 2010).
2. NPSA (2007). *Patient Safety Alert: Safer Practice with Epidural Injections and Infusions* March 2007. London: National Patient Safety Agency. www.nrls.npsa.nhs.uk.

## Bibliography

SPC Intralipid 10%, 20%, 30% (accessed 11 May 2010).

# Iron dextran (CosmoFer)

**Iron (as iron dextran) 50 mg/mL solution in 2-mL, 5-mL and 10-mL ampoules**

* Iron is an essential element, being necessary for haemoglobin formation and the storage of oxygen in living cells. Iron deficiency results in defective erythropoiesis and anaemia.
* Iron dextran complex is used to treat iron deficiency when oral iron preparations cannot be used (for example owing to intolerance), when oral preparations have had a demonstrated lack of effect, or when rapid replenishment of iron stores is necessary.
* Each millilitre of CosmoFer injection contains 50 mg of ferric iron as iron(III)-hydroxide dextran complex.

## Pre-treatment checks

* Not to be given in: history of allergic disorders including asthma and eczema; infection; active rheumatoid arthritis; severe hepatic impairment; acute renal failure.
* Not be used in the first trimester of pregnancy.
* Do not use in non-iron-deficiency anaemias, e.g. haemolytic anaemias, iron overload or disturbances in utilisation of iron.
* Owing to the potential risk of anaphylactoid reactions, resuscitation equipment and staff trained to evaluate and treat anaphylaxis should be available whenever a dose of iron dextran is administered.

*Biochemical and other tests*

Bodyweight

FBC (including Hb)

LFTs

Renal function: U, Cr, CrCl (or eGFR)

## Dose

The total dose required to treat iron-deficiency anaemia and replenish iron stores is dependent on the initial Hb level and bodyweight (see Dose calculation below).

**Standard dose:** give 100–200 mg (2–4 mL) by IV injection or infusion 2–3 times weekly until the calculated dose has been given.

Alternatively, give doses of 100–200 mg (2–4 mL) by IM injection. For moderately active patients, give injections daily into alternate buttocks; in relatively inactive or frail patients, give injections once or twice weekly. Continue administration until the calculated dose has been given.

**Total dose infusion for rapid replenishment of iron stores (hospital use only):** up to 20 mg/kg/day by IV infusion may be given. If the calculated total dose required exceeds 20 mg/kg/day, the administration must be split over two days (see Table I6 below).

**Dose calculation for iron-deficiency anaemia:** the desired dose may be calculated from the following equations (dependent on the unit of measure for Hb), which apply to a bodyweight >35 kg; or use Table I6 below. The dose should be rounded to the nearest easily measurable volume.

*For Hb reported in g/dL:*

Total dose required (mg iron) = [bodyweight (kg) × (target Hb − actual Hb) × 2.4] + 500

*For Hb reported in mmol/L:*

Total dose required (mg iron) = [bodyweight (kg) × (target Hb − actual Hb) × 3.84] + 500

**Iron replacement for blood loss:** the aim is to replace the iron content of the estimated blood loss. Giving 200 mg (4 mL) by IV injection or infusion results in an increase in Hb roughly equivalent to that supplied by one unit of blood.

## Intermittent intravenous infusion (preferred route)

*Preparation and administration*

1. Withdraw the required dose and add to a suitable volume of NaCl 0.9% (100 mL for standard dose; 500 mL for total dose infusion).
2. The solution should be dark brown. Inspect visually for particulate matter or discoloration prior to administration and discard if present.
3. Initial test dose (prior to first dose only): Give the first 25 mg by IV infusion over 15 minutes; stop the infusion and observe the patient carefully for signs of allergic reaction for at least 60 minutes; if no adverse effects are seen give the remainder of the infusion.
4. For the standard dose give the dose by IV infusion over 30 minutes; for a total dose infusion give the dose by IV infusion over 4–6 hours.
5. Observe the patient carefully for a minimum of 1 hour after total dose infusion.

## Intramuscular injection

*Preparation and administration*

1. Initial test dose (prior to first dose only): Withdraw 25 mg (0.5 mL) and give by IM injection following the procedure outlined in points 2–6 below. Observe the patient carefully for signs of allergic reaction for at least 60 minutes; if no adverse effects are seen give the remainder of the dose.
2. Withdraw the required dose (or the remainder of the dose if a test dose has been given). Up to 2 mL may be given at each administration (total dose required is determined by dosage calculation).

*(continued)*

**Table 16** Total dose of CosmoFer for iron-deficiency anaemia in mL (based on bodyweight and initial Hb)

| Bodyweight (kg) | Initial Hb | | | | | | | |
|---|---|---|---|---|---|---|---|---|
| | 6.0 g/dL 3.7 mmol/L | | 7.5 g/dL 4.7 mmol/L | | 9.0 g/dL 5.6 mmol/L | | 10.5 g/dL 6.5 mmol/L | |
| | Total dose (mL) | For TDI: split infusions required? | Total dose (mL) | For TDI: split infusions required? | Total dose (mL) | For TDI: split infusions required? | Total dose (mL) | For TDI: split infusions required? |
| 35 | 25 | Yes | 23 | Yes | 20 | Yes | 18 | Yes |
| 40 | 27 | Yes | 24 | Yes | 22 | Yes | 19 | Yes |
| 45 | 29 | Yes | 26 | Yes | 23 | Yes | 20 | Yes |
| 50 | 32 | Yes | 28 | Yes | 24 | Yes | 21 | Yes |
| 55 | 34 | Yes | 30 | Yes | 26 | Yes | 22 | No |
| 60 | 36 | Yes | 32 | Yes | 27 | Yes | 23 | No |
| 65 | 38 | Yes | 33 | Yes | 29 | Yes | 24 | No |
| 70 | 40 | Yes | 35 | Yes | 30 | Yes | 25 | No |
| 75 | 42 | Yes | 37 | Yes | 32 | Yes | 26 | No |
| 80 | 45 | Yes | 39 | Yes | 33 | Yes | 27 | No |
| 85 | 47 | Yes | 41 | Yes | 34 | No | 28 | No |
| 90 | 49 | Yes | 42 | Yes | 36 | No | 29 | No |

3. Attach a 20–21G × 50-mm needle for average-sized adults (use 23G × 32-mm needle for smaller adults; 20–21G × 80–100-mm needle for obese adults).
4. The patient should be positioned in the lateral position with the injection site uppermost, or standing bearing their weight on the leg opposite the injection site.
5. Using the Z-track technique, give the dose smoothly and slowly by deep IM injection into the muscle mass of the upper outer quadrant of the buttock. It must never be given into the arm or other exposed areas as there is a risk of SC staining.
6. Leave the needle *in situ* for a few seconds before withdrawal to allow the muscle mass to accommodate the injection volume. To minimise leakage up the injection track, the patient should be advised not to rub the injection site. Rotate injection sites for subsequent injections.

## Intravenous injection (or injection into the venous limb of a dialyser)

*Preparation and administration*

1. Withdraw the required dose (2–4 mL) and dilute to a final volume of 10–20 mL with NaCl 0.9% to produce a solution containing 10 mg/mL.
2. The solution should be dark brown. Inspect visually for particulate matter or discoloration prior to administration and discard if present.
3. Initial test dose (prior to first dose only): Give 2.5 mL (25 mg) of the diluted injection by IV injection over 1–2 minutes. Observe the patient carefully for signs of allergic reaction for at least 15 minutes; if no adverse effects are seen, give the remainder of the injection.
4. Give the diluted injection by IV injection at a maximum rate of 1 mL/minute.

## Technical information

| | |
|---|---|
| Incompatible with | No Information |
| Compatible with | **Flush**: NaCl 0.9%<br>**Solutions**: NaCl 0.9% (preferred), Gluc 5% (↑risk of thrombophlebitis)<br>**Y-site**: No information but likely to be unstable |
| pH | 5.2–6.5 |
| Sodium content | Negligible |
| Storage | Store below 25°C in original packaging. |
| Stability after preparation | From a microbiological point of view, should be used immediately; however, prepared infusions may be stored at 2–8°C and infused (at room temperature) within 24 hours. |

## Monitoring

| Measure | Frequency | Rationale |
|---|---|---|
| Hypersensitivity or intolerance | Throughout administration | • Discontinue therapy immediately if this occurs. |
| Blood pressure | | • ↓BP can occur if IV administration is too rapid. |
| Respiratory observations | Throughout administration | • Respiratory difficulties such as dyspnoea have been reported – discontinue treatment if they occur. |

*(continued)*

## Monitoring (continued)

| Measure | Frequency | Rationale |
|---|---|---|
| Reticulocyte count | Every 3–5 days in acute phase | • Indicative of response (should observe ↑reticulocyte counts within a few days of treatment). |
| Haematocrit and Hb levels | | • Indicative of response. |
| Serum ferritin | | • Indicative of response. |
| Mean cell volume | | • Indicative of response. |
| Total iron-binding capacity | Periodically | • Useful to assess saturation of the system when the treatment cycle completed, to decide whether response has been satisfactory, and also to assess iron overload. |

## Additional information

| | |
|---|---|
| Common and serious undesirable effects | *Immediate:* Anaphylactoid and other hypersensitivity reactions have been reported.<br>*Injection/infusion-related:*<br>• Too rapid administration: ↓BP.<br>• Local: Injection-site reactions (soreness, phlebitis, staining of the skin, bleeding, sterile abscesses, tissue necrosis or atrophy).<br><br>*Other:* ↑risk of allergic reactions in patients with immune or inflammatory conditions (e.g. SLE, rheumatoid arthritis), also in patients receiving total dose infusions. Reactions may be delayed for up to 4 days post dose. Symptoms include arthralgia, myalgia, pyrexia, urticaria, rashes, itching, nausea, shivering (rarely respiratory difficulty, angioedema and cardiovascular collapse); cramps; blurred vision.<br>Chronic repeated administration of iron at high doses can cause liver accumulation, leading to fibrosis as a result of inflammation.<br>GI disturbances, pyrexia, flushing, dyspnoea, chest pain; ↑pulse and arrhythmias; ↑ or ↓BP; headache; dizziness; seizure; loss of consciousness; haemolysis. |
| Pharmacokinetics | Elimination half-life is 5 hours for circulating iron; 20 hours for total iron (bound and circulating). |
| Significant interactions | • Iron dextran may ↑levels or effect (or ↑side-effects) of dimercaprol (avoid combination - may result in serious toxicity).<br>• Iron dextran may ↓levels or effect of oral iron salts (↓absorption - do not start within 5 days of parenteral treatment).<br>• Iron dextran may affect the following tests:<br>Doses >5 mL have been reported to give a brown colour to serum from blood samples taken up to 4 hours after administration. Falsely ↑bilirubin levels. Falsely ↓Ca levels. |

*(continued)*

## Additional information (*continued*)

| | |
|---|---|
| Action in case of overdose | *Symptoms to watch for:* Acute iron overload which may appear as haemosiderosis.<br>*Antidote:* Iron chelation therapy can be used. |
| Counselling | Advise patient to report any hypersensitivity reactions. |

| | |
|---|---|
| Risk rating: **AMBER** | Score = 5<br>Moderate-risk product: Risk-reduction strategies are recommended. |

This assessment is based on the full range of preparation and administration options described in the monograph. These may not all be applicable in some clinical situations.

## Bibliography

SPC CosmoFer (accessed 24 August 2009).

# Iron sucrose (Venofer)

### 20 mg/mL solution in 5-mL ampoules

* Iron is an essential element, being necessary for haemoglobin formation and the storage of oxygen in living cells. Iron deficiency results in defective erythropoiesis and anaemia.
* Iron sucrose complex is used to treat iron deficiency when oral iron preparations cannot be used (for example owing to intolerance), when oral preparations have had a demonstrated lack of effect, or when rapid replenishment of iron stores is necessary.
* Some patients who have had prior hypersensitivity reactions to iron dextran may tolerate iron sucrose better. Should treatment with iron sucrose be contemplated in these patients, a full treatment plan (including monitoring and treatment of hypersensitivity reactions) should be prepared.
* Each millilitre of Venofer injection contains 20 mg of ferric iron as iron (III)-hydroxide sucrose complex.

## Pre-treatment checks

* Not to be given in: history of allergic disorders including asthma and eczema.
* Not be used in the first trimester of pregnancy.
* Do not use in non-iron-deficiency anaemias, e.g. haemolytic anaemias, iron overload or disturbances in utilisation of iron.
* Caution in hepatic impairment; in case of acute or chronic infection (the manufacturer recommends that the administration is stopped in patients with ongoing bacteraemia).
* Owing to the potential risk of anaphylactoid reactions, resuscitation equipment and staff trained to evaluate and treat anaphylaxis should be available whenever a dose of iron sucrose is administered.

*Biochemical and other tests*

Bodyweight

FBC (including Hb)

LFTs

## Dose

The total dose required to treat iron-deficiency anaemia and replenish iron stores is dependent on the initial Hb level and bodyweight (see Dose calculation below).

**Standard dose**: 100–200 mg by IV injection or infusion up to 2–3 times a week until the calculated dose has been given.

**Dose calculation for iron-deficiency anaemia:** the desired dose may be calculated from the following equations (dependent on the unit of measure for Hb) which apply to a bodyweight >35 kg; or use Table I7 below. The dose should be rounded to the nearest easily measurable volume.

*For Hb reported in g/dL:*

Total dose required (mg iron) = [bodyweight (kg) × (target Hb − actual Hb) × 2.4] + 500

*For Hb reported in mmol/L:*

Total dose required (mg iron) = [bodyweight (kg) × (target Hb − actual Hb) × 3.84] + 500

## Intermittent intravenous infusion

*Preparation and administration*

1. Withdraw the required dose and add to a suitable volume of NaCl 0.9% to produce a solution containing no less than 1 mg/mL (i.e. add 100 mg to 50–100 mL; add 200 mg to 100–200 mL).
2. The solution should be brown and clear. Inspect visually for particulate matter or discoloration prior to administration and discard if present.
3. Initial test dose (prior to first dose only): give the first 25 mg by IV infusion over 15 minutes; stop the infusion and observe the patient carefully for signs of allergic reaction; if no adverse effects are seen, give the remainder of the infusion.
4. Give by IV infusion via a volumetric infusion device as follows: give 100 mg over at least 15 minutes; give 200 mg over at least 30 minutes.

## Intravenous injection (or injection into the venous limb of a dialyser)

*Preparation and administration*

1. Withdraw the required dose.
2. The solution should be brown and free of sediment. Inspect visually for particulate matter or discoloration prior to administration and discard if present.
3. Initial test dose (prior to first dose only): give 1 mL of undiluted injection by IV injection over 1–2 minutes. Observe the patient carefully for signs of allergic reaction for at least 15 minutes; if no adverse effects are seen, give the remainder of the injection.
4. Give undiluted injection by IV injection at a maximum rate of 1 mL/minute (i.e. 5 minutes per ampoule).

Table 17  Total dose of venofer for iron-deficiency anaemia in mg (based on bodyweight and initial Hb)

| Bodyweight (kg) | Initial Hb | | | | | | | |
| --- | --- | --- | --- | --- | --- | --- | --- | --- |
| | 6.0 g/dL 3.7 mmol/L | | 7.5 g/dL 4.7 mmol/L | | 9.0 g/dL 5.6 mmol/L | | 10.5 g/dL 6.5 mmol/L | |
| | Total dose (mg iron) | Approx. no. 200-mg doses required | Total dose (mg iron) | Approx. no. 200-mg doses required | Total dose (mg iron) | Approx. no. 200-mg doses required | Total dose (mg iron) | Approx. no. 200-mg doses required |
| 35 | 1250 | 6 | 1150 | 6 | 1000 | 5 | 900 | 5 |
| 40 | 1350 | 7 | 1200 | 6 | 1100 | 6 | 950 | 5 |
| 45 | 1500 | 8 | 1300 | 7 | 1150 | 6 | 1000 | 5 |
| 50 | 1600 | 8 | 1400 | 7 | 1200 | 6 | 1050 | 5 |
| 55 | 1700 | 9 | 1500 | 8 | 1300 | 7 | 1100 | 6 |
| 60 | 1800 | 9 | 1600 | 8 | 1350 | 7 | 1150 | 6 |
| 65 | 1900 | 10 | 1650 | 8 | 1450 | 7 | 1200 | 6 |
| 70 | 2000 | 10 | 1750 | 9 | 1500 | 8 | 1250 | 6 |
| 75 | 2100 | 11 | 1850 | 9 | 1600 | 8 | 1300 | 7 |
| 80 | 2250 | 11 | 1950 | 10 | 1650 | 8 | 1350 | 7 |
| 85 | 2350 | 12 | 2050 | 10 | 1700 | 9 | 1400 | 7 |
| 90 | 2450 | 12 | 2150 | 11 | 1800 | 9 | 1450 | 7 |

## Technical information

| | |
|---|---|
| Incompatible with | No information |
| Compatible with | **Flush**: NaCl 0.9%<br>**Solutions**: NaCl 0.9% (but only at the concentration specified)<br>**Y-site**: No information but likely to be unstable. |
| pH | 10.5-11.1 |
| Sodium content | Negligible |
| Storage | Store below 25°C in original packaging. Do not freeze. |
| Stability after preparation | Use prepared infusions immediately. |

## Monitoring

| Measure | Frequency | Rationale |
|---|---|---|
| Hypersensitivity or intolerance | Throughout administration | • Discontinue therapy immediately if this occurs. |
| Blood pressure | | • ↓BP can occur if IV administration is too rapid. |
| Respiratory observations | | • Respiratory difficulties such as dyspnoea reported. Discontinue treatment if this occurs. |
| Reticulocyte count | Every 3-5 days in acute phase | • Indicative of response (should observe ↑reticulocyte counts within a few days of treatment). |
| Haematocrit and Hb levels | | • Indicative of response. |
| Serum ferritin | | • Indicative of response. |
| Mean cell volume | | • Indicative of response. |
| Total iron-binding capacity | Periodically | • Useful to assess saturation of system when treatment cycle completed, to decide whether response has been satisfactory, and also to assess iron overload. |

## Additional information

| | |
|---|---|
| Common and serious undesirable effects | *Immediate:* Anaphylaxis and other hypersensitivity reactions have been reported.<br>*Injection/infusion-related:*<br>• Too rapid administration: ↓BP.<br>• Local: Injection-site reactions (pain, inflammation, tissue necrosis and brown discoloration of the skin). |

*(continued)*

## Additional information *(continued)*

| | |
|---|---|
| Common and serious undesirable effects | *Other:* Pruritus; urticaria; rash; exanthema; erythema; arthralgia (more common if recommended dose exceeded); headache; dizziness; confusion; metallic taste; pyrexia; shivering; GI disturbances (nausea, vomiting, abdominal pain, diarrhoea); ↑pulse and palpitations; chest pain; peripheral oedema; hyperhidrosis.<br>Chronic repeated administration of iron at high doses can cause liver accumulation, leading to fibrosis as a result of inflammation. |
| Pharmacokinetics | Elimination half-life is 6 hours. |
| Significant interactions | • Iron sucrose may ↑levels or effect of the following drugs (or ↑side-effects): dimercaprol (avoid combination – may result in serious toxicity).<br>• Iron sucrose may ↓levels or effect of oral iron salts (↓absorption – do not start within 5 days of parenteral treatment). |
| Action in case of overdose | *Symptoms to watch for:* Acute iron overload which may appear as haemosiderosis.<br>*Antidote:* Iron chelation therapy can be used. |
| Counselling | Advise the patient to report any hypersensitivity reactions. |

| Risk rating: **AMBER** | Score = 5<br>Moderate-risk product: Risk-reduction strategies are recommended. |
|---|---|

This assessment is based on the full range of preparation and administration options described in the monograph. These may not all be applicable in some clinical situations.

### Bibliography

SPC Venofer (accessed 24 August 2009).

# Isoniazid

### 25 mg/mL solution in 2-mL ampoules

* Isoniazid is a hydrazide derivative that is bactericidal against actively dividing *Mycobacterium tuberculosis*.
* It is used as part of multidrug regimens in the primary treatment of pulmonary and extrapulmonary tuberculosis and for tuberculosis prophylaxis in high-risk subjects.
* Isoniazid is well absorbed from the GI tract following oral dosing, so parenteral routes should be used only when the oral route is unavailable.

- Pyridoxine (10–50 mg daily) is commonly co-prescribed with isoniazid to those predisposed to peripheral neuropathy, e.g. malnourishment, chronic renal impairment, diabetes, HIV infection, and in alcohol dependence.
- Isoniazid injection is also licensed for intrapleural use (50–250 mg is instilled intrapleurally after aspiration of pus; the oral dose is correspondingly reduced on the same day) and for intrathecal use. It may also be used to treat infected ulcers and irrigate fistulae.

## Pre-treatment checks

- Caution if there is a history of seizures or psychotic reactions (↑risk).
- Check drug interactions if the patient is on antiepileptic drugs.
- If the patient is a 'slow acetylator' (genetically determined metabolic pathway) they may be more susceptible to drug-induced peripheral neuropathy (in rare instances this may require a dose reduction to 200 mg daily).
- Caution also in alcohol dependence, malnutrition, diabetes mellitus, HIV infection (risk of peripheral neuropathy) and acute porphyria.

*Biochemical and other tests*

LFTs (use cautiously in chronic alcoholism and pre-existing hepatitis)
Renal function: U, Cr, CrCl (or eGFR)

## Dose

**Dose for 2-month initial and 4-month continuation phases:** 300 mg as a single daily dose.
**Dose for intermittent supervised 6-month treatment:** 15 mg/kg (max. 900 mg) 3 times a week.
**Dose in renal impairment:** in patients with CrCl <10 mL/minute the dose *may* need to be reduced to 200 mg daily (see Monitoring below).

## Intramuscular injection

*Preparation and administration*

1. Withdraw the required dose.
2. Give by IM injection. Volumes > 4 mL should be distributed between two or more injection sites.

## Intravenous injection

*Preparation and administration*

Isoniazid is incompatible with Gluc 5%.

1. Withdraw the required dose.
2. The solution should be clear and colourless. Inspect visually for particulate matter or discoloration prior to administration and discard if present.
3. Give by IV injection over 3–5 minutes.

| Technical information | |
|---|---|
| Incompatible with | Isoniazid is incompatible with Gluc 5%. |
| Compatible with | **Flush**: NaCl 0.9%<br>**Solutions**: NaCl 0.9%<br>**Y-site**: No information |
| pH | 5.6-7 |

*(continued)*

## Technical information (continued)

| | |
|---|---|
| Sodium content | Nil |
| Storage | Store below 25°C in original packaging. |

## Monitoring

| Measure | Frequency | Rationale |
|---|---|---|
| LFTs | Monthly | • May induce abnormalities in LFTs especially if given with rifampicin, in patients with pre-existing liver disorders, and in elderly, very young and malnourished patients.<br>• Stop therapy if ALT and AST exceed 3 times the ULN. |
| Signs of hepatic toxicity | Throughout treatment | • Discontinue treatment if symptoms develop: persistent fatigue, weakness or fever exceeding 3 days, malaise, nausea, vomiting, unexplained anorexia or jaundice. |
| Signs of peripheral neuritis | | • The first sign is usually paraesthesia of the feet and hands.<br>• Use pyridoxine 50 mg three times daily. |
| Signs of optic neuritis | | • Symptoms may include blurred or loss of vision and require investigation.<br>• Some authorities recommend that baseline and follow-up visual evoked potentials (VEP) should be performed in patients receiving concomitant ethambutol. |
| Signs of hypersensitivity reaction | | • Symptoms may include fever, skin eruptions (morbilliform, maculopapular, purpuric, exfoliative), lymphadenopathy, vasculitis, and (rarely) ↓BP.<br>• Discontinue therapy (and other antituberculous drugs).<br>• If reinstituted, it should be in small, gradually increasing doses only after symptoms have cleared. If there is any sign of hypersensitivity recurrence, isoniazid should be discontinued immediately. |
| Renal function | Periodically | • Changes in renal function may require a dose adjustment. |
| Plasma isoniazid concentration | If indicated | • Rarely required; may be necessary to check that dose is appropriate in severe renal impairment.<br>• Target trough plasma level <1 microgram/mL. |

## Additional information

| | |
|---|---|
| Common and serious undesirable effects | Nausea, vomiting, constipation, fever, peripheral neuropathy (preventable with pyridoxine), optic neuritis and atrophy, allergic skin conditions, hyperglycaemia, gynaecomastia |
| Pharmacokinetics | Elimination half-life is 0.7-2 hours in 'rapid acetylators'; 2.3-3.5 hours in 'slow acetylators'. |

(continued)

| **Additional information** *(continued)* | |
|---|---|
| Significant interactions | • Carbamazepine may ↑risk of isoniazid-related hepatotoxicity.<br>• Isoniazid may ↑levels of the following drugs (or ↑side-effects): carbamazepine (monitor levels), ethosuximide, phenytoin (monitor levels). |
| Action in case of overdose | *Symptoms to watch for:* Large doses have been associated with seizures.<br>*Antidote:* No known antidote but haemodialysis may be effective. Stop administration and give supportive therapy as appropriate to control seizures (use of phenytoin is not advised), pyridoxine may control other symptoms. |
| Counselling | Patients should be warned to report any signs of hepatic toxicity or neuritis immediately. |

| Risk rating: **GREEN** | Score = 1<br>Lower-risk product: Risk-reduction strategies should be considered. |
|---|---|

This assessment is based on the full range of preparation and administration options described in the monograph. These may not all be applicable in some clinical situations.

## Bibliography

SPC Isoniazid ampoules 50 mg/2 mL, Cambridge Laboratories (accessed 24 March 2009).

# Isosorbide dinitrate (ISDN)

**500 micrograms/mL (0.05%) solution in 50-mL vials**
**1 mg/mL (0.1%) solution in 10-mL ampoules; 50-mL and 100-mL vials**

• Isosorbide dinitrate is a vasodilator that relaxes smooth vascular muscle, reducing cardiac filling pressure and volume (pre-load) and lowering myocardial oxygen demand.
• It is used in the treatment of unresponsive left ventricular failure of various aetiologies and severe to unstable angina pectoris.
• It is also is used during percutaneous transluminal coronary angioplasty to facilitate prolongation of balloon inflation and to prevent or relieve coronary spasm.

## Pre-treatment checks

• Contraindicated in severe anaemia, ↑intracranial pressure due to head trauma or cerebral haemorrhage, uncorrected hypovolaemia and hypotensive shock, arterial hypoxaemia and angina caused by hypertrophic obstructive cardiomyopathy, constrictive pericarditis, pericardial tamponade or toxic pulmonary oedema.
• Caution in severe renal/hepatic impairment, hypothyroidism, malnutrition, or hypothermia.

*Biochemical and other tests (not all are necessary in an emergency situation)*

| | |
|---|---|
| Blood pressure | LFTs |
| Electrolytes: serum Na, K | Renal function: U, Cr, CrCl (or eGFR) |
| Heart rate | TFTs |

## Dose

**Unresponsive left ventricular failure of various aetiologies and severe angina pectoris**: initially 2 mg/hour titrated against individual clinical response (usual range is 2–12 mg/hour but up to 20 mg/hour may be required).

## Continuous intravenous infusion via syringe pump

*Preparation and administration*

> Avoid use of PVC infusion containers, administration sets and in-line filters if possible. Rigid plastics, i.e. polyethylene or polypropylene administration sets and syringes, should be used if available.

1. Withdraw 50 mL of the 500 micrograms/mL strength into a syringe suitable for use with a syringe pump. Alternatively, withdraw 25 mL of the 1 mg/mL strength and make up to 50 mL with NaCl 0.9%. Cap the syringe and mix well to give a solution containing 500 micrograms/mL.
2. The solution should be clear and colourless. Inspect visually for particulate matter or discoloration prior to administration and discard if present.
3. Give by IV infusion using a syringe pump. For most indications the starting infusion rate is 2 mg/hour (4 mL/hour). Adjust dose to clinical response as indicated above.

## Technical information

| | |
|---|---|
| Incompatible with | Avoid use of PVC infusion containers, administration sets and in-line filters if possible. Rigid plastics, i.e. polyethylene or polypropylene administration sets and syringes, should be used if available.<br>Heparin sodium. |
| Compatible with | **Flush**: NaCl 0.9%<br>**Solutions**: NaCl 0.9%, Gluc 5%<br>**Y-site**: Furosemide |
| pH | 3.5-7.0 |
| Sodium content | 7.5 mmol/50 mL |
| Storage | Store below 30°C in original packaging.<br>All ampoules/vials are single use only - discard any unused portion. |
| Stability after preparation | From a microbiological point of view, should be used immediately; however, prepared infusions may be stored at 2-8°C and infused (at room temperature) within 24 hours provided use of PVC containers is avoided. |

## Monitoring

| Measure | Frequency | Rationale |
|---|---|---|
| Blood pressure | Continuously | • ↓BP may occur. |
| Heart rate | | • ↑Pulse may occur (↓pulse occurs very rarely). |

*(continued)*

## Monitoring (continued)

| Measure | Frequency | Rationale |
|---------|-----------|-----------|
| Angina pain and symptoms | Continuously | • To monitor therapeutic response. |
| Pulmonary capillary wedge pressure, cardiac output and precordial ECG (depending on the clinical picture) | | • To monitor therapeutic response. |
| Response to therapy | Daily | • Relative haemodynamic and antianginal tolerance may develop during prolonged infusions; titrate the dose accordingly. |

## Additional information

| | |
|---|---|
| Common and serious undesirable effects | All effects are reversible on infusion rate reduction or discontinuation. Headache, dizziness, flushing, ↓BP, ↑pulse (all these are especially likely if the infusion is too rapid). Also nausea, diaphoresis, restlessness, retrosternal discomfort, abdominal pain and paradoxical ↓pulse. |
| Pharmacokinetics | Serum half-life is about 20 minutes. Active metabolites are longer acting. |
| Significant interactions | • The following may ↑ isosorbide dinitrate levels or effect (or ↑side-effects): other hypotensive drugs; phosphodiesterase type-5 inhibitors (sildenafil is contraindicated). |
| Action in case of overdose | Symptoms are rapidly reversed by discontinuing treatment; if ↓BP persists, raising the foot of the bed and the use of a vasoconstrictor such as IV phenylephrine are recommended. |
| Counselling | Advise of risk of headache and symptoms of ↓BP. |

| | |
|---|---|
| Risk rating: **AMBER** | Score = 4<br>Moderate-risk product: Risk-reduction strategies are recommended. |

This assessment is based on the full range of preparation and administration options described in the monograph. These may not all be applicable in some clinical situations.

## Bibliography

SPC Isoket 0.05%, Isoket 0.1% (accessed 28 April 2009).

# Itraconazole

**10 mg/mL solution in 25-mL vials (with 50 mL NaCl 0.9% infusion bag and in-line filter)**
* Itraconazole is a triazole antifungal drug.
* It is used in the treatment of systemic aspergillosis, candidiasis and cryptococcosis including cryptococcal meningitis where other antifungal drugs are inappropriate or ineffective, and also in histoplasmosis.

## Pre-treatment checks

* Check drug interactions for contraindications.
* The UK CSM has advised caution in patients at high risk of heart failure, i.e. patients receiving high doses and longer treatment courses, older patients and those with cardiac disease, and patients receiving treatment with negative inotropic drugs, e.g. calcium channel antagonists.
* Oral absorption is reduced in AIDS and neutropenia (↑dose if necessary).

*Biochemical tests*

| | |
|---|---|
| Electrolytes: serum K | LFTs |
| FBC | Renal function: U, Cr, CrCl (or eGFR) |

## Dose

**Standard dose**: 200-mg by IV infusion twice daily for 2 days, then 200 mg daily by IV infusion for up to 12 days.
**Dose in renal impairment:** do not use if CrCl < 30 mL/minute.
**Dose in hepatic impairment**: use with caution only if benefit exceeds the risk of hepatic injury.

## Intermittent intravenous infusion

Vials (and prepared infusions) contain an overage. When the infusion is prepared as directed, a 200-mg dose is contained in 60 mL.
The infusion must be stopped after 200 mg (60 mL) has been given.

*Preparation*

1. Withdraw the entire vial contents and add to the 50-mL bag of NaCl 0.9% provided (no other bag should be used).
2. Gently mix the contents of the infusion bag to give a solution containing 3.33 mg/mL (200 mg/ 60 mL).
3. The solution should be clear and colourless. Inspect visually for particulate matter or discoloration prior to administration and discard if present.

*Administration*

1. Attach a standard infusion line to the infusion bag and fill the drip chamber to half full by squeezing (pumping) it.
2. Connect the infusion line to the two-way stop cock provided, which includes a 0.2 micron in-line filter, and prime the line. Exposure to normal room light during infusion is acceptable, but protect from direct sunlight.
3. Give by IV infusion via a volumetric infusion device at a rate of 60 mL/hour. Administer 60 mL only of the solution over 60 minutes then stop the infusion (this provides the 200-mg dose).
4. Flush the extension line with 15–20 mL NaCl 0.9% at the two-way stop cock (just before the in-line filter), allowing the flush to run continuously for between 30 seconds and 15 minutes.

## Technical information

| | |
|---|---|
| Incompatible with | Itraconazole is incompatible with Gluc 5%, Gluc-NaCl, Hartmann's, Ringer's (precipitation likely).<br>Do not mix with other drugs during infusion. |
| Compatible with | **Flush**: NaCl 0.9%<br>**Solutions**: NaCl 0.9%<br>**Y-site**: No information but likely to be unstable. |
| pH | 4.5 |
| Sodium content | 7.7 mmol (from 50-mL infusion bag) |
| Excipients | Contains propylene glycol (adverse effects seen in ↓renal function, may interact with disulfiram and metronidazole). |
| Storage | Store below 25°C in original packaging. |
| Stability after preparation | Protect from direct sunlight during infusion - exposure to normal room light is acceptable.<br>From a microbiological point of view, should be used immediately; however, prepared infusions may be stored at 2-8°C and infused (at room temperature) within 24 hours. |

## Monitoring

| Measure | Frequency | Rationale |
|---|---|---|
| Renal function | 2-3 times weekly | • A component of the formulation, hydroxypropyl-$\beta$-cyclodextrin, is eliminated through glomerular filtration and this causes the caution in renal impairment.<br>• In mild and moderate renal impairment serum Cr levels should be closely monitored - if renal toxicity is suspected consider switching to the oral formulation.<br>• ↓K commonly occurs - if severe it may require potassium replacement and/or cessation of treatment. |
| LFTs | 2-3 times weekly in first week then weekly | • Hepatitis, jaundice, ↑liver enzymes occur commonly.<br>• Very rarely serious hepatotoxicity including fatal acute liver failure has occurred, sometimes within the first week of treatment.<br>• Patients reporting signs and symptoms suggestive of hepatitis should have treatment stopped immediately. |
| Signs and symptoms of neuropathy or congestive heart failure | Throughout treatment | • If these occur, stop treatment immediately. |

## Additional information

| | |
|---|---|
| Common and serious undesirable effects | Headache, dizziness, nausea, abdominal pain, vomiting, diarrhoea, constipation, rash, pruritus, oedema, ↓K, nephrotoxicity, hepatitis, jaundice, ↑LFTs, severe hepatotoxicity |
| Pharmacokinetics | Elimination half-life is 35–64 hours. |
| Significant interactions | • Ritonavir may ↑itraconazole levels or effect (or ↑side-effects).<br>• The following may ↓itraconazole levels or effect: phenytoin (avoid combination), rifabutin (avoid combination), rifampicin.<br>• Avoid combination of itraconazole with the following drugs: artemether-lumefantrine, atorvastatin (↑risk of myopathy), disopyramide, eletriptan, eplerenone, ergotamine, ivabradine, lapatinib, methysergide, mizolastine, nilotinib, pimozide (↑risk of ventricular arrhythmias), ranolazine, reboxetine, rifabutin (↑risk of uveitis), simvastatin (↑risk of myopathy), sertindole (↑risk of ventricular arrhythmias), sirolimus, vardenafil<br>• Itraconazole may ↑levels or effect of the following drugs (or ↑side-effects): aripiprazole (↓dose aripiprazole), ciclosporin (monitor levels), coumarin anticoagulants (monitor INR), digoxin, felodipine, indinavir (consider ↓dose indinavir), midazolam (risk of prolonged sedation), ritonavir, tacrolimus (↑plasma levels), vincristine (↑risk of neurotoxicity). |
| Action in case of overdose | There is no specific antidote and it is not removed by haemodialysis. General supportive methods should be employed. |
| Counselling | Patients should be told how to recognise signs of liver disorder and advised to seek prompt medical attention if symptoms such as anorexia, nausea, vomiting, fatigue, abdominal pain or dark urine develop. |

Risk rating: **AMBER**  Score = 4
Moderate-risk product: Risk-reduction strategies are recommended.

This assessment is based on the full range of preparation and administration options described in the monograph. These may not all be applicable in some clinical situations.

## Bibliography

SPC Sporanox IV (accessed 24 March 2009).

# Ketamine

**10 mg/mL solution in 20-mL vials; 50 mg/mL solution in 10-mL vials; 100 mg/mL solution in 10-mL vials**

* Ketamine hydrochloride is a general anaesthetic agent.
* It is used for the induction and maintenance of anaesthesia and as a supplementary anaesthetic.
* It may also be used (unlicensed) for its analgesic action in neuropathic and other pain unresponsive to conventional analgesics. Routes of administration and doses used vary widely.
* Ketamine has abuse potential; if it is used regularly for a few weeks, dependence and tolerance may develop.
* Doses are expressed in terms of the base:
  Ketamine 1 mg ≅ 15 mg ketamine hydrochloride.

## Pre-treatment checks

* Avoid in patients where ↑BP may be dangerous, patients with eclampsia or pre-eclampsia, severe coronary or myocardial disease, cerebrovascular accident or cerebral trauma.
* Caution in patients with mild to moderate ↑BP, those with ↑cerebrospinal fluid pressure, and those with chronic alcoholism or acutely alcohol intoxicated.
* If it is being used for elective surgery, ensure that the patient has been nil by mouth for 6 hours prior to anaesthesia.

*Biochemical and other tests*

Blood pressure
Bodyweight

## Dose

**Short procedures by IM injection:** initially 6.5–13 mg/kg. A dose of 4 mg/kg is used for diagnostic manoeuvres and procedures not involving intense pain. A dose of 10 mg/kg will usually produce 12–25 minutes of surgical anaesthesia.

**Short procedures by IV injection:** initially 1–4.5 mg/kg. A dose of 2 mg/kg will usually produce 5–10 minutes of surgical anaesthesia.

**For induction and longer procedures by IV infusion**: at induction use a total dose of 0.5–2 mg/kg; for maintenance use 10–45 micrograms/kg/minute adjusted according to patient response.

## Intramuscular injection

*Preparation and administration*

Check that you have selected the correct strength of vial.

1. Withdraw the required dose.
2. Give by IM injection.

## Intravenous injection

*Preparation and administration*

Check that you have selected the correct strength of vial.

1. Withdraw the required dose.
2. If using the 100 mg/mL strength dilute with an equal volume of WFI, NaCl 0.9% or Gluc 5%.
3. The solution should be clear and colourless to slightly yellow. Inspect visually for particulate matter or discoloration prior to administration and discard if present.
4. Give by IV injection over at least 60 seconds.

## Continuous intravenous infusion

*Preparation and administration*

Check that you have selected the correct strength of vial.

1. Withdraw 500 mg of ketamine.
2. Remove an equivalent volume of infusion fluid from a 500-mL bag of NaCl 0.9% or Gluc 5%.
3. Add the ketamine to the prepared infusion bag to give a solution containing 1 mg/mL. Mix well. (Alternatively, following the same procedure, add 500 mg to 250 mL infusion fluid to give a solution containing 2 mg/mL.)
4. The solution should be clear and colourless to slightly yellow. Inspect visually for particulate matter or discoloration prior to administration and discard if present.
5. Give by continuous IV infusion via a volumetric infusion device. The rate of infusion is dependent on the patient's reaction and response to anaesthesia.

**Fluid restriction:** solutions containing up to 50 mg/mL have been used (unlicensed).

## Technical information

| | |
|---|---|
| Incompatible with | Barbiturates, diazepam. |
| Compatible with | **Flush**: NaCl 0.9%<br>**Solutions**: Gluc 5%, NaCl 0.9%<br>**Y-site**: Propofol |
| pH | 3.5-5.5 |
| Sodium content | Negligible |
| Storage | Store below 30°C in original packaging. Do not freeze. The drug may darken on prolonged exposure to light; this darkening does not appear to affect potency. |
| Stability after preparation | Use prepared infusions immediately. |

## Monitoring

| Measure | Frequency | Rationale |
|---------|-----------|-----------|
| Cardiac function | Continually during procedure | • Monitor during the procedure in patients with ↑BP or cardiac decompensation. |
| Respiratory depression | Post administration | • May occur with over-rapid administration or overdosage of ketamine. |
| Blood pressure and pulse | Postoperative | • May cause ↑BP and ↑pulse. |
| Emergence of psychiatric symptoms | | • High incidence of symptoms such as hallucinations, anxiety, dysphoria, insomnia or disorientation. Less common in children and elderly patients. |

## Additional information

| | |
|---|---|
| Common and serious undesirable effects | *Immediate:* Anaphylaxis has been reported rarely.<br>*Injection-related:*<br>• Too rapid administration: Respiratory depression.<br>• Local: Injection-site reactions; extravasation may cause tissue damage.<br><br>*Other:* Arrhythmias, ↑ or ↓pulse, ↑ or ↓BP, ↑salivation, laryngospasm; anxiety, insomnia; diplopia, nystagmus, ↑intraocular pressure; rashes, ↑muscle tone. Vivid dreams and psychiatric symptoms on emergence from anaesthesia. |
| Pharmacokinetics | Elimination half-life is approximately 2–3 hours. |
| Significant interactions | Barbiturates or narcotics may ↑ketamine levels or effect (or ↑side-effects) (prolonged recovery time). |
| Action in case of overdose | *Symptoms to watch for:* Respiratory depression.<br>*Antidote:* No known antidote; stop administration and give supportive therapy as appropriate. |

| Risk rating: **AMBER** | Score = 4<br>Moderate-risk product. Risk-reduction strategies are recommended. |
|---|---|

This assessment is based on the full range of preparation and administration options described in the monograph. These may not all be applicable in some clinical situations.

## Bibliography

SPC Ketalar (accessed 11 November 2008).

# Ketoprofen

**50 mg/mL solution in 2-mL ampoules**
* Ketoprofen is a non-steroidal anti-inflammatory drug (NSAID).
* It may be given by the IM route for the management of pain and inflammation in acute exacerbations of rheumatic disease and other musculoskeletal disorders.

## Pre-treatment checks

* Do not administer to patients with active peptic ulceration or a history of recurrent peptic ulceration or chronic dyspepsia, severe renal failure, sensitivity to aspirin or other NSAIDs, severe heart failure.
* Use with caution in renal impairment.

*Biochemical and other tests*

Blood pressure
Renal function: U, Cr, CrCl (or eGFR)

## Dose

**All indications**: 50–100 mg every 4 hours up to a maximum of 200 mg in 24 hours. The injection should not normally be used for more than 3 days.
**Dose in renal impairment:** dose as in normal renal function but avoid if possible.

## Intramuscular injection

*Preparation and administration*

1. Withdraw the required dose.
2. Give by deep IM injection into the gluteal muscle.

## Technical information

| | |
|---|---|
| Incompatible with | Not relevant |
| Compatible with | Not relevant |
| pH | Not relevant |
| Sodium content | Nil |
| Excipients | Contains benzyl alcohol. |
| Storage | Store below 30°C in original packaging. |

## Monitoring

| Measure | Frequency | Rationale |
|---------|-----------|-----------|
| Pain | Post injection | • To ensure that treatment is effective. |
| Injection site | | • Injection-site reactions have occurred. |
| Blood pressure | Periodically | • May cause ↑BP. |
| Renal function | | • In patients with renal impairment or if on long-term NSAIDs. |

## Additional information

| | |
|---|---|
| Common and serious undesirable effects | *Immediate:* Anaphylaxis and other hypersensitivity reactions may occur. <br> *Injection-related:* Local: Temporary pain on injection. <br> *Other:* GI side-effects, skin reactions, oedema, ↑BP, cardiac failure. |
| Pharmacokinetics | Elimination half-life is approximately 1.88 hours. |
| Significant interactions | • The following may ↑risk of bleeding with ketoprofen: antidepressants-SSRIs, aspirin, dabigatran, erlotinib, ketorolac, NSAIDs, venlafaxine. <br> • Ketoprofen may ↑levels or effect of the following drugs (or ↑side-effects): ciclosporin (↑risk of nephrotoxicity), coumarin anticoagulants (monitor INR), lithium (monitor levels), methotrexate (↑toxicity, avoid combination), phenindione (monitor INR), phenytoin (monitor levels), quinolones (↑risk of seizures), sulfonylureas. <br> • Probenecid may ↑ketoprofen levels or effect (or ↑side-effects): avoid combination. |
| Action in case of overdose | *Antidote:* No known antidote; stop administration and give supportive therapy as appropriate. |

| | |
|---|---|
| Risk rating: **GREEN** | Score = 1 <br> Lower-risk product. Risk-reduction strategies should be considered. |

This assessment is based on the full range of preparation and administration options described in the monograph. These may not all be applicable in some clinical situations.

## Bibliography

SPC Oruvail IM injection (accessed 15 October 2008).

# Ketorolac trometamol

**10 mg/mL and 30 mg/mL solution in 1-mL ampoules**
* Ketorolac trometamol is a non-steroidal anti-inflammatory drug (NSAID).
* It is used for the short-term management of moderate to severe acute postoperative pain.

## Pre-treatment checks

* Avoid in active or previous peptic ulcer, cerebrovascular bleeding, haemorrhagic diatheses, the complete or partial syndrome of nasal polyps, angioedema or bronchospasm, hypovolaemia or dehydration, moderate or severe renal impairment (Cr >160 micromol/L) and severe heart failure.
* Do not use in patients who have had operations with a high risk of haemorrhage or incomplete haemostasis or during pregnancy, labour, delivery or lactation.
* Do not give to women attempting to conceive as the use of ketorolac may impair female fertility.
* Do not give with aspirin or other NSAIDs (including COX 2 inhibitors), pentoxifylline, probenecid, lithium or patients on anticoagulants (including low-dose heparin).
* Caution in uncontrolled ↑BP, heart failure, ischaemic heart disease and cerebrovascular disease.

*Biochemical and other tests (not all are necessary in an emergency situation)*

| | |
|---|---|
| Blood pressure | FBC |
| Bodyweight | Renal function: U, Cr, CrCl (or eGFR) |

## Dose

**Postoperative pain**: 10 mg by IM or IV injection followed by 10–30 mg every 4–6 hours as required.
* In the initial postoperative period ketorolac may be given every 2 hours if needed.
* Maximum daily dose: 90 mg (60 mg for elderly patients and patients <50 kg bodyweight; 40 mg for oral therapy).
* Convert to oral medication as soon as practicable; the oral dose should not exceed 40 mg on the day the formulation is changed and the combined daily dose should not exceed the maximum daily dose.
* Because of the high incidence of reported adverse effects, in the UK the maximum licensed duration of therapy is: parenteral therapy 2 days; oral therapy 7 days.

**Dose in renal impairment**: adjusted according to creatinine clearance.
* CrCl >20–50 mL/minute: maximum 60 mg daily.
* CrCl <10–20 mL/minute: avoid if possible.

## Intramuscular Injection

*Preparation and administration*

1. Withdraw the required dose.
2. Give by IM injection.

## Intravenous injection

*Preparation and administration*

1. Withdraw the required dose.
2. The solution should be clear and colourless or slightly yellow. Inspect visually for particulate matter or discoloration prior to administration and discard if present.
3. Give by IV injection over at least 15 seconds.

## Technical information

| | |
|---|---|
| Incompatible with | No information |
| Compatible with | **Flush**: NaCl 0.9%<br>**Solutions**: NaCl 0.9%, Gluc 5%, Gluc-NaCl, Hartmann's, Ringer's<br>**Y-site**: Cisatracurium, fentanyl, remifentanil |
| pH | 6.9-7.9 |
| Sodium content | Negligible |
| Excipients | Contains ethanol (may interact with metronidazole; possible religious objections). |
| Storage | Store below 30°C in original packaging. Do not refrigerate or freeze. |

## Monitoring

| Measure | Frequency | Rationale |
|---|---|---|
| Reduction of pain | Postoperative | • To ensure that treatment is effective.<br>• For some patients pain relief may not occur until 30 minutes after administration. |
| Blood pressure | Postoperative and periodically | • May ↑BP. |
| FBC, U&Es | Daily for 2 days (then 6–12 months if on long-term therapy) | • May cause ↑K, ↓Na.<br>• May affect renal function.<br>• May cause ↓Hb due to gastric bleeding. |

## Additional information

| | |
|---|---|
| Common and serious undesirable effects | *Immediate:* Anaphylaxis and other hypersensitivity reactions may occur.<br>*Injection-related:* Local: Temporary pain on injection.<br>*Other:* GI side-effects, skin reactions, oedema, ↑BP, cardiac failure, postoperative bleeding. |
| Pharmacokinetics | Elimination half-life is about 5 hours. |
| Significant interactions | • The following may ↑risk of bleeding with ketorolac: antidepressants-SSRIs, aspirin, dabigatran, erlotinib, heparin (low dose), NSAIDs, pentoxifylline, venlafaxine.<br>• Ketorolac may ↑levels or effect of the following drugs (or ↑side-effects): ciclosporin (↑risk of nephrotoxicity), coumarin anticoagulants (monitor INR), lithium (monitor levels), methotrexate (↑toxicity, avoid combination), phenindione (monitor INR), phenytoin (monitor levels), quinolones (↑risk of seizures), sulfonylureas.<br>• Probenecid may ↑ketorolac levels or effect (or ↑side-effects): avoid concomitant use. |
| Action in case of overdose | *Antidote:* No known antidote. Stop administration and give supportive therapy as appropriate. |

| Risk rating: **GREEN** | Score = 1<br>Lower-risk product. Risk-reduction strategies should be considered. |
|---|---|

This assessment is based on the full range of preparation and administration options described in the monograph. These may not all be applicable in some clinical situations.

## Bibliography

SPC Toradol (accessed 14 November 2008).
SPC Ketorolac 30 mg/mL, Beacon Pharmaceuticals (accessed 14 November 2008).

# Labetalol hydrochloride

**5 mg/mL solution in 20-mL ampoules**

* Labetalol hydrochloride is a mixed alpha- and beta-adrenoceptor blocker that lowers BP by decreasing peripheral vascular resistance.
* It is used IV for rapid control of severe ↑BP, including severe ↑BP of pregnancy.
* Patients should always receive the drug while in the supine or left lateral position. Raising the patient into the upright position within 3 hours of dosing should be avoided since excessive postural ↓BP may occur.

## Pre-treatment checks

* Treatment should be avoided in sick sinus syndrome, ↓BP, heart block greater than first degree, ↓pulse (<45–50 bpm), cardiogenic shock and overt heart failure.
* Use with caution in patients with a history of wheezing or asthma and peripheral circulatory conditions.

*Biochemical and other tests (not all are necessary in an emergency situation)*

Blood pressure
LFTs
Pulse

## Dose

**For rapid reduction of BP:** 50 mg by IV injection repeated at 5-minute intervals as necessary until a satisfactory response occurs. The total dose should not exceed 200 mg.

**Hypotensive anaesthesia:** the recommended starting dose is 10–20 mg by IV injection depending on the age and condition of the patient. Patients for whom halothane is contraindicated usually require a higher initial dose of 25–30 mg. If satisfactory ↓BP is not achieved after 5 minutes, additional doses of 5–10 mg should be given at 5-minute intervals until the desired response is achieved.

**Hypertension of pregnancy:** initially 20 mg/hour by IV infusion. The dose may be doubled every 30 minutes until a satisfactory response or a dosage of 160 mg/hour is reached. Occasionally, higher doses may be necessary.

**Hypertensive episodes following acute MI:** 15 mg/hour by IV infusion, gradually increased to a maximum of 120 mg/hour as necessary.

**Hypertension due to other causes:** 2 mg/minute by IV infusion until a satisfactory response is obtained; the infusion should then be stopped. The effective cumulative dose is usually in the range of 50–200 mg depending on the severity of the ↑BP. Larger doses may be required particularly in patients with phaeochromocytoma.

## Intravenous injection

*Preparation and administration*

1. Withdraw the required dose.
2. The solution should be clear and colourless. Inspect visually for particulate matter or discoloration prior to administration. Discard if present.
3. Give by IV injection over at least 1 minute.

## Continuous intravenous infusion

*Preparation of a 1 mg/mL solution (other strengths may be used)*

1. Withdraw and discard 10 mL from a 250-mL infusion bag containing compatible infusion fluid (usually Gluc 5%).

2. Withdraw 300 mg (60 mL) of labetalol injection solution from three ampoules using a syringe and add to the remaining 240 mL of infusion fluid and mix well. This gives a solution containing 1 mg/mL.
3. The solution should be clear and colourless. Inspect visually for particulate matter or discoloration prior to administration and discard if present.

*Administration*

Give by IV infusion via a volumetric infusion device at a rate appropriate to dosing regimen.

**Fluid restriction:** there are anecdotal reports of undiluted injection solution being given (unlicensed) via syringe pump in critical care situations.

## Technical information

| Incompatible with | Sodium bicarbonate.<br>Amphotericin, ceftriaxone, furosemide, heparin sodium, insulin (soluble), micafungin. |
|---|---|
| Compatible with | **Flush**: NaCl 0.9%<br>**Solutions**: Gluc 5%, Gluc-NaCl, NaCl 0.9%, Hartmann's, Ringer's (all with added KCl)<br>**Y-site**: Adrenaline (epinephrine), amikacin, aminophylline, ampicillin, benzylpenicillin, calcium gluconate, ceftazidime, chloramphenicol sodium succinate, clindamycin phosphate, co-trimoxazole, dobutamine, dopamine, erythromycin lactobionate, fentanyl, gentamicin, glyceryl trinitrate, linezolid, magnesium sulfate, metronidazole, midazolam, noradrenaline (norepinephrine), propofol, ranitidine, tobramycin, vancomycin, vecuronium |
| pH | 3-4.5 |
| Sodium content | Negligible |
| Storage | Store below 30°C in original packaging. |
| Stability after preparation | From a microbiological point of view, should be used immediately; however, prepared infusions may be stored at 2-8°C and infused (at room temperature) within 24 hours. |

## Monitoring

| Measure | Frequency | Rationale |
|---|---|---|
| Blood pressure | 5 minutes after IV injection, and continuously during infusion if possible | • Response to therapy.<br>• After IV injection the duration of action is usually about 6 hours but may be as long as 18 hours. |
| Heart rate | | • In most patients, there is a small decrease in heart rate.<br>• Excessive ↓pulse can be countered with IV atropine sulfate in doses of 600 micrograms repeated every 3-5 minutes up to a maximum of 2.4 mg. |
| Respiratory function or oxygen saturation in at risk individuals | After initial dosing | • May cause bronchoconstriction in susceptible individuals, e.g. patients with history of bronchospasm or respiratory disease. |
| Infusion site | Every 30 minutes | • Extravasation may cause tissue damage. |

*(continued)*

## Monitoring (continued)

| Measure | Frequency | Rationale |
|---------|-----------|-----------|
| LFTs | Periodically | • Severe hepatocellular damage has been reported after both short-term and long-term treatment.<br>• Check at first symptom of liver dysfunction and if there is laboratory evidence of damage (or if there is jaundice) therapy should be stopped and not restarted. |

## Additional information

| | |
|---|---|
| Common and serious undesirable effects | *Common:* Headache, tiredness, dizziness, orthostatic ↓BP. Paraesthesia, usually mild, transient tingling of the scalp or skin. Bronchospasm may occur in patients with asthma or other respiratory disease.<br>*Rare:* Hepatocellular injury; LFTs should be checked at the first sign or symptom of liver dysfunction. |
| Elimination half-life | The plasma half-life of labetalol is about 4 hours. |
| Significant drug interactions | • The following may ↑labetalol levels or effect (or ↑side-effects): adrenaline (risk of severe ↑BP and ↓pulse), alpha-blockers (severe ↓BP), amiodarone (risk of ↓pulse and AV block), antiarrhythmics (risk of myocardial depression), clonidine (↑risk of withdrawal ↑BP), diltiazem (risk of ↓pulse and AV block), dobutamine (risk of severe ↑BP and ↓pulse), flecainide (risk of myocardial depression and ↓pulse), moxisylyte (severe ↓BP), nifedipine (severe ↓BP and heart failure), noradrenaline (risk of severe ↑BP and ↓pulse), verapamil (risk of asystole and severe ↓BP). |
| Overdose | *Symptoms to watch for:* ↓Pulse, ↓BP, acute cardiac insufficiency and bronchospasm.<br>*Antidote:* Excessive ↓pulse can be countered with IV atropine sulfate (see Monitoring above and the Atropine monograph). Glucagon or dobutamine are further options for unresponsive ↓pulse – seek specialist advice. Bronchospasm can usually be reversed by bronchodilators. |
| Counselling | Patients may experience fatigue and cold extremities during maintenance therapy, and should report wheezing. |

| Risk rating: **AMBER** | Score = 3<br>Moderate-risk product: Risk-reduction strategies are recommended. |
|---|---|

This assessment is based on the full range of preparation and administration options described in the monograph. These may not all be applicable in some clinical situations.

## Bibliography

SPC Trandate injection (accessed 16 February 2010).

# Lacosamide

**10 mg/mL solution in 20-mL vials**

- Lacosamide is an antiepileptic agent.
- It is used as adjunctive therapy in partial seizures with or without secondary generalisation in patients aged 16 years and older.
- It is used parenterally in patients normally maintained on lacosamide when the oral route is temporarily unavailable.

## Pre-treatment checks

- Avoid in known second- or third-degree atrioventricular (AV) block.
- Caution in patients with known conduction problems or severe cardiac disease such as a history of myocardial infarction or heart failure (prolongations in PR interval have been observed).

*Biochemical and other tests (not all are necessary in an emergency situation)*

LFTs
Renal function: U, Cr, CrCl (or eGFR)

## Dose

For existing patients with epilepsy switched from oral maintenance to parenteral dosing, no adjustment of dose or frequency of lacosamide is necessary.

There is no experience of parenteral treatment extending beyond 5 days.

**Patients previously established on oral therapy:** doses are given by IV infusion at the same dose and frequency as previous oral therapy.

**Initiation of treatment in patients temporarily unable to tolerate oral therapy:** 50 mg twice daily by IV infusion increased every 7 days by 50 mg twice daily to a maximum of 200 mg twice daily.

**Dose in renal impairment:** adjusted according to creatinine clearance,

- CrCl ≤30 mL/minute: maximum daily dose 250 mg.
- Haemodialysis: a supplement of up to 50% of the divided daily dose should be given directly after the end of the session.

**Dose in hepatic impairment:** no adjustment for mild to moderate hepatic impairment. Not studied in severe hepatic impairment.

## Intravenous infusion

*Preparation and administration*

1. Withdraw the required dose. Infuse undiluted or mix with a convenient volume of compatible infusion fluid, e.g. 100 mL NaCl 0.9%.
2. The solution should be clear and colourless. Inspect visually for particulate matter or discoloration prior to administration and discard if present.
3. Give by IV infusion over 15–60 minutes.

## Technical information

| | |
|---|---|
| Incompatible with | No information |
| Compatible with | **Flush**: NaCl 0.9%<br>**Solutions**: NaCl 0.9%, Gluc 5%, Hartmann's<br>**Y-site**: No information |
| pH[1] | 3.5-5.0 |
| Sodium content | 2.6 mmol/20 mL |
| Storage | Store below 25°C in original packaging. |
| Stability after preparation | From a microbiological point of view, should be used immediately; however, prepared infusions may be stored at 2-8°C and infused (at room temperature) within 24 hours. |

## Monitoring

| Measure | Frequency | Rationale |
|---|---|---|
| Signs of suicidal ideation and behaviours | Throughout treatment | • There is potential for this.<br>• Patients and carers should be advised to seek medical advice should this emerge. |
| Renal function and LFTs | Periodically | • Changes in renal or hepatic function may require a review of the dosing regimen. |

## Additional information

| | |
|---|---|
| Common and serious undesirable effects | *Common:* Depression, dizziness, headache, balance disorder, coordination abnormal, memory impairment, cognitive disorder, somnolence, tremor, nystagmus, diplopia, vision blurred, nausea, vomiting, constipation, flatulence, pruritus, gait disturbance, asthenia, fatigue, falls. |
| Pharmacokinetics | Elimination half-life is about 13 hours; the major metabolite has an elimination half-life of 15-23 hours. |
| Significant interactions | • The following may ↓lacosamide levels or effect: antidepressants-SSRIs (↓convulsive threshold), antidepressants-tricyclic (↓convulsive threshold), antidepressants-tricyclic, related (↓convulsive threshold), mefloquine, St John's wort (avoid combination). |
| Action in case of overdose | There is no specific antidote. Use general supportive measures, which may include haemodialysis if necessary. |
| Counselling | Treatment with lacosamide has been associated with dizziness that could ↑risk of accidental injury or falls. Counsel patient to exercise caution until they are familiar with the potential effects. |

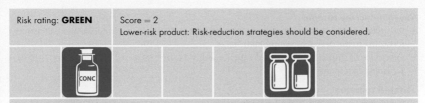

Risk rating: **GREEN**   Score = 2
Lower-risk product: Risk-reduction strategies should be considered.

This assessment is based on the full range of preparation and administration options described in the monograph. These may not all be applicable in some clinical situations.

## Reference

1. Personal communication with UCB Pharma Ltd; 12 October 2009.

## Bibliography

SPC Vimpat 50 mg, 100 mg, 150 mg and 200 mg film-coated tablets, 15 mg/mL syrup and 10 mg/mL solution for infusion (accessed 10 October 2009).

# Lanreotide

**60 mg, 90 mg, 120 mg viscous solution in pre-filled syringes, 30-mg dry powder vials with solvent**

* Lanreotide acetate is a somatostatin analogue with similar properties to octreotide.
* It is used in the symptomatic management of neuroendocrine tumours, particularly carcinoid syndrome, and also in the treatment of acromegaly and thyrotrophic adenomas.
* Doses are usually expressed in terms of lanreotide base.

## Pre-treatment checks

* Do not give if the patient is hypersensitive to lanreotide or related peptides.
* Use with caution in diabetes mellitus and if there is a history of gall stones (consider gall bladder echography).

*Biochemical tests*

LFTs
Renal function: U, Cr, CrCl (or eGFR)
TFTs (possibly)

## Dose

**Acromegaly:**

* *Somatuline Autogel:* initially 60 mg every 28 days by SC injection (if a somatostatin analogue not previously given), adjusted according to response. For patients previously treated with a somatostatin analogue, consult product literature for initial dose.
* *Somatuline LA:* initially 30 mg by IM injection every 14 days, increased to 30 mg every 7–10 days according to response.

**Neuroendocrine tumour:**
* *Somatuline Autogel:* initially 60–120 mg every 28 days by SC injection with subsequent adjustment according to the degree of symptomatic relief.
* *Somatuline LA:* initially 30 mg by IM injection every 14 days, increased to 30 mg every 7–10 days according to response.

**Thyroid tumours:**
* *Somatuline LA:* initially 30 mg by IM injection every 14 days, increased to 30 mg every 10 days according to response.

## Intramuscular injection (Somatuline LA depot injection only)

*Preparation and administration (see package insert for full details)*

1. Attach one of the needles to syringe supplied and reconstitute the vial with the solvent provided (**do not remove the syringe** at this stage).
2. Shake the vial gently from side to side 20–30 times to obtain a homogenous suspension with a milky appearance.
3. **Do not invert the vial**. Withdraw the entire contents of the vial (there is an overage in the vial to account for the small amount remaining in the vial).
4. **Without delay**, give by IM injection into the buttock.

## Subcutaneous injection (Somatuline Autogel pre-filled syringe only)

*Preparation and administration (see package insert for full details)*

1. Remove the correct strength of pre-filled syringe from the fridge 30 minutes prior to use.
2. Upon opening the package, use immediately.
3. Give by deep SC injection (at 90° to the skin and inserting the needle to its full length) into the upper outer quadrant of the buttock. The upper outer thigh may be used if the patient is self-administering. Use alternate sides for subsequent injections.

| Technical information | |
|---|---|
| Incompatible with | Not relevant |
| Compatible with | Not relevant. Use solvent provided with pack (depot only). |
| Sodium content | Negligible |
| Storage | Store at 2-8°C in original packaging. Do not freeze. |

| Monitoring | | |
|---|---|---|
| **Measure** | **Frequency** | **Rationale** |
| Circulating growth hormones (GH) or insulin-like growth factor (IGF-1) | Monthly | • Adjust the dose according to response as above. |
| Blood glucose | Frequently initially, then as required | • Can produce transient inhibition of insulin and glucagon secretion.<br>• Check to determine whether antidiabetic treatment needs to be adjusted. |

*(continued)*

## Monitoring (continued)

| Measure | Frequency | Rationale |
|---------|-----------|-----------|
| Thyroid function | If clinically indicated, and periodically for thyroid tumour treatment | • Hypothyroidism is rare but ↓thyroid function has been seen in patients treated for acromegaly. |
| Symptoms of gallstones | On presentation | • May reduce gall bladder motility. Treat if symptomatic. |
| Renal function, LFTs | Periodically | • If renal or hepatic function deteriorates, the dose interval may need adjusting only if clinically necessary. |

## Additional information

| | |
|---|---|
| Common and serious undesirable effects | *Injection-related:* Local: Mild pain, redness, itching and induration at injection site 30 minutes after the dose that decreases with frequency. *Other:* Diarrhoea, abdominal pain, nausea, constipation, flatulence, gallstones, gall bladder sludge, lethargy, ↑bilirubin. |
| Pharmacokinetics | Apparent elimination half-life is 5 to 30 days. |
| Significant interactions | No significant interactions |
| Action in case of overdose | No specific antidote. Treat symptomatically. |
| Counselling | How to store and dispose of correctly. |

Risk rating: **GREEN**  Score = 1
Lower-risk product: Risk-reduction strategies should be considered.

This assessment is based on the full range of preparation and administration options described in the monograph. These may not all be applicable in some clinical situations.

## Bibliography

SPC Somatuline Autogel 60 mg, Somatuline Autogel 90 mg, Somatuline Autogel 120 mg (accessed 24 February 2010).
SPC Somatuline LA (accessed 24 February 2010).

# Lenograstim (recombinant human granulocyte colony-stimulating factor, rHuG-CSF)

**13.4 million units (105 micrograms) and 33.6 million units (263 micrograms) dry powder vials with solvent (WFI)**

- Lenograstim is a recombinant glycosylated human granulocyte-colony stimulating factor (rHuG-CSF) that acts primarily on neutrophil precursors to increase neutrophil levels.
- It is used to treat or prevent neutropenia in patients receiving myelosuppressive cancer chemotherapy, to reduce the duration of neutropenia in patients undergoing bone marrow transplantation and to mobilise peripheral blood progenitor cells in blood stem cell transplantation.

## Pre-treatment checks

- Contraindicated in myeloid malignancy (other than *de novo* AML); in patients with *de novo* AML aged <55 years; and/or in patients with *de novo* AML with good cytogenetics.
- Not be used in patients with secondary AML, myelodysplasia or chronic myelogenous leukaemia.
- Use with extreme caution in any pre-malignant myeloid condition such as myelodysplastic syndrome.
- Check recent pulmonary history (recent history of pulmonary infiltrates or pneumonia ↑risk of pulmonary adverse events).
- Confirm whether women of child-bearing potential are pregnant or breast feeding (contraindicated unless benefit outweighs risk, at discretion of clinician).
- Prior treatment with certain cytotoxic agents and/or radiotherapy may compromise effectiveness of lenograstim in generating mobilisation of sufficient PBPCs, and alternative forms of treatment may be needed.
- Potential PBPC donors should be <60 years of age and cannot undergo apheresis if anticoagulated, or if they have known problems with haemostasis; therefore confirm relevant history prior to lenograstim treatment.
- If the patient is receiving cytotoxic chemotherapy, the first dose of lenograstim must not given in the first 24 hours following the completion of the cycle of chemotherapy.

*Biochemical and other tests*

Body surface area for certain indications (and therefore height and bodyweight)
FBC

## Dose

**Cytotoxic-induced neutropenia:** 19.2 million units (150 micrograms) per m$^2$ by SC injection once daily.
Give the first dose a minimum of 24 hours after cytotoxic therapy and continue until the neutrophil count is within the acceptable range.

**Following bone marrow transplantation:** 19.2 million units (150 micrograms) per m$^2$ by IV infusion once daily. Give the first dose the day after transplantation and continue until the neutrophil count is within the acceptable range. For timing of leucopheresis, consult product literature.

**Mobilisation of PBPCs (used alone):** 1.28 million units (10 micrograms) per kg by SC injection once daily for 4–6 consecutive days.

**Mobilisation of PBPCs after myeloablative therapy:** 19.2 million units (150 micrograms) per m² by SC injection once daily. Give the first dose a minimum of 24 hours after cytotoxic therapy and continue until the neutrophil count is within the acceptable range. For timing of leucopheresis, consult product literature.

## Subcutaneous injection

*Preparation and administration*

1. Withdraw the entire contents of the solvent ampoule and add to the vial using the 19G needle provided.
2. Agitate the vial gently until the powder has completely dissolved but do not shake vigorously. The solution then contains either 13.4 million units (105 micrograms)/mL or 33.6 million units (263 micrograms)/mL, depending on the vial size used.
3. Withdraw the required dose using the 19G needle then change to the 26G needle provided.
4. Give by SC injection. Rotate injection sites for subsequent injections to avoid bruising/bleeding.

## Intermittent intravenous infusion

*Preparation and administration*

1. Withdraw the entire contents of the solvent ampoule and add to the vial using the 19G needle provided.
2. Agitate the vial gently until the powder has completely dissolved but do not shake vigorously. The solution then contains either 13.4 million units (105 micrograms)/mL or 33.6 million units (263 micrograms)/mL, depending on the vial size used.
3. Withdraw the required dose using the 19G needle and add to a suitable volume of NaCl 0.9% or Gluc 5% (use a maximum of 50 mL for 13.4 million unit vial; use a maximum of 100 mL for 33.6 million unit vial).
4. The solution should be clear and colourless. Inspect visually for particulate matter or discoloration prior to administration and discard if present.
5. Give by IV infusion over 30 minutes.

## Technical information

| | |
|---|---|
| Incompatible with | No information |
| Compatible with | **Solutions**: NaCl 0.9%, Gluc 5%<br>**Y-site**: No information |
| pH | 6.5 |
| Sodium content | Nil |
| Storage | Store below 30°C. Do not freeze. |
| Displacement value | Not relevant. The vials contain an overage so that the final solution contains either 13.4 million units (105 micrograms)/mL or 33.6 million units (263 micrograms)/mL when reconstituted as directed. |
| Stability after preparation | From a microbiological point of view, should be used immediately; however:<br>• Reconstituted vials may be stored at 2–8°C for 24 hours.<br>• Prepared infusions may be stored at 2–8°C and infused (at room temperature) within 24 hours. |

## Monitoring

| Measure | Frequency | Rationale |
|---|---|---|
| WBC | Initially 2-3 times weekly, reducing in frequency if clinically appropriate | • ANC to assess patient response.<br>• Severe leucocytosis may occur, and treatment should be discontinued if leucocytes are >50 000 cells/mm³ (>50 × 10⁹/L) after expected nadir; and discontinued or dose reduced if leucocytes are >70 000 cells/mm³ (>70 × 10⁹/L) in PBPC mobilisation. |
| Overall FBC | | • Especially if receiving cytotoxic chemotherapy, the patient may be at higher risk of thrombocytopenia and anaemia.<br>• PBPC donors may develop thrombocytopenia – potentially due to apheresis procedure. Apheresis should not be performed if platelets are <75 000/mm³ (<75 × 10⁹/L).<br>• Consider discontinuation if thrombocytopenia develops in patients with severe chronic neutropenia. |
| Signs of respiratory distress (cough, dyspnoea) | Throughout course of treatment | • May be initial signs of ARDS; discontinue at discretion of clinician. |
| Tumour re-growth | | • Although rare, some tumours can express a G-CSF receptor and care should be taken to monitor for signs of unexpected tumour growth during treatment. |
| Physical examination of spleen size (and ultrasound scan if appropriate) | Regularly through treatment, and urgently if the patient presents with left upper abdominal pain or shoulder tip pain | • Splenomegaly is a direct effect of lenograstim therapy, but splenic rupture may occur. Dose reduction has been noted to slow or stop progression of enlargement. |
| LFTs | Monthly | • ↑Alk Phos and GGT have been reported (reversible and dose dependent). |
| Serum lactate dehydrogenase and uric acid | | • ↑Levels have been reported (reversible and dose-dependent). |
| Morphological and cytogenetic bone marrow examinations | Annually | • Any cytogenetic changes observed during treatment should prompt a review of the risks and benefits of continuing treatment. |

## Additional information

| | |
|---|---|
| Common and serious undesirable effects | *Injection-related:* Local: Injection-site reactions.<br>*Other:* Nausea, diarrhoea, anorexia, headache, asthenia, fever, bone pain, rash, alopecia, thrombocytopenia, leucocytosis, chest pain, hypersensitivity reactions, arthralgia. |
| Pharmacokinetics | Elimination half-life is about 3–4 hours (SC administration), or 1–1.5 hours (IV administration). |
| Significant interactions | • Lenograstim may ↑side-effects of:<br>myelosuppressive cytotoxic chemotherapy (may exacerbate neutropenia – do not administer lenograstim in the 24 hours prior to chemotherapy and 24 hours after final dose of chemotherapy). |
| Action in case of overdose | Effects not established. Discontinuation of treatment usually results in a 50% decrease in circulating neutrophils within 1–2 days, returning to normal levels in 1–7 days. |

Risk rating: **AMBER**

Score = 3
Moderate-risk product. Risk-reduction strategies are recommended.

This assessment is based on the full range of preparation and administration options described in the monograph. These may not all be applicable in some clinical situations.

## Bibliography

SPC Granocyte 13 million IU, and 34 million IU (accessed 5 August 2009)

# Lepirudin

**50-mg dry powder vial**

- Lepirudin is a recombinant hirudin that is a direct inhibitor of thrombin.
- It is used as an anticoagulant in the management of thromboembolic disorders in patients with HIT type II requiring parenteral therapy.

## Pre-treatment checks

- Diagnosis should be confirmed by the HIPAA (heparin induced platelet activation assay) or an equivalent test.
- It is inadvisable to use if there is active bleeding.
- Caution should be taken in the following conditions with a careful balance of risk versus benefit: recent puncture of large vessels or organ biopsy; anomaly of vessels or organs; recent

cerebrovascular accident, stroke, or intracerebral surgery; severe uncontrolled ↑BP; bacterial endo-carditis; advanced renal impairment; haemorrhagic diathesis; recent major surgery; recent bleed-ing (e.g. intracranial, GI, intraocular, pulmonary); overt signs of bleeding; recent active peptic ulcer; age >65 years.

* Anaphylaxis is more likely if the patient has had previous exposure to lepirudin.
* Ensure that resuscitation facilities are available.

*Biochemical and other tests (not all are necessary in an emergency situation)*

| | |
|---|---|
| APTT ratio | LFTs (serious impairment may result in enhance-ment of the anticoagulant effect of lepirudin due to impaired production of vitamin K-dependent coagulation factors) |
| Blood pressure | |
| Body weight | |
| FBC | |
| | Renal function: U, Cr, CrCl (or eGFR) |

## Dose

**Standard dose**: 0.4 mg/kg by slow IV injection (see Table L1). This is followed by 0.15 mg/kg/hour (maximum 16.5 mg/hour) by IV infusion for 2–10 days or longer (see Table L1). Check APTT ratio 4 hours after the start of therapy and adjust the infusion rate according to APTT ratio (see Monitoring below).

**Dose in renal impairment:** the dose is adjusted according to creatinine clearance (see Table L1):
* CrCl 45–60 mL/minute: reduce loading dose to 0.2 mg/kg and infusion rate to 50% of original.
* CrCl 30–44 mL/minute: reduce loading dose to 0.2 mg/kg and infusion rate to 30% of original.
* CrCl 15–29 mL/minute: reduce loading dose to 0.2 mg/kg and infusion rate to 15% of original.
* CrCl <15 mL/minute: avoid using or stop infusion if already started.

In haemodialysis patients or cases of acute renal failure, IV bolus doses of 0.1 mg/kg may be used on alternate days, according to response.[1]

**Dose in hepatic impairment:** there is no experience in patients with significant liver impairment.

## Conversion to oral anticoagulant therapy

* Initiate oral anticoagulants only after substantial recovery from acute HIT has occurred and platelet counts are normalising.
* When converting to oral anticoagulant therapy, the dose of lepirudin should be reduced gradually until the APTT ratio is just above 1.5, after which therapy with, for example, warfarin can be started.
* Start with modest doses of warfarin (e.g. 2.5–5 mg daily) and do not use a loading dose.
* Overlap lepirudin and warfarin therapy for a minimum of 4–5 days until the desired INR has been achieved.

## Intravenous injection

*Preparation and administration*

1. Reconstitute one 50-mg vial with 1 mL WFI or NaCl 0.9 % and shake gently for up to 3 minutes to obtain a clear, colourless solution containing 50 mg/mL.
2. Withdraw 1 mL into a 10-mL syringe and dilute to 10 mL with NaCl 0.9% or Gluc 5% to give a solution containing 5 mg/mL.
3. The solution should be clear and colourless. Inspect visually for particulate matter or discolor-ation prior to administration and discard if present.
4. Expel any excess lepirudin to give the required dose (see Table L1).
5. Give by IV injection over 3–5 minutes then follow with the continuous infusion.

**Table L1** Lepirudin dose adjusted according to bodyweight and renal function

| Bodyweight (kg) | Loading dose (mL of 5 mg/mL solution) | | Continuous IV infusion rate (mL/hour of 2 mg/mL solution) | | | |
|---|---|---|---|---|---|---|
| Dose: | 0.4 mg/kg | 0.2 mg/kg | 100% | 50% | 30% | 15% |
| CrCl (mL/minute): | >60 | 15–60[a] | >60 | 45–60 | 30–44 | 15–29 |
| 50 | 4.0 | 2.0 | 3.8 | 1.9 | 1.1 | 0.6 |
| 55 | 4.4 | 2.2 | 4.1 | 2.1 | 1.2 | 0.6 |
| 60 | 4.8 | 2.4 | 4.5 | 2.3 | 1.4 | 0.7 |
| 65 | 5.2 | 2.6 | 4.9 | 2.4 | 1.5 | 0.7 |
| 70 | 5.6 | 2.8 | 5.3 | 2.6 | 1.6 | 0.8 |
| 75 | 6.0 | 3.0 | 5.6 | 2.8 | 1.7 | 0.8 |
| 80 | 6.4 | 3.2 | 6.0 | 3.0 | 1.8 | 0.9 |
| 85 | 6.8 | 3.4 | 6.4 | 3.2 | 1.9 | 1.0 |
| 90 | 7.2 | 3.6 | 6.8 | 3.4 | 2.0 | 1.0 |
| 95 | 7.6 | 3.8 | 7.1 | 3.6 | 2.1 | 1.1 |
| 100 | 8.0 | 4.0 | 7.5 | 3.8 | 2.3 | 1.1 |
| 105 | 8.4 | 4.2 | 7.9 | 3.9 | 2.4 | 1.2 |
| ≥110 | 8.8 | 4.4 | 8.3 | 4.1 | 2.5 | 1.2 |

[a] If CrCl < 15 mL/minute, avoid using lepirudin or stop infusion if already started.

## Continuous intravenous infusion via syringe pump

*Preparation and administration*

1. Reconstitute each of two 50-mg vials with 1 mL WFI or NaCl 0.9 % and shake gently for up to 3 minutes to obtain a clear, colourless solution containing 50 mg/mL.
2. Make 100 mg (2 mL) up to 50 mL in a syringe pump with NaCl 0.9% or Gluc 5%.
3. Cap the syringe and mix well to give a solution containing 2 mg/mL.
4. The solution should be clear and colourless. Inspect visually for particulate matter or discoloration prior to administration and discard if present.
5. Give by continuous IV infusion at the correct rate for the patient's weight and renal function (see Table L1).
6. Prepare a fresh syringe every 12 hours.

## Technical information

| | |
|---|---|
| Incompatible with | No information |
| Compatible with | **Flush**: NaCl 0.9%<br>**Solutions**: NaCl 0.9%, Gluc 5%<br>**Y-site**: No information |
| pH | 7 |
| Sodium content | Negligible |
| Storage | Store below 25°C in original packaging. Do not freeze. |
| Displacement value | Negligible |
| Stability after preparation | Use prepared infusions immediately. |

## Monitoring

| Measure | Frequency | Rationale |
|---|---|---|
| APTT | Initially 4 hours after commencing the infusion or if the infusion rate is changed.<br>If stable check daily.<br>Check more frequently in patients with renal impairment or with ↑risk of bleeding. | • Check with the local laboratory concerning the target range for the APTT ratio in a patient on lepirudin.<br>• If a confirmed APTT ratio is above the target range, stop the infusion for 2 hours. After this, decrease infusion rate by 50% (with no additional IV bolus) and check APTT ratio again after 4 hours.<br>• If the confirmed APTT ratio is below the target range, increase infusion rate by 20 % and check APTT ratio again after 4 hours. Seek Haematology advice if a further increase appears to be necessary. |
| Renal function | Periodically | • Changes in renal function may require an adjustment in infusion rate, but check APTT ratio first. |

(continued)

## Monitoring (continued)

| Measure | Frequency | Rationale |
|---------|-----------|-----------|
| FBC and blood pressure | Periodically | • Unexplained ↓haematocrit, Hb or BP may indicate haemorrhage.<br>• Treatment should be stopped if bleeding is observed or suspected.<br>• Consider testing stool for occult blood. |

## Additional information

| | |
|---|---|
| Common and serious undesirable effects | *Immediate:* Anaphylaxis has been reported rarely, more frequently on re-exposure.<br>*Common:* Anaemia or ↓Hb value without obvious source of bleeding, minor bleeding at any site, major haemorrhage at any site, bruising. |
| Pharmacokinetics | Elimination half-life is 0.8–2 hours. Increased in severe renal impairment to about 2 days. |
| Significant interactions | The following may ↑lepirudin levels or effect (or ↑side-effects): thrombolytics, coumarin anticoagulants, antiplatelet drugs. |
| Action in case of overdose | *Symptoms to watch for:* Bleeding.<br>*Antidote:* No specific antidote. Immediately stop administration. Determine APTT ratio and other coagulation parameters. Check Hb and prepare for blood transfusion. Follow local guidelines for shock therapy. Haemofiltration or haemodialysis may be useful. |
| Counselling | Patients should be informed that they have received lepirudin (owing to risk associated with future re-exposure). |

| | |
|---|---|
| Risk rating: **RED** | Score = 6<br>High-risk product: Risk-reduction strategies are required to minimise these risks. |

This assessment is based on the full range of preparation and administration options described in the monograph. These may not all be applicable in some clinical situations.

## Reference

1. Ashley C, Currie A, eds. *The Renal Drug Handbook*, 3rd edn. Oxford: Radcliffe Medical Press, 2009.

## Bibliography

SPC Refludan 50 mg powder for solution for injection or infusion (accessed 19 August 2009).

# Leuprorelin acetate (leuprolide acetate)

**3.75-mg dry powder vial with 1 mL solvent in prefilled syringe (Prostap SR)**
**11.25-mg dry powder vial with 2 mL solvent in prefilled syringe (Prostap 3)**

* Leuprorelin acetate is a synthetic analogue of gonadorelin (gonadotrophin-releasing hormone).
* It is used for the suppression of testosterone in the treatment of prostate cancer.
* It is used in the treatment of endometriosis and uterine fibroids and may also be given before surgery for endometrial ablation.
* Doses are expressed as leuprorelin acetate.

## Pre-treatment checks

Caution in diabetes and osteoporosis (or those at risk, i.e. chronic alcohol and/or tobacco use, strong family history of osteoporosis, or chronic use of drugs that can reduce bone mass, e.g. anticonvulsants or corticosteroids).

*Biochemical and other tests*

Blood pressure
Female patients: confirm that the patient is not pregnant
LFTs

## Dose

**Prostate cancer**: 3.75 mg by SC or IM injection every 28 days or 11.25 mg by SC injection every 12 weeks. An antiandrogen agent may be given for 3 days before until 2–3 weeks after commencement to ↓risk of disease flare, e.g. cyproterone acetate 100 mg three times daily.
**Endometriosis**: 3.75 mg by SC or IM injection every 28 days or 11.25 mg by SC injection every 12 weeks for a maximum of 6 months. Treatment should be initiated during the first 5 days of the menstrual cycle. Supplementary combined HRT may ↓bone mineral density loss and vasomotor symptoms.
**Endometrial preparation prior to intrauterine surgery**: 3.75 mg by SC or IM injection 5–6 weeks prior to surgery. Therapy should be initiated during days 3–5 of the menstrual cycle.
**Preoperative management of uterine fibroids**: 3.75 mg by SC or IM injection every 28 days usually for 3–4 months but for a maximum of 6 months. If anaemia is present due to uterine fibroids, ensure that iron supplementation is prescribed.

## Subcutaneous injection

*Preparation and administration*

1. Remove the cap from the vial of powder and from the pre-filled syringe containing the solvent.
2. Attach a 23G needle securely to the syringe and inject the whole contents of the syringe into vial of powder. Remove the syringe/needle and keep aseptic.
3. Shake the vial gently for 15–20 seconds to produce a uniform cloudy suspension.
4. Immediately withdraw the whole vial contents, taking care to exclude air bubbles. The injection should be given as soon as possible after mixing. If any settling of suspension occurs in the vial or syringe, shake gently to re-suspend.
5. Attach a new 23G needle and give by SC injection. Aspirate before injection to avoid inadvertent intravascular injection.

## Intramuscular injection (Prostap SR only)

*Preparation and administration*

1. Remove the cap from the vial of powder and from the pre-filled syringe containing the solvent.
2. Attach a 23G needle securely to the syringe and inject the whole contents of the syringe into vial of powder. Remove the syringe/needle and keep aseptic.
3. Shake the vial gently for 15–20 seconds to produce a uniform cloudy suspension.
4. Immediately withdraw the whole vial contents, taking care to exclude air bubbles. The injection should be given as soon as possible after mixing. If any settling of suspension occurs in the vial or syringe, shake gently to re-suspend.
5. Attach a 21G needle and give by IM injection. Aspirate before injection to avoid inadvertent intravascular injection.

## Technical information

| | |
|---|---|
| Incompatible with | Not relevant |
| Compatible with | Solvent is provided with each pack. |
| pH | Not relevant |
| Sodium content | Nil |
| Storage | Store below 25°C in original packaging. |
| Stability after preparation | From a microbiological point of view, should be used immediately; however, the reconstituted preparation may be stored at 2-8°C and given (at room temperature) within 24 hours. |

## Monitoring

| Measure | Frequency | Rationale |
|---|---|---|
| Blood glucose in diabetic patients | Regularly | • ↑Blood glucose levels can occur (↓glucose tolerance). |
| Prostate-specific antigen (PSA) serum levels and plasma testosterone level | Periodically | • Monitor during treatment to assess efficacy. There is no standard level to aim for, but in one study serum testosterone levels fell from 350 to 21 nanograms/dL after 4 weeks and 20 nanograms/dL after 45 months.[1] |
| LFTs | | • Hepatic dysfunction and jaundice with ↑liver enzyme levels have been reported. |
| Blood lipid levels | | • Lipid levels can be lowered and raised. |
| FBC | | • Thrombocytopenia and leucopenia sometimes occur. |
| Blood pressure | | • ↓ or ↑BP can occur (rarely) and may require medical intervention or withdrawal of treatment. |
| Bone mineral density | Consider if treatment is prolonged | • May lead to bone loss, which enhances the risk of osteoporosis. The generally accepted level of bone loss with LHRH analogues is 5%. |

## Additional information

| | |
|---|---|
| Common and serious undesirable effects | *Immediate:* Rarely anaphylaxis and other hypersensitivity reactions.<br>*Injection/infusion-related:* Local: Injection-site pain, redness or local inflammation.<br>*Other:* ↓BMD, hot flushes, sweating, ↓libido, breast tenderness (infrequently).<br>Women: Headaches, mood changes, depression, vaginal dryness, change in breast size. |
| Pharmacokinetics | Elimination half-life is 3 hours. |
| Significant interactions | No significant interactions. |
| Action in case of overdose | There is no specific antidote and treatment should be symptomatic. |
| Counselling | The ability to drive and use machines may be impaired owing to visual disturbances and dizziness.<br>Women to be treated because of submucous fibroids should be warned of the possibility of abnormal bleeding or pain (earlier surgical intervention may be required).<br>Fertile women should use non-hormonal, barrier methods of contraception during the entire treatment period. |

| Risk rating: **GREEN** | Score = 2<br>Lower-risk product: Risk-reduction strategies should be considered. |
|---|---|

This assessment is based on the full range of preparation and administration options described in the monograph. These may not all be applicable in some clinical situations.

## Reference

1. Kienle E, Lübben G. Efficacy and safety of leuprorelin acetate depot for prostate cancer. The German Leuprorelin Study Group. *Urol Int* 1996; 56(Suppl 1): 23–30.

## Bibliography

SPC Prostap 3 Leuprorelin acetate depot injection 11.25 mg (accessed 24 February 2010).
SPC Prostap SR accessed 24 February 2010

# Levetiracetam

**100 mg/mL solution in 5-mL vials**

- Levetiracetam is an antiepileptic drug.
- It is used as monotherapy of partial seizures with or without secondary generalisation, and as adjunctive therapy in various types of epilepsy.
- It is usually used parenterally in patients normally maintained on levetiracetam when the oral route is temporarily unavailable.

## Pre-treatment checks

Pregnancy test if possible.

*Biochemical and other tests (not all are necessary in an emergency situation)*

Bodyweight
LFTs
Renal function: U, Cr, CrCl (or eGFR)

## Dose

> For existing patients with epilepsy switched from oral maintenance to parenteral dosing, no adjustment of dose or frequency of levetiracetam is necessary.
> There is no experience of parenteral treatment extending beyond 4 days.

**Patients previously established on oral therapy:** doses are given by IV infusion at the same dose and frequency as in previous oral therapy.

**Initiation of treatment in patients temporarily unable to tolerate oral therapy:**

- *Monotherapy for partial seizures with or without secondary generalisation:* initially 250 mg by IV infusion twice daily (increased according to response every 2 weeks).
- *Adjunctive therapy:* initially 500 mg by IV infusion twice daily (increased according to response every 2 weeks).

**Dose in renal impairment**: the maximum dose is adjusted according to creatinine clearance:

- CrCl 50–79 mL/minute: maximum dose 1 g twice daily.
- CrCl 30–49 mL/minute: maximum dose 750 mg twice daily.
- CrCl <30 mL/minute: maximum dose 500 mg twice daily.
- CrCl <10 mL/minute in patients undergoing dialysis: maximum dose 1 g once daily.

**Dose in hepatic impairment:** no dose adjustment is needed in patients with mild to moderate hepatic impairment.

## Intermittent intravenous infusion

*Preparation and administration*

1. Withdraw the required dose and add to a suitable volume of compatible infusion fluid, e.g. a minimum of 100 mL NaCl 0.9%).
2. The solution should be clear and colourless. Inspect visually for particulate matter or discoloration prior to administration and discard if present.
3. Give by IV infusion over 15 minutes.

## Technical information

| | |
|---|---|
| Incompatible with | No information |
| Compatible with | **Flush**: NaCl 0.9%<br>**Solutions**: NaCl 0.9%, Gluc 5%, Hartmann's<br>**Y-site**: No information |
| pH | 5–6 |
| Sodium content | Negligible |
| Storage | Store below 25°C in original packaging. |
| Stability after preparation | From a microbiological point of view, should be used immediately; however, prepared infusions may be stored at 2–8°C and infused (at room temperature) within 24 hours. |

## Monitoring

| Measure | Frequency | Rationale |
|---|---|---|
| Infusion solution, rate of infusion and infusion site | During administration | • Discard if the solution forms precipitates or becomes discoloured.<br>• Injection-site reactions may occur. |
| Seizures frequency | Throughout treatment | • For therapeutic effect. |
| Pregnancy test | Periodically | • The effect on the neonate is not fully known; there may be a risk congenital malformations in the neonate. |
| Bodyweight | | • May cause ↑or↓ bodyweight. |
| FBC | | • May cause thrombocytopenia, leucopenia, neutropenia, and pancytopenia. |
| Mental health | At review consultation and if required | • Suicide, suicidal behaviour and suicidal ideation have been reported in patients treated with levetiracetam. |

## Additional information

| | |
|---|---|
| Common and serious undesirable effects | *Infusion-related:* Local: Injection-site reactions.<br>*Other:* Abdominal pain, agitation, amnesia, anxiety, asthenia, ataxia, confusion, convulsion, cough, diarrhoea, diplopia, dizziness, fatigue, headache, hostility, hyperkinesia, ↑LFTs, nausea, myalgia, thrombocytopenia, tremor, pruritus, rash, somnolence. |
| Pharmacokinetics | Elimination half-life is 6–8 hours. |
| Significant interactions | • The following may ↓levetiracetam levels or effect: antidepressants-SSRI (↓convulsive threshold), antidepressants-tricyclic (↓convulsive threshold), antidepressants-tricyclic, related (↓convulsive threshold), mefloquine, St John's wort (avoid combination). |

*(continued)*

## Additional information (continued)

| | |
|---|---|
| Action in case of overdose | *Symptoms to watch for:* Somnolence, agitation, aggression, ↓consciousness, respiratory depression, coma.<br>*Antidote:* No known antidote but haemodialysis may be effective. Stop administration and give supportive therapy as appropriate. |
| Counselling | Do not stop suddenly without consulting a doctor.<br>Ensure that adequate contraception is used.<br>This medicine causes drowsiness. |

Risk rating: **AMBER**   Score = 3
Moderate-risk product: Risk-reduction strategies are recommended.

This assessment is based on the full range of preparation and administration options described in the monograph. These may not all be applicable in some clinical situations.

### Bibliography

SPC Keppra 250, 500, 750 and 1000 mg film-coated tablets, 100 mg/ml oral solution and 100 mg/ml concentrate for solution for infusion (accessed 21 April 2008).

# Levocarnitine (L-carnitine)

### 200 mg/mL solution in 5-mL ampoules

- Carnitine is an amino acid derivative that is an essential co-factor of fatty acid metabolism. It occurs as distinct L- and D-isomers, although only the L-isomer is believed to be biologically active.
- Levocarnitine is used in the treatment of primary carnitine deficiency and in carnitine deficiency resulting from various defects of intermediary metabolism.
- It has been used to treat carnitine deficiency in haemodialysis patients. The first 3 months of therapy is usually given IV to replenish normal muscle levels, after which maintenance doses may be given orally. All doses are given at the end of haemodialysis sessions.
- Levocarnitine has also been used in cases of valproate toxicity (unlicensed indication).

### Pre-treatment checks

- Caution should be exercised in diabetic patients receiving insulin or oral treatment.
- Patients with severe renal impairment should not be given high oral doses for prolonged periods owing to accumulation of toxic metabolites (not shown to occur to the same extent after IV doses).

*Biochemical tests*

Free and acyl carnitine levels in plasma and urine.

## Dose

**Primary deficiency:** up to 25 mg/kg four times daily.
**Secondary deficiency:** 20 mg/kg after each dialysis session (dosage adjusted according to carnitine concentration). Treatment should be continued for at least 3 months.
**For valproate toxicity in patients who have hyperammonaemia or hepatotoxicity (unlicensed):**

It is essential to consult a poisons information service, e.g. Toxbase at www.toxbase.org (password or registration required) for full details of the management of valproate toxicity.

Consider IV administration of levocarnitine in patients who have taken a massive valproate overdose and who have hyperammonaemia or hepatotoxicity.[1] Discuss with your local poisons information service.

### Intravenous injection

*Preparation and administration*

1. Withdraw the required dose.
2. The solution should be clear and colourless to light straw coloured. Inspect visually for particulate matter or discoloration prior to administration and discard if present.
3. Give by IV injection over 2–3 minutes.

### Intermittent intravenous infusion (unlicensed use for valproate toxicity)

*Preparation and administration*

1. Withdraw the required dose.
2. May be infused undiluted, or added to a suitable volume of compatible infusion fluid.
3. The solution should be clear and colourless to light straw coloured. Inspect visually for particulate matter or discoloration prior to administration and discard if present.
4. Give by IV infusion over 30 minutes (loading dose) or 10–30 minutes (subsequent doses).

## Technical information

| | |
|---|---|
| Incompatible with | No information |
| Compatible with | **Flush**: NaCl 0.9%<br>**Solutions**: NaCl 0.9%, Hartmann's<br>**Y-site**: No information |
| pH | 6–6.5 |
| Sodium content | Nil |
| Storage | Store below 25°C in original packaging. |
| Stability after preparation | Use opened ampoules immediately.<br>Use prepared infusions immediately. |

## Monitoring

| Measure | Frequency | Rationale |
|---|---|---|
| Carnitine levels (acyl and free) in plasma and urine | Prior to, during and after treatment | • To assess response to treatment.<br>• Secondary carnitine deficiency is suggested by a plasma ratio of acyl to free carnitine greater than 0.4 and/or when free carnitine concentrations are <20 micromol/L. |
| Blood glucose | Throughout treatment | • Improved glucose utilisation may cause hypoglycaemia to occur in diabetic patients receiving insulin or oral hypoglycaemic treatment. |
| Symptoms of deficiency | | • Patients with primary carnitine deficiency have presented with hypoglycaemia and encephalopathy, skeletal myopathy and cardiomyopathy.<br>• The dialysis-related secondary carnitine deficiency manifests notably as anaemia, intradialytic ↓BP, cardiomyopathy, and muscle weakness and fatigability. |

## Additional information

| | |
|---|---|
| Common and serious undesirable effects | *Injection/infusion-related:* None.<br>*Other:*<br>• Common: Body odour, GI disturbances including nausea, vomiting, diarrhoea, and abdominal cramps, hypoglycaemia in patients receiving insulin or oral hypoglycaemic agents (due to ↑glucose utilisation).<br>• Rare: Seizures. |
| Pharmacokinetics | Elimination half-life is 17.4 hours. |
| Significant interactions | • Levocarnitine may ↑levels or effect of the following drugs (or ↑side-effects): insulins, oral hypoglycaemic agents. |
| Action in case of overdose | There have been no reports of levocarnitine overdosage. If necessary, stop administration and give supportive therapy as appropriate. |

| Risk rating: **GREEN** | Score = 1<br>Lower-risk product: Risk-reduction strategies should be considered. |
|---|---|

This assessment is based on the full range of preparation and administration options described in the monograph. These may not all be applicable in some clinical situations.

## Reference

1. Toxbase. www.toxbase.org (accessed 12 July 2010).

## Bibliography

SPC Carnitor 1 g solution for injection (accessed 16 February 2010).

# Levofloxacin

**5 mg/mL solution in 100-mL infusion bottles**

* Levofloxacin hemihydrate is an isomer of the fluorinated quinolone antibacterial ofloxacin.
* It is used to treat infections cause by susceptible Gram-positive and Gram-negative bacteria.
* Levofloxacin is rapidly and well absorbed from the GI tract following oral dosing so the IV route should be used only when the oral route is unavailable.
* Doses are expressed in terms of the base:
  Levofloxacin 250 mg ≡ 256 mg levofloxacin hemihydrate.

## Pre-treatment checks

* Do not give if there is known hypersensitivity to quinolone antibacterials.
* Avoid in patients with a past history of tendinitis or a history of epilepsy, or in pregnant or breast-feeding women.
* Use with caution if there is a history of psychiatric disease or in patients with latent or actual defects in G6PD activity.
* Patients should be well hydrated and asked to drink fluids liberally.

*Biochemical and other tests*

Blood pressure
LFTs
Renal function: U, Cr, CrCl (or eGFR)

## Dose

**Community-acquired pneumonia**: 500 mg once or twice daily.
**Complicated urinary tract infections (including pyelonephritis)**: 250 mg daily, increased in severe infections.
**Skin and soft-tissue infections**: 500 mg twice daily.
**Dose in renal impairment**: adjusted according to creatinine clearance:

* CrCl >20–50 mL/minute: initial dose 250–500 mg then reduce dose by 50%.
* CrCl 10–20 mL/minute: initial dose 250–500 mg then 125 mg every 12–24 hours.
* CrCl <10 mL/minute: initial dose 250–500 mg then 125 mg every 24–48 hours.

## Intermittent intravenous infusion

*Preparation and administration*

1. The infusion is pre-prepared for use. It should be clear and greenish yellow. Inspect visually for particulate matter or discoloration prior to administration and discard if present.
2. Give by IV infusion over at least 30 minutes for 250 mg (at least 60 minutes for 500 mg).

## Technical information

| | |
|---|---|
| Incompatible with | Aciclovir, drotrecogin alfa (activated), furosemide, glyceryl trinitrate, heparin sodium, insulin (soluble), propofol. |
| Compatible with | **Flush**: NaCl 0.9%<br>**Solutions**: NaCl 0.9%, Gluc 5%, Gluc-NaCl (with added KCl)<br>**Y-site**: Adrenaline (epinephrine), amikacin, aminophylline, clindamycin, dexamethasone, dobutamine, dopamine, linezolid, metoclopramide, vancomycin |

*(continued)*

## Technical information (continued)

| pH | 4.8 |
|---|---|
| Sodium content | 15.4 mmol/100 mL |
| Storage | Store below 25°C in original packaging.<br>Use opened vials immediately and discard any unused solution. |

## Monitoring

| Measure | Frequency | Rationale |
|---|---|---|
| Blood pressure | Check during infusion | • BP can drop suddenly, especially if the patient is taking hypotensive agents.<br>• In rare cases circulatory collapse may occur – if a conspicuous drop occurs, stop the infusion immediately. |
| Renal function | Periodically | • Changes in renal function may necessitate a dose adjustment. |
| LFTs | | • Mild ↑AST, ↑ALT commonly and ↑bilirubin occasionally. |
| FBC | | • Eosinophilia and leucopenia are the most common effects although other dyscrasias may occur.<br>• WCC: for signs of the infection resolving. |
| Signs of tendon damage (including rupture) | Throughout treatment | • Although rare, rupture may occur within 48 hours of starting treatment.<br>• There is a higher risk in elderly patients and with concomitant use of corticosteroids.<br>• If tendinitis is suspected, discontinue immediately; the affected limb should not be exerted and should be made non-weight-bearing. |
| Signs of CNS disorders | | • Use with caution in patients with epilepsy or patients with tendency to spasms, previous seizures, vascular disorders in the brain, alterations in brain structure or stroke.<br>• If self-destructive behaviour is demonstrated or seizures occur, discontinue treatment. |
| Symptoms of neuropathy | | • Due to axonal polyneuropathy and may be irreversible, although incidence is rare.<br>• Discontinue if such symptoms occur, e.g. pain, burning, tingling, numbness; or deficits in light touch, pain, temperature, position sense, vibratory sensation, motor strength. |
| Signs of supra-infection or superinfection | | • May result in the overgrowth of non-susceptible organisms – appropriate therapy should be commenced; treatment may need to be interrupted. |

*(continued)*

## Monitoring (continued)

| Measure | Frequency | Rationale |
|---|---|---|
| Blood glucose concentration | Increased frequency in patients with diabetes | • Symptomatic hyperglycaemia and/or hypoglycaemia have been reported, requiring closer monitoring<br>• If signs or symptoms of glucose disturbances develop, therapy should be stopped. |
| Development of diarrhoea | Throughout and up to 2 months after treatment | • Development of severe, persistent diarrhoea may be suggestive of *Clostridium difficile*-associated diarrhoea and colitis (pseudomembranous colitis). Discontinue drug and treat. Do not use drugs that inhibit peristalsis. |

## Additional information

| | |
|---|---|
| Common and serious undesirable effects | *Infusion-related:* Local: reddening of the infusion site and phlebitis.<br>*Other:* Nausea and vomiting, headache, dizziness, sleep disorders, restlessness, skin rash, itching. |
| Pharmacokinetics | Elimination half-life is 6–8 hours. |
| Significant interactions | • Levofloxacin may ↑levels or effect of the following drugs (or ↑side-effects): artemether with lumefantrine (avoid combination), amiodarone (↑risk of ventricular arrhythmias - avoid combination), ciclosporin (↑risk of nephrotoxicity), NSAIDs (↑risk of seizures), theophylline (↑risk of seizures).<br>• Levofloxacin may ↓levels or effect of antiepileptic drugs (↓seizure threshold). |
| Action in case of overdose | *Symptoms to watch for:* CNS side-effects are the biggest concern. Monitor pulse, BP and cardiac rhythm. Perform 12-lead ECG and measure QT interval. Measure U&Es, LFTs, creatine kinase in symptomatic patients.<br>*Antidote:* If seizures are frequent or prolonged, control with IV diazepam (10–20 mg) or lorazepam (4 mg). Give oxygen and correct acid-base and metabolic disturbances as required. Consider IV phenytoin if convulsions continue to be unresponsive to above measures. |
| Counselling | Photosensitivity may develop on exposure to strong sunlight and ultraviolet rays, e.g. sunlamps, solaria - patients should avoid unnecessary exposure. |

| Risk rating: **GREEN** | Score = 2<br>Lower-risk product: Risk-reduction strategies should be considered. |
|---|---|

This assessment is based on the full range of preparation and administration options described in the monograph. These may not all be applicable in some clinical situations.

## Bibliography

SPC Tavanic IV (accessed 24 March 2009).

# Levomepromazine (methotrimeprazine)

### 25 mg/mL solution in 1-mL ampoules

- Levomepromazine hydrochloride is a phenothiazine derivative.
- It is used as an antiemetic, antihistamine and sedative in palliative care.
- It may also be given by continuous SC infusion in palliative care for the management of pain, nausea and vomiting, and the accompanying restlessness or distress.
- Doses below are expressed in terms of levomepromazine hydrochloride.

## Pre-treatment checks

- Avoid or use with caution in patients with liver dysfunction or cardiac disease.
- Patients receiving large initial doses should be kept in bed as it may have a hypotensive effect.

*Biochemical and other tests (not all are necessary in an emergency situation)*

Blood pressure                          Electrolytes: serum Ca, Mg, K
ECG                                     LFTs

## Dose

**Standard dose**: 12.5–25 mg by IM or IV injection every 6 to 8 hours. In cases of severe agitation the dose may be increased to 50 mg.

## Intramuscular injection

*Preparation and administration*

1. Withdraw the required dose.
2. Give by IM injection.

## Intravenous injection

*Preparation and administration*

1. Withdraw the required dose and dilute with an equal volume of NaCl 0.9%.
2. The solution should be clear and colourless. Inspect visually for particulate matter or discoloration prior to administration and discard if present.
3. Give by IV injection over 3–5 minutes.

## Technical information

| Incompatible with | Heparin sodium |
|---|---|
| Compatible with | **Flush**: NaCl 0.9%<br>**Solutions**: NaCl 0.9%<br>**Y-site**: Diamorphine, fentanyl |
| pH | 3–5 |
| Sodium content | Negligible |
| Excipients | Contains sulfites (may cause hypersensitivity reactions) |

*(continued)*

## Technical information (*continued*)

| | |
|---|---|
| Storage | Store below 25°C in original packaging. On exposure to light, levomepromazine rapidly discolours; such solutions should be discarded. |

## Monitoring

| Measure | Frequency | Rationale |
|---|---|---|
| ECG | Whenever dose escalation is proposed and when the maximum therapeutic dose is reached | • QT interval prolongation may occur.<br>• There is ↑risk of arrhythmias if used with drugs that prolong the QT interval. |
| Serum Ca, Mg, K | Periodically | • Owing to the potential QT prolongation these electrolytes should be monitored and corrected, especially where long-term use is anticipated. |
| LFTs | | • Use with caution in people with liver dysfunction.<br>• Phenothiazines are hepatotoxic; can precipitate coma. |
| Blood pressure | | • Can cause ↓BP. |

## Additional information

| | |
|---|---|
| Common and serious undesirable effects | *Immediate:* EPSEs, ↓BP.<br>*Other:* ↓BP, drowsiness, asthenia, neuroleptic malignant syndrome – these may be experienced on long-term therapy. |
| Pharmacokinetics | Elimination half-life is about 30 hours. |
| Significant interactions | • The following may ↑levomepromazine levels or effect (or ↑side-effects): anaesthetics-general (↑risk of ↓BP), antidepressants-tricyclic, artemether with lumefantrine (avoid combination), ritonavir, sibutramine (avoid combination).<br>• Levomepromazine may ↓levels or effect of levodopa.<br>• Levomepromazine may ↑risk of ventricular arrhythmias with the following drugs: amiodarone (avoid combination), antidepressants-tricyclic, atomoxetine, disopyramide, droperidol (avoid combination), methadone, moxifloxacin (avoid combination), pentamidine isetionate, pimozide (avoid combination), sotalol.<br>• Levomepromazine ↓convulsive threshold and may ↓effect of the following drugs:<br>barbiturates, carbamazepine, ethosuximide, oxcarbazepine, phenytoin, primidone, valproate. |
| Action in case of overdose | *Symptoms to watch for:* Drowsiness or loss of consciousness, ↓BP, ↑pulse.<br>Treatment is supportive and symptomatic:<br>Severe dystonic reactions may be treated with 5–10 mg procyclidine or 20–40 mg orphenadrine.<br>Convulsions may be treated with IV diazepam.<br>Neuroleptic malignant syndrome should be treated with cooling. Dantrolene sodium may be required.<br>Do not give adrenaline. |

| Risk rating: **GREEN** | Score = 1<br>Lower-risk product. Risk-reduction strategies should be considered. |

This assessment is based on use by IM administration. This may not be applicable in some clinical situations.

## Bibliography

SPC Nozinan (accessed 26 August 2008).

---

# Lidocaine (lignocaine) hydrochloride – intravenous administration

**10 mg/mL (1%) in 10-mL pre-filled syringes; 20 mg/mL (2%) in 5-mL pre-filled syringes**
**10 mg/mL (1%) solution and 20 mg/mL (2%) solution in 2-mL, 5-mL, 10-mL and 20-mL ampoules**
**1 mg/mL (0.1%) and 2 mg/mL (0.2%) in Gluc 5% in 500-mL infusion bags**

- Lidocaine is a local anaesthetic and it also has class 1b antiarrhythmic effects.
- It is used IV to treat ventricular arrhythmias, especially after MI.
- Doses are expressed in terms of lidocaine hydrochloride.

Products containing adrenaline (epinephrine) or preservatives **must not** be given by IV injection.

## Pre-treatment checks

- Caution in patients with porphyria.
- In IV therapy resuscitative equipment and drugs should be immediately available for the management of severe adverse cardiovascular, respiratory or central nervous system effects.

*Biochemical and other tests (not all are necessary in an emergency situation)*

Possibly prior to IV treatment:
  ECG
  Electrolytes: serum K (correct ↓K before
  commencing therapy)

Renal function: U, Cr, CrCl (or eGFR)

## Dose

**Ventricular arrhythmias:** 100 mg by IV injection in patients without gross circulatory impairment (50 mg in lighter patients or those whose circulation is severely impaired); followed immediately by 4 mg/minute by IV infusion for 30 minutes, then 2 mg/minute for 2 hours, then 1 mg/minute. Reduce the rate further if infusion is continued beyond 24 hours (rarely required).

* The IV injection dose can be repeated once or twice at intervals of not less than 10 minutes if an infusion is not immediately available.
* Stop the infusion as soon as the basic cardiac rhythm appears to be stable or at the earliest signs of toxicity.

## Intravenous injection

*Preparation and administration*

1. Select the appropriate pre-filled syringe. Expel any excess lidocaine if necessary. Alternatively, withdraw the required dose.
2. The solution should be clear and colourless. Inspect visually for particulate matter or discoloration prior to administration and discard if present.
3. Give by IV injection at a rate of 25–50 mg/minute, i.e. give 1% injection at 2.5–5 mL/minute; give 2% injection at 1.25–2.5 mL/minute.

## Continuous intravenous infusion

*Preparation and administration*

1. Select the correct pre-prepared infusion bag. Alternatively, withdraw the required dose of 1% or 2% injection and add to a suitable volume (usually 500 mL) of Gluc 5% to give a solution containing between 1 mg/mL and 4 mg/mL. Mix well.
2. The solution should be clear and colourless. Inspect visually for particulate matter or discoloration prior to administration and discard if present.
3. Give by IV infusion via a volumetric infusion device at the appropriate rate (see Dose above).

## Technical information

| Incompatible with | Amphotericin, thiopental sodium. |
|---|---|
| Compatible with | **Flush**: NaCl 0.9%<br>**Solutions**: Gluc 5%, NaCl 0.9%, Hartmann's (all with added KCl)<br>**Y-site**: Alteplase, bivalirudin, cisatracurium, ciprofloxacin, clarithromycin, dobutamine, dopamine, glyceryl trinitrate, linezolid, micafungin, propofol, remifentanil, streptokinase, tirofiban |
| pH | 5-7 for injection solutions; 3.5-7 for infusions in Gluc |
| Sodium content | Negligible |
| Storage | Store below 25°C in original packaging. |
| Stability after preparation | From a microbiological point of view, should be used immediately; however, prepared infusions may be stored at 2-8°C and infused (at room temperature) within 24 hours. |

## Monitoring

| Measure | Frequency | Rationale |
|---|---|---|
| ECG, heart rate and blood pressure | Continuously | • Response to therapy.<br>• ↓BP and ↓pulse may lead to cardiac arrest. |
| CNS toxicity | | • Convulsions, respiratory depression may occur. |
| Infusion site | Half-hourly | • Extravasation may cause tissue damage. |

## Additional information

| | |
|---|---|
| Common and serious undesirable effects | *Immediate:* Anaphylaxis and other hypersensitivity reactions have rarely been reported.<br>*Injection/infusion-related:*<br>• Too rapid administration: Dizziness, paraesthesia, drowsiness, ↓BP, ↓pulse.<br>• Local: Extravasation may cause tissue damage.<br><br>*Other:* Apprehension, nervousness, euphoria, tinnitus, blurred or double vision, nystagmus, vomiting, sensations of heat, cold or numbness, twitching, tremors. |
| Pharmacokinetics | Plasma concentrations decline rapidly after an IV dose with an initial half-life of less than 30 minutes.<br>Elimination half-life is 1–2 hours but may be prolonged if infusions are given for longer than 24 hours or if hepatic blood flow is reduced. |
| Significant interactions | • The following may ↑lidocaine levels or effect (or ↑side-effects):<br>antiarrhythmics (↑risk of myocardial depression), antipsychotics (↑risk of ventricular arrhythmias), atazanavir, beta-blockers (↑risk of myocardial depression), cimetidine (↑risk of toxicity), fosamprenavir (avoid combination), quinupristin with dalfopristin (↑risk of ventricular arrhythmias).<br>• ↓K caused by the following may ↓lidocaine levels or effect: acetazolamide, diuretics-loop, diuretics-thiazide. |
| Action in case of overdose | *Symptoms to watch for:* Medullary depression, seizures, cardiovascular collapse.<br>*Antidote:* No specific antidote; stop administration and give supportive therapy as appropriate, which may include diazepam for seizures and metaraminol for ↓BP. |

| | |
|---|---|
| Risk rating: **AMBER** | Score = 5<br>Moderate-risk product: Risk-reduction strategies are recommended. |

This assessment is based on the full range of preparation and administration options described in the monograph. These may not all be applicable in some clinical situations.

## Bibliography

SPC Lidocaine Hydrochloride Injection BP Minijet 1% and 2% (accessed 3 May 2010).
SPC Lidocaine Injection BP 1% and 2% w/v, Hameln (accessed 3 May 2010).

# Lidocaine (lignocaine) hydrochloride – local anaesthetic use

**10 mg/mL (1%) and 20 mg/mL (2%) solution in 2-mL, 5-mL, 10-mL and 20-mL ampoules**
**10 mg/mL (1%) with adrenaline (epinephrine) 1 : 200 000 solution in 20-mL and 50-mL vials**
**20 mg/mL (2%) with adrenaline (epinephrine) 1 : 200 000 solution in 20-mL and 50-mL vials**

* Lidocaine is a local anaesthetic and it also has class 1b antiarrhythmic effects.
* It is used for infiltration anaesthesia and for regional nerve blocks. It has a rapid onset and anaesthesia is usually effective within a few minutes.
* In some preparations a local vasoconstrictor such as adrenaline (epinephrine) is added to ↑speed of onset and duration of action and also to ↓toxicity of lidocaine by limiting absorption into the general circulation.
* Some multidose vials contain preservatives and these preparations must not be used for spinal, epidural, caudal or IV regional anaesthesia.
* Lidocaine is included in some injections such as depot corticosteroids to prevent pain, itching, and other local irritation; it may also be use to reconstitute IM injections of some antibacterials to reduce injection site pain.
* A wide range of formulations exists and the listing above is not exhaustive.

## Pre-treatment checks

Caution in patients with porphyria.

*Biochemical and other tests (not all are necessary in an emergency situation)*

Nil for local anaesthetic use

## Dose

> Products containing adrenaline or preservatives **must not** be given by IV injection.
> **Important:** When lidocaine is used for local anaesthesia, rapid and extensive absorption may occur resulting in systemic side-effects.

**Infiltration anaesthesia:** dose is determined by patient's weight and the site and nature of the procedure:
* Maximum dose without adrenaline: 200 mg.
* Maximum dose with adrenaline: 500 mg.

**IV regional anaesthesia and nerve blocks:** seek expert advice.

| Technical information | |
|---|---|
| Incompatible with | Not relevant |
| Compatible with | Not relevant |
| pH | 5-7 |
| Sodium content | Negligible |

*(continued)*

## Technical information (*continued*)

| | |
|---|---|
| Excipients | Some products contain preservatives. These products must not be used for spinal, epidural, caudal or IV regional anaesthesia. |
| Storage | As specified in the individual product literature. |

## Monitoring

There is little need for monitoring when used for local anaesthesia. If it is accidentally given intravenously, see the separate monograph on intravenous administration for monitoring requirements.

## Additional information

| | |
|---|---|
| Common and serious undesirable effects | Inadvertent IV dosing during local anaesthetic procedures can cause dizziness, paraesthesia and drowsiness. ↓BP and ↓pulse may lead to cardiac arrest. |
| Pharmacokinetics | Serum lidocaine concentrations are usually insignificant following local use. |
| Significant interactions | None expected when used for local anaesthesia. |
| Action in case of overdose | *Symptoms to watch for:* Cardiovascular collapse, seizure, medullary depression. *Antidote:* No specific antidote; stop administration and give supportive therapy as appropriate, which may include diazepam for seizures and metaraminol for ↓BP. |

| Risk rating: **GREEN** | Score = 2 Lower-risk product. Risk-reduction strategies should be considered. |
|---|---|

This assessment is based on the full range of preparation and administration options described in the monograph. These may not all be applicable in some clinical situations.

## Bibliography

SPC Lidocaine Injection BP with preservative 1% and 2%, Hameln Pharmaceuticals Ltd (accessed 3 May 2010).
SPC Xylocaine 1% and 2% with adrenaline, AstraZeneca UK Ltd (accessed 3 May 2010).

# Linezolid

**2 mg/mL solution in 300-mL infusion bags**

- Linezolid is an oxazolidinone antibacterial.
- It is used for the treatment of Gram-positive infections of the skin and respiratory tract, including those due to vancomycin-resistant enterococci and MRSA. It is not effective against Gram-negative organisms.

- It is also a reversible, non-selective inhibitor of monoamine oxidase (MAOI), although it does not exert an antidepressive effect in antibacterial dose (see Pre-treatment checks and Significant interactions below).
- Linezolid has an oral bioavailability of approximately 100%. The parenteral formulation should be used only if the oral route is unavailable.

## Pre-treatment checks

- Only give to patients with the following conditions if facilities are available to closely monitor BP: uncontrolled ↑BP, phaeochromocytoma, carcinoid, thyrotoxicosis, bipolar depression, schizo-affective disorder, acute confusional states; or patients taking the following medication: SSRIs, tricyclic antidepressants, 5HT1 agonists (triptans), sympathomimetics, buspirone, pethidine and possibly other opioid analgesics).
- ↑Risk of seizures in patients with a history of seizures.

*Biochemical and other tests*

Blood pressure
Electrolytes: serum Na, K
FBC

LFTs
Renal function: U, Cr, CrCl (or eGFR)

## Dose

**Standard dose**: 600 mg twice daily usually for 10–14 days.
**Dose in renal impairment**: adjusted according to creatinine clearance:[1]

- CrCl 10–50 mL/minute: dose as in normal renal function
- CrCl <10 mL/minute: dose as in normal renal function. If platelet count drops on a dose of 600 mg twice daily, consider reducing to 600 mg once daily. The two primary metabolites accumulate and have MAOI activity but no antibacterial activity – monitor the patient closely. For patients under-going dialysis, give the dose after dialysis.

## Intermittent intravenous infusion

*Preparation and administration*

1. Remove the overwrap only when ready to use. Check for minute leaks by squeezing the bag firmly – if the bag leaks, do not use.
2. The solution is pre-prepared for use. It should be clear and colourless to yellow. Inspect visually for particulate matter or discoloration prior to administration and discard if present.
3. Give by IV infusion over 30–120 minutes.

| Technical information | |
|---|---|
| Incompatible with | Amphotericin, ceftriaxone, co-trimoxazole, diazepam, erythromycin, pentamidine isetionate, phenytoin sodium. |
| Compatible with | **Flush**: NaCl 0.9%<br>**Solutions**: NaCl 0.9%, Gluc 5% (with added KCl), Gluc-NaCl, Hartmann's, Ringer's<br>**Y-site**: Aciclovir, alfentanil, amikacin, aminophylline, aztreonam, calcium gluconate, ceftazidime, cefuroxime, ciprofloxacin, cisatracurium, clindamycin, dexamethasone, digoxin, esmolol, fluconazole, furosemide, ganciclovir, gentamicin, glyceryl trinitrate, granisetron, hydrocortisone sodium succinate, imipenem with cilastatin, labetalol, magnesium sulfate, meropenem, methylprednisolone sodium succinate, metoclopramide, metronidazole, midazolam, naloxone, ondansetron, piperacillin with tazobactam, ranitidine, tigecycline, tobramycin, vancomycin, vecuronium bromide |

*(continued)*

## Technical information (continued)

| | |
|---|---|
| pH | 4.8 |
| Sodium content | 5 mmol/300 mL |
| Excipients | Each 300 mL contains 13.7 g glucose. |
| Storage | Store below 25°C. Protect from light and freezing.<br>The solution may exhibit a yellow colour, which can intensify over time. This does not affect potency or stability.<br>Once opened, use immediately. Discard any unused solution. |

## Monitoring

| Measure | Frequency | Rationale |
|---|---|---|
| FBC (including haemoglobin, platelets, total and differentiated leucocyte counts) | Weekly | • Myelosuppression may occur (including anaemia, leucopenia, pancytopenia and thrombocytopenia).<br>• More common if treatment is long duration and/or in patients with severe renal impairment.<br>• Blood transfusions have been used if anaemia is severe.<br>• Neutrophil and eosinophil counts commonly rise. |
| Signs of metabolic acidosis | Throughout treatment | • Symptoms include recurrent nausea, vomiting, abdominal pain, low bicarbonate level or hyperventilation.<br>• Immediate medical attention is required. |
| Signs of supra-infection or superinfection | | • May result in the overgrowth of non-susceptible organisms - appropriate therapy should be commenced; treatment may need to be interrupted. |
| Signs of visual impairment | | • Can cause peripheral and optic neuropathy: monitor for blurred vision, visual field defects, changes in visual acuity and colour vision. Evaluate promptly and refer to an ophthalmologist as necessary.<br>• Formally check visual function if treatment is longer than 28 days.<br>• If this occurs, weigh continued use against potential risks |
| LFTs | Periodically | • ↑AST, ↑ALT, ↑LDH, ↑Alk Phos levels and ↓albumin and ↓total protein are commonly seen. |
| U&Es | | • ↑U, ↓Na and ↓↑K levels are commonly seen. |
| Development of diarrhoea | Throughout and up to 2 months after treatment | • Development of severe, persistent diarrhoea may be suggestive of *Clostridium difficile*-associated diarrhoea and colitis (pseudomembranous colitis). Discontinue drug and treat. Do not use drugs that inhibit peristalsis. |

## Additional information

| | |
|---|---|
| Common and serious undesirable effects | Candidiasis (particularly oral and vaginal candidiasis) or fungal infections, headache, taste perversion (metallic taste), diarrhoea, nausea, vomiting, abnormal LFTs. |
| Pharmacokinetics | Elimination half-life is 5 hours. The two primary metabolites accumulate and have MAOI activity but no antibacterial activity. |
| Significant interactions | • Linezolid is a reversible non-selective MAOI.<br>• Avoid concurrent use of linezolid with the following (see above and BNF for details):<br>anaesthetics-general, antidepressants-tricyclic, antidepressants-tricyclic related, atomoxetine, bupropion, carbamazepine, duloxetine, entacapone, indoramin, methyldopa, mirtazapine, moclobemide, nefopam, opioid analgesics, rizatriptan, sibutramine, sumatriptan.<br>• ↑Risk of hypertensive crisis if linezolid is given with:<br>levodopa, MAOIs, methylphenidate, rasagiline, reboxetine, sympathomimetics.<br>• ↑Risk of CNS toxicity if linezolid if given with:<br>antidepressants-SSRI, antidepressants-tricyclic, clozapine, MAOIs, tetrabenazine, tryptophan, venlafaxine, zolmitriptan.<br>• Linezolid may ↓levels or effect of carbamazepine. |
| Action in case of overdose | No cases of overdose have been reported.<br>*Antidote:* No known antidote but haemodialysis is known to remove the two primary metabolites. Stop administration and give supportive therapy as appropriate. |
| Counselling | Linezolid is a reversible non-selective MAOI. Advise against consuming large amounts of tyramine-rich foods, e.g. mature cheese, yeast extracts, undistilled alcoholic beverages and fermented soya-bean products such as soy sauce. |

| | |
|---|---|
| Risk rating: **GREEN** | Score = 0<br>Lower-risk product: Risk-reduction strategies should be considered. |

This assessment is based on the full range of preparation and administration options described in the monograph. These may not all be applicable in some clinical situations.

### Reference

1. Ashley C, Currie A, eds. *The Renal Drug Handbook*, 3rd edn. Oxford: Radcliffe Medical Press, 2009.

### Bibliography

SPC Zyvox 2 mg/mL solution for infusion (accessed 24 March 2009).

# Liothyronine sodium (L-tri-iodothyronine)

**20 micrograms dry powder ampoules**

- Liothyronine sodium has a similar action to levothyroxine but is more rapidly metabolised and has a faster effect.
- Given IV it is the treatment of choice in severe hypothyroid states and hypothyroid coma when a rapid response is desired.
- Doses may be expressed as liothyronine sodium or liothyronine. Doses below are expressed in terms of liothyronine sodium:
  Liothyronine 10 micrograms ≡ 10.3 micrograms liothyronine sodium.

## Pre-treatment checks

- Caution in myxoedema coma as a large dose can precipitate heart failure, especially in elderly patients and those with ischaemic heart disease.
- In severe and prolonged hypothyroidism there may be decreased adrenocortical activity. When thyroid replacement therapy is started, metabolism is raised at a greater rate than adrenocortical activity; this can result in adrenocortical insufficiency so that additional corticosteroid therapy may be required.
- An increase in hypoglycaemic therapy may be necessary in patients with diabetes mellitus started on thyroid replacement therapy.

*Biochemical and other tests*

Blood pressure
Pulse
TFTs

## Dose

Liothyronine 20 micrograms IV ≅ levothyroxine 100 micrograms orally.
Oral therapy should be instituted as soon as possible.
When changing from IV to oral therapy, levothyroxine should be introduced gradually, particularly in elderly patients and patients with pre-existing ischaemic heart disease.
Liothyronine must not be given by IM injection (the solution is very alkaline).

**Hypothyroid coma:** 5–20 micrograms by IV injection every 12 hours or more frequently if necessary. No more than 12 hours should elapse between doses to avoid fluctuations in hormone levels. Administration more frequently than every 4 hours does not allow for assessment of therapeutic response between doses.

## Intravenous injection

*Preparation and administration*

1. Add 1–2 mL WFI to the ampoule and shake gently until the plug has dissolved.
2. Withdraw the required dose.
3. The solution should be clear and colourless. Inspect visually for particulate matter or discoloration prior to administration.
4. Give by IV injection over 3–5 minutes.

## Technical information

| Incompatible with | No information |
|---|---|
| Compatible with | **Flush**:NaCl 0.9%<br>**Solutions**: WFI<br>**Y-site**: No information |
| pH | 9.8–11.2 |
| Sodium content | Negligible |
| Storage | Store below 25°C in original packaging. |
| Stability after preparation | Use prepared solutions immediately. |

## Monitoring

| Measure | Frequency | Rationale |
|---|---|---|
| Blood pressure and pulse | Periodically through treatment | • ↑Pulse and anginal pain can occur, particularly in elderly patients and in patients with pre-existing IHD. |
| ECG | | • Treatment of myxoedema coma can precipitate heart failure, particularly elderly patients and in patients with pre-existing IHD. |
| TFTs | Periodically | • To monitor therapeutic response. |

## Additional information

| Common and serious undesirable effects | The following are indicative of overdosage, and disappear after reduction of dosage or stopping treatment for a day or more: anginal pain, cardiac arrhythmias, palpitations, ↑pulse, cramps, diarrhoea, muscular weakness, flushing, sweating, restlessness, excitability, headache. |
|---|---|
| Pharmacokinetics | Liothyronine has a plasma half-life in euthyroidism of about 1–2 days; the half-life is prolonged in hypothyroidism and reduced in hyperthyroidism.<br>Following a single IV dose of liothyronine sodium, a detectable metabolic response occurs within as little as 2–4 hours, with a maximum therapeutic response within 2 days. |
| Significant interactions | • Liothyronine may ↑levels or effect of the following drugs (or ↑side-effects): acenocoumarol (monitor INR), warfarin (monitor INR), phenindione (monitor INR). |
| Action in case of overdose | Symptoms of overdosage disappear after reduction in dose or stopping treatment for a day or more. Give supportive therapy as appropriate. |

| Risk rating: **GREEN** | Score = 2<br>Lower-risk product: Risk-reduction strategies should be considered. |

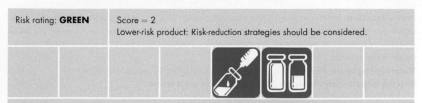

This assessment is based on the full range of preparation and administration options described in the monograph. These may not all be applicable in some clinical situations.

## Reference

1. Jeevanandam V *et al.* Reversal of donor myocardial dysfunction by triiodothyronine replacement therapy. *J Heart Lung Transplant* 1994; 13: 681–687.

## Bibliography

SPC Triiodothyronine, Goldshield (received by e-mail 26 January 2009).

# Lorazepam

### 4 mg/mL solution in 1-mL ampoules

* Lorazepam is a short-acting benzodiazepine with anxiolytic, anticonvulsant and central muscle relaxant properties.
* It is used parenterally to provide sedation prior to procedures such as endoscopy, as a premedication before general anaesthesia, to treat status epilepticus and to manage severe acute anxiety or agitation.
* It is also used for rapid tranquillisation in the treatment of acutely disturbed behaviour.

## Pre-treatment checks

* Avoid in acute pulmonary insufficiency, sleep apnoea syndrome, myasthenia gravis and severe hepatic insufficiency.
* Caution should be used in acute narrow-angle glaucoma.
* Equipment necessary to maintain a patent airway and to support respiration/ventilation should be available in the event of a respiratory arrest.
* Do not give within 1 hour of olanzapine IM injection.

*Biochemical and other tests (not all are necessary in an emergency)*

| | |
|---|---|
| Blood pressure | Renal function: U, Cr, CrCl (or eGFR) |
| Bodyweight | Respiratory rate |
| LFTs | |

## Dose

**Acute anxiety and acute panic attacks**: 25–30 micrograms/kg (usual range 1.5–2.5 mg) repeated every 6 hours if necessary.

**Premedication:** 50 micrograms/kg (3.5 mg for an average 70 kg man) by IV injection 30–45 minutes before procedure. Sedation will be evident after 5–10 minutes and maximal loss of recall will occur after 30–45 minutes. If the IV and oral routes are not available, give by IM injection 60–90 minutes before the procedure.

**Status epilepticus:** 4 mg by IV injection. Repeat once after 10 minutes if necessary.

**Dose in hepatic impairment:** reduce dose and avoid if severe.

## Intravenous injection (preferred route)

*Preparation and administration*

> IV injection should be performed with extreme care to avoid inadvertent intra-arterial injection, which can cause arteriospasm possibly resulting in gangrene.

1. Add 1 mL NaCl 0.9% or WFI to the lorazepam ampoule and mix the contents gently to give a solution containing 2 mg/mL.
2. Withdraw the required dose.
3. Immediately return the remainder of the lorazepam box to the refrigerator (not stable at room temperature for longer than 30 minutes).
4. The solution should be clear and colourless. Inspect visually for particulate matter or discoloration prior to administration and discard if present.
5. If treating status epilepticus give by rapid IV injection into a large vein, otherwise give by slow IV injection into a large vein over 3–5 minutes.

## Intramuscular injection

*Preparation and administration*

> IM injection is not recommended; it works no more rapidly than oral administration.

1. Add 1 mL NaCl 0.9% or WFI to the lorazepam ampoule and mix the contents gently to give a solution containing 2 mg/mL.
2. Withdraw the required dose.
3. Immediately return the remainder of the lorazepam box to the refrigerator (not stable at room temperature for longer than 30 minutes).
4. Give by deep IM injection into a large muscle.

## Technical information

| | |
|---|---|
| Incompatible with | Do not mix with other drugs in the same syringe.<br>Aztreonam, flucloxacillin, foscarnet, imipenem with cilastatin, omeprazole, ondansetron. |
| Compatible with | **Flush**: NaCl 0.9%<br>**Solutions**: NaCl 0.9%, WFI (for dilution - injection is viscous when cold)<br>**Y-site**: Aciclovir, adrenaline (epinephrine), amikacin, amoxicillin, atracurium, bumetanide, cefotaxime, cisatracurium, co-amoxiclav, co-trimoxazole, dexamethasone, dobutamine, dopamine, erythromycin, fentanyl, fluconazole, fosphenytoin sodium, furosemide, gentamicin, glyceryl trinitrate, granisetron, hydrocortisone sodium succinate, labetalol, metronidazole, micafungin, noradrenaline (norepinephrine), piperacillin with tazobactam, potassium chloride, propofol, ranitidine, remifentanil, vancomycin, vecuronium bromide |

*(continued)*

## Technical information (continued)

| | |
|---|---|
| pH | Not relevant - non-aqueous solution |
| Sodium content | Nil |
| Excipients | Contains benzyl alcohol and propylene glycol (adverse effects seen in ↓renal function, may interact with disulfiram and metronidazole). |
| Storage | Store at 2-8°C. Product degrades quickly on exposure to higher temperatures. The manufacturer currently recommends that the injection should not be raised to room temperature for longer than 30 minutes. Do not freeze. |

## Monitoring

| Measure | Frequency | Rationale |
|---|---|---|
| Respiratory rate | Monitor every 15 minutes for 2 hours after the injection | • Can cause respiratory depression.<br>• Keep under observation for 8 hours after the injection and preferably overnight. |
| Mental state | Post injection | • Excessive central nervous system depression may develop, e.g. drowsiness, lethargy. |
| Blood pressure | | • ↓BP occurs rarely, but if a patient is predisposed, e.g. elderly, closer monitoring is required. |
| Injection-site reaction (IM) | | • Pain and redness can occur but is rarely reported. |

## Additional information

| | |
|---|---|
| Common and serious undesirable effects | *Immediate:* Anaphylaxis and other hypersensitivity reactions have been reported.<br>*Injection-related:* Local: Rarely pain and redness.<br>*Other:* Sedation, drowsiness, unsteadiness, muscle weakness, ataxia. Rarely respiratory depression, ↓BP. |
| Pharmacokinetics | Elimination half-life is 12-16 hours. |
| Significant interactions | • Olanzapine IM may ↑lorazepam levels or effect (or ↑side-effects): ↓BP, ↓pulse, respiratory depression.<br>• Lorazepam may ↑levels or effect (or ↑side-effects) of sodium oxybate (avoid combination). |
| Action in case of overdose | *Symptoms to watch for:* ↑sedation, respiratory depression, ↓BP.<br>*Antidote:* Flumazenil (use with caution in patients with a history of seizures, head injury or chronic benzodiazepine use including for the control of epilepsy).<br>Stop administration and give supportive therapy as appropriate. |

*(continued)*

**Additional information** (*continued*)

| Counselling | Alcoholic drinks should not be consumed for at least 24–48 hours after receiving lorazepam.<br>If applicable the patient should be accompanied home by a responsible adult and should not drive or operate machinery for 24 hours. |

Risk rating: **AMBER**

Score = 3
Moderate-risk product: Risk-reduction strategies are recommended.

This assessment is based on the full range of preparation and administration options described in the monograph. These may not all be applicable in some clinical situations.

## Bibliography

SPC Ativan (accessed 22 January 2008).

# Magnesium sulfate

**10% solution in 10-mL and 50-mL ampoules: 20% solution in 20-mL ampoules**
**50% solution in 2-mL, 5-mL and 10-mL ampoules; 4-mL and 10-mL pre-filled syringes**
**20 mmol in 100 mL NaCl 0.9% (a 'specials' product)**

* Magnesium is the second most abundant cation in the intracellular fluid; it is an essential electrolyte and a co-factor in many enzyme systems.
* Normal range for plasma magnesium is 0.75–0.95 mmol/L.
* Magnesium sulfate injection is used to treat hypomagnesaemia.
* It may also be used in the emergency management of severe asthma and also in eclampsia and pre-eclampsia (all unlicensed).

| | |
|---|---|
| 10% magnesium sulfate injection contains | 0.1 g/mL ≅ Mg²⁺ 0.4 mmol/mL. |
| 20% magnesium sulfate injection contains | 0.2 g/mL ≅ Mg²⁺ 0.8 mmol/mL. |
| 50% magnesium sulfate injection contains | 0.5 g/mL ≅ Mg²⁺ 2 mmol/mL. |

## Pre-treatment checks

* Avoid in renal failure, heart block and myocardial damage.
* Avoid in hepatic coma if there is a risk of renal failure.
* Do not give with high doses of barbiturates, opioids or hypnotics (risk of respiratory depression).
* Caution if patient is taking cardiac glycosides.

*Biochemical and other tests (not all are necessary in an emergency situation)*

Bodyweight
Electrolytes: serum Mg
Renal function: U, Cr, CrCl (or eGFR)

## Dose

Doses should be tailored to individual requirements.

**Mild hypomagnesaemia:** a dose of 4 mmol (1 g) by IM injection every 6 hours for 4 doses has been used, but injections are painful.

**Symptomatic hypomagnesaemia:** 1–2 mmol/kg by IV infusion. Up to a total of 160 mmol may be required over 5 days.

One regimen is to give 0.5 mmol/kg by IV infusion on day 1; then 0.25 mmol/kg by IV infusion on days 2–5, rounding the doses to conveniently measurable volumes.

**Asthma (unlicensed):** 4.8–8 mmol (1.2–2 g) by IV infusion over 20 minutes.

**Ventricular fibrillation in the presence of ↓Mg; arrhythmias including torsade de pointes:** 8 mmol (2 g) by slow IV injection.

**Prevention of recurrent seizures in pregnant women with eclampsia (unlicensed):** 16 mmol (4 g) by IV injection or small-volume infusion over 10–15 minutes followed by 4 mmol (1 g)/hour by IV infusion for at least 24 hours after last seizure. If seizures recur then an additional dose of 8–16 mmol (2–4 g) may be given by IV injection or small-volume infusion.

**Dose in renal impairment:** monitor levels closely and reduce dose as appropriate.

**Fluid restriction:** solutions containing up to 0.4 mmol/mL magnesium sulfate may be given by IV infusion via a peripheral vein; solutions containing up to 0.8 mmol/mL magnesium sulfate may be given by IV infusion via a central line.

## Intravenous infusion (preferred method)

*Preparation and administration*

1. Withdraw the required dose and add to a suitable volume NaCl 0.9% or Gluc 5% to give a solution containing a maximum of 0.4 mmol/mL.
2. The solution should be clear and colourless. Inspect visually for particulate matter or discoloration prior to administration and discard if present.
3. Infuse via a volumetric infusion device at a rate appropriate to the indication (usually 4–8 mmol/hour).

## Intravenous injection

*Preparation and administration*

1. Withdraw the required dose and dilute if necessary with NaCl 0.9% or Gluc 5% to give a solution containing a maximum of 0.8 mmol/mL (i.e. a maximum concentration of 20%).
2. The solution should be clear and colourless. Inspect visually for particulate matter or discoloration prior to administration and discard if present.
3. Give by slow IV injection at a rate not exceeding 0.6 mmol/minute (dose is typically given over 5–15 minutes).

## Intramuscular injection (painful, avoid if possible)

*Preparation and administration*

1. Withdraw the required dose.
2. If the injection solution used contains more than 20% magnesium sulfate dilute to 20% before administration, e.g. dilute the 50% injection with at least 1.5 parts WFI.
3. Give by deep IM injection.

## Technical information

| | |
|---|---|
| Incompatible with | Amiodarone, amphotericin, ciprofloxacin, drotrecogin alfa (activated). |
| Compatible with | **Flush**: NaCl 0.9%<br>**Solutions**: NaCl 0.9%, Gluc 5% (both with added KCl)<br>**Y-site**: Aciclovir, amikacin, ampicillin, aztreonam, benzylpenicillin, cefotaxime, chloramphenicol sodium succinate, cisatracurium, clindamycin, dobutamine, erythromycin, esmolol, gentamicin, granisetron, hydrocortisone sodium succinate, labetalol, linezolid, metronidazole, ondansetron, piperacillin with tazobactam, propofol, remifentanil, tobramycin, vancomycin |
| pH | 5.5-7.0 |
| Electrolyte content | See box above. |
| Osmolarity (plasma osmolality = 280-300 mOsmol/L)[1] | Magnesium sulfate 10% ≅ 812 mOsmol/L.<br>Magnesium sulfate 20% ≅ 1624 mOsmol/L.<br>Magnesium sulfate 50% ≅ 4060 mOsmol/L. |
| Storage | Store below 25°C in original packaging. |
| Stability after preparation | From a microbiological point of view, should be used immediately; however, prepared infusions may be stored at 2-8°C and infused (at room temperature) within 24 hours. |

## Monitoring

| Measure | Frequency | Rationale |
| --- | --- | --- |
| Serum Mg | Throughout therapy | • For signs of clinical improvement. |
| Blood pressure | | • May produce vasodilatation and result in ↓BP if administered quickly. |
| Respiratory rate | | • Risk of respiratory depression. |
| Urinary output | | • Mg is renally excreted. |
| CrCl or eGFR | Periodically | • ↑Risk of Mg toxicity in renal impairment. |
| Patellar reflex | | • Loss of patellar reflex is indicative of Mg toxicity. |

## Additional information

| | |
| --- | --- |
| Common and serious undesirable effects | *Injection/infusion-related:*<br>• Too rapid administration: Vasodilatation, ↓BP.<br>• Local: May be irritant to veins; extravasation may cause tissue damage.<br><br>*Other:* Other side-effects are associated with ↑Mg (see overdose below). |
| Pharmacokinetics | Following IV administration the onset of action is immediate and lasts for approximately 30 minutes. Following IM administration the onset of action is approximately 1 hour later and the duration of action is 3-4 hours. |
| Significant interactions | ↓BP with calcium channel blockers.<br>Risk of respiratory depression if given with high doses of barbiturates, opioids or hypnotics. |
| Action in case of overdose | *Symptoms to watch for:* Respiratory depression, loss of deep tendon reflexes, flushing, thirst, ↓BP, drowsiness, nausea, vomiting, confusion, arrhythmias, coma and cardiac arrest.<br>*Antidote:* Calcium gluconate by IV injection. It is essential to consult a poisons information service, e.g. Toxbase at www.toxbase.org (password or registration required) for full details of the management of magnesium toxicity. |

| | |
| --- | --- |
| Risk rating: **AMBER** | Score = 4<br>Moderate-risk product: Risk-reduction strategies are recommended. |

This assessment is based on the full range of preparation and administration options described in the monograph. These may not all be applicable in some clinical situations.

## Reference

1. Longmore M *et al.*, eds. *Oxford Handbook of Clinical Medicine*, 6th edn. Oxford: Oxford University Press, 2004.

## Bibliography

SPC Magnesium Sulphate Injection 50%, UCB Pharma Ltd (accessed 30 March 2010).
SPC Magnesium Sulphate Injection BP Minijet 50% w/v, International Medication Systems (accessed 30 March 2010).

# Mannitol

**100 mg/mL (10%) solution in 250-mL and 500-mL infusion bags**
**200 mg/mL (20%) solution in 250-mL and 500-mL infusion bags**
* Mannitol is a hexahydric alcohol that is an isomer of sorbitol. When infused it increases serum osmolality, which in turn removes fluid from tissues and promotes diuresis.
* It is used as an osmotic diuretic in the treatment of cerebral oedema and in ↑intraocular pressure.

## Pre-treatment checks

Do not give in congestive cardiac failure, pulmonary oedema and active intracranial bleeding (except during craniotomy).

*Biochemical and other tests (not all are necessary in an emergency situation)*

Bodyweight
Electrolytes: serum Na, K

Plasma volume
Renal function: U, Cr, CrCl (or eGFR)

## Dose

**Cerebral oedema and raised intraocular pressure**: 0.25–2 g/kg by IV infusion (preferably via a central line) over 30–60 minutes repeated if necessary 1 or 2 times after 4–8 hours.

## Intravenous infusion

Infusion via a central venous catheter is preferable because of the risk of damage to veins (see Osmolarity below).

1. The infusion is pre-prepared for use. It should be clear and colourless. Inspect visually for particulate matter (particularly crystals) or discoloration prior to administration and discard if present.
2. Give the required dose by IV infusion over 30–60 minutes using a giving set with an in-line filter.

| Technical information | |
|---|---|
| Incompatible with | Pantoprazole, potassium chloride. |
| Compatible with | **Flush**: NaCl 0.9%<br>**Solutions**: NaCl 0.9%, Gluc 5%<br>**Y-site**: Aztreonam, cisatracurium, linezolid, ondansetron, piperacillin with tazobactam, remifentanil |
| pH | 4.5-7 |

*(continued)*

## Technical information (continued)

| | |
|---|---|
| Sodium content | Nil |
| Osmolarity (plasma osmolality = 280-300 mOsmol/L)[1] | Mannitol 10% ≅ 550 mOsmol/L.<br>Mannitol 20% ≅ 1100 mOsmol/L. |
| Storage | Store at 20-30°C. Avoid lower temperatures because of the risk of crystallisation. |

## Monitoring

| Measure | Frequency | Rationale |
|---|---|---|
| Observation of infusion site | Consider every 30 minutes | • Extravasation can lead to necrosis and thrombosis. |
| Renal function, serum electrolytes and urine output | Consider 2-4 hourly | • Fluid imbalance and worsening renal function may be precipitated.<br>• ↓or ↑Na and ↓or ↑K may occur.<br>• May obscure and intensify inadequate hydration or hypovolaemia. |
| Cardiovascular status | | • May intensify existing or latent congestive heart failure due to expansion of extracellular fluid volume. |
| Respiratory function | | • May precipitate pulmonary oedema. |

## Additional information

| | |
|---|---|
| Common and serious undesirable effects | *Infusion-related:*<br>• Too rapid administration: ↑pulse, ↑ or ↓BP, chest pain.<br>• Local: Phlebitis, thrombophlebitis. Extravasation may cause tissue damage.<br><br>*Other:* Fluid and electrolyte imbalance, circulatory overload, acidosis at high doses, ↑extracellular volume can precipitate pulmonary oedema. Chills, fever, nausea, vomiting, thirst, headache. |
| Pharmacokinetics | Elimination half-life is about 100 minutes.<br>CSF and intraocular fluid pressure fall within 15 minutes of the start of a mannitol infusion and this lasts for 3-8 hours after the infusion is stopped; diuresis occurs after 1-3 hours. |
| Significant interactions | No significant interactions. |
| Action in case of overdose | Give supportive measures and observe the recommendations in Monitoring above. |

| Risk rating: **AMBER** | Score = 3 Moderate-risk product: Risk-reduction strategies are recommended. |

This assessment is based on the full range of preparation and administration options described in the monograph. These may not all be applicable in some clinical situations.

## Reference

1. Longmore M *et al.*, eds. *Oxford Handbook of Clinical Medicine*, 6th edn. Oxford: Oxford University Press, 2004.

## Bibliography

SPC Mannitol 10% and 20%. www.baxterhealthcare.co.uk (accessed 03 March 2010).

# Meptazinol

### 100 mg/mL solution in 1-mL ampoules

* Meptazinol hydrochloride is an opioid agonist-antagonist analgesic, with central cholinergic activity. It is reported to have a low incidence of respiratory depression.
* It is used for the acute treatment of moderate to severe pain.
* Doses are expressed in terms of the base:
  Meptazinol 100 mg ≅ 116 mg meptazinol hydrochloride.

## Pre-treatment checks

* Do not use in acute respiratory depression, where there is a risk of paralytic ileus, in ↑intracranial pressure and in head injury, in comatose patients, in acute abdomen, in delayed gastric emptying, in chronic constipation, in cor pulmonale or in acute porphyria.
* Caution in ↓BP, shock, convulsive disorders, supraventricular tachycardias, atrial flutter, chronic obstructive pulmonary disease and acute asthma attack, obstructive or inflammatory bowel diseases, biliary tract diseases, alcoholism, prostatic hyperplasia, myasthenia gravis, hypothyroidism (reduce dose), adrenocortical insufficiency (reduce dose).
* Caution in toxic psychosis and pancreatitis.
* Ensure that resuscitation equipment and naloxone are available especially for IV administration.

*Biochemical and other tests (not all are necessary in an emergency situation)*

| | |
|---|---|
| Blood pressure and pulse | Pain score |
| Bodyweight (for obstetric pain) | Renal function: U, Cr, CrCl (or eGFR) |
| LFTs | Respiratory rate |

## Dose

**Acute pain**: 75–100 mg by IM injection, or 50–100 mg by IV injection every 2–4 hours when required.
**Obstetric pain:** 100–150 mg by IM injection based on bodyweight (approximately 2 mg/kg).

**Dose in renal impairment:** reduce dose or avoid.
**Dose in hepatic impairment:** reduce dose or avoid.

## Intramuscular injection

*Preparation and administration*

1. Withdraw the required dose.
2. Give by deep IM injection.
3. Close monitoring of respiratory rate and consciousness is recommended for 30 minutes in patients receiving an initial dose, especially elderly patients or those of low bodyweight.

## Intravenous injection

*Preparation and administration*

1. Withdraw the required dose.
2. The solution should be clear and colourless to slightly yellow. Inspect visually for particulate matter or discoloration prior to administration and discard if present.
3. Give by slow IV injection over 3–5 minutes.
4. Close monitoring of respiratory rate and consciousness is recommended for 30 minutes in patients receiving an initial dose, especially elderly patients or those of low bodyweight.

## Technical information

| Incompatible with | No information |
|---|---|
| Compatible with | **Flush**: NaCl 0.9%<br>**Solutions**: NaCl 0.9%<br>**Y-site**: No information |
| pH | 3.5-6 |
| Sodium content | Nil |
| Storage | Store below 25°C in original packaging. |

## Monitoring

Close monitoring of respiratory rate and consciousness is recommended for 30 minutes in patients receiving initial dose, especially elderly patients or those of low bodyweight

| Measure | Frequency | Rationale |
|---|---|---|
| Pain | At regular intervals | • To ensure therapeutic response. |
| Blood pressure, pulse and respiratory rate | | • ↓BP, ↓pulse, ↑pulse, palpitations and respiratory depression can occur. |
| Sedation | | • Can cause sedation. |
| Monitor for side-effects and toxicity | | • May cause side-effects such as nausea and constipation, which may need treating.<br>• Signs of toxicity includes dysphoria. |

## Additional information

| | |
|---|---|
| Common and serious undesirable effects | *Common:* Nausea and vomiting (particularly initially), constipation, dry mouth, urticaria, pruritus, biliary spasm, ↑ or ↓pulse, hallucinations, euphoria, drowsiness, withdrawal symptoms in opioid-dependent patients.<br>*At higher doses:* ↓BP, sedation, respiratory depression, muscle rigidity. |
| Pharmacokinetics | Elimination half-life is 2 hours. |
| Significant interactions | • The following may ↑meptazinol levels or effect (or ↑side-effects): antihistamines-sedating (↑sedation), MAOIs (avoid combination and for 2 weeks after stopping MAOI), moclobemide.<br>• Meptazinol may ↑levels or effect (or ↑side-effects) of sodium oxybate (avoid combination). |
| Action in case of overdose | *Symptoms to watch for:* ↑Sedation, respiratory depression.<br>*Antidote:* Naloxone (see the Naloxone monograph), but may only partially reverse toxicity.<br>Stop administration and give supportive therapy as appropriate. |
| Counselling | May cause drowsiness that may affect the ability to perform skilled tasks; if affected do not drive or operate machinery, avoid alcoholic drink (the effects of alcohol are enhanced).<br>Inform the patient of possible side-effects: see above.<br>Drink plenty of fluids to help avoid constipation. |

| Risk rating: **GREEN** | Score = 2<br>Lower-risk product: Risk-reduction strategies should be considered. |
|---|---|

This assessment is based on the full range of preparation and administration options described in the monograph. These may not all be applicable in some clinical situations.

## Bibliography

SPC Meptid injections (accessed 13 July 2009).

# Meropenem

**500-mg, 1-g dry powder vials**

• Meropenem trihydrate is a carbapenem beta-lactam antibacterial.
• It is used in the treatment of infections caused by susceptible Gram-negative and Gram-positive organisms including neutropenic sepsis, meningitis and infections in immune-compromised patients.

- Doses are expressed in terms of the base:
  Meropenem 1g $\cong$ 1.14 g of meropenem trihydrate.

## Pre-treatment checks

- Do not give if there is known hypersensitivity to any carbapenem antibacterial agent or previous immediate hypersensitivity reaction to penicillins or cephalosporins.
- Caution if predisposed to seizures (antiepileptic agents should be continued in those with known seizure disorders).

*Biochemical tests*

FBC
LFTs
Renal function: U, Cr, CrCl (or eGFR)

## Dose

**Standard dose:** 500 mg by IV injection or infusion every 8 hours.
**Severe infections:** 1 g by IV injection or infusion every 8 hours.
**Meningitis:** 2 g by IV injection or infusion every 8 hours.
**Exacerbations of chronic lower respiratory tract infection in cystic fibrosis**: 2 g by IV injection or infusion every 8 hours.
**Dose in renal impairment**: adjusted according to creatinine clearance:[1]

- CrCl >20–50 mL/minute: 500 mg–2 g every 12 hours.
- CrCl 10–20 mL/minute: 500 mg–1 g every 12 hours or 500 mg every 8 hours.
- CrCl <10 mL/minute: 500 mg–1 g every 24 hours.

## Intravenous injection

*Preparation and administration*

1. Reconstitute each 500-mg vial with 10 mL WFI (use 20 mL for each 1-g vial).
2. Shake well until dissolved then allow to stand until solution is clear.
3. Withdraw the required dose.
4. Give by IV injection over 5 minutes

## Intermittent intravenous infusion

*Preparation and administration*

1. Reconstitute each 500-mg vial with 10 mL WFI (use 20 mL for each 1-g vial).
2. Shake well until dissolved then allow to stand until the solution is clear.
3. Withdraw the required dose and add to a suitable volume of compatible infusion fluid (usually 50–200 mL NaCl 0.9%).
4. Give by IV infusion over 15–30 minutes.

| Technical information | |
|---|---|
| Incompatible with | Amphotericin, calcium gluconate, diazepam, ondansetron, pantoprazole. |
| Compatible with | **Flush**: NaCl 0.9%<br>**Solutions**: NaCl 0.9%, Gluc 5% (with added KCl)<br>**Y-site**: Aminophylline, dexamethasone, fluconazole, furosemide, gentamicin, metoclopramide, noradrenaline (norepinephrine), vancomycin |
| pH | 7.3–8.3 |

*(continued)*

## Technical information (continued)

| | |
|---|---|
| Sodium content | 3.9 mmol/g |
| Storage | Store below 30°C in original packaging. Do not freeze. |
| Displacement value | Negligible |
| Stability after preparation | Reconstituted vials and prepared infusions should be used immediately. |

## Monitoring

| Measure | Frequency | Rationale |
|---|---|---|
| Temperature | Minimum daily | • For clinical signs of fever declining. |
| LFTs | Periodically in prolonged therapy | • ↑ALT, ↑ AST, ↑Alk Phos and ↑bilirubin commonly occur. |
| Renal function | | • If renal function changes a dose adjustment may be necessary. |
| FBC | | • Commonly causes thrombocytopenia.<br>• WCC: for signs of the infection resolving. |
| Sensitivity testing in *Pseudomonas aeruginosa* infection | | • To ensure microorganism remains sensitive to therapy. |
| Signs of supra-infection or superinfection | Throughout treatment | • May result in the overgrowth of non-susceptible organisms - appropriate therapy should be commenced; treatment may need to be interrupted. |
| Development of diarrhoea | Throughout and up to 2 months after treatment | • Development of severe, persistent diarrhoea may be suggestive of *Clostridium difficile*-associated diarrhoea and colitis (pseudomembranous colitis). Discontinue drug and treat. Do not use drugs that inhibit peristalsis. |

## Additional information

| | |
|---|---|
| Common and serious undesirable effects | *Immediate:* Anaphylaxis and other hypersensitivity reactions have been reported.<br>*Injection/infusion-related:* Local: Thrombophlebitis<br>*Other:* Headache, nausea, vomiting, diarrhoea, abdominal pain, rash, pruritus. |
| Pharmacokinetics | Elimination half-life is 1 hour (>6 hours if CrCl <50 mL/minute; >20 hours if CrCl <20 mL/minute). |
| Significant interactions | No significant interactions. |
| Action in case of overdose | *Antidote:* No known antidote but haemodialysis may be effective. Stop administration and give supportive therapy as appropriate. |

| Risk rating: **GREEN** | Score = 2<br>Lower-risk product: Risk-reduction strategies should be considered. |
|---|---|

This assessment is based on the full range of preparation and administration options described in the monograph. These may not all be applicable in some clinical situations.

### Reference

1. Ashley C, Currie A, eds. *The Renal Drug Handbook*, 3rd edn. Oxford: Radcliffe Medical Press, 2009.

### Bibliography

SPC Meronem IV 500 mg and 1 g (accessed 25 March 2009).

# Mesna

### 100 mg/mL solution in 4-mL and 10-mL ampoules

* Mesna is given systemically to protect the urinary tract from toxic urinary metabolites in patients being treated with oxazaphosphorine derivatives (ifosfamide, cyclophosphamide).
* The aim of treatment is to ensure that there are adequate levels of mesna in the bladder throughout the period that the toxic metabolites are present. Duration of mesna treatment should therefore equal that of the oxazaphosphorine treatment plus about 8–12 hours (the time it takes for the urinary metabolites to fall to non-toxic levels).
* Mesna has also been used as a mucolytic in the management of some respiratory tract disorders.

### Pre-treatment checks

Patients receiving mesna for the prevention of ifosfamide-induced hemorrhagic cystitis should be adequately hydrated (at least 1 L of oral or IV fluid daily, prior to and during ifosfamide therapy).

### Dose

In all cases be guided by the oncology team responsible for treating the patient.

**Intermittent injection or infusion**: the total dose of mesna is 60% (w/w) of the oxazapho-sphorine dose in three divided doses; the first dose is concomitant with the oxazaphosphorine with the remaining doses after 4 and 8 hours.

**Where ifosfamide is used as a 24-hour or long-term infusion**: once administration of the ifosfamide dose is complete, a further 12-hour infusion of mesna is given at a dose of 60% (w/w) of the ifosfamide dose. Alternatively, the final 12-hour infusion of mesna may be replaced by three IV or oral doses, each of 20% (w/w) of the ifosfamide dose.

**Mucolytic (unlicensed)**: the usual daily dose is 600 mg–1.2 g given by a nebuliser; it may also be given by direct endotracheal instillation.

## Intravenous injection

*Preparation and administration*

1. Withdraw the required dose.
2. The solution should be clear and colourless. Inspect visually for particulate matter or discoloration prior to administration and discard if present.
3. Give by IV injection over 3 minutes or as recommended by your oncology team.

## Intermittent intravenous infusion

*Preparation and administration*

1. Withdraw the required dose and add to a convenient volume of compatible infusion fluid (usually NaCl 0.9% or Gluc 5%) to give a solution containing approximately 20 mg/mL.
2. The solution should be clear and colourless. Inspect visually for particulate matter or discoloration prior to administration and discard if present.
3. Give by IV infusion over 15–30 minutes or as recommended by your oncology team.

## Continuous intravenous infusion

*Preparation and administration*

1. Withdraw the required dose and add to a convenient volume of compatible infusion fluid (usually NaCl 0.9% or Gluc 5%) to give a solution containing approximately 20 mg/mL. Mix well.
2. The solution should be clear and colourless. Inspect visually for particulate matter or discoloration prior to administration and discard if present.
3. Give by IV infusion as recommended by your oncology team.

## Oral (tablets are also available)

Measure the required dose and add to a flavoured soft drink (e.g. orange juice, cola). This mixture is stable when refrigerated in a sealed container for 24 hours.

| Technical information | |
|---|---|
| Incompatible with | Amphotericin |
| Compatible with | **Flush**: NaCl 0.9%<br>**Solutions**: NaCl 0.9%, Gluc 5%, Gluc-NaCl, Hartmann's<br>**Y-site**: Aztreonam, granisetron, linezolid, ondansetron, piperacillin with tazobactam, sodium bicarbonate |
| pH | 6.5-8.5 |
| Sodium content | Negligible |
| Storage | Store below 30°C in original packaging.<br>Use opened ampoules immediately and discard any unused solution. |
| Stability after preparation | From a microbiological point of view, should be used immediately; however, prepared infusions are stable at room temperature for 24 hours. |

## Monitoring

| Measure | Frequency | Rationale |
|---|---|---|
| Observe for infusion-related reactions | During administration | See list below for potential reactions, but because patients also receive cytotoxic drugs it is difficult to determine the true side-effect profile. |

## Additional information

| | |
|---|---|
| Common and serious undesirable effects | Nausea, vomiting, colic, diarrhoea, headache, fatigue, limb and joint pains, depression, irritability, lack of energy, rash, ↓BP and ↑pulse. Rarely pseudo-allergic reactions including ↓BP and ↑pulse have been reported. |
| Pharmacokinetics | Elimination half-life is about 20 minutes. |
| Significant interactions | • Mesna may affect the following tests:<br>urine dipstick for ketones (false-positive), urine dipstick tests for erythrocytes (false-positive or false-negative). |
| Action in case of overdose | No evidence of toxic effects even at extremely high doses. |

Risk rating: **AMBER**    Score = 3
Moderate-risk product: Risk-reduction strategies are recommended.

This assessment is based on the full range of preparation and administration options described in the monograph. These may not all be applicable in some clinical situations

### Bibliography

SPC Uromitexan injection. www.ecomm.baxter.com/ecatalog/loadResource.do?bid=25410 (accessed 22 February 2010).

# Metaraminol

### 10 mg/mL solution in 1-mL ampoules

- Metaraminol tartrate is a sympathomimetic which exerts an inotropic effect and acts as a peripheral vasoconstrictor, thus ↑cardiac output, peripheral resistance and BP.
- It is used to treat acute ↓BP where other measures have failed. It has also been used for its pressor action in hypotensive states such as those that may occur after spinal anaesthesia.

- Doses are expressed in terms of the base:
  Metaraminol 5 mg ≅ 9.5 mg metaraminol tartrate.

## Pre-treatment checks

- Do not use in pregnancy.
- Do not use with cyclopropane or halothane anaesthesia.
- Extreme caution in ↑BP (monitor BP and rate of flow frequently).
- Caution in coronary, mesenteric, or peripheral vascular thrombosis; following myocardial infarction, Prinzmetal's variant angina, hyperthyroidism, diabetes mellitus; hypoxia or hypercapnia; uncorrected hypovolaemia; elderly patients; a history of malaria; and cirrhosis.
- Hypoxia, hypercapnia, and acidosis should be corrected prior to or concurrently with administration of metaraminol (they may reduce the effectiveness and/or ↑adverse effects).
- Blood volume depletion should be corrected as fully as possible before therapy commences. In an emergency, it may be used as an adjunct to fluid volume replacement or as a temporary supportive measure to maintain coronary and cerebral artery perfusion until volume replacement therapy can be completed, but must not be used as sole therapy in hypovolaemic patients.
- Extravasation at injection site may cause necrosis.

*Biochemical and other tests (not all are necessary in an emergency situation)*

Blood pressure
TFTs

## Dose

Avoid SC and IM injection (associated with local tissue necrosis and sloughing).

**Standard dose:** 15–100 mg by IV infusion, adjusted according to response.
**In an emergency**: 0.5–5 mg by IV injection, then 15–100 mg by IV infusion, adjusted according to response.

### Intravenous injection

*Preparation and administration*

1. Withdraw the required dose.
2. The solution should be clear and colourless. Inspect visually for particulate matter or discoloration prior to administration and discard if present.
3. Give by IV injection preferably into a large vein of the antecubital fossa or the thigh (veins in the ankle or hand should be avoided).

### Continuous intravenous infusion

*Preparation and administration*

1. Withdraw the required dose and add to a suitable volume of compatible infusion fluid (usually 15–100 mg in 500 mL; however, up to 500 mg per 500 mL has been used). Mix well.
2. The solution should be clear and colourless. Inspect visually for particulate matter or discoloration prior to administration and discard if present.
3. Give by IV infusion via a volumetric infusion device, adjusting rate to clinical response. Maximum effects are not immediately apparent: at least 10 minutes should elapse between dose increases. The possibility of a cumulative effect should be borne in mind. The patient should not be left unattended and the infusion flow rate must be closely monitored (severe ↓BP may develop).

## Technical information

| | |
|---|---|
| Incompatible with | No information |
| Compatible with | **Flush**: NaCl 0.9%.<br>**Solutions**: NaCl 0.9%, Gluc 5%<br>**Solutions**: No information |
| pH | 3.2–4.5 |
| Sodium content | Negligible |
| Excipients | May contain sulfites (may cause hypersensitivity reactions). |
| Storage | Store below 30°C in original packaging. Protect from light. |
| Stability after preparation | Use prepared infusions immediately.<br>Prepare a fresh infusion bag every 24 hours. |

## Monitoring

| Measure | Frequency | Rationale |
|---|---|---|
| Improvement in clinical condition | Throughout treatment | • Perfusion of extremities as seen through warming, coloration and strengthening of pulse.<br>• Improvement of mental status.<br>• Improved urine output providing the patient has good renal function. |
| Blood pressure | Frequently (especially when given IV) | • In previously normotensive patients, systolic BP should be maintained at 80–100 mmHg.<br>• In previously hypertensive patients, the systolic BP should be maintained at 30–40 mmHg below usual BP. |
| Central venous pressure or left ventricular filling pressure | If indicated | • May be helpful in detecting and treating hypovolaemia.<br>• Monitoring of central venous or pulmonary arterial diastolic pressure is necessary to avoid overloading the cardiovascular system and precipitating congestive heart failure. |

## Additional information

| | |
|---|---|
| Common and serious undesirable effects | ↑BP, headache, ↑or↓ pulse, arrhythmias, peripheral ischaemia; fatal ventricular arrhythmia reported in Laennec's cirrhosis. |
| Pharmacokinetics | Elimination half-life is not known. |
| Significant interactions | • The following may ↑metaraminol levels or effect (or ↑side-effects):<br>MAOIs (risk of hypertensive crisis), moclobemide (risk of hypertensive crisis), rasagiline (avoid combination).<br>• Metaraminol may ↓levels or effect of guanethidine (↓hypotensive effect). |
| Action in case of overdose | Reduce infusion rate or stop administration and give supportive therapy as appropriate. |

Risk rating: **AMBER**   Score = 4
Moderate-risk product: Risk-reduction strategies are recommended.

This assessment is based on the full range of preparation and administration options described in the monograph. These may not all be applicable in some clinical situations.

# Methadone hydrochloride

**10 mg/mL solution in 1-mL, 2-mL, 3.5-mL and 5-mL ampoules**
* Methadone hydrochloride is an opioid analgesic.
* It is used to treat moderate to severe pain.
* It is also used in the management of opioid withdrawal because withdrawal symptoms from methadone develop more slowly than with other opioids.

## Pre-treatment checks

* Do not use in acute respiratory depression, where there is a risk of paralytic ileus, in ↑intracranial pressure and in head injury, in comatose patients; in acute abdomen; delayed gastric emptying; chronic constipation; cor pulmonale; acute porphyria.
* Caution in ↓BP, shock, convulsive disorders, supraventricular tachycardias, atrial flutter, chronic obstructive pulmonary disease and acute asthma attack, obstructive or inflammatory bowel diseases, biliary tract diseases, alcoholism, prostatic hyperplasia, myasthenia gravis, hypothyroidism (reduce dose), adrenocortical insufficiency (reduce dose).
* Caution in toxic psychosis and pancreatitis.
* Ensure resuscitation equipment and naloxone are available.

*Biochemical and other tests (not all are necessary in an every situation)*

Blood pressure and pulse
ECG in patients at risk of QT prolongation (if the dose is increased above 100 mg/day in any patient an ECG should be carried out before the increase and 7 days after)

LFTs
Pain score
Renal function: U, Cr, CrCl (or eGFR)
Respiratory rate

## Dose

**Moderate to severe pain**: 5–10 mg by IM or SC injection every 6–8 hours when necessary. If required for longer than 2 days then give by IM injection twice daily to avoid accumulation.
**Opioid dependence**: 10–20 mg by IM injection once daily. Increase the dose by 10–20 mg a day until there are no signs of withdrawal or toxicity (usual range 40–60 mg in 24 hours). Reduce the dose gradually to zero, usually as part of a managed regimen.
**Dose in renal impairment:** reduce dose or avoid.
**Dose in hepatic impairment:** reduce dose or avoid.

## Intramuscular injection (preferred route if repeated doses are to be given)

*Preparation and administration*

1. Withdraw the required dose.
2. Give by deep IM injection. Volumes >2 mL (20 mg) should be distributed between injection sites.
3. Close monitoring of respiratory rate and consciousness is recommended for 30 minutes in patients receiving an initial dose, especially elderly patients or those of low bodyweight.

## Subcutaneous injection

*Preparation and administration*

1. Withdraw the required dose.
2. Give by SC injection.
3. Close monitoring of respiratory rate and consciousness is recommended for 30 minutes in patients receiving initial dose, especially elderly patients or those of low bodyweight.

## Technical information

| | |
|---|---|
| Incompatible with | Not relevant |
| Compatible with | Not relevant |
| pH | 4.5–6.5 |
| Sodium content | Negligible |
| Storage | Store below 25°C in original packaging. Controlled Drug. |

## Monitoring

Close monitoring of respiratory rate and consciousness is recommended for 30 minutes in patients receiving initial dose, especially elderly patients or those of low bodyweight

| Measure | Frequency | Rationale |
|---|---|---|
| Signs of withdrawal | At regular intervals | • To ensure therapeutic response. |
| Pain | | • To ensure therapeutic response. |
| Blood pressure, pulse and respiratory rate | | • ↓BP, ↓pulse, ↑pulse, palpitations and respiratory depression with ↓oxygen saturation can occur. |
| Sedation | At regular intervals | • May cause sedation. |
| Monitor for side-effects and toxicity | | • May cause side-effects such as nausea and constipation, which may need treating.<br>• Can cause respiratory depression (may be delayed) and CNS depression. |

## Additional information

| | |
|---|---|
| Common and serious undesirable effects | *Injection/infusion-related:* Local: Injection-site irritation, pain, induration (following SC injection).<br>*Other:* Nausea and vomiting (particularly initially), constipation, dry mouth, urticaria, pruritus, biliary spasm, ↑ or ↓pulse, ↑QT interval, hallucinations, euphoria, drowsiness, histamine release (caution in asthmatics).<br>At higher doses ↓BP, torsade de pointes, sedation, respiratory depression, muscle rigidity. |
| Pharmacokinetics | The half-life is variable, following a single IM dose it is around 6-8 hours. After regular dosing it increases to 13-47 hours. |
| Significant interactions | • The following may ↑methadone levels or effect (or ↑side-effects): antihistamines-sedating (↑sedation), MAOIs (avoid combination and for 2 weeks after stopping MAOI), moclobemide, voriconazole (↓methadone dose).<br>• Methadone may ↑risk of ventricular arrhythmias with the following drugs:<br>amisulpride (avoid combination), antipsychotics (if prolong QT interval), atomoxetine.<br>• Methadone may ↑levels or effect (or ↑side-effects) of sodium oxybate (avoid combination). |
| Action in case of overdose | *Symptoms to watch for:* ↑Sedation, respiratory depression.<br>*Antidote:* Naloxone (see the Naloxone monograph). Stop administration and give supportive therapy as appropriate. |
| Counselling | May cause drowsiness that may affect the ability to perform skilled tasks; if affected do not drive or operate machinery, avoid alcoholic drink (the effects of alcohol are enhanced).<br>Drink plenty of fluids to help avoid constipation use a laxative if required. |

| | |
|---|---|
| Risk rating: **GREEN** | Score = 2<br>Lower-risk product: Risk-reduction strategies should be considered. |

This assessment is based on the full range of preparation and administration options described in the monograph. These may not all be applicable in some clinical situations.

## Bibliography

SPC Methadone 10 mg/mL solution for injection, Wockhardt UK Ltd (accessed 3 March 2009).

# Methylprednisolone acetate

**40 mg/mL aqueous suspension in 1-mL, 2-mL and 3-mL vials**

This preparation must not be confused with the combined preparation that includes lidocaine.

* Methylprednisolone acetate is a corticosteroid with mainly glucocorticoid activity.
* It is used in inflammatory conditions of the joints, particularly rheumatoid arthritis.
* It is used in the treatment of conditions for which systemic corticosteroid therapy is indicated (except adrenal-deficiency states). Deep IM injections have a depot effect and may provide cover for up to 2 weeks.
* It may also be given by intra-articular, intrasynovial or intralesional injection for various inflammatory conditions.

## Pre-treatment checks

* Avoid where systemic infection is present (unless specific therapy given).
* Avoid live virus vaccines in those receiving immunosuppressive doses.
* May activate or exacerbate amoebiasis or strongyloidiasis (exclude before initiating a corticosteroid in those at risk or with suggestive symptoms). Fungal or viral ocular infections may also be exacerbated.
* Caution in patients predisposed to psychiatric reactions, including those who have previously suffered corticosteroid-induced psychosis, or who have a personal or family history of psychiatric disorders.

**Intra-articular:**
* Do not inject into unstable joints.
* Do not give in the presence of active infection in or near joints.

## Dose

**Intramuscular:** 40–120 mg. The dose depends on the severity of the condition and may be repeated as indicated by the patient's response and clinical condition. The effect of a single 80-mg injection may be expected to last approximately 2 weeks.

**Intra-articular or intrasynovial or intradermal injection:** large joints: up to 20–80 mg; medium joints: 10–40 mg; small joints: 4–10 mg; intra-bursal: 4–30 mg; intralesional: 20–60 mg depending on the size of the lesion (for large lesions the dose may be distributed by repeated local injections of 20–40 mg); tendon sheath: 4–30 mg.

In recurrent or chronic conditions, repeat doses may be necessary.

## Intramuscular injection

*Preparation and administration*

1. Withdraw the required dose.
2. Give by IM injection deep into the upper outer quadrant of the gluteal muscle (avoid the deltoid). Use alternate sides for subsequent injections.

## Other routes

*Preparation and administration*

1. Withdraw the required dose.
2. Inject into the affected area.

- In tenosynovitis care should be taken to inject into the tendon sheath rather than into the substance of the tendon.
- After intra-articular injections treatment failure is usually the result of not entering the joint space.

## Technical information

| | |
|---|---|
| Incompatible with | Not relevant |
| Compatible with | Not relevant |
| pH | Not relevant |
| Sodium content | Negligible |
| Storage | Store below 25°C in original packaging. Do not freeze. |

## Monitoring

| Measure | Frequency | Rationale |
|---|---|---|
| Serum Na, K, Ca | Throughout systemic treatment | • May cause fluid and electrolyte disturbances. |
| Withdrawal symptoms and signs | During withdrawal and after stopping systemic treatment | • During prolonged therapy with corticosteroids, adrenal atrophy develops and can persist for years after stopping. Abrupt withdrawal after a prolonged period can lead to acute adrenal insufficiency, ↓BP or death.<br>• The CSM has recommended that gradual withdrawal of systemic corticosteroids should be considered in patients whose disease is unlikely to relapse. Full details can be found in the BNF. |
| Signs of infection | During systemic treatment | • Prolonged courses ↑susceptibility to infections and severity of infections. Serious infections may reach an advanced stage before being recognised. |
| Signs of chickenpox | | • Unless they have had chickenpox, patients receiving corticosteroids for purposes other than replacement should be regarded as being at risk of severe chickenpox.<br>• Confirmed chickenpox requires urgent treatment; corticosteroids should not be stopped and dosage may need to be increased. |
| Exposure to measles | During systemic treatment | • Patients should be advised to take particular care to avoid exposure to measles and to seek immediate medical advice if exposure occurs.<br>• Prophylaxis with IM normal immunoglobulin may be needed. |
| Symptoms of septic arthritis | Following intra-articular injection | • A marked increase in pain accompanied by local swelling, further restriction of joint motion, fever, and malaise are suggestive of septic arthritis. |

## Additional information

| | |
|---|---|
| Common and serious undesirable effects | *Immediate:* Anaphylaxis and other hypersensitivity reactions have been reported. <br> *Injection-related:* <br> • IM and intradermal: Severe local pain, sterile abscess, cutaneous and subcutaneous atrophy, hyper/hypopigmentation. <br> • Intra-articular: Transient pain, sterile abscess, hyper/ hypopigmentation, Charcot-like arthropathy and occasional increase in joint discomfort. <br> *Short-term use:* Undesirable effects that may result from short-term use (minimise by using the lowest effective dose for the shortest time): ↑BP, Na and water retention, ↓K, ↓Ca, ↑blood glucose, peptic ulceration and perforation, psychiatric reactions, ↑susceptibility to infection, muscle weakness, tendon rupture, insomnia, ↑intracranial pressure, ↓seizure threshold, impaired healing. For undesirable effects resulting from long-term corticosteroid use refer to the BNF. |
| Pharmacokinetics | Elimination half-life is 2.4-3.5 hours. |
| Significant interactions | • The following may ↓corticosteroid levels or effect: barbiturates, carbamazepine, phenytoin, primidone, rifabutin, rifampicin. <br> • Corticosteroids may ↑levels or effect of the following drugs (or ↑side-effects): anticoagulants (monitor INR), methotrexate (↑risk of blood dyscrasias). If using amphotericin IV monitor fluid balance and K level closely. <br> • Corticosteroids may ↓levels or effect of vaccines (↓immunological response, ↑risk of infection with live vaccines). |
| Action in case of overdose | No known antidote but haemodialysis may be effective. Give supportive therapy as appropriate. Following chronic overdose the possibility of adrenal suppression should be considered. |
| Counselling | Patients on long-term corticosteroid treatment should read and carry a Steroid Treatment Card. |

| | |
|---|---|
| Risk rating: **GREEN** | Score = 2 <br> Lower-risk product: Risk-reduction strategies should be considered. |

This assessment is based on the full range of preparation and administration options described in the monograph. These may not all be applicable in some clinical situations.

## Bibliography

SPC Depo-Medrone 40 mg/mL (accessed 12 July 2009).

# Methylprednisolone sodium succinate

**40-mg, 125-mg, 500-mg, 1-g and 2-g dry powder vials all with solvent (WFI)**

* Methylprednisolone sodium succinate is a corticosteroid with mainly glucocorticoid activity.
* It is used in the treatment of conditions for which systemic corticosteroid therapy is indicated.
* It is used parenterally when a rapid effect is required in emergencies, and also when the oral route is temporarily unavailable or inappropriate.
* Doses are expressed in terms of the base:
  Methylprednisolone 100 mg $\cong$ 133 mg methylprednisolone sodium succinate.

## Pre-treatment checks

* Do not use in the treatment of cerebral oedema associated with malaria.
* Avoid where systemic infection is present (unless specific therapy is given).
* Avoid live virus vaccines in those receiving immunosuppressive doses.
* May activate or exacerbate amoebiasis or strongyloidiasis (exclude before initiating a corticosteroid in those at risk or with suggestive symptoms). Fungal or viral ocular infections may also be exacerbated.
* Caution in patients predisposed to psychiatric reactions, including those who have previously suffered corticosteroid-induced psychosis, or who have a personal or family history of psychiatric disorders.
* Rapid IV administration of large doses is associated with cardiovascular collapse.

*Biochemical and other tests (not all are necessary in an emergency situation)*

Electrolytes: serum Na, K, Ca

## Dose

**Standard dose:** depending on the indication, 10–500 mg given by IM injection or by IV injection or infusion. The dose depends on the severity of the condition and may be repeated as indicated by the patient's response and clinical condition.

**Acute exacerbations of multiple sclerosis**: 1 g daily for 3 days.

**Acute graft rejection reactions**: 1 g daily for up to 3 days.

## Intramuscular injection

*Preparation and administration*

1. Reconstitute with the diluent provided.
2. Withdraw the required dose.
3. Give by IM injection.

## Intravenous injection (for doses up to 250 mg only)

*Preparation and administration*

1. Reconstitute each vial with the diluent provided.
2. The solution should be clear and colourless. Inspect visually for particulate matter or discoloration prior to administration. Discard if present.
3. Give by IV injection over a minimum of 5 minutes.

## Intermittent intravenous infusion (for doses more than 250 mg)

*Preparation and administration*

1. Reconstitute each vial with the diluent provided.
2. Withdraw the required dose and add to a suitable volume of compatible infusion solution (usually 100–250 mL NaCl 0.9%)

3. The solution should be clear and colourless. Inspect visually for particulate matter or discoloration prior to administration. Discard if present.
4. Give by IV infusion over a minimum of 30 minutes.

## Technical information

| | |
|---|---|
| Incompatible with | Ciprofloxacin, cisatracurium, ondansetron, propofol, tigecycline. |
| Compatible with | **Flush**: NaCl 0.9%<br>**Solutions**: NaCl 0.9%, Gluc 5% (with added KCl), Gluc-NaCl, Hartmann's<br>**Y-site**: Aciclovir, aztreonam, ceftazidime, dopamine, granisetron, linezolid, metronidazole, midazolam, piperacillin with tazobactam, remifentanil, sodium bicarbonate |
| pH | 7.4–8 |
| Sodium content | 2 mmol/g |
| Storage | Store below 25°C in original packaging. |
| Displacement value | Negligible |
| Stability after preparation | From a microbiological point of view, should be used immediately; however, prepared infusions (in NaCl 0.9% only) may be stored at 2–8°C and infused (at room temperature) within 24 hours. |

## Monitoring

| Measure | Frequency | Rationale |
|---|---|---|
| Serum Na, K, Ca | Throughout treatment | • May cause fluid and electrolyte disturbances. |
| LFTs | Periodically | • May cause a rise, reversible upon stopping. |
| Withdrawal symptoms and signs | During withdrawal and after stopping treatment | • During prolonged therapy with corticosteroids, adrenal atrophy develops and can persist for years after stopping. Abrupt withdrawal after a prolonged period can lead to acute adrenal insufficiency, ↓BP or death.<br>• The CSM has recommended that gradual withdrawal of systemic corticosteroids should be considered in patients whose disease is unlikely to relapse. Full details can be found in the BNF |
| Signs of infection | During treatment | • Prolonged courses ↑susceptibility to infections and severity of infections. Serious infections may reach an advanced stage before being recognised. |
| Signs of chickenpox | | • Unless they have had chickenpox, patients receiving corticosteroids for purposes other than replacement should be regarded as being at risk of severe chickenpox.<br>• Confirmed chickenpox requires urgent treatment; corticosteroids should not be stopped and dosage may need to be increased. |

## Additional information

| | |
|---|---|
| Common and serious undesirable effects | *Immediate:* Anaphylaxis and other hypersensitivity reactions have been reported.<br>*Injection/infusion-related:* Too rapid administration: Cardiovascular collapse.<br>*Short-term use:* Undesirable effects that may result from short-term use (minimise by using the lowest effective dose for the shortest time):<br>↑BP, Na and water retention, ↓K, ↓Ca, ↑blood glucose, peptic ulceration and perforation, psychiatric reactions, ↑susceptibility to infection, muscle weakness, tendon rupture, insomnia, ↑intracranial pressure, ↓seizure threshold, impaired healing. For undesirable effects resulting from long-term corticosteroid use refer to the BNF. |
| Pharmacokinetics | Elimination half-life is 2.4-3.5 hours. |
| Significant interactions | • Methylprednisolone may ↑levels or effect (or ↑side-effects) of ciclosporin (↑levels, risk of convulsions).<br>• The following may ↓corticosteroid levels or effect: barbiturates, carbamazepine, phenytoin, primidone, rifabutin, rifampicin.<br>• Corticosteroids may ↑levels or effect of the following drugs (or ↑side-effects):<br>  anticoagulants (monitor INR), methotrexate (↑risk of blood dyscrasias). If using amphotericin IV monitor fluid balance and K level closely.<br>• Corticosteroids may ↓levels or effect of vaccines (↓immunological response, ↑risk of infection with live vaccines). |
| Action in case of overdose | No known antidote but haemodialysis may be effective.<br>Give supportive therapy as appropriate. Following chronic overdose the possibility of adrenal suppression should be considered. |
| Counselling | Patients on long-term corticosteroid treatment should read and carry a Steroid Treatment Card. |

| | |
|---|---|
| Risk rating: **AMBER** | Score = 4<br>Moderate-risk product: Risk-reduction strategies are recommended. |

This assessment is based on the full range of preparation and administration options described in the monograph. These may not all be applicable in some clinical situations.

## Bibliography

SPC Solu-Medrone (accessed 12 July 2009).

# Metoclopramide hydrochloride

**5 mg/mL solution in 2-mL and 20-mL ampoules**

* Metoclopramide hydrochloride is a substituted benzamide that has prokinetic and antiemetic activity.
* It is used to treat nausea and vomiting of various aetiologies and to restore normal co-ordination and tone to the upper GI tract and it may also be given prior to various GI procedures. High-dose metoclopramide is now less commonly used for cytotoxic-induced nausea and vomiting.
* It may be given (unlicensed) by SC infusion in palliative care to treat nausea and vomiting and also to treat hiccups due to gastric distension.
* Doses below are expressed in terms of metoclopramide hydrochloride.

## Pre-treatment checks

* Avoid in patients with phaeochromocytoma as it may induce an acute hypertensive response.
* Do not give during the first 3–4 days following operations such as pyloroplasty or gut anastomosis as vigorous muscular contractions may inhibit healing.
* Do not give in GI obstruction, perforation or haemorrhage.
* Caution in epilepsy and patients treated with other centrally acting drugs.
* Care should be taken in patients with a history of atopy (including asthma) or porphyria.

*Biochemical and other tests (not all are necessary in an emergency situation)*

Bodyweight (if using in association with chemotherapy)
LFTs
Renal function: U, Cr, CrCl (or eGFR)

## Dose

Because of the ↑risk of dystonic reactions (including oculogyric crises) in elderly and in young patients, particularly girls and young women, use of metoclopramide should be restricted to those situations for which there is no safer alternative. Lower doses should be used in these patient groups (maximum 500 micrograms/kg for high-dose therapy).

**Treatment of nausea and vomiting:** 10 mg (5 mg in young adults 15–19 years < 60 kg) by IV or IM injection three times a day.

**Diagnostic procedures:** 10–20 mg (10 mg in young adults 15–19 years) by IV or IM injection 5–10 minutes before procedure.

**Nausea and vomiting associated with cytotoxic chemotherapy:** 2–4 mg/kg by IV infusion before commencing chemotherapy followed by a continuous IV infusion of 3–5 mg/kg over 8–12 hours. Alternatively, give up to 2 mg/kg by IV infusion before commencing chemotherapy and repeat every 2 hours as necessary. Maximum dose by either method: 10 mg/kg in 24 hours.

**Dose in renal impairment:** avoid or reduce dose if CrCl <10 mL/minute (↑risk of dystonic reactions).
**Dose in hepatic impairment:** reduce dose.

## Intramuscular injection

*Preparation and administration*

1. Withdraw the required dose.
2. Give by IM injection.

## Intravenous injection

*Preparation and administration*

1. Withdraw the required dose.
2. The solution should be clear and colourless. Inspect visually for particulate matter or discoloration (degradation is indicated by yellow discoloration) prior to administration and discard if present.
3. Give by slow IV injection over 2 minutes. Rapid administration may cause intense feelings of anxiety and restlessness which pass quickly and are then followed by drowsiness.

## Intermittent intravenous infusion (for cytotoxic chemotherapy only)

*Preparation and administration*

1. Withdraw the required dose and add to 50 mL of compatible infusion fluid.
2. The solution should be clear and colourless. Inspect visually for particulate matter or discoloration (degradation is indicated by yellow discoloration) prior to administration and discard if present.
3. Give by IV infusion over at least 15 minutes.

## Continuous intravenous infusion

*Preparation and administration*

1. Withdraw the required dose and add to 500 mL of compatible infusion fluid. Mix well.
2. The solution should be clear and colourless. Inspect visually for particulate matter or discoloration (degradation is indicated by yellow discoloration) prior to administration and discard if present.
3. Give by IV infusion over 8–12 hours.

| Technical information | |
|---|---|
| Incompatible with | Amphotericin, furosemide, propofol. |
| Compatible with | **Flush**: NaCl 0.9%<br>**Solutions**: Gluc 5%, NaCl 0.9%, Gluc-NaCl, Hartmann's, Ringer's<br>**Y-site**: Aciclovir, aztreonam, calcium folinate, ciprofloxacin, cisatracurium, clarithromycin, fentanyl, fluconazole, foscarnet, linezolid, meropenem, piperacillin with tazobactam, remifentanil, tigecycline |
| pH | 2.5-6.5 |
| Sodium content | Negligible |
| Excipients | Some preparations contain sulfites (may cause hypersensitivity reactions). |
| Storage | Store below 25°C in original packaging. Do not use discoloured solutions. |
| Stability after preparation | From a microbiological point of view, should be used immediately; however, prepared infusions may be stored at room temperature and infused within 24 hours. |

## Monitoring

| Measure | Frequency | Rationale |
|---|---|---|
| Clinical improvement | Periodically | • To ensure improvement in nausea/vomiting.<br>• If vomiting persists the patient should be reassessed to exclude the possibility of an underlying disorder. |
| Blood pressure | | • May ↑BP. |
| EPSE | | • May cause EPSE. |

## Additional information

| | |
|---|---|
| Common and serious undesirable effects | *Immediate:* Anaphylaxis and other hypersensitivity reactions have been reported.<br>*Injection/infusion-related:* Too rapid administration: Intense feelings of anxiety and restlessness that pass quickly and are then followed by drowsiness.<br>*Other:* Dystonias (especially in young adults) including oculogyric crisis, other EPSE, hyperprolactinaemia, rarely NMS, very rarely cardiac conduction abnormalities, red cell disorders particularly at high dose (extremely rare). |
| Pharmacokinetics | Elimination half-life is 4–6 hours, longer in renal impairment. |
| Significant interactions | Metoclopramide may ↑levels or effect (or ↑side effects) of ciclosporin. |
| Action in case of overdose | Stop administration and give supportive therapy as appropriate. |

Risk rating: **GREEN**    Score = 2
Moderate-risk product: Risk-reduction strategies are recommended.

This assessment is based on the full range of preparation and administration options described in the monograph. These may not all be applicable in some clinical situations.

## Bibliography

SPC Maxalon injection (accessed 24 September 2008).
SPC Metoclopramide 5 mg/mL injection, Hameln (accessed 24 August 2009).

# Metoprolol tartrate

**1 mg/mL injection solution in 5-mL ampoules**
* Metoprolol is a cardioselective beta-blocker.
* It is used parenterally for the early management of suspected acute myocardial infarction, within 12 hours of onset of chest pain.
* It may also be used in the management of tachyarrhythmias, particularly supraventricular tachyarrhythmias and to prevent or treat arrhythmias occurring during anaesthesia.

## Pre-treatment checks

* Treatment should be avoided in sick sinus syndrome, ↓BP (use with caution in systolic BP <100 mmHg), heart block greater than first degree, ↓pulse (<45–50 bpm), cardiogenic shock and overt heart failure.
* Use with caution in patients with a history of wheezing or asthma.

*Biochemical and other tests (not all are necessary in an emergency situation)*

LFTs

## Dose

**Cardiac arrhythmias**: up to 5 mg by IV injection repeated at 5-minute intervals until a satisfactory response has been obtained. A total dose of 10–15 mg generally proves sufficient.

**During anaesthesia**: 2–4 mg IV at induction to prevent arrhythmias or to control arrhythmias developing during anaesthesia. Further injections of 2 mg may be given as required to a maximum overall dose of 10 mg.

**Myocardial infarction**: 5 mg by IV injection every 2 minutes to a maximum of 15 mg total dose as determined by BP and heart rate. Doses subsequent to the initial dose should not be given if systolic BP is <90 mmHg, the heart rate is <40 beats/minute and the P-Q time is >0.26 seconds, or if there is any aggravation of dyspnoea or cold sweating.

Oral therapy should commence 15 minutes after the last injection. Patients who fail to tolerate the full IV dose should be given a reduced oral dose when their condition permits.

**Dose in hepatic impairment:** reduce dose in severe impairment.

## Intravenous injection

*Preparation and administration*

1. Withdraw the required dose.
2. The solution should be clear and colourless. Inspect visually for particulate matter or discoloration prior to administration and discard if present.
3. Give by IV injection at a rate of 1–2 mg per minute.

| Technical information | |
|---|---|
| Incompatible with | Amphotericin |
| Compatible with | **Flush**: NaCl 0.9%<br>**Solutions**: NaCl 0.9%, Gluc 5%<br>**Y-site**: Abciximab, alteplase, bivalirudin |
| pH | 5-8 |

*(continued)*

## Technical information (continued)

| | |
|---|---|
| Sodium content | Negligible |
| Storage | Store below 25°C, protected from light. |

## Monitoring

| Measure | Frequency | Rationale |
|---|---|---|
| ECG/heart rate | Continuously | • Response to treatment.<br>• Consider withholding therapy if heart rate drops to 50-55 bpm or lower.<br>• Excessive ↓pulse can be countered with IV atropine sulfate in doses of 600 micrograms repeated every 3-5 minutes up to a maximum of 2.4 mg. |
| Blood pressure | | • Stop dosing if ↓BP occurs that requires corrective measures. |
| Respiratory function or oxygen saturation in at risk individuals | After initial dosing | • May cause bronchoconstriction in susceptible individuals, e.g. patients with history of bronchospasm or respiratory disease. |

## Additional information

| | |
|---|---|
| Common and serious undesirable effects | ↓Pulse, ↓BP.<br>Cold extremities.<br>Bronchospasm may occur in patients with asthma or other respiratory disease. |
| Pharmacokinetics | Elimination half-life is 1-9 hours. |
| Significant interactions | • The following may ↑metoprolol levels or effect (or ↑side-effects): adrenaline (risk of severe ↑BP and ↓pulse), alpha-blockers (severe ↓BP), amiodarone (risk of ↓pulse and AV block), anti-arrhythmics (risk of myocardial depression), artemether with lumefantrine (avoid combination), clonidine (↑risk of withdrawal ↑BP), diltiazem (risk of ↓pulse and AV block), dobutamine (risk of severe ↑BP and ↓pulse), flecainide (risk of myocardial depression and ↓pulse), moxisylyte (severe ↓BP), nifedipine (severe ↓BP and heart failure), noradrenaline (risk of severe ↑BP and ↓pulse), verapamil (risk of asystole and severe ↓BP). |
| Action in case of overdose | *Symptoms to watch for:* ↓Pulse, ↓BP, acute cardiac insufficiency and bronchospasm.<br>*Antidote:* Excessive ↓pulse can be countered with IV atropine sulfate (see Monitoring above and the Atropine monograph).<br>Glucagon or dobutamine are further options for unresponsive ↓pulse - seek specialist advice.<br>Bronchospasm can usually be reversed by bronchodilators. |
| Counselling | Patients may experience fatigue and cold extremities during maintenance therapy, and should report wheezing. |

| Risk rating: **GREEN** | Score = 2<br>Lower-risk product. Risk-reduction strategies should be considered. |

This assessment is based on the full range of preparation and administration options described in the monograph. These may not all be applicable in some clinical situations.

## Bibliography

SPC Betaloc IV injection (accessed 8 February 2009).

# Metronidazole

**5 mg/mL solution in 100-mL infusion bags**
- Metronidazole is a synthetic, nitroimidazole-derivative antibacterial with activity against anaerobes, facultative anaerobes and protozoa.
- It is used in the treatment and prophylaxis of anaerobic infections and in the treatment of susceptible protozoal infections such as amoebiasis, giardiasis and trichomoniasis.

## Pre-treatment checks

- Avoid in acute porphyria.
- Caution in hepatic impairment and hepatic encephalopathy.

*Biochemical tests*

LFTs
FBC

## Dose

**Anaerobic infections (if oral therapy is inappropriate):** 500 mg by IV infusion every 8 hours (usually for 7 days; for 10 days in antibiotic-associated colitis). Oral medication should be substituted as soon as is practical.

**Surgical prophylaxis (if oral or rectal administration is inappropriate):** 500 mg by IV infusion at induction, with up to three further doses of 500 mg given every 8 hours for high-risk procedures. Check local policies.

**Dose in hepatic encephalopathy:** 500 mg once daily - this is usually only when hepatic function is very poor, and particularly when renal function is also impaired.

## Intermittent intravenous infusion

*Preparation and administration*

Metronidazole is incompatible with Gluc 10% and Hartmann's.

1. The infusion is pre-prepared for use and should be clear and colourless to pale yellow. Inspect visually for particulate matter or discoloration prior to administration and discard if present.
2. Give by IV infusion at a rate of about 5 mL/minute (i.e. 500 mg over 20 minutes).

## Technical information

| | |
|---|---|
| Incompatible with | Metronidazole is incompatible with Gluc 10% and Hartmann's. Amphotericin, aztreonam, benzylpenicillin, drotrecogin alfa (activated), filgrastim, pantoprazole. |
| Compatible with | **Flush**: NaCl 0.9%<br>**Solutions**: NaCl 0.9%, Gluc 5%, Gluc-NaCl<br>**Y-site**: Aciclovir, cefotaxime (in the same bag), ceftazidime (in the same bag), cefuroxime (in the same bag), cisatracurium, clarithromycin, dopamine, esmolol, fluconazole, foscarnet, granisetron, labetalol, linezolid, magnesium sulfate, methylprednisolone sodium succinate, midazolam, piperacillin with tazobactam, remifentanil |
| pH | 4.5-7 |
| Sodium content | 13-14 mmol/100 mL |
| Storage | Store below 25°C in original packaging. Do not refrigerate. Once opened, use immediately. Discard any unused solution. |

## Monitoring

| Measure | Frequency | Rationale |
|---|---|---|
| LFTs | Periodically | • Significant accumulation may occur in patients with hepatic encephalopathy and the resulting high plasma concentrations of metronidazole may contribute to the symptoms of the encephalopathy. |
| FBC | | • Leucopenia, agranulocytosis, neutropenia, thrombocytopenia and pancytopenia have occurred rarely and usually reversibly. |
| Signs of supra-infection or superinfection | Throughout treatment | • May result in oral, vaginal, or intestinal candidiasis – appropriate therapy should be commenced. |
| Symptoms of peripheral neuropathy or transient seizures | | • Incidence is rare and therapy should be discontinued. Symptoms usually reverse. |

## Additional information

| | |
|---|---|
| Common and serious undesirable effects | *Infusion-related:* Local: Thrombophlebitis may occur (rarely) and can be minimised by avoiding prolonged use of in-dwelling IV catheters.<br>*Other:* Taste disorders (metallic taste), oral mucositis, furred tongue, nausea, vomiting, GI disturbances, anorexia, pruritus, rash, urticaria. |
| Pharmacokinetics | Elimination half-life is 8.5 hours. |

*(continued)*

| **Additional information** (*continued*) | |
|---|---|
| Significant interactions | • Metronidazole may ↑levels or effect of the following drugs (or ↑side-effects): busulfan (↑risk of toxicity), coumarin anticoagulants (monitor INR), phenytoin (monitor levels). |
| Action in case of overdose | *Antidote:* No known antidote, stop administration and give supportive therapy as appropriate. |
| Counselling | Avoid alcoholic beverages for up to 2 days after completing a course: risk of flushing, nausea, vomiting, ↑pulse and shortness of breath. Urine may become dark or reddish-brown owing to the presence of water-soluble pigments resulting from its metabolism. Patients should be warned about the potential for drowsiness, dizziness, confusion, hallucinations, convulsions, transient visual disorders and advised not to drive or operate machinery (if in a position to do so) if these symptoms present. |

| Risk rating: **GREEN** | Score = 0 Lower-risk product: Risk-reduction strategies should be considered. |
|---|---|
| | | | | | |

This assessment is based on the full range of preparation and administration options described in the monograph. These may not all be applicable in some clinical situations.

### Bibliography

SPC Flagyl 500 mg/100 mL solution for infusion (accessed 1 April 2009).

# Mexiletine hydrochloride

### 25 mg/mL solution in 10-mL ampoules

- Mexiletine hydrochloride is a class Ib antiarrhythmic with actions similar to those of lidocaine.
- It has been used for the treatment of life-threatening ventricular arrhythmias.
- It is no longer marketed in the UK as toxicity is common even at therapeutic blood concentrations, but it is available from 'special-order' manufacturers or specialist-importing companies.

### Pre-treatment checks

- Do not give in cardiogenic shock and in second- or third-degree AV block (unless the patient has a pacemaker).
- Caution in patients with sinus node dysfunction, other conduction disorders, ↓pulse, ↓BP, heart failure, or hepatic impairment.

*Biochemical and other tests (not all are necessary in an emergency situation)*

Blood pressure and pulse
ECG
LFTs

## Dose (no longer licensed in UK; doses specified are previously licensed doses)

**Loading doses:**

1. Give 100–250 mg (4–10 mL) by slow IV injection at a maximum rate of 25 mg/minute.
2. Add 500 mg to 500 mL infusion fluid and give 250 mg (250 mL) by IV infusion over the first hour, then 250 mg (250 mL) over the next 2 hours.

**Maintenance infusion:** add 250 mg to 500 mL infusion fluid and give by IV infusion at an initial rate of 500 micrograms/minute (1 mL/minute) and adjust according to clinical response. Switch to oral therapy as soon as possible.

**Alternative method using combined IV and oral loading:** give 200 mg (4 mL) by slow IV injection at a maximum rate of 25 mg/minute. Give 400 mg orally on completion of the injection, then regular oral therapy thereafter.

**Dose in renal impairment:** adjusted according to creatinine clearance:[1]

* CrCl >20–50 mL/minute: dose as in normal renal function.
* CrCl 10–20 mL/minute: dose as in normal renal function.
* CrCl <10 mL/minute: 50–75% of normal dose and titrate according to response.

### Intravenous injection (initial loading dose only)

*Preparation and administration*

1. Withdraw the required dose.
2. The solution should be clear and colourless. Inspect visually for particulate matter or discoloration prior to administration and discard if present.
3. Give by slow IV injection at a maximum rate of 25 mg/minute (1 mL/minute). May be diluted with NaCl 0.9% or Gluc 5% to facilitate slow administration.

### Intravenous infusion (subsequent doses)

*Preparation and administration*

1. Withdraw the required dose (see Dose above) and add to 500 mL NaCl 0.9% or Gluc 5%.
2. The solution should be clear and colourless. Inspect visually for particulate matter or discoloration prior to administration and discard if present.
3. Give by IV infusion via a volumetric infusion device at the rate specified above.
4. Prepare a fresh infusion every 8 hours if required.

| Technical information | |
|---|---|
| Incompatible with | Heparin sodium |
| Compatible with | **Flush**: NaCl 0.9%<br>**Solutions**: NaCl 0.9%, Gluc 5%<br>**Y-site**: No information |
| pH | 5–6 |
| Sodium content | Negligible |
| Storage | Store below 25°C in original packaging. Protect from light. |
| Stability after preparation | Use prepared infusions immediately. Solutions are stable for up to 8 hours |

## Monitoring

| Measure | Frequency | Rationale |
|---------|-----------|-----------|
| ECG | Continuously | • Response to therapy.<br>• Cardiac adverse effects include sinus ↓pulse, heart block and AV dissociation, and atrial fibrillation. |
| Blood pressure | | • May cause ↓BP. |

## Additional information

| | |
|---|---|
| Common and serious undesirable effects | *Injection/infusion-related:* Too rapid administration: ↓BP, sinus ↓pulse, atrial fibrillation, AV dissociation, exacerbation of arrhythmias.<br>*Other:* Nausea, vomiting, diarrhoea. May rarely cause tremor or convulsions. |
| Pharmacokinetics | Elimination half-life: 10 hours in healthy subjects but this may be prolonged in patients with heart disease, hepatic impairment, or severe renal impairment. |
| Significant interactions | Caution with other antiarrhythmic drugs. |
| Action in case of overdose | Stop infusion and provide supportive measures. |

| | |
|---|---|
| Risk rating: **AMBER** | Score = 4<br>Moderate-risk product: Risk-reduction strategies are recommended. |

This assessment is based on the full range of preparation and administration options described in the monograph. These may not all be applicable in some clinical situations.

### Reference

1. Ashley C, Currie A, eds. *The Renal Drug Handbook*, 3rd edn. Oxford: Radcliffe Medical Press, 2009.

### Bibliography

SPC Mexitil ampoules. www.boehringer-ingelheim.co.uk (accessed 21 January 2009).

# Micafungin

#### 50-mg and 100-mg dry powder vials

• Micafungin sodium is a semi-synthetic, echinocandin antifungal agent with properties similar to caspofungin.
• It is used in the treatment of invasive candidiasis and also for prophylaxis of candidal infection in patients who are to undergo stem cell transplantation or who are likely to develop neutropenia.
• Doses are expressed in terms of micafungin base.

## Pre-treatment checks

Do not give to patients with galactose intolerance, the Lapp lactase deficiency or glucose-galactose malabsorption (lactose is an excipient).

*Biochemical and other tests (not all are necessary in an emergency situation)*

| | |
|---|---|
| Bodyweight | LFTs |
| Electrolytes: serum Na, K, (consider Mg, Ca, PO$_4$) | Renal function: U, Cr |
| FBC | |
| Fungal culture to identify causative organism, although therapy may be commenced before these results are known | |

## Dose

**Invasive candidiasis:** adults >40 kg, 100 mg once daily (increased to 200 mg daily if inadequate response) for at least 14 days; adults ≤40 kg, 2 mg/kg once daily (increased to 4 mg/kg daily if inadequate response) for at least 14 days.

**Oesophageal candidiasis where IV therapy is appropriate:** adults >40 kg, 150 mg once daily; adults ≤40 kg, 3 mg/kg once daily; for at least one week after resolution of symptoms.

**Prophylaxis of candidiasis in patients undergoing bone-marrow transplantation or who are expected to become neutropenic for over 10 days:** adults >40 kg, 50 mg once daily; adults ≤40 kg, 1 mg/kg once daily. Continue for at least 7 days after neutrophil count in desirable range.

**Dose in hepatic impairment:** use with caution in mild to moderate hepatic impairment; avoid in severe hepatic impairment—no information available.

## Intermittent intravenous infusion

Protect from light after reconstitution and during infusion.

*Preparation and administration*

* Reconstitute each vial with 5 mL NaCl 0.9% or Gluc 5% by injecting the fluid slowly against the side of the inner wall of the vial to minimise foaming.
* Swirl gently to dissolve the contents (vigorous shaking will cause foaming) to give a solution containing 10 mg/mL (50-mg vial) or 20 mg/mL (100-mg vial).
* Withdraw the required dose and add to 100 mL NaCl 0.9% or Gluc 5%. Gently invert to disperse the diluted solution but **do not** agitate in order to avoid foaming.
* The solution should be clear and colourless. Inspect visually for particulate matter or discoloration prior to administration and discard if present.
* Insert the infusion bag/bottle into a closable opaque bag to protect it from light (it is not necessary to cover the giving set).
* Give by IV infusion over 60 minutes.

## Technical information

| | |
|---|---|
| Incompatible with | Adrenaline (epinephrine), amiodarone, cisatracurium, dobutamine, insulin (soluble), labetalol, midazolam, ondansetron, phenytoin sodium, vecuronium bromide. |
| Compatible with | **Flush**: NaCl 0.9%<br>**Solutions**: NaCl 0.9%, Gluc 5%<br>**Y-site**: Aminophylline, bumetanide, calcium gluconate, dopamine, esmolol, furosemide, glyceryl trinitrate, magnesium sulfate, noradrenaline (norepinephrine), potassium chloride |

*(continued)*

## Technical information (*continued*)

| | |
|---|---|
| pH | 5.0–7.0 |
| Sodium content | Negligible |
| Storage | Store below 25°C in original packaging. |
| Displacement value | Negligible |
| Stability after preparation | Must be protected from light after reconstitution and during infusion. From a microbiological point of view, should be used immediately; however:<br>• Reconstituted vials may be stored at 2–8°C for 24 hours.<br>• Prepared infusions may be stored at 2–8°C and infused (at room temperature) within 24 hours. |

## Monitoring

| Measure | Frequency | Rationale |
|---|---|---|
| Candida blood cultures | At least weekly in the treatment of invasive candidiasis | • Treatment should continue for at least one week after two sequential negative blood cultures have been obtained and after resolution of clinical signs and symptoms of infection. |
| LFTs | Periodically | • Monitor closely if ↑ALT, ↑AST, ↑total bilirubin to >3 times ULN.<br>• Potentially life-threatening hepatotoxicity has been reported. |
| FBC | | • Leucopenia, neutropenia, anaemia occur commonly.<br>• Haemolysis or haemolytic anaemia occurs rarely but requires monitoring for. |
| U&Es | | • ↓K, ↓Mg, ↓Ca occur commonly.<br>• ↓Na, ↓PO₄, ↑K occur less commonly.<br>• Renal failure occurs rarely: monitor for ↑U, ↑Cr. |

## Additional information

| | |
|---|---|
| Common and serious undesirable effects | *Immediate:* Anaphylaxis has been reported rarely.<br>*Injection/infusion-related:*<br>• Too rapid administration: Rapid infusions can result in allergic reactions.<br>• Local: Injection-site pain, inflammation or thrombosis.<br><br>*Other:* Headache, nausea, vomiting, diarrhoea, abdominal pain, rash, pyrexia, rigors, peripheral oedema. |
| Pharmacokinetics | Elimination half-life is 10–17 hours. |
| Significant interactions | No significant interactions. |
| Action in case of overdose | No antidote: give supportive therapy as appropriate. Micafungin is not dialysable. |
| Counselling | Warn patient to report any symptoms consistent with liver toxicity, e.g. nausea, vomiting, loss of appetite, pain in upper stomach, yellowing of skin or the whites of the eyes. |

| Risk rating: **RED** | Score = 6<br>High-risk product: Risk-reduction strategies are required to minimise these risks. |

This assessment is based on the full range of preparation and administration options described in the monograph. These may not all be applicable in some clinical situations.

## Bibliography

SPC Mycamine 50 mg and 100 mg powder for solution for infusion (accessed 13 April 2009).

# Midazolam

**1 mg/mL solution in 2-mL and 5-mL ampoules**

*High-strength preparations:*

**2 mg/mL solution in 5-mL ampoules**

**5 mg/mL solution in 2-mL and 10-mL ampoules**

* Midazolam hydrochloride is a benzodiazepine with anxiolytic and amnesic activity in addition to sedative and hypnotic properties.
* It is used as a short-acting sleep-inducing drug in anaesthesia, conscious sedation and for sedation in critical care units.
* The injection solution may be given (unlicensed) by buccal administration in the treatment of status epilepticus.
* Midazolam may also be given (unlicensed) by SC injection or infusion in palliative care to calm very restless patients.
* Doses are expressed in terms of the base:
  Midazolam 1 mg ≅ 1.1 mg midazolam hydrochloride.

### NPSA Rapid Response Report (December 2008)

In order to reduce the risk of overdose with midazolam injection in adults the UK NPSA has stipulated that:

* Use of high-strength midazolam preparations is restricted to clinical areas/situations where its use has been risk-assessed.
* Other clinical areas should only routinely stock low-strength midazolam.
* Staff involved in sedation techniques must have the necessary skills.
* Flumazenil should be available wherever midazolam is used.

## Pre-treatment checks

* Avoid use for conscious sedation in patients with severe respiratory failure or acute respiratory depression.
* Caution in high-risk patients, e.g. >60 years old, chronically ill or debilitated – closer monitoring will be required.

- Caution in patients with myasthenia gravis.
- Facilities for resuscitation should always be available when IV midazolam is administered.
- When midazolam and an opioid are used together, the opioid should be given first.

*Biochemical and other tests (not all are necessary in an emergency situation)*

Bodyweight (in certain indications)
LFTs
Renal function: U, Cr, CrCl (or eGFR)

## Dose

**Conscious sedation in adults <60 years**: initial dose 2–2.5 mg by IV injection 5–10 minutes before the procedure. If required additional doses of 1 mg by IV injection may be given up to a maximum of 7.5 mg (usual total dose: 3.5–5 mg).

**Conscious sedation in adults ≥60 years/debilitated or chronically ill**: initial dose 0.5–1 mg by IV injection 5–10 minutes before the procedure. If required additional doses of 0.5–1 mg by IV injection may be given up to a maximum of 3.5 mg.

**Premedication in adults <60 years**: 1–2 mg by IV injection repeated as required or 70–100 micrograms/kg by deep IM injection. The IM injection should be given 20–60 minutes before induction.

**Premedication in adults ≥60 years/debilitated or chronically ill:** 0.5 mg by IV injection repeated as required; or 25–50 micrograms/kg by deep IM injection. The IM injection should be given 20–60 minutes before induction.

**Anaesthesia induction in adults <60 years**: 150–200 micrograms/kg (300–350 if no premedication) by IV injection.

**Anaesthesia induction in adults ≥60 years/debilitated or chronically ill:** 50–150 micrograms/kg (150–300 if no premedication) by IV injection.

**Sedative component in combined anaesthesia**: 30–100 micrograms/kg by IV injection repeated as necessary; or 30–100 micrograms/kg/hour by continuous IV infusion. Use lower doses in adults ≥60 years and the debilitated or chronically ill.

**Sedation in critical care:** initially 30–300 micrograms/kg given in increments of 1–2.5 mg by IV injection every 2 minutes followed by a maintenance dose of 30–200 micrograms/kg/hour by continuous IV infusion.

**Status epilepticus (unlicensed):** 10 mg by buccal administration, repeated once if necessary.

**Dose in renal impairment:** a lower dose may be required; monitor carefully during continuous infusion.

**Dose in hepatic impairment:** a lower dose may be required.

## Intravenous injection

*Preparation and administration*

Make sure that you have selected the correct strength of midazolam ampoule.

1. Withdraw the required dose.
2. The solution should be clear and colourless to light yellow. Inspect visually for particulate matter or discoloration prior to administration and discard if present.
3. Give by slow IV injection at a rate of approximately 1 mg per 30 seconds (dependent on individual age, weight and response).

## Continuous intravenous infusion via syringe pump

*Preparation and administration*

Make sure that you have selected the correct strength of midazolam ampoule.

1. Withdraw the required dose and dilute to a suitable volume in a syringe pump with NaCl 0.9% or Gluc 5%. (The recommended concentration for infusion in a critically ill adult patient is 1 mg/mL but it may be administered undiluted.)
2. Cap the syringe and mix well.
3. The solution should be clear and colourless to light yellow. Inspect visually for particulate matter or discoloration prior to administration and discard if present.
4. Give by IV infusion at a rate appropriate to indication. Adjust rate to clinical response.

## Intramuscular injection (painful – use only if no other route is available)

*Preparation and administration*

Make sure that you have selected the correct strength of midazolam ampoule.

1. Withdraw the required dose.
2. Give by deep IM injection into a large muscle mass.

## Buccal administration (unlicensed use in status epilepticus)

*Preparation and administration*

Make sure that you have selected the correct strength of midazolam ampoule (usually the 10 mg/ 2 mL strength is used).

1. Withdraw the required dose from the ampoule using a filter straw attached to a 2-mL oral syringe.
2. Remove the filter straw from the syringe.
3. Open the patient's lips and drip the midazolam solution into the buccal area of the mouth (between the cheek and gum of the lower jaw).
4. Once the dose has been given, hold the lips gently shut for 1–2 minutes to prevent leakage.

## Technical information

| | |
|---|---|
| Incompatible with | Midazolam is incompatible with Hartmann's solution. Amoxicillin, bumetanide, ceftazidime, cefuroxime, co-amoxiclav, co-trimoxazole, dexamethasone sodium phosphate, dobutamine, drotrecogin alfa (activated), flucloxacillin, foscarnet, fosphenytoin sodium, furosemide, hydrocortisone sodium succinate, imipenem with cilastatin, micafungin, omeprazole, pantoprazole, propofol, sodium bicarbonate. |
| Compatible with | **Flush**: NaCl 0.9% <br> **Solutions**: NaCl 0.9%, Gluc 5% Gluc-NaCl <br> **Y-site**: Adrenaline (epinephrine), amikacin, atracurium, cefotaxime, cisatracurium, clindamycin, digoxin, dopamine, erythromycin, esmolol, fentanyl, fluconazole, gentamicin, glyceryl trinitrate, labetalol, methylprednisolone sodium succinate, metronidazole, noradrenaline (norepinephrine), ranitidine, remifentanil, tobramycin, vancomycin, vecuronium bromide |
| pH | 2.9–3.7 |
| Sodium content | Negligible |
| Storage | Store below 25°C in original packaging. Controlled Drug. |
| Stability after preparation | From a microbiological point of view, should be used immediately; however, prepared infusions may be stored at 2-8°C and infused (at room temperature) within 24 hours. |

## Monitoring

| Measure | Frequency | Rationale |
|---------|-----------|-----------|
| Injection-site reactions | Post administration | • Reactions have been reported. |
| Sedation | Continuously | • To ensure that treatment is effective. |
| Cardiac function | | • May cause ↓pulse, chest pain and ↓cardiac output, stroke volume and systemic vascular resistance. |
| Respiratory rate | Continuously | • May cause respiratory depression. There is ↑risk if given with opioids or other sedatives. |
| BP | Periodically | • ↓BP may be observed in critically ill patients. |

## Additional information

| | |
|---|---|
| Common and serious undesirable effects | *Immediate:* Anaphylaxis has been reported very rarely.<br>*Injection/infusion-related:* Local: Erythema and pain on injection site.<br>*Other:*<br>• Common: Nausea, vomiting.<br>• Rare: Cardiac arrest, respiratory arrest. |
| Pharmacokinetics | Elimination half-life is approximately 2 hours, although half-lives longer than 7 hours have been reported in some patients. |
| Significant interactions | • The following may ↑midazolam levels or effect (↑risk of prolonged sedation): atazanavir, clarithromycin, efavirenz (avoid combination), erythromycin, fluconazole, fosamprenavir, indinavir, itraconazole, ketoconazole, nelfinavir, posaconazole, quinupristin with dalfopristin, ritonavir, saquinavir, telithromycin.<br>• Olanzapine IM may ↑midazolam levels or effect (or ↑side-effects): ↓BP, ↓pulse, respiratory depression.<br>• Midazolam may ↑levels or effect (or ↑side-effects) of sodium oxybate (avoid combination). |
| Action in case of overdose | *Symptoms to watch for:* ↑sedation, respiratory depression, ↓BP.<br>*Antidote:* Flumazenil (use with caution in patients with a history of seizures, head injury or chronic benzodiazepine use including for the control of epilepsy).<br>Stop administration and give supportive therapy as appropriate. |

| | |
|---|---|
| Risk rating: **RED** | Score = 6<br>High-risk product: Risk-reduction strategies are required to minimise these risks. |

This assessment is based on the full range of preparation and administration options described in the monograph. These may not all be applicable in some clinical situations.

## Bibliography

SPC Hypnovel ampoules 10 mg/5 mL (accessed 30 March 2010).

SPC Hypnovel 10 mg/2 mL (accessed 30 March 2010).

SPC Midazolam 2 mg/mL, solution for injection, Hameln Pharmaceuticals Ltd (accessed 20 January 2010).

SPC Midazolam 5 mg/mL, solution for injection, Hameln Pharmaceuticals Ltd (accessed 20 January 2010)

# Milrinone

### 1 mg/mL solution in 10-mL ampoules

- Milrinone lactate is a phosphodiesterase type 3 inhibitor with positive inotropic and vasodilator activity.
- It is used for short-term management of heart failure unresponsive to other treatments, including low-output states following heart surgery.
- Doses are expressed in terms of the base:
  Milrinone 1 mg ≡ 1.43 mg milrinone lactate.

## Pre-treatment checks

Use with caution in heart failure associated with hypertrophic cardiomyopathy, stenotic or obstructive valvular disease or other outlet obstruction.

*Biochemical and other tests (not all are necessary in an emergency situation)*

Bodyweight

Electrolytes: serum K

Renal function: U, Cr, CrCl (or eGFR)

## Dose

**Loading dose:** 50 micrograms/kg usually followed by maintenance infusion.

**Maintenance infusion:** at 0.375–0.75 microgram/kg/minute according to haemodynamic and clinical response.

**Dose in renal impairment**: renal impairment significantly reduces the terminal elimination half-life of milrinone. The following are maximum recommended maintenance infusion rates adjusted according to creatinine clearance:

- CrCl 50 mL/minute: 0.43 microgram/kg/minute.
- CrCl 40 mL/minute: 0.38 microgram/kg/minute.
- CrCl 30 mL/minute: 0.33 microgram/kg/minute.
- CrCl 20 mL/minute: 0.28 microgram/kg/minute.
- CrCl 10 mL/minute: 0.23 microgram/kg/minute.
- CrCl 5 mL/minute: 0.20 microgram/kg/minute.

## Intravenous injection (loading dose only)

*Preparation and administration*

1. Withdraw the required dose.
2. The solution should be clear and colourless to pale yellow. Inspect visually for particulate matter or discoloration prior to administration and discard if present.
3. Give by IV injection over 10 minutes. May be diluted to 10 mL with NaCl 0.9% or Gluc 5% to facilitate slow administration.

## Continuous intravenous infusion via a syringe pump

*Preparation of a 200 micrograms/mL solution*

1. Withdraw 10 mg (10 mL) of injection and make up to 50 mL in a syringe pump with NaCl 0.9% or Gluc 5% fluid.
2. Cap the syringe and mix well to give a solution containing 200 micrograms/mL.
3. The solution should be clear and colourless to pale yellow. Inspect visually for particulate matter or discoloration prior to administration and discard if present.

*Administration*

Give by IV infusion via a syringe pump at an initial rate of 0.375 microgram/kg/minute. Adjust the dose according to clinical response. Prepare a fresh syringe every 24 hours.

**Calculation of infusion rate:**

$$\text{Infusion rate (mL/hour)} = \frac{\text{Weight (kg)} \times \text{required rate (micrograms/minute)} \times 60}{\text{Concentration of prepared infusion (micrograms/mL)}}$$

See Table M1 below for a dosage chart detailing pre-calculated infusion rates for each bodyweight using a 200 micrograms/mL solution.

## Technical information

| | |
|---|---|
| Incompatible with | Sodium bicarbonate.<br>Bumetanide, furosemide, imipenem with cilastatin. |
| Compatible with | **Flush**: NaCl 0.9%<br>**Solutions**: NaCl 0.9%, Gluc 5%<br>**Y-site**: Aciclovir, adrenaline (epinephrine), amikacin, ampicillin, atracurium, calcium gluconate, cefotaxime, ceftazidime, cefuroxime, ciprofloxacin, clindamycin, dexamethasone, digoxin, dobutamine, dopamine, fentanyl, gentamicin, glyceryl trinitrate, magnesium sulfate, meropenem, methylprednisolone sodium succinate, metronidazole, micafungin, midazolam, noradrenaline (norepinephrine), piperacillin with tazobactam, propofol, ranitidine, ticarcillin with clavulanate, tobramycin, vancomycin, vecuronium. |
| pH | 3.2–4 |
| Sodium content | Negligible |
| Storage | Store below 25°C in original packaging. Do not freeze. |
| Stability after preparation | From a microbiological point of view, should be used immediately; however, prepared infusions may be stored at 2–8°C and infused (at room temperature) within 24 hours. |

## Monitoring

| Measure | Frequency | Rationale |
|---------|-----------|-----------|
| Signs and symptoms of congestive heart failure | Throughout therapy | • For signs of clinical improvement. |
| Ventricular arrhythmias and exacerbation of anginal symptoms | | • May ↑ventricular response rate in patients with uncontrolled atrial flutter or fibrillation.<br>• Stop infusion if arrhythmias occur.<br>• ↑Myocardial oxygen consumption. |
| BP and pulse | | • May reduce BP through vasodilatation. |

## Additional information

| | |
|---|---|
| Common and serious undesirable effects | *Immediate:* Anaphylaxis has rarely been reported.<br>*Other:* Headache, ventricular ectopic activity, supraventricular arrhythmias, ventricular tachycardia, ↓BP. |
| Pharmacokinetics | Elimination half-life is 1–3 hours. |
| Significant interactions | Milrinone should not be used with anagrelide. |
| Action in case of overdose | *Symptoms to watch for:* ↓BP.<br>Reduce dose and provide general circulatory support. |

Risk rating: **RED**

Score = 6
High-risk product: Risk-reduction strategies are required to minimise these risks.

This assessment is based on the full range of preparation and administration options described in the monograph. These may not all be applicable in some clinical situations.

## Bibliography

SPC Primacor 1 mg/mL 10-mL ampoules (accessed 20 August 2008).

**Table M1** Milrinone rate of infusion using milrinone 10 mg (10 mL) made up to 50 mL in a 50-mL syringe pump, i.e. 200 micrograms/mL)

| Weight (kg) | Infusion rate (micrograms/kg/minute) | | | | | |
|---|---|---|---|---|---|---|
| | **0.375** | **0.400** | **0.500** | **0.600** | **0.700** | **0.750** |
| | Rate of infusion in mL/hour | | | | | |
| 40 | 4.5 | 4.8 | 6.0 | 7.2 | 8.4 | 9.0 |
| 45 | 5.1 | 5.4 | 6.8 | 8.1 | 9.5 | 10.1 |
| 50 | 5.6 | 6.0 | 7.5 | 9.0 | 10.5 | 11.3 |
| 55 | 6.2 | 6.6 | 8.3 | 9.9 | 11.6 | 12.4 |
| 60 | 6.8 | 7.2 | 9.0 | 10.8 | 12.6 | 13.5 |
| 65 | 7.3 | 7.8 | 9.8 | 11.7 | 13.7 | 14.6 |
| 70 | 7.9 | 8.4 | 10.5 | 12.6 | 14.7 | 15.8 |
| 75 | 8.4 | 9.0 | 11.3 | 13.5 | 15.8 | 16.9 |
| 80 | 9.0 | 9.6 | 12.0 | 14.4 | 16.8 | 18.0 |
| 85 | 9.6 | 10.2 | 12.8 | 15.3 | 17.9 | 19.1 |
| 90 | 10.1 | 10.8 | 13.5 | 16.2 | 18.9 | 20.3 |
| 95 | 10.7 | 11.4 | 14.3 | 17.1 | 20.0 | 21.4 |
| 100 | 11.3 | 12.0 | 15.0 | 18.0 | 21.0 | 22.5 |
| 110 | 12.4 | 13.2 | 16.5 | 19.8 | 23.1 | 24.8 |
| 120 | 13.5 | 14.4 | 18.0 | 21.6 | 25.2 | 27.0 |
| 130 | 14.6 | 15.6 | 19.5 | 23.4 | 27.3 | 29.3 |
| 140 | 15.8 | 16.8 | 21.0 | 25.2 | 29.4 | 31.5 |

# Morphine sulfate

**10 mg/mL, 15 mg/mL, 20 mg/mL, 30 mg/mL solution in 1-mL and 2-mL ampoules**
**1 mg/mL solution in 10-mL pre-filled syringe; 1 mg/mL and 2 mg/mL solution in 50-mL vials**

* Morphine sulfate is a potent opioid analgesic.
* It is used parenterally for the treatment of moderate to severe pain; relief of dyspnoea of left ventricular failure and pulmonary oedema; pre-operative and postoperative care.
* Morphine may also be given by SC infusion to control pain in palliative care.
* Doses below are expressed in terms of morphine sulfate.

## Pre-treatment checks

* Do not use in acute respiratory depression, where there is a risk of paralytic ileus, in ↑intracranial pressure and in head injury, in comatose patients; in acute abdomen; delayed gastric emptying; chronic constipation; acute porphyria; heart failure secondary to chronic lung disease; and phaeochromocytoma.
* Caution in ↓BP, shock, convulsive disorders, cardiac arrhythmias, e.g. supraventricular tachycardias and atrial flutter, chronic obstructive pulmonary disease and acute asthma attack, obstructive or inflammatory bowel diseases, biliary tract diseases, alcoholism, prostatic hyperplasia, myasthenia gravis, hypothyroidism (reduce dose), adrenocortical insufficiency (reduce dose), pancreatitis, severe cor pulmonale.
* Ensure resuscitation equipment and naloxone are available especially for IV administration.

*Biochemical and other tests (not all are necessary in an emergency situation)*

| | |
|---|---|
| Blood pressure and pulse | Renal function: U, Cr, CrCl (or eGFR) |
| LFTs | Respiratory rate |
| Pain score | |

## Dose

> Note: Doses above those stated must not be given to opioid naive patients.

**Acute pain**: 10 mg by SC or IM injection or 2.5 mg by slow IV injection every 4 hours when required. Halve the initial dose in elderly or frail patients. Doses may be given more frequently during initial titration of requirements but the patient must be very closely monitored.
**Chronic pain**: 5–20 mg by SC or IM injection or 2.5–15 mg by slow IV injection regularly every 4 hours adjusted according to requirements. Initial dose is dependent on previous opioid exposure – see below.

> **Approximate equivalents for patients switched from oral to parenteral**
>
> 10 mg orally every 4 hours (or 60 mg daily as oral modified release) is equivalent to:
> * 5 mg by IM injection every 4 hours (total 30 mg daily)
> * 5 mg by SC injection every 4 hours (total 30 mg daily)
> * 2.5 mg by IV injection every 4 hours (total 15 mg daily)

Alternatively, give 1–5 mg every hour by IV infusion adjusted according to requirements. Similar doses have been given by SC infusion (unlicensed).
**Premedication**: up to 10 mg by SC or IM injection 60–90 minutes before procedure.

**Myocardial infarction**: 10 mg by slow IV injection followed by a further 5–10 mg if necessary (halve dose in elderly or frail patients).

**Acute pulmonary oedema**: 5–10 mg by slow IV injection.

**Patient-controlled analgesia** (PCA): consult local hospital protocol.

**Dose in hepatic impairment**: reduce dose or avoid (may precipitate coma).

**Dose in renal impairment:** reduce dose or avoid (prolonged effect, and ↑cerebral sensitivity).

## Subcutaneous injection (not suitable for oedematous patients)

*Preparation and administration*

> Check that you have selected the correct strength of ampoule. High-strength ampoules are available for use in PCA and palliative care. These are not suitable for use in acute situations.

1. Withdraw the required dose.
2. Give by SC injection.
3. Close monitoring of respiratory rate and consciousness is recommended for 30 minutes in patients receiving initial dose, especially elderly patients or those of low bodyweight.

## Intramuscular injection

*Preparation and administration*

> Check that you have selected the correct strength of ampoule. High-strength ampoules are available for use in PCA and palliative care. These are not suitable for use in acute situations.

1. Withdraw the required dose.
2. Give by IM injection.
3. Close monitoring of respiratory rate and consciousness is recommended for 30 minutes in patients receiving initial dose, especially elderly patients or those of low bodyweight.

## Intravenous injection

*Preparation and administration*

> Check that you have selected the correct strength of ampoule. High-strength ampoules are available for use in PCA and palliative care. These are not suitable for use in acute situations.

1. Withdraw the required dose. It may be further diluted with NaCl 0.9% or Gluc 5% to facilitate slow administration (10 mg is often diluted to 10 mL).
2. The solution should be clear and colourless. Inspect visually for particulate matter or discoloration prior to administration and discard if present.
3. Give by slow IV injection at a maximum rate of 2 mg/minute (1 mg/minute in opioid naive patients).
4. Close monitoring of respiratory rate and consciousness is recommended for 30 minutes in patients receiving initial dose, especially elderly patients or those of low bodyweight.

## Patient-controlled analgesia[1]

*Preparation and administration*

> Strength used may vary depending on local policies.

1. Make 50 mg morphine sulfate up to 50 mL with NaCl 0.9% in a PCA syringe to give a solution containing 1 mg/mL or use a pre-prepared solution.
2. Cap the syringe and mix well.
3. The solution should be clear and colourless. Inspect visually for particulate matter or discoloration prior to administration and discard if present.
4. The usual setting for the PCA device is to deliver a 1-mg bolus with a 5-minute lock-out period. Lower doses are used in patients with renal failure.

## Continuous intravenous infusion

*Preparation and administration*

1. Withdraw the required dose and further dilute with NaCl 0.9% or other compatible diluent to a convenient volume.
2. The solution should be clear and colourless. Inspect visually for particulate matter or discoloration prior to administration and discard if present.
3. Give by continuous IV infusion via a volumetric infusion device.

| Technical information | |
|---|---|
| Incompatible with | Aciclovir, amphotericin, furosemide, micafungin, phenytoin sodium, propofol. |
| Compatible with | **Flush**: NaCl 0.9%<br>**Solutions**: NaCl 0.9%, Gluc 5% (both with added KCl)<br>**Y-site**: Adrenaline (epinephrine), amikacin, aminophylline, ampicillin, atenolol, atracurium, aztreonam, benzylpenicillin, bumetanide, cefotaxime, ceftazidime, ceftriaxone, cefuroxime, chloramphenicol sodium succinate, cisatracurium, clindamycin, co-trimoxazole, dexamethasone, digoxin, dobutamine, erythromycin, esmolol, fluconazole, foscarnet, gentamicin, glyceryl trinitrate, granisetron, hydrocortisone sodium succinate, labetalol, linezolid, magnesium sulfate, meropenem, methylprednisolone sodium succinate, metoclopramide, metronidazole, midazolam, noradrenaline (norepinephrine), ondansetron, pantoprazole, piperacillin with tazobactam, ranitidine, remifentanil, ticarcillin with clavulanate, tobramycin, vancomycin, vecuronium bromide |
| pH | 2.5–6.5 |
| Sodium content | Negligible |
| Excipients | Some products contain sulfites (may cause hypersensitivity reactions). |
| Storage | Store below 25°C in original packaging. Controlled Drug. |
| Stability after preparation | From a microbiological point of view, should be used immediately; however, prepared infusions may be stored at 2–8°C and infused (at room temperature) within 24 hours. |

## Monitoring

Close monitoring of respiratory rate and consciousness is recommended for 30 minutes in patients receiving initial dose, especially elderly patients or those of low bodyweight.

| Measure | Frequency | Rationale |
|---------|-----------|-----------|
| Pain | At regular intervals | • To ensure therapeutic response. |
| Blood pressure, pulse and respiratory rate | | • ↓BP, ↑ or ↓pulse, palpitations and respiratory depression can occur. |
| Sedation | | • Morphine can cause sedation. |
| Monitor for side-effects and toxicity | | • Can cause side-effects such as itching, nausea, vomiting and constipation, which may need treating. |

## Additional information

| | |
|---|---|
| Common and serious undesirable effects | *Immediate:* Anaphylaxis has been reported following IV injection.<br>*Injection/infusion-related:* Local: Pain and irritation at injection site.<br>*Other:* Nausea and vomiting (particularly initially), constipation, dry mouth, urticaria, pruritus, biliary spasm, ↑ or ↓pulse, hallucinations, euphoria, drowsiness.<br>At higher doses: ↑ or ↓BP, sedation, respiratory depression, muscle rigidity. |
| Pharmacokinetics | Elimination half-life is about 2 hours; 2.4–6.7 hours for morphine-3-glucuronide (active metabolite). |
| Significant interactions | • The following may ↑morphine levels or effect (or ↑side-effects): antihistamines-sedating (↑sedation), MAOIs (avoid combination and for 2 weeks after stopping MAOI), moclobemide.<br>• Morphine may ↑levels or effect (or ↑side-effects) of sodium oxybate (avoid combination). |
| Action in case of overdose | *Symptoms to watch for:* ↑Sedation, respiratory depression.<br>*Antidote:* Naloxone (see the Naloxone monograph).<br>Stop administration and give supportive therapy as appropriate. |
| Counselling | Avoid drinking alcohol while using morphine.<br>If you are pregnant or breast feeding inform your doctor.<br>Inform the patient of possible side-effects: See above.<br>May cause drowsiness and dizziness that may affect the ability to perform skilled tasks; if affected do not drive or operate machinery. To help avoid dizziness, get up slowly from a sitting or lying position.<br>Drink plenty of fluids to help avoid constipation and use a laxative if required. |

| Risk rating: **AMBER** | Score = 5<br>Moderate-risk product: Risk-reduction strategies are recommended. |
|---|---|

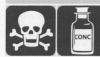   

This assessment is based on the full range of preparation and administration options described in the monograph. These may not all be applicable in some clinical situations.

## Reference

1. Walder B *et al* 2001;Efficacy and safety of patient controlled opioid analgesia for acute postoperative pain. *Acta Anaesthesiol Scand*. 45: 795–804.

## Bibliography

SPC Morphine Sulphate Injection BP Minijet 1 mg/mL, International Medication Systems (accessed 29 June 2008).

SPCs Morphine Sulphate Injection 10 mg/mL, 15 mg/mL and 30 mg/mL Injection BP, Wockhardt UK Ltd (accessed 29 June 2008).

SPC Morphine Sulphate Injection 10 mg/mL, Hameln Pharmaceuticals Ltd (accessed 29 June 2008).

SPC Morphine Sulphate Injection BP 10 mg/mL, 15 mg/mL and 30 mg/1mL, UCB Pharma Ltd (accessed 29 June 2008).

# Morphine tartrate with cyclizine (Cyclimorph)

**Cyclimorph 10 solution in 1-mL ampoules (≅ morphine tartrate 10 mg plus cyclizine tartrate 40 mg)**
**Cyclimorph 15 solution in 1-mL ampoules (≅ morphine tartrate 15 mg plus cyclizine tartrate 40 mg)**

* Cyclimorph injection contains the potent opioid analgesic morphine tartrate combined with the antiemetic antihistamine cyclizine tartrate.
* It is used to treat moderate to severe pain where an additional antiemetic effect is helpful.
* Cyclimorph is intended for short-term use only and is not recommended for palliative care.
* Doses below are quoted in millilitres of either of the combined products:
  Cyclizine tartrate 40 mg ≅ 50 mg cyclizine lactate in effect.

## Pre-treatment checks

* Do not use in acute respiratory depression, where there is a risk of paralytic ileus, in ↑intracranial pressure and in head injury, in comatose patients; in acute abdomen; delayed gastric emptying; chronic constipation; acute porphyria; heart failure secondary to chronic lung disease; and phaeochromocytoma.
* Caution in ↓BP, shock, convulsive disorders, cardiac arrhythmias, e.g. supraventricular tachycardias and atrial flutter, chronic obstructive pulmonary disease and acute asthma attack, obstructive

or inflammatory bowel diseases, biliary tract diseases, alcoholism, prostatic hyperplasia, myasthenia gravis, hypothyroidism (reduce dose), adrenocortical insufficiency (reduce dose), pancreatitis, severe cor pulmonale.
* Caution also in severe heart failure and myocardial infarction as cyclizine lowers cardiac output and counteract the haemodynamic benefits of opioids.
* Ensure resuscitation equipment and naloxone are available especially for IV administration.

*Biochemical and other tests (not all are necessary in an emergency situation)*

Blood pressure and pulse
LFTs
Pain score

Renal function: U, Cr, CrCl (or eGFR)
Respiratory rate

## Dose

**Moderate to severe pain**: 1 mL (i.e. 10 or 15 mg of morphine tartrate) by SC, IM, or IV injection every 4 hours as required up to a maximum three doses in 24 hours. Use reduced doses in elderly or frail patients.
**Dose in hepatic impairment:** reduce the dose or avoid (may precipitate coma).
**Dose in renal impairment:** avoid if CrCl <20 mL/minute.

## Subcutaneous injection

*Preparation and administration*

1. Withdraw the required dose.
2. Give by SC injection.

## Intramuscular injection

*Preparation and administration*

1. Withdraw the required dose.
2. Give by IM injection.
3. Close monitoring of respiratory rate and consciousness is recommended for 30 minutes in patients receiving initial dose, especially elderly patients or those of low bodyweight.

## Intravenous injection

*Preparation and administration*

1. Withdraw the required dose. May be diluted with an equal volume of WFI to facilitate slow administration.
2. The solution should be clear and colourless. Inspect visually for particulate matter or discoloration prior to administration and discard if present.
3. Give by slow IV injection at a rate of 2 mg/minute of morphine (1 mg/minute in opioid naive patients).
4. Close monitoring of respiratory rate and consciousness is recommended for 30 minutes in patients receiving initial dose, especially elderly patients or those of low bodyweight.

| Technical information | |
|---|---|
| Incompatible with | No information but likely to precipitate. |
| Compatible with | **Flush**: WFI or NaCl 0.9%<br>**Solutions**: WFI, Gluc 5% (via Y-site), less stable in NaCl 0.9%<br>**Y-site**: No information but likely to precipitate |

*(continued)*

## Technical information (continued)

| | |
|---|---|
| pH | 4.3-5.0 |
| Sodium content | Negligible |
| Excipients | Contains sulfites (may cause hypersensitivity reactions). |
| Storage | Store below 30°C in original packaging. Do not freeze. Controlled Drug. |

## Monitoring

Close monitoring of respiratory rate and consciousness is recommended for 30 minutes in patients receiving initial dose, especially elderly patients or those of low bodyweight.

| Measure | Frequency | Rationale |
|---|---|---|
| Pain | At regular intervals | • To ensure therapeutic response. |
| Blood pressure, pulse and respiratory rate | | • ↓BP, ↑ or ↓pulse, palpitations and respiratory depression can occur. |
| Sedation | | • Morphine can cause sedation. |
| Monitor for side-effects and toxicity | | • Can cause side-effects such as itching, nausea, vomiting and constipation which may need treating. |

## Additional information

| | |
|---|---|
| Common and serious undesirable effects | *Immediate:* Anaphylaxis has been reported following IV injection.<br>*Injection/infusion related:* Local: Pain at injection site, vein tracking, erythema and thrombophlebitis.<br>*Other:* Nausea and vomiting (particularly initially), constipation, dry mouth, urticaria, pruritus, biliary spasm, ↑ or ↓pulse, hallucinations, euphoria, drowsiness.<br>At higher doses: ↑ or ↓BP, sedation, respiratory depression, muscle rigidity. |
| Pharmacokinetics | Elimination half-life is about 2 hours for morphine; 2.4-6.7 hours for morphine-3-glucuronide (active metabolite of morphine).<br>Cyclizine: Around 20 hours. |
| Significant interactions | • The following may ↑morphine levels or effect (or ↑side-effects): antihistamines-sedating (↑sedation), MAOIs (avoid combination and for 2 weeks after stopping MAOI), moclobemide.<br>• Morphine may ↑levels or effect (or ↑side-effects) of sodium oxybate (avoid combination).<br>• Cyclizine may ↑sedative effect of opioid analgesics. |
| Action in case of overdose | *Symptoms to watch for (morphine tartrate):* ↑Sedation, respiratory depression.<br>*Antidote (morphine tartrate):* Naloxone (see the Naloxone monograph). Stop administration and give supportive therapy as appropriate. |

| Risk rating: **GREEN** | Score = 1 Lower-risk product: Risk-reduction strategies should be considered. |
| --- | --- |

This assessment is based on the full range of preparation and administration options described in the monograph. These may not all be applicable in some clinical situations.

## Bibliography

SPC Cyclimorph 10 injection, Amdipharm (accessed 4 January 2010).

# Mycophenolate mofetil

### 500-mg dry powder vials

- Mycophenolate mofetil hydrochloride is an immunosuppressant derived from *Penicillium stoloniferum*. It is a reversible inhibitor of inosine monophosphate dehydrogenase and inhibits purine synthesis with potent effects on both T- and B-lymphocytes.
- It is given with other immunosuppressants for the prevention of graft rejection and it has also been used (unlicensed) in various autoimmune diseases.
- The parenteral form is used when oral therapy is not possible and is licensed for up to 14 days use.
- Doses are expressed in terms of mycophenolate mofetil:
Mycophenolate mofetil 1 g $\cong$ 1.08 g mycophenolate mofetil hydrochloride.

## Pre-treatment checks

- Do not give in pregnancy or breast feeding.
- Caution in elderly patients ($\uparrow$risk of infection, GI haemorrhage and pulmonary oedema), active serious GI disease (risk of haemorrhage, ulceration and perforation) and delayed graft function.

*Biochemical and other tests*

Blood glucose
Blood pressure and pulse
Electrolytes: serum K, Mg, Ca, $PO_4$

Lipid profile
Renal function: U, Cr, CrCl (or eGFR)

## Dose

The initial dose of parenteral therapy should be given within 24 hours of transplantation.

**Renal transplantation**: 1 g by IV infusion twice daily.

**Hepatic transplantation**: 1 g by IV infusion twice daily for the first 4 days following hepatic transplantation, followed by oral therapy (1.5 g twice daily mycophenolate mofetil) as soon as it can be tolerated.

**Dose in renal impairment:** outside the immediate post-transplantation period doses >1 g twice daily of mycophenolate mofetil should be avoided if CrCl <20 mL/minute.

## Intermittent intravenous infusion

*Preparation and administration*

See Special handling and Spillage below.
Mycophenolate mofetil is incompatible with NaCl 0.9%, Hartmann's, Ringer's.

1. Reconstitute each 500-mg vial with 14 mL Gluc 5% and shake gently to give a solution containing 500 mg/15 mL.
2. Withdraw the required dose and add to a suitable volume of Gluc 5% to give a solution containing approximately 6 mg/mL (i.e. add each 1-g dose to 140 mL Gluc 5%; add each 1.5-g dose to 210 mL Gluc 5%).
3. The solution should be clear and colourless to slightly yellow. Inspect visually for particulate matter or discoloration prior to administration and discard if present.
4. Give by IV infusion over 2 hours.

## Technical information

| | |
|---|---|
| Incompatible with | Mycophenolate mofetil is incompatible with NaCl 0.9%, Hartmann's, Ringer's.<br>Ciclosporin, micafungin. |
| Compatible with | **Flush**: Gluc 5%<br>**Solutions**: Gluc 5%<br>**Y-site**: No information |
| pH | 2.4–4.1 |
| Sodium content | Negligible |
| Storage | Store below 30°C. |
| Displacement value | Approximately 1 mL/500 mg |
| Special handling | Teratogenic: handle with care and not at all if pregnant. |
| Spillage | If contact with skin or mucous membranes occurs, wash thoroughly with soap and water; rinse the eyes with water. Wipe up any spillage with a wet paper towel. |
| Stability after preparation | From a microbiological point of view, should be used immediately; however, reconstituted vials and prepared infusions may be stored at 15–30°C provided that administration is started within 3 hours of initial reconstitution. |

## Monitoring

| Measure | Frequency | Rationale |
|---------|-----------|-----------|
| Mycophenolate serum concentration | If considered necessary | • A trough concentration of 1-3.5 mg/L has been proposed, but there is great patient variability and other drugs may affect this.<br>• It is probably necessary to measure the level if ciclosporin, sirolimus or tacrolimus are concomitantly prescribed and possibly to assess compliance. |
| FBC | Weekly for the first month, fortnightly for the next 2 months, then monthly | • Leucopenia, thrombocytopenia, anaemia, pancytopenia, neutropenia may occur.<br>• Consideration should be given to interrupting treatment, reducing the dose or stopping therapy in these circumstances. |
| Patient experiencing infection, unexpected bruising, bleeding | Report immediately | • Signs of bone marrow depression. |
| LFTs | Periodically | • Hepatic enzymes commonly increase. |
| Renal function | | • ↑K, ↓K, ↑Cr commonly occur. |
| Blood glucose | | • Hyperglycaemia commonly occurs. |
| Lipid profile | | • Hypercholesterolaemia, hyperlipidaemia commonly occur. |
| Serum Mg, Ca, PO$_4$ | | • ↓Mg, ↓Ca, ↓PO4 commonly occur. |
| Blood pressure and pulse | | • ↑Pulse, ↓BP, ↑BP commonly occur. |

## Additional information

| | |
|---|---|
| Common and serious undesirable effects | *Infusion-related:* Local: Phlebitis and thrombosis<br>*Other:* Common: Include infections, benign and malignant neoplasms, blood dyscrasias, metabolism and nutrition disorders, psychiatric disorders, GI upset and nervous system disorders. See manufacturer's literature for full information. |
| Pharmacokinetics | Elimination half-life is 16.6 hours. |
| Significant interactions | Rifampicin may ↓mycophenolate levels or effect. |
| Action in case of overdose | *Antidote:* Bile acid sequestrants reduce serum concentration, e.g. colestyramine. |

*(continued)*

## Additional information (*continued*)

| Counselling | Exposure to sunlight and UV light should be limited by wearing protective clothing and using a sunscreen with a high protection factor to minimise the risk for skin cancer. |
| | Effective contraception must be used before commencing therapy, during therapy and for 6 weeks following cessation of therapy. |

| Risk rating: **AMBER** | Score = 5 |
| | Moderate-risk product: Risk-reduction strategies are recommended. |

This assessment is based on the full range of preparation and administration options described in the monograph. These may not all be applicable in some clinical situations.

## Bibliography

SPC Cellcept 500 mg powder (accessed 5 March 2010).

# Naloxone hydrochloride

**400 micrograms/mL solution in 1-mL ampoules; 1-mL, 2-mL and 5-mL pre-filled syringes**
**1 mg/mL solution in 2-mL pre-filled syringe**

* Naloxone hydrochloride is a specific opioid antagonist that acts competitively at opioid receptors.
* It is used in the treatment of respiratory depression induced by opioids, partial opioid agonists or in suspected opioid overdose.
* It is also used to treat asphyxia in neonates after the administration of opioid analgesics to the mother during labour.
* Naloxone has been used (unlicensed) to treat cholestatic pruritus.
* It has also been given (unlicensed) to treat severe constipation resulting from opioid use in critical care.
* Naloxone has also been given by endotracheal, intranasal and intraosseous routes (all unlicensed).

## Pre-treatment checks

* Caution in cardiovascular disease, it has caused serious adverse effects, e.g. ventricular tachycardia and fibrillation in postoperative patients.
* Caution in patients who may be physically dependent on opioids as this may precipitate severe withdrawal symptoms.

*Biochemical and other tests (not all are necessary in an emergency situation)*

Bodyweight                                    Pulse
Blood pressure                               Respiratory rate

## Dose

Naloxone onset of action: 1–2 minutes following IV injection; 2–5 minutes following SC or IM injection. It is rapidly metabolised in the liver.

**Opioid overdose (known or suspected):** 400 micrograms – 2 mg by IV injection repeated at intervals of 2–3 minutes to the required degree of reversal. Maximum dose 10 mg. If respiratory function does not improve, reconsider diagnosis. If the IV route is unavailable, may be given by IM or SC injection but onset is slower.
**Continuous IV infusion:** for opioid overdose use the syringe pump method below. The rate is set to deliver 60% of the initial effective IV injection dose over 1 hour and adjusted according to response.
**Postoperative use:** 100–200 micrograms (1.5–3 micrograms/kg) by IV injection. Titrate the dose to patient response. Allow a full 2 minutes to elapse between 100-microgram increments. Be aware that analgesia will also be reversed.
**Cholestatic pruritus (unlicensed):** 400 micrograms by IV injection followed by 0.2 micrograms/kg/minute by IV infusion.
**Severe constipation due to opioid use in critical care (unlicensed):** 4 mg via nasogastric tube. Warning: this can be *very* effective!

## Intravenous injection (preferred route)

*Preparation and administration*

1. Withdraw the required dose.
2. The solution should be clear and colourless. Inspect visually for particulate matter or discoloration prior to administration and discard if present.
3. Give by IV injection into a large vein.

## Continuous intravenous infusion via a syringe pump (unlicensed concentration)

*Preparation and administration*

1. Withdraw 4 mg and make up to 20 mL with NaCl 0.9% in a syringe pump
2. Cap the syringe and mix well to give a solution containing 200 micrograms/mL.
3. The solution should be clear and colourless. Inspect visually for particulate matter or discoloration prior to administration and discard if present.
4. Give by IV infusion. Rate is set to deliver 60% of the initial effective IV injection dose over 1 hour and adjusted according to response. Be aware that some opioids may be relatively long-acting.
5. Prepare a fresh syringe at least every 24 hours if necessary.

## Continuous intravenous infusion (large volume infusion)

*Preparation and administration*

1. Withdraw 2 mg of naloxone and add to 500 mL NaCl 0.9% or Gluc 5%.
2. Mix well to give a solution containing 4 micrograms/mL.
3. The solution should be clear and colourless. Inspect visually for particulate matter or discoloration prior to administration and discard if present.
4. Give by IV infusion. Adjust the rate according to clinical response.
5. Prepare a fresh infusion at least every 24 hours if necessary.

## Intramuscular injection

*Preparation and administration*

1. Withdraw the required dose.
2. Give by IM injection.

## Subcutaneous injection

*Preparation and administration*

1. Withdraw the required dose.
2. Give by SC injection.

| Technical information | |
|---|---|
| Incompatible with | No information |
| Compatible with | **Flush**: NaCl 0.9%<br>**Solutions**: NaCl 0.9%, Gluc 5%, WFI<br>**Y-site**: Linezolid, propofol |
| pH | 3-6.5 |
| Sodium content | Negligible |

*(continued)*

## Technical information (continued)

| | |
|---|---|
| Storage | Store below 25°C in original packaging. |
| Stability after preparation | From a microbiological point of view, should be used immediately; however, prepared infusions may be stored at 2-8°C and infused (at room temperature) within 24 hours. |

## Monitoring

| Measure | Frequency | Rationale |
|---|---|---|
| Blood pressure | Close monitoring even after a satisfactory response | • May cause ↓ or ↑ BP. |
| Pulse | | • May cause ↑pulse. |
| Respiratory rate | | • To check effectiveness.<br>• NB: for all these measures be aware that the duration of action of some opioids may exceed that of naloxone. |
| Reduction in opioid drug effects | Close monitoring for up to 4 hours post dose | • May cause clinically important reversal of analgesia post surgery if high doses of naloxone are used. |
| Signs and symptoms of opioid withdrawal | | • May precipitate withdrawal symptoms in patients physically dependent on opioids. |

## Additional information

| | |
|---|---|
| Common and serious undesirable effects | *Injection/infusion-related:* Local: irritation and inflammation after IM injection. *Other:* ↑ or ↓BP, ventricular tachycardia and fibrillation, hyperventilation. Abrupt reversal of narcotic depression may result in nausea, vomiting, sweating, ↑pulse, hyperventilation, ↑BP, tremulousness and reversal of opioid analgesia. |
| Pharmacokinetics | Onset of action: 1-2 minutes by IV injection; 2-5 minutes by SC or IM injection. Elimination half-life is 30-81 minutes. |
| Significant drug interactions | No significant interactions. |
| Overdose | Due to broad therapeutic margin, adverse effects are not expected. |

| | |
|---|---|
| Risk rating: **AMBER** | Score = 4<br>Moderate-risk product. Risk-reduction strategies are recommended. |

This assessment is based on the full range of preparation and administration options described in the monograph. These may not all be applicable in some clinical situations.

## Bibliography

SPC Naloxone injection (accessed 30 March 2010).
SPC Miniject Naloxone (accessed 30 March 2010).

# Nandrolone

**50 mg/mL solution in ampoule or disposable syringe**

* Nandrolone decanoate is an anabolic steroid with some androgenic properties.
* It is licensed for use in treating osteoporosis in postmenopausal women, but its use has been superseded.
* It has been used to ↑lean body mass in various conditions where muscle wasting may occur such as debilitating illness, pre-dialysis chronic renal impairment and HIV-associated wasting. It has also been used to treat aplastic anaemia and anaemia of chronic renal failure (all unlicensed).

## Pre-treatment checks

* Do not use in patients with peanut allergy as the injection contains arachis oil.
* Do not use in patients with an allergy to soya.
* Avoid in porphyria.
* Avoid in known or suspected carcinoma of prostate or mammary carcinoma in the male.
* Avoid in patients with skeletal metastases, since anabolic steroids may cause ↑Ca and hypercalciuria in these patients.

*Biochemical and other tests*

| | |
|---|---|
| Baseline prothrombin time | Lipids: baseline cholesterol |
| Electrolytes: serum Na, K, Ca, $PO_4$ | Renal function: U, Cr, CrCl (or eGFR) |
| LFTs | |

## Dose

**Osteoporosis:** 50 mg every 3 weeks.
**As an anabolic steroid in debilitating illness (unlicensed):** 25–100 mg every 3–4 weeks has been used.
**In anaemia of chronic renal failure (unlicensed):** female patients have received 50–100 mg once weekly; male patients have received 100–200 mg once weekly.

## Intramuscular injection

Contains arachis oil – should not be given in peanut allergy.

*Preparation and administration*

1. Withdraw the required dose.
2. Give by deep IM injection.

## Technical information

| | |
|---|---|
| Incompatible with | Not relevant |
| Compatible with | Not relevant |
| pH | Not relevant |
| Sodium content | None |
| Excipients | Contains arachis oil (should not be used in peanut allergy). Contains benzyl alcohol. |
| Storage | Store below 30°C in original packaging. Do not refrigerate or freeze. |

## Monitoring

| Measure | Frequency | Rationale |
|---|---|---|
| LFTs | Periodically | • May cause abnormal liver function tests. |
| Serum lipids | | • May cause dyslipidaemias. |
| Blood glucose | | • May cause hypoglycaemia, particularly in treated diabetes mellitus. |
| Serum Ca and PO$_4$ | | • Can cause derangement particularly in patients with skeletal metastases. |
| Renal function | | • May cause electrolyte imbalance and exacerbate pre-existing cardiac failure and renal impairment. |
| Prothrombin time | | • May increase prothrombin time, particularly in patients treated with anticoagulants. |

## Additional information

| | |
|---|---|
| Common and serious undesirable effects | Virilisation may occur (hoarseness, acne, hirsutism, ↑libido) but is unlikely at the dose licensed for osteoporosis. If virilisation does occur then consider stopping treatment. Amenorrhoea and inhibition of spermatogenesis (at higher doses). Sodium and water retention - may exacerbate pre-existing cardiac failure, renal failure, hypertension, epilepsy or migraine. Abnormal LFTs have been reported in patients treated with (high doses) of nandrolone decanoate. Dyslipidaemias have been observed. |
| Pharmacokinetics | The half-life for the combined process of hydrolysis of nandrolone decanoate and of distribution and elimination of nandrolone is 4.3 hours. |
| Significant interactions | • Nandrolone may ↑levels or effect of the following drugs (or ↑side-effects): coumarin anticoagulants (monitor INR), phenindione (monitor INR). |
| Action in case of overdose | There are no reports of acute overdosage with nandrolone decanoate in humans. |

*(continued)*

| **Additional information** (*continued*) | |
|---|---|
| Counselling | Instructions on how to self-administer and correct disposal of equipment (if appropriate). |
| | For female patients: report changes in menstrual cycle or masculinisation such as hoarseness/deepening of voice or hair growth. |
| | For male patients: report new or worsening acne or persistent erections. |
| | Report swelling in hands, ankles, or feet, rapid weight gain. |
| | Report unexplained or unusual fever, bleeding, or bruising. |
| | Report yellow skin or eyes, dark-coloured urine or pale stools. |

| Risk rating: **GREEN** | Score = 1 |
|---|---|
| | Lower-risk product: Risk-reduction strategies should be considered. |

This assessment is based on the full range of preparation and administration options described in the monograph. These may not all be applicable in some clinical situations.

## Bibliography

SPC Deca-Durabolin 50 mg/mL (accessed 2 February 2009).

# Natalizumab

**20 mg/mL solution in 15 mL vials**

- Natalizumab is an alpha-4 integrin-specific humanised monoclonal antibody.
- It is used as monotherapy to reduce the frequency of clinical exacerbations, and delay the accumulation of physical disability, in patients with highly active relapsing-remitting forms of multiple sclerosis.
- As there is ↑risk of progressive multifocal leucoencephalopathy (PML; an opportunistic viral infection of the brain that usually leads to death or severe disability), its availability is restricted and its use limited to patients who have had an inadequate response to, or are unable to tolerate, other therapies.
- In the USA all doctors, pharmacies, infusion centres and patients must be registered with the TOUCH Prescribing Program before they can use or receive the drug (more information at www.tysabri.com).
- Continued therapy must be carefully reconsidered in any patients showing no evidence of therapeutic benefit beyond 6 months.

## Pre-treatment checks

- Do not use in PML (a recent – usually within 3 months – MRI scan should be available), active infection (see notes above), concomitantly with interferon beta or glatiramer acetate, in immunosuppression, in active malignancies and pregnancy or breast feeding.
- Resources for the management of hypersensitivity reactions and access to MRI should be available.

*Biochemical and other tests*

FBC (there should be no signs of neutropenia before commencement and no evidence that the patient is immunocompromised)

LFTs

## Dose

**Standard dose:** 300 mg by IV infusion every 4 weeks.

## Intravenous infusion through a dedicated line

*Preparation and administration*

1. Inspect the vial contents prior to use. The solution should be clear and colourless to slightly opalescent. Discard if particulate matter or discoloration is present.
2. Withdraw the required dose, i.e. 300 mg (15 mL) and add to 100 mL NaCl 0.9%.
3. Invert the solution gently (do not shake) to mix completely.
4. The solution should be clear and colourless. Inspect visually for particulate matter or discoloration prior to administration and discard if present.
5. Give by IV infusion over 1 hour at a rate of approximately 2 mL/minute.
6. After the infusion is complete, flush the line with NaCl 0.9%.
7. Observe the patient (see monitoring below).

## Technical information

| | |
|---|---|
| Incompatible with | No information but do not mix with any other drug. |
| Compatible with | **Flush**: NaCl 0.9%<br>**Solutions**: NaCl 0.9%<br>**Y-site**: No information but likely to be unstable |
| pH | 6.1 |
| Sodium content | Approximately 2 mmol/15 mL |
| Storage | Store at 2-8°C in original packaging. Do not freeze. |
| Stability after preparation | From a microbiological point of view, should be used immediately; however, prepared infusions may be stored at 2-8°C and infused (at room temperature) within 8 hours. |

## Monitoring

| Measure | Frequency | Rationale |
|---|---|---|
| Signs and symptoms of hypersensitivity reactions | During the infusion and for 1 hour after completion for each infusion | • Occurs in <1% of patients.<br>• Symptoms may include: hypotension, hypertension, chest pain, chest discomfort, dyspnoea, angioedema, as well as the more usual symptoms, e.g. rash and urticaria. |

*(continued)*

## Monitoring (*continued*)

| Measure | Frequency | Rationale |
|---|---|---|
| If new neurological symptoms occur, suspend treatment until PML has been excluded | Upon assessment | • If any doubt exists, further evaluation, including MRI scan (compared with pre-treatment MRI), CSF testing for JC Viral DNA and repeat neurological assessments, should be considered. If PML is excluded, treatment may resume.<br>• If a patient develops PML, natalizumab must be permanently discontinued. |
| Disease exacerbations or infusion-related events | Upon presentation | • May indicate the development of antibodies against natalizumab.<br>• Presence of antibodies should be evaluated; if these remain positive in a confirmatory test after 6 weeks, treatment should be discontinued. |
| FBC | Periodically | • Pharmacodynamic effects, e.g. ↑lymphocyte counts can persist for up to 12 weeks following the last dose. |
| LFTs | | • There have been reports of serious liver injury. Doctors are advised to cease therapy if any significant liver injury occurs. |

## Additional information

| | |
|---|---|
| Common and serious undesirable effects | *Immediate:* Hypersensitivity and anaphylaxis reported.<br>*Infusion-related:* Nausea, vomiting, flushing, headache, dizziness, fatigue, rigors, pyrexia, arthralgia, urticaria, and pruritus.<br>*Other:* opportunistic infection and progressive multifocal leucoencephalopathy. |
| Pharmacokinetics | Elimination half-life is 11 days. |
| Significant interactions | • The following may ↑side-effects of natalizumab:<br>immunosuppressive and anti-neoplastic drugs are contraindicated as they ↑risk of opportunistic infections, although short courses of corticosteroids may be used. |
| Action in case of overdose | No cases have been reported and there is no specific antidote: manage symptomatically. |
| Counselling | Each patient must be given a Tysabri Patient Alert Card. They should also inform their partner or carer about their treatment as they may notice symptoms the patient is unaware of.<br>Patients should be told of the importance of uninterrupted dosing; particularly in the early months of treatment (intermittent therapy may ↑risk of sensitisation). |

| Risk rating: **GREEN** | Score = 2 Lower-risk product: Risk-reduction strategies should be considered. | | | | |
|---|---|---|---|---|---|

This assessment is based on the full range of preparation and administration options described in the monograph. These may not all be applicable in some clinical situations.

## Bibliography

SPC TYSABRI 300 mg concentrate for solution for infusion (accessed 1 April 2009).

# Neostigmine metilsulfate (neostigmine methylsulfate)

**2.5 mg/mL solution 1-mL ampoules**

- Neostigmine is a compound with anticholinesterase activity that prolongs and intensifies the actions of acetylcholine.
- It is used to treat myasthenia gravis and as an antagonist to non-depolarising neuromuscular blockade. It has also been used to treat paralytic ileus, postoperative urinary retention and paroxysmal SVT.

## Pre-treatment checks

- Do not give to patients with mechanical obstruction of intestinal or urinary tract or patients with peritonitis.
- Use with caution in patients with bronchial asthma, ↓pulse, cardiac arrhythmias, epilepsy, recent coronary occlusion, hyperthyroidism, peptic ulcer, vagotonia or parkinsonism.

*Biochemical and other tests*

Bodyweight (if using for reversal of non-depolarising neuromuscular blockade)
Pulse

## Dose

**For existing myasthenia gravis patients switched from maintenance to parenteral dosing:**

Neostigmine bromide 15 mg orally ≅ neostigmine metilsulfate 1–1.5 mg by IM or SC injection.

**Myasthenia gravis:** 1–2.5 mg by IM or SC injection at periodic intervals throughout the day (each dose will last 2–4 hours). The usual total daily dose is 5–20 mg but some patients may require more.
**Reversal of non-depolarising neuromuscular blockade:** a single dose of 50–70 micrograms/kg (maximum dose 5 mg) by IV injection after or with glycopyrronium or atropine (in ↓pulse, the pulse rate should be increased to 80 bpm before administering neostigmine).
**Other indications:** 0.5–2.5 mg by IM or SC injection.

**Dose in renal impairment:** adjusted according to creatinine clearance:[1]
* CrCl >20–50 mL/minute: 50–100% of normal dose.
* CrCl 10–20 mL/minute: 50–100% of normal dose.
* CrCl <10 mL/minute: 50–100% of normal dose.

## Intramuscular injection

*Preparation and administration*

1. Withdraw the required dose.
2. Give by IM injection.

## Subcutaneous injection

*Preparation and administration*

1. Withdraw the required dose.
2. Give by SC injection.

## Intravenous injection

*Preparation and administration*

1. Withdraw the required dose.
2. The solution should be clear and colourless. Inspect visually for particulate matter or discoloration prior to administration and discard if present.
3. Give by slow IV injection over 1 minute.

## Technical information

| | |
|---|---|
| Incompatible with | No information |
| Compatible with | **Flush:** NaCl 0.9%<br>**Solutions**: May be diluted with WFI but stability cannot be guaranteed<br>**Y-site**: Glycopyrronium (in-syringe compatible), hydrocortisone sodium succinate |
| pH | 5–6.5 |
| Sodium content | Negligible |
| Storage | Store below 25°C in original packaging. |

## Monitoring

| Measure | Frequency | Rationale |
|---|---|---|
| Clinical improvement | Post administration | • To ensure that treatment is effective. |
| Signs and symptoms of cholinergic crisis | | • Overdose of neostigmine may cause cholinergic crisis. |

## Additional information

| | |
|---|---|
| Common and serious undesirable effects | Nausea, vomiting, diarrhoea, miosis, abdominal cramps, ↓pulse. |
| Pharmacokinetics | Elimination half-life is 1–2 hours. |

*(continued)*

| **Additional information** (*continued*) | |
|---|---|
| Significant interactions | • The following may ↓neostigmine levels or effect: aminoglycosides (neostigmine dose in myasthenia gravis may need adjustment). |
| Action in case of overdose | *Symptoms to watch for:* Respiratory compromise. *Antidote:* Atropine can be used to control muscarinic symptoms (take care to avoid atropine overdose). Respiration can be assisted mechanically or with oxygen, if necessary. |

| Risk rating: **GREEN** | Score = 1 Lower-risk product. Risk-reduction strategies should be considered. |
|---|---|

This assessment is based on the full range of preparation and administration options described in the monograph. These may not all be applicable in some clinical situations.

## Reference

1. Ashley C, Currie A, eds. *The Renal Drug Handbook*, 3rd edn. Oxford: Radcliffe Medical Press, 2009.

## Bibliography

SPC Neostigmine Metilsulphate BP (accessed 30 March 2010).

# Nimodipine

### 200 micrograms/mL solution in 50-mL (10 mg) vials

* Nimodipine is a calcium-channel blocker acting primarily on cerebral blood vessels.
* It is used in treatment of aneurismal subarachnoid haemorrhage. Efficacy and safety have not been assessed in traumatic subarachnoid haemorrhage.
* Nimodipine infusion contains 23.7% ethanol by volume.
* A 250-mL average daily dose supplies 50 g ethanol ≅ 6 units (1 UK unit = 8 g).

### Pre-treatment checks

* Avoid within 1 month of ACS.
* Do not use concurrently with oral nimodipine.
* Caution in cerebral oedema, ↑intracranial pressure, ↓BP, cirrhosis, renal disease.

*Biochemical and other tests (not all are necessary in an emergency situation)*

Blood pressure
Bodyweight
Electrolytes: serum Na, K

LFTs
Renal function: U, Cr, CrCl (or eGFR)

## Dose

**Standard dose for patients > 70 kg with stable BP:** 1 mg/hour (5 mL/hour) by IV infusion via a central line for the first 2 hours; if tolerated, increase to 2 mg/hour (10 mL/hour).

**Standard dose for patients < 70 kg or with unstable BP:** 0.5 mg/hour (2.5 mL/hour) or less by IV infusion via a central line for the first 2 hours; if tolerated, increase gradually to 2 mg/hour (10 mL/hour).

**Duration of treatment:** treat for at least 5 days up to a maximum of 14 days. Continue for at least 5 days after neurological surgery. Where treatment is sequential with oral nimodipine, the total course should not exceed 21 days.

## Intravenous infusion via central line

*Preparation and administration*

Use only the infusion container and the infusion line provided by the manufacturer.
Protect the infusion and giving set from direct sunlight.

1. Attach the infusion line provided by the manufacturer to the vial and prime the line. Do not use other lines, or other infusion containers.
2. The solution should be clear and yellow in colour. Inspect visually for particulate matter or discoloration prior to administration and discard if present.
3. Attach the proximal end of the infusion line to a three-way tap such that a second infusion may run simultaneously into the central line.
4. The co-infusion must be set to run at 40 mL/hour (see Y-site below for suitable solutions).
5. Give nimodipine by IV infusion at the initial rate specified under Dose above and increase the rate as tolerated.
6. Protect the infusion and giving set from direct sunlight. The drug is stable in diffuse daylight and artificial light for up to 10 hours. Prepare a fresh infusion if required once 10 hours has elapsed.

## Technical information

| | |
|---|---|
| Incompatible with | Nimodipine is incompatible with some soft plastics used in infusion containers, administration sets and in-line filters, e.g. PVC. Avoid use of these materials. |
| Compatible with | **Flush**: NaCl 0.9%<br>**Solutions**: Do not dilute<br>**Y-site**: NaCl 0.9%, Gluc 5%, Hartmann's (for other options see product literature) |
| pH | Not relevant |
| Sodium content | Negligible |
| Excipients | Contains ethanol (may interact with metronidazole, possible religious objections) |
| Storage | Store below 25°C in original packaging. Protect from light. |
| Stability after preparation | Infusion must not be delayed once the infusion line is primed. |

## Monitoring

| Measure | Frequency | Rationale |
|---------|-----------|-----------|
| Blood pressure | Continuously | • ↓BP may necessitate dose reduction. ↑Risk in impaired renal and hepatic function. |
| Renal function | Daily | • Consider dose reduction in ↓renal function. |
| Alcohol intoxication | | • Vials contain alcohol, which could accumulate in impaired hepatic function. |

## Additional information

| | |
|---|---|
| Common and serious undesirable effects | *Injection/infusion-related:* Local: Rarely thrombophlebitis.<br>*Other:* ↓BP, variation in heart rate, flushing, headache, GI disorders, nausea, sweating feeling of warmth. |
| Pharmacokinetics | Elimination half-life is 1.1–1.7 hours. |
| Significant interactions | • The following may ↑nimodipine levels or effect (or ↑side-effects): alpha blockers (↑hypotensive effect), ritonavir.<br>• The following may ↓nimodipine levels or effect: barbiturates, primidone, rifampicin.<br>• Nimodipine may ↑levels or effect (or ↑side-effects) of theophylline.<br>• Injectable preparation contains ethanol: may interact with disulfiram and metronidazole. |
| Action in case of overdose | *Symptoms to watch for:* ↓BP.<br>*Antidote:* None specific. Consider dopamine or noradrenaline IV if serious ↓BP. |
| Counselling | Advise of risk of headache and symptoms of ↓BP. |

| | |
|---|---|
| Risk rating: **AMBER** | Score = 3<br>Moderate-risk product: Risk-reduction strategies are recommended. |

This assessment is based on the full range of preparation and administration options described in the monograph. These may not all be applicable in some clinical situations.

## Bibliography

SPC Nimotop 0.02% solution for infusion (accessed 30 March 2010).

# Noradrenaline acid tartrate (norepinephrine bitartrate)

**1 mg/mL (as base) solution in 2-mL, 4-mL and 20-mL ampoules**

* Noradrenaline acid tartrate is an extremely potent peripheral vasoconstrictor used as an emergency measure in the restoration of BP in acute hypotension, usually in critical care.
* Ampoules are labelled in terms of the acid tartrate, but doses are expressed in terms of the base: Noradrenaline 1 mg $\cong$ 2 mg noradrenaline acid tartrate.

## Pre-treatment checks

* An inadequate circulating blood volume should be restored prior to treatment with noradrenaline.

*Extreme caution in patients with:*

* Coronary, mesenteric or peripheral vascular thrombosis; noradrenaline may extend the area of infarction.
* ↑BP following MI and in patients with Prinzmetal's variant angina.
* Hyperthyroidism, diabetes mellitus.
* Hypoxia or hypercapnia.

*Biochemical and other tests*

Electrolytes: serum Na, K
Renal function: U, Cr, CrCl (or eGFR)

## Dose

Dosing regimens in the literature vary and may include weight-adjusted dosing.

There is a wide inter-individual variation in response and titration to response is fundamental. This is an example of a simple regimen:

* Initially 8–12 micrograms/minute adjusted according to BP response.
* Average maintenance dose is 2–4 micrograms/minute.
* Do not be stop suddenly – withdraw gradually to avoid ↓BP.

## Continuous intravenous infusion via syringe pump

> Infusion into a peripheral vein is not recommended owing to the high risk of extravasation and tissue necrosis.

*Preparation of a 40 micrograms/mL solution*

(Higher strength solutions using, e.g. 4 mg, 8 mg or 16 mg noradrenaline base may be prepared).

1. Make 2 mg (2 mL) up to 50 mL in a syringe pump with Gluc 5% to give a solution containing 40 micrograms/mL (as base).
2. The solution should be clear and colourless. Inspect visually for particulate matter or discoloration prior to administration and discard if present.

*Administration*

1. Give by IV infusion via a central venous catheter adjusting rate to clinical response, e.g. using a 40 micrograms/mL solution, an initial rate of 8–12 micrograms/minute equates to 12–18 mL/hour.
2. Prepare a fresh infusion every 24 hours. Discard if a brown colour or precipitate develops.

## Technical information

| | |
|---|---|
| Incompatible with | Sodium bicarbonate.<br>Drotrecogin alfa (activated), insulin (soluble), pantoprazole, phenytoin sodium. |
| Compatible with | **Flush**: NaCl 0.9%<br>**Solutions**: Gluc 5%, Gluc-NaCl (both with added KCl)<br>**Y-site**: Adrenaline (epinephrine), cisatracurium, dobutamine, dopamine, fentanyl, furosemide, glyceryl trinitrate, hydrocortisone sodium succinate, meropenem, micafungin, midazolam, milrinone, propofol, ranitidine, remifentanil, vecuronium |
| pH | 3–4.5 |
| Sodium content | 0.145 mmol/mL |
| Storage | Store below 25°C in original packaging. |
| Stability after preparation | From a microbiological point of view, should be used immediately; however, prepared infusions may be stored at 2–8°C and infused (at room temperature) within 24 hours. |

## Monitoring

| Measure | Frequency | Rationale |
|---|---|---|
| Blood pressure | Initially every 2 min | • Response to therapy. The aim should be to establish a low normal systolic BP (100–120 mmHg) or to achieve an adequate mean arterial BP (>80 mmHg).<br>• Risk of ↑BP. |
| ECG/pulse | Continuously | • Ectopic beats and arrhythmias.<br>• ↓Pulse. |
| Peripheral circulation (extremities) | Hourly | • Monitor for ischaemia. |
| Infusion site (if peripheral) | | • Risk of necrosis if extravasation occurs. |

## Additional information

| | |
|---|---|
| Common and serious undesirable effects | *Infusion-related:* Local: Extravasation when given via peripheral vein – necrosis and sloughing of the surrounding tissue. Ischaemia can be reversed by infiltration of the affected area with phentolamine (see the Phentolamine monograph).<br>*Other:* Ectopic heart beats, ↓pulse, anginal pain, palpitation, ↑BP, vasoconstriction. Gangrene in extremities in patients with pre-existing vascular disease. ↑Risk of arrhythmias in patients with hypercapnia and hypoxia. Nausea, vomiting. Headache. |
| Pharmacokinetics | The pressor response subsides within 2–3 minutes of discontinuation. |

*(continued)*

| **Additional information** (continued) | |
|---|---|
| Significant interactions | • The following may ↑noradrenaline levels or effect (or ↑side-effects): dopexamine, MAOIs (risk of hypertensive crisis), moclobemide (risk of hypertensive crisis), rasagiline (avoid combination).<br>• Noradrenaline may ↑levels or effect of the following drugs (or ↑side-effects): antidepressants-tricyclic (risk of arrhythmias and ↑BP), beta-blockers (risk of severe ↑BP and ↓pulse).<br>• Noradrenaline may ↓levels or effect of guanethidine (↓hypotensive effect). |
| Action in case of overdose | Effects are short lived and typically require supportive measures only. |
| Counselling | Headache, nausea, report pain at infusion site. |

| Risk rating: **RED** | Score = 6<br>High-risk product: Risk-reduction strategies are required to minimise these risks. |
|---|---|

This assessment is based on the full range of preparation and administration options described in the monograph. These may not all be applicable in some clinical situations.

## Bibliography

SPC Noradrenaline (Norepinephrine) 1 : 1000 or Levophed (Hospira UK Ltd) (accessed 30 May 2009).

# Norethisterone enantate

### 200 mg/mL oily solution in 1-mL ampoules

• Norethisterone enantate is a progestogen formulated as a depot injection.
• It is given IM as an oily injection to provide short-term interim contraception.

## Pre-treatment checks

• Do not give in history of undiagnosed vaginal bleeding, or of breast or endometrial cancer (within the last 5 years; can be considered if incidence was >5 years ago with no current evidence of disease and non-hormonal methods of contraception are unacceptable).
• Contraindicated in women with a history of idiopathic jaundice, pruritus, herpes gestationis or deterioration of otosclerosis during pregnancy; in Dubin–Johnson and Rotor syndromes; in severe diabetes with vascular complications; in patients with ↑BP, current thromboembolic disease (or in periods of high risk of thromboembolic disease, e.g. immobilisation or surgery).
• Patients with a history of diabetes should be carefully monitored during treatment, as a reduction in glucose tolerance may occur.
• Do not give during pregnancy.

*Biochemical and other tests*

FBC – contraindicated in sickle-cell anaemia
LFTs
Lipid profile

## Dose

**Standard dose**: 200 mg by IM injection within first 5 days of cycle (the first day of menstruation counting as day 1); or immediately after delivery or abortion (so that no possibility for pregnancy exists). It may be repeated once after 8 weeks.

## Intramuscular injection

*Preparation and administration*

1. Immerse the ampoule in warm water before injection to reduce the viscosity, making it easier to inject.
2. Withdraw the 1 mL dose from the ampoule.
3. The injection requires significant force to administer due to its oily nature: firmly attach at least a medium-bore needle to the syringe before administration.
4. Give very slowly by deep IM injection into the gluteal muscle (coughing, dyspnoea and circulatory irregularities have been reported on administration, which can all be minimised by very slow administration).

| Technical information | |
|---|---|
| Incompatible with | Not relevant |
| Compatible with | Not relevant |
| pH | Not relevant – oily injection |
| Sodium content | Nil |
| Storage | Store below 25°C in original packaging. |

| Monitoring | | |
|---|---|---|
| **Measure** | **Frequency** | **Rationale** |
| Occurrence of migraine | Post administration | • No further injection should be given if the patient develops severe or migranous headaches. |
| BP | Monthly during treatment | • May cause ↑BP, no further injection should be given if this occurs. |
| LFTs and lipid profile | | • Progestogen therapy can cause jaundice, acute porphyrias and deranged lipid profile – no further injection should be given. |
| Blood glucose in diabetic patients | As clinically indicated | • ↓Glucose tolerance may be seen, necessitating amendment in glycaemic control. |

*(continued)*

## Monitoring (continued)

| Measure | Frequency | Rationale |
|---------|-----------|-----------|
| Signs of thromboembolic disease | Ongoing through treatment | • Patients should be advised to report any physical signs of thromboembolic disease, such as a loss of visual acuity, breathlessness, leg pain. |
| Patients mood | Ongoing | • Predisposition to depression may be exacerbated by progestogen therapy. |

## Additional information

| | |
|---|---|
| Common and serious undesirable effects | *Injection/infusion-related:* Local: Injection-site reactions.<br>*Other:* Menstrual irregularities; nausea and vomiting; headache; dizziness; breast discomfort; depression; skin disorders; appetite disturbance; weight changes; disturbances of lipid metabolism; jaundice; porphyria; changes in libido; hypersensitivity reactions; potentially ↑risk in thromboembolic disease; potential ↑risk of breast and cervical cancer incidence in women taking progestogen contraceptives. |
| Pharmacokinetics | There are two elimination half-lives (biphasic release from the depot): 4-5 days, and 15-20 days. |
| Significant interactions | • The following may ↓contraceptive effect of norethisterone (consider an alternative):<br>aprepitant, barbiturates, bosentan, carbamazepine, griseofulvin, nevirapine, oxcarbazepine, phenytoin, primidone, rifamycins, St John's wort (avoid combination), topiramate.<br>• Norethisterone may ↑levels or effect of the following drugs (or ↑side-effects): ciclosporin (monitor levels), coumarin anticoagulants (monitor INR).<br>• Norethisterone may ↓levels or effect of the following drugs:<br>coumarin anticoagulants (monitor INR), lamotrigine, phenindione (monitor INR). |
| Action in case of overdose | Studies have indicated that no acute toxicity is to be expected in overdose. |
| Counselling | Inform the patient that her menstrual pattern is likely to alter, and changes in the form of spotting, breakthrough bleeding and delayed menstruation are relatively frequent. |

| Risk rating: **GREEN** | Score = 1<br>Lower-risk product: Risk-reduction strategies should be considered. |
|---|---|

This assessment is based on the full range of preparation and administration options described in the monograph. These may not all be applicable in some clinical situations.

## Bibliography

SPC Noristerat (accessed 19 February 2010).

# Octreotide

**50, 100, 200, 500 micrograms/mL solution in 1-mL ampoules**
**200 micrograms/mL solution in 5-mL vials**
**10-mg, 20-mg and 30-mg dry powder vials**

- Octreotide acetate is a synthetic polypeptide analogue of somatostatin with similar properties but a longer duration of action.
- It is used for the symptomatic management of neuroendocrine tumours (GEP tumours) such as carcinoid tumours, VIPomas and glucagonomas.
- It is also used in the treatment of acromegaly and the prevention of complications after pancreatic surgery, and in other disorders including variceal haemorrhage, reduction of intestinal secretions and HIV-associated diarrhoea.
- Octreotide may also be given (unlicensed) by SC infusion in palliative care to reduce intestinal secretions and vomiting.
- Doses are expressed as octreotide base.

## Pre-treatment checks

A test dose of 50–100 micrograms SC octreotide if commencing depot injections in patients with no previous exposure to octreotide.

*Biochemical and other tests*

| | |
|---|---|
| Blood glucose | LFTs |
| Electrolytes: serum Zn (if receiving TPN) | TFTs (if to be long term) |

## Dose

> Give all doses between meals or before bedtime to reduce flatulence, abdominal pain and bloating.

**Neuroendocrine tumours:** initially 50 micrograms once or twice daily by SC injection gradually increased to 100–200 micrograms three times daily according to clinical response (exceptionally higher doses may be used). If a rapid response is required, e.g. carcinoid crises, the initial dose can be given by IV injection.

*Sandostatin LAR:* for patients whose symptoms are adequately controlled by SC injection, initially 20 mg Sandostatin LAR by IM injection every 4 weeks for 3 months, increasing to a maximum of 30 mg every 4 weeks if symptoms are only partially controlled. SC octreotide should be continued at the previously effective dose for 2 weeks after the first depot injection.

**Acromegaly:** initially 100–200 micrograms three times daily by SC injection. Discontinue if there is no improvement in 3 months.

*Sandostatin LAR:* patients new to octreotide must receive a test dose of 50–100 micrograms by SC injection to assess tolerability on the day before depot injections are commenced.

Initially, give 20 mg by IM injection every 4 weeks for 3 months, commencing on the day after the last SC injection. Adjust the dose according to response.

**Prevention of complications following pancreatic surgery:** 100 micrograms three times daily by SC injection for 7 consecutive days, starting on the day of the operation at least 1 hour before laparotomy.

**Variceal haemorrhage in patients with cirrhosis (unlicensed):** 25 micrograms/hour by continuous IV infusion for 48 hours. Doses up to 50 micrograms/hour have been used. Patients at high risk of re-bleeding may continue for up to 5 days.

**HIV-associated diarrhoea (unlicensed):** 100 micrograms three times daily by SC injection. If the diarrhoea is not controlled after a week the dose may be increased to 250 micrograms three times daily. Stop if not effective after a further week.

## Subcutaneous injection (preferred route)

*Preparation and administration*

1. Allow the injection to reach room temperature before administration.
2. Withdraw the required dose, taking care to select the smallest volume that will deliver the dose (this minimises the pain associated with SC injection).
3. Give by SC injection into the upper arm, thigh or abdomen. Injection-site rotation should be planned for subsequent injections to minimise discomfort.

## Intravenous injection (for use only when a rapid response is required)

*Preparation and administration*

1. Allow the injection to reach room temperature before administration.
2. Withdraw the required dose and dilute each mL to 2–10 mL with NaCl 0.9%.
3. The solution should be clear and colourless. Inspect visually for particulate matter or discoloration prior to administration and discard if present.
4. Give by IV injection over 3–5 minutes with ECG monitoring.

## Intramuscular injection (Sandostatin LAR depot injection only)

*Preparation and administration*

1. Allow the vial to reach room temperature before administration, but do not prepare until immediately before administration.
2. Lightly tap the vial to settle the powder at the bottom of the vial.
3. Attach one of the supplied needles to the solvent syringe and insert needle through the centre of the rubber stopper of the Sandostatin LAR vial.
4. Without disturbing the powder, gently inject the solvent into the vial by running it down the inside wall of the vial. Do not inject the solvent directly into the powder.
5. When complete, withdraw any excess air present in the vial.
6. Do not disturb the vial until the solvent has wetted all the powder (usually takes about 2–5 minutes).
7. Swirl the vial moderately until a uniform suspension is formed. Do not shake vigorously.
8. Inject 2 mL of air into the vial then, with the bevel down and the vial tipped at a 45° angle, slowly withdraw the entire contents of the vial into the syringe.
9. Change the needle (supplied) then gently invert the syringe to maintain a uniform suspension and eliminate air from syringe.
10. Give by IM injection into the gluteus muscle. Aspirate before injection to avoid inadvertent intravascular injection.

## Intravenous infusion (unlicensed)

*Preparation and administration*

1. Withdraw the required dose and add to 50–200 mL NaCl 0.9%.
2. The solution should be clear and colourless. Inspect visually for particulate matter or discoloration prior to administration and discard if present.
3. Give by IV infusion via volumetric infusion device or syringe pump over 15–30 minutes (or continuously depending upon indication) with ECG monitoring.

## Technical information

| Incompatible with | Micafungin, pantoprazole. |
|---|---|
| Compatible with | **Flush**: NaCl 0.9%<br>**Solutions**: NaCl 0.9%<br>**Y-site**: No information |
| pH | 3.9–4.6 |
| Sodium content | Negligible |
| Storage | Store at 2–8°C in original packaging. Do not freeze.<br>*In use:* Ampoules and vials may be stored at room temperature for up to 2 weeks – do not puncture vials more than 10 times, to reduce contamination. |
| Stability after preparation | From a microbiological point of view, should be used immediately; however, prepared infusions may be stored at 2–8°C and infused (at room temperature) within 24 hours. |

## Monitoring

| Measure | Frequency | Rationale |
|---|---|---|
| Circulating growth hormones (GH) or insulin-like growth factor (IGF-1) | Monthly | • In acromegaly dose adjustments should be made based on these measurements (target: GH less than 2.5 nanograms/mL (5 mU/L) and IGF-1 within normal range). If no significant reduction GH levels and no improvement of clinical symptoms have been achieved within 3 months of starting octreotide, therapy should be discontinued. |
| LFTs | | • The half-life may be increased in impairment requiring an adjustment of the maintenance dose. |
| Zinc serum concentration | Monthly in patients receiving TPN | • Its ability to reverse GI fluid loss may cause ↑serum zinc concentration. |
| Blood glucose | Daily initially then after a dose change | • It is relatively more potent in inhibiting glucagon secretion rather than inhibiting insulin secretion. Unstable blood sugar concentrations may be avoided by dividing the daily dose into several injections.<br>• Insulin requirements in Type 1 diabetes may be reduced. In Type 2 and non-diabetic patients there may be prandial increases in glycaemia.<br>• Monitor closely when discontinuing therapy in Type 1 and 2 diabetes. |
| TFTs | 6-monthly | • Thyroid function should be monitored in patients receiving long-term octreotide therapy. It can reduce thyrotropin secretion, leading to ↓plasma $T_4$ concentration (levothyroxine dose adjustment may be necessary for patients on supplementation). |

*(continued)*

## Monitoring (continued)

| Measure | Frequency | Rationale |
|---------|-----------|-----------|
| Ultrasonic examination for gallstones | 6- to 12-monthly | • The presence of gallstones during prolonged octreotide treatment occurs in up to 30% of patients (usually asymptomatically); symptomatic stones should be treated in the normal manner. |

## Additional information

| | |
|---|---|
| Common and serious undesirable effects | *Immediate:* Anaphylaxis has very rarely been reported.<br>*Injection-related:* Local: Pain at the administration site (stinging, throbbing or burning with redness, swelling and rash).<br>*Other:* Diarrhoea, steatorrhoea, loose stools, nausea, flatulence, abdominal pain and bloating, hyperglycaemia (sometimes persistent), impaired post-prandial glucose tolerance, hypoglycaemia, gallstones. |
| Pharmacokinetics | Elimination half-life is 100 minutes after SC administration; 10 and 90 minutes after IV administration (the elimination is biphasic). |
| Significant interactions | Octreotide may ↓levels or effect of ciclosporin (monitor levels; may require ciclosporin dose increase of up to 50%). |
| Action in case of overdose | *Antidote:* No known antidote; stop administration and give supportive therapy as appropriate. |
| Counselling | Explain how to store and dispose of injections and paraphernalia correctly. |

Risk rating: **AMBER**     Score = 5
Moderate-risk product: Risk reduction strategies are recommended.

This assessment is based on the full range of preparation and administration options described in the monograph. These may not all be applicable in some clinical situations.

## Bibliography

SPC Octreotide 500 micrograms/mL solution for injection, Hospira UK Ltd (accessed 1 April 2009).

SPC Octreotide 100 microgram/mL solution for injection, Sun Pharmaceuticals UK Ltd (accessed 1 April 2009)

SPC Sandostatin 0.05 mg/mL, 0.1 mg/mL, 0.5 mg/mL ampoules and multi-dose vial 1 mg/5 mL (accessed 1 April 2009).

SPC Sandostatin Lar (accessed 1 April 2009).

# Ofloxacin

**2 mg/mL solution in 100-mL infusion bottles**

* Ofloxacin hydrochloride is a fluorinated quinolone antibacterial.
* It is used to treat infections caused by susceptible Gram-positive and Gram-negative bacteria.
* Ofloxacin is rapidly and well absorbed from the GI tract following oral dosing so the IV route should be used only when the oral route is unavailable.
* Doses are expressed in terms of the base:
  Ofloxacin 200 mg $\cong$ 220 mg ofloxacin hydrochloride.

## Pre-treatment checks

* Do not give if there is known hypersensitivity to quinolone antibacterials.
* Avoid in patients with a past history of tendinitis, with a history of epilepsy or with a lowered seizure threshold, in pregnant or breast-feeding women.
* Use with caution if there is a history of psychiatric disease or in patients with latent or actual defects in G6PD activity.
* Patients should be well hydrated and asked to drink fluids liberally.

*Biochemical and other tests (not all are necessary in an emergency situation)*

Blood pressure
LFTs
Renal function: U, Cr, CrCl (or eGFR)

## Dose

**Complicated urinary tract infection:** 200 mg daily.
**Lower respiratory tract infection and septicaemia:** 200 mg every 12 hours.
**In severe or complicated infections:** the dose may be increased to 400 mg every 12 hours.
**Skin and soft-tissue infections:** 400 mg every 12 hours.
**Dose in renal impairment:** adjusted according to creatinine clearance:[1]

* CrCl >20–50 mL/minute: 200–400 mg every 24 hours.
* CrCl 10–20 mL/minute: 200–400 mg every 24 hours.
* CrCl <10 mL/minute: 200 mg every 24 hours

**Dose in hepatic impairment:** in severe impairment or cirrhosis a maximum daily dose of 400 mg has been recommended.

## Intermittent intravenous infusion

*Preparation and administration*

1. The infusion is pre-prepared for use. It should be clear and light yellow to amber. Inspect visually for particulate matter or discoloration prior to administration and discard if present.
2. Give by IV infusion over at least 30 minutes for 200 mg (at least 60 minutes for 400 mg).

## Technical information

| | |
|---|---|
| Incompatible with | Amphotericin, heparin sodium. |
| Compatible with | **Flush**: NaCl 0.9%<br>**Solutions**: NaCl 0.9%, Gluc 5%, Gluc-NaCl, Ringer's<br>**Y-site**: Cisatracurium, granisetron, linezolid, propofol, remifentanil |
| pH[2] | 4.0–5.0 |
| Sodium content[1] | 15 mmol/100 mL |
| Storage | Store below 25°C in original packaging.<br>Use opened vials immediately and discard any unused solution. |

## Monitoring

| Measure | Frequency | Rationale |
|---|---|---|
| Blood pressure | Check during infusion | • BP can suddenly drop, especially if taking hypotensive agents.<br>• In rare cases circulatory collapse occurs – if BP significantly drops stop the infusion immediately. |
| Signs of tendon damage (including rupture) | Throughout treatment | • Although rare, rupture may occur within 48 hours of starting treatment.<br>• Risk is higher in elderly patients and with concomitant use of corticosteroids.<br>• If tendinitis is suspected, discontinue immediately; the affected limb should be made non-weight-bearing and not exerted. |
| Signs of CNS disorders | | • Use with caution in epileptics or patients with tendency to spasms, previous seizures, vascular disorders in the brain, alterations in brain structure or stroke.<br>• If self-destructive behaviour is demonstrated or seizures occur, discontinue treatment. |
| Symptoms of neuropathy | | • Discontinue if symptoms occur, e.g. pain, burning, tingling, numbness; or deficits in: light touch, pain, temperature, position sense, vibratory sensation, motor strength.<br>• Due to axonal polyneuropathy and may be irreversible, although incidence is rare. |
| Signs of supra-Infection or superinfection | | • May result in the overgrowth of non-susceptible organisms – appropriate therapy should be commenced; treatment may need to be interrupted. |
| Blood glucose concentration | Increased frequency in diabetic patients | • Symptomatic hyperglycaemia and/or hypoglycaemia have been reported, requiring closer monitoring.<br>• If signs or symptoms of glucose disturbances develop, therapy should be stopped. |

*(continued)*

## Monitoring (continued)

| Measure | Frequency | Rationale |
|---------|-----------|-----------|
| LFTs | Periodically | • Mild rises in AST, ALT, Alk Phos, bilirubin and GGT may occur.<br>• Very rarely severe liver damage, hepatitis or cholestatic jaundice may occur - stop therapy. |
| U&Es | | • Changes in renal function may necessitate a dose adjustment. |
| FBC | | • Blood dyscrasias occur rarely.<br>• WCC: For signs of the infection resolving. |
| Development of diarrhoea | Throughout and up to 2 months after treatment | • Development of severe, persistent diarrhoea may be suggestive of *Clostridium difficile*-associated diarrhoea and colitis (pseudomembranous colitis). Discontinue drug and treat. Do not use drugs that inhibit peristalsis. |

## Additional information

| | |
|---|---|
| Common and serious undesirable effects | *Infusion-related:* Local: reddening of the infusion site and phlebitis.<br>*Other:* Nausea and vomiting, headache, dizziness, sleep disorders, restlessness, skin rash, itching. |
| Pharmacokinetics | Elimination half-life is about 5 hours. |
| Significant interactions | Ofloxacin may ↑levels or effect of the following drugs (or ↑side-effects): artemether with lumefantrine (avoid combination), ciclosporin (↑risk of nephrotoxicity), coumarin anticoagulants (monitor INR), NSAIDs (↑risk of seizures), theophylline (↑risk of seizures). |
| Action in case of overdose | *Symptoms to watch for:* CNS side-effects are of most concern. Ensure good urinary output (forced diuresis).<br>*Antidote:* If seizures are frequent or prolonged, control with IV diazepam (10-20 mg) or lorazepam (4 mg). Give oxygen and correct acid-base and metabolic disturbances as required. Consider IV phenytoin if convulsions continue to be unresponsive to above measures. |
| Counselling | A rash may develop on exposure to strong sunlight and ultraviolet rays, e.g. sunlamps, solaria - patients should avoid unnecessary exposure. |

| Risk rating: **GREEN** | Score = 1<br>Lower-risk product: Risk-reduction strategies should be considered. |
|---|---|

This assessment is based on the full range of preparation and administration options described in the monograph. These may not all be applicable in some clinical situations.

## Reference

1. Ashley C, Currie A, eds. *The Renal Drug Handbook*, 3rd edn. Oxford: Radcliffe Medical Press, 2009.
2. Communication with Sanofi-Aventis, 20 April 2009.

### Bibliography

SPC Tarivid IV infusion solution (accessed 2 April 2009).

# Olanzapine

**10-mg dry powder vials**

This preparation must not be confused with the depot preparation.

* Olanzapine is a thienobenzodiazepine atypical antipsychotic. It has affinity for serotonin, muscarinic, histamine ($H_1$), and adrenergic (alpha$_1$, $\alpha_1$) receptors as well as various dopamine receptors.
* It is given IM for the rapid control of agitation and disturbed behaviours in patients with schizophrenia or mania, when oral therapy is not appropriate.

## Pre-treatment checks

* Do not give to patients with known risk of narrow-angle glaucoma.
* Do not give in cardiac illness: acute myocardial infarction, unstable angina, severe hypotension or bradycardia, sick sinus syndrome, recent heart surgery.
* If parenteral benzodiazepine treatment is also required, do not give until at least 1 hour after the IM olanzapine.
* Review the physical health of patient.

*Biochemical and other tests (not all are necessary in an emergency situation)*

Blood pressure and pulse          Renal function: U, Cr, CrCl (or eGFR)
LFTs                              Respiratory rate

## Dose

The maximum dose in 24 hours is 20 mg by all routes.

**Standard dose:** usually 5–10 mg (2.5–5 mg in elderly patients). An effect would be expected in 15–45 minutes. A second dose of 5–10 mg may be given after 2 hours if necessary. The number of injections should not exceed 3 daily for a maximum of 3 days.
**Dose in renal impairment:** consider a lower starting dose of 5 mg.
**Dose in liver impairment:** consider a lower starting dose of 5 mg in cirrhosis (Child–Pugh class A or B).

## Intramuscular injection

*Preparation and administration*

1. Add 2.1 mL WFI to the vial and rotate until the contents have completely dissolved to give a clear yellow solution containing 5 mg/mL.
2. Withdraw the required dose.
3. Give by IM injection.

### Technical information

| | |
|---|---|
| Incompatible with | Diazepam, haloperidol, lorazepam. |
| Compatible with | Solutions: WFI |
| pH | Not relevant |
| Sodium content | Negligible |
| Storage | Store below 25°C in original packaging. |
| Displacement value | Not relevant. The vial contains an overage so that the final solution contains 5 mg/mL when reconstituted as directed. |
| Stability after preparation | Reconstituted vials must be used within 1 hour. |

### Monitoring

| Measure | Frequency | Rationale |
|---|---|---|
| Blood pressure | For at least 4 hours after injection, e.g. at 15 minute intervals. | • May cause ↓BP. |
| Pulse | | • May cause ↓pulse. |
| Respiratory rate | | • May cause respiratory depression. |
| Observe for signs of EPSE or NMS | Throughout treatment | • May cause EPSE, e.g. muscles shakes and tremor, or very rarely NMS. |

### Additional information

| | |
|---|---|
| Common and serious undesirable effects | *Infusion-related:* Local: Injection-site discomfort. <br> *Other:* Drowsiness, respiratory depression, ↓BP, ↓pulse. May worsen symptoms of Parkinson disease. |
| Pharmacokinetics | Elimination half-life is 32-50 hours. The effect of an IM dose could be expected in 15-45 minutes. |

*(continued)*

| **Additional information** *(continued)* | |
|---|---|
| Significant interactions | • The following may ↑olanzapine levels or effect (or ↑side-effects): anaesthetics-general (↑risk of ↓BP), antidepressants-tricyclic, artemether with lumefantrine (avoid combination), benzodiazepines (↑risk of ↓BP, ↓pulse and respiratory depression), ritonavir, sibutramine (avoid combination), valproate (↑risk of neutropenia). <br>• Olanzapine may ↓levels or effect of levodopa. <br>• Olanzapine may ↑risk of ventricular arrhythmias with the following drugs: antiarrhythmics, antidepressants-tricyclic, atomoxetine, methadone. <br>• Olanzapine ↓convulsive threshold and may ↓effect of the following drugs: barbiturates, carbamazepine, ethosuximide, oxcarbazepine, phenytoin, primidone, valproate. |
| Action in case of overdose | Treatment is symptomatic and supportive. Do not use adrenaline, dopamine or other sympathomimetic agents with beta-agonist activity (beta agonists may further ↓BP). |

| Risk rating: **GREEN** | Score = 1 <br> Lower-risk product: Risk-reduction strategies should be considered. |
|---|---|

This assessment is based on the full range of preparation and administration options described in the monograph. These may not all be applicable in some clinical situations.

## Bibliography

SPC Zyprexa (accessed 4 April 2009).

# Olanzapine embonate (olanzapine pamoate)

**210-mg, 300-mg and 405-mg dry powder vials with solvent (150 mg/mL after reconstitution)**

This preparation is a depot preparation and must not be confused with olanzapine injection for rapid tranquillisation.

• Olanzapine embonate is a thienobenzodiazepine atypical antipsychotic. It has affinity for serotonin, muscarinic, histamine ($H_1$), and adrenergic (alpha$_1$, $\alpha_1$) receptors as well as various dopamine receptors.
• It is used for the maintenance treatment of adult patients with schizophrenia sufficiently stabilised during acute treatment with oral olanzapine.

## Pre-treatment checks

- Avoid in patients with Parkinson disease or with a known risk of narrow-angle glaucoma.
- Caution in patients with a low leucocyte and/or neutrophil count.
- Caution in patients on other medication known to ↑QTc interval, patients with congenital long QT syndrome, congestive heart failure, heart failure, heart hypertrophy, ↓K or ↓Mg.
- Caution in patients with a history of seizures as olanzapine may reduce the seizure threshold.
- Patients should be treated initially with oral olanzapine before administering prolonged-release injection to establish tolerability and response.
- Check that the patient will not travel alone to their destination after each injection.

*Biochemical and other tests*

| | |
|---|---|
| Blood glucose | FBC |
| Blood pressure | LFTs |
| Bodyweight | Lipid profile |
| ECG | Prolactin |
| Electrolytes: serum Mg, K | Renal function: U, Cr, CrCl (or eGFR) |

## Dose

**Starting dose:** the patient should be treated with oral olanzapine initially to establish tolerability and response. The initial depot dose is dependent on the target oral olanzapine dose and is shown in Table O1.

**Maintenance dose:** after 2 months of treatment the recommended maintenance dose is as shown in Table O1.

**Table O1** Olanzapine depot maintenance dosing regimen

| Target oral olanzapine dose | Recommended starting dose | Maintenance after 2 months |
|---|---|---|
| 10 mg/day | 210 mg/2 weeks or 405 mg/4 weeks | 150 mg/2 weeks or 300 mg/4 weeks |
| 15 mg/day | 300 mg/2 weeks | 210 mg/2 weeks or 405 mg/4 weeks |
| 20 mg/day | 300 mg/2 weeks | 300 mg/2 weeks |

**Dose in renal impairment:** a lower starting dose of 150 mg every 4 weeks should be considered.
**Dose in hepatic impairment:** in moderate hepatic impairment (cirrhosis, Child–Pugh class A or B) start with 150 mg every 4 weeks and only increase with caution.

## Intramuscular injection

See Special handling below.

*Preparation and administration*

1. Loosen the powder by gently tapping the vial.
2. Follow the manufacturer's detailed instructions included in the pack and withdraw the required volume of solvent. This is dependent on the strength of the vial being reconstituted, i.e. 1.3 mL (210 mg), 1.8 mL (300 mg) or 2.3 mL (405 mg). NB: There is more solvent in the vial than is needed for reconstitution.
3. Continue to follow the instruction card carefully until a yellow, opaque suspension is formed containing 150 mg/mL.

4. Continue to follow the instruction card carefully to determine which of the needles supplied should be used to withdraw the dose, and which to administer the injection.
5. Give by deep IM injection into the gluteal muscle. Do not massage the injection site.

## Technical information

| Incompatible with | Not relevant |
|---|---|
| Compatible with | Not relevant |
| pH | Not relevant |
| Sodium content | Negligible |
| Storage | Store below 25°C in original packaging. Do not refrigerate or freeze. |
| Special handling | Wear gloves as this product may irritate the skin. |
| Stability after preparation | Any suspension withdrawn into a syringe must be used immediately. From a microbiological point of view, reconstituted vials should be used immediately; however, they may be stored at 20-25°C and used within 24 hours. If the product is not used straight away, the vial should be shaken vigorously to re-suspend. |

## Monitoring

| Measure | Frequency | Rationale |
|---|---|---|
| Signs and symptoms consistent with olanzapine overdose | After each injection, patients should be observed in a healthcare facility by appropriately qualified personnel for at least 3 hours | • The injection can sometimes be released into the bloodstream too quickly.<br>• It should be confirmed that the patient is alert, oriented, and absent of any signs and symptoms of overdose.<br>• If an overdose is suspected, close medical supervision and monitoring should continue until examination indicates that signs and symptoms have resolved. |
| Therapeutic effect | During dose adjustment and periodically | • To ensure reduction/elimination of psychotic symptoms. |
| U&Es, LFTs | At least annually | • To check renal and hepatic function as part of regular health check. |
| Prolactin | | • May cause ↑serum prolactin. |
| Glucose | | • May cause hyperglycaemia. |
| BP | | • May cause ↓BP. |
| EPSEs | During dose adjustment and every 3 months | • May cause EPSEs. |
| Bodyweight | At least annually | • Can cause weight gain.<br>• Measure waist hip ratio or waist circumference. |
| Lipid profile | | • As part of regular health check.<br>• Include cholesterol, HDL, LDL and triglycerides. |

## Additional information

| | |
|---|---|
| Common and serious undesirable effects | *Injection-related:* Injection-site reactions, sinus pause, hypoventilation.<br>*Common:* ↑Weight; ↑prolactin; mild, transient antimuscarinic effects (*very rarely* precipitation of angle-closure glaucoma); drowsiness, speech difficulty, exacerbation of Parkinson's disease, abnormal gait, hallucinations, akathisia, asthenia, fatigue, increased appetite, increased body temperature, raised triglyceride concentration, oedema, hyperprolactinaemia (but clinical manifestations rare); urinary incontinence; eosinophilia.<br>*Rare:* Hypotension, bradycardia, QT interval prolongation, photosensitivity; *rarely* seizures, leucopenia, rash; *very rarely* thromboembolism, hypercholesterolaemia, hypothermia, urinary retention, priapism, thrombocytopenia, neutropenia, rhabdomyolysis, hepatitis, pancreatitis and alopecia. |
| Pharmacokinetics | The olanzapine embonate salt dissolves very slowly to provide a slow continuous release of olanzapine that is complete approximately 6–8 months after the last injection. |
| Significant interactions | • The following may ↑olanzapine levels or effect (or ↑side-effects): anaesthetics-general (↑risk of ↓BP), antidepressants-tricyclic, artemether with lumefantrine (avoid combination), benzodiazepines (↑risk of ↓BP, ↓pulse and respiratory depression), ritonavir, sibutramine (avoid combination), valproate (↑risk of neutropenia).<br>• Olanzapine may ↓levels or effect of levodopa.<br>• Olanzapine may ↑risk of ventricular arrhythmias with the following drugs: antiarrhythmics, antidepressants-tricyclic, atomoxetine, methadone.<br>• Olanzapine ↓convulsive threshold and may ↓effect of the following drugs: barbiturates, carbamazepine, ethosuximide, oxcarbazepine, phenytoin, primidone, valproate. |
| Action in case of overdose | Treat symptomatically. Do **not** use adrenaline (epinephrine), dopamine or other sympathomimetic agents with beta-agonist activity since this may worsen ↓BP. Cardiovascular monitoring is necessary to detect possible arrhythmias. |
| Counselling | Do not drive or operate machinery for the remainder of the day on which the injection is administered. Do not travel alone after receiving the injection. |

| Risk rating: **AMBER** | Score = 4<br>Moderate-risk product: Risk-reduction strategies are recommended. |
|---|---|

This assessment is based on the full range of preparation and administration options described in the monograph. These may not all be applicable in some clinical situations.

## Bibliography

SPC Zypadhera (accessed 1 May 2009).

# Omeprazole

**40-mg dry powder vials**

* Omeprazole sodium is a proton pump inhibitor (PPI).
* It is used IV when the oral route is temporarily unavailable, to treat conditions where inhibition of gastric acid secretion may be beneficial: treatment and prevention of gastric and duodenal ulcers, gastro-oesophageal reflux disease (GORD) and Zollinger–Ellison syndrome.
* It is also used (unlicensed) for acute GI bleeding and to prevent re-bleeding following therapeutic endoscopy for acute bleeding gastric or duodenal ulcers.
* There are two preparations available: IV injection and IV infusion. The IV injection preparation is accompanied by 10 mL special solvent containing macrogol 400, citric acid and WFI.
* Doses are expressed in terms of omeprazole:
Omeprazole 40 mg ≡ 42.6 mg omeprazole sodium.

## Pre-treatment checks

PPIs may mask symptoms of gastric cancer (and delay diagnosis); when a gastric ulcer is suspected the possibility of malignancy should be excluded before treatment is instituted.

*Biochemical and other tests*

LFTs

## Dose

**Prophylaxis of acid aspiration:** 40 mg by IV injection or infusion completed 1 hour before surgery.
**Benign gastric ulcer, duodenal ulcer and gastro-oesophageal reflux:** 40 mg by IV injection or infusion once daily, until oral administration is possible (recommended duration of treatment is up to 5 days).
**Zollinger–Ellison syndrome:** 60 mg by IV injection or infusion twice daily.
**Gastrointestinal haemorrhage following successful haemostasis of bleeding peptic ulcers (unlicensed):** 80 mg by IV injection followed by a continuous IV infusion of 8 mg/hour for 72 hours.[1]
**Dose in hepatic impairment:** 20 mg daily by IV injection or infusion may be sufficient.

## Intermittent intravenous infusion (using the preparation for IV infusion)

*Preparation and administration*

1. Add approximately 5 mL NaCl 0.9% or Gluc 5% from a 100-mL bag to each omeprazole vial.
2. Mix thoroughly to dissolve and transfer the required dose to the infusion bag.
3. Repeat steps 1–2 to ensure the full dose is transferred or use a double-ended transfer needle device for the whole process.
4. The solution should be clear and colourless. Inspect visually for particulate matter or discoloration prior to administration and discard if present.
5. Give by IV infusion over 20–30 minutes.

## Intravenous injection

*Preparation and administration*

1. Withdraw 10 mL solvent from the ampoule and add approximately 5 mL to the omeprazole vial.
2. Immediately withdraw as much air as possible from the vial back into the syringe in order to reduce positive pressure and add the remaining solvent into the vial.
3. Rotate and shake the vial to ensure all the powder has dissolved.

(continued)

4. The solution should be clear and colourless. Inspect visually for particulate matter or discoloration prior to administration and discard if present.
5. Give by IV injection over 5 minutes.

## Continuous intravenous infusion (using the preparation for IV infusion)

Various (unlicensed) regimens are used.

*Preparation of a 200 mg/500mL solution (other strengths may be used)*

1. Reconstitute each of 5 vials (total 200 mg) with 5 mL of NaCl 0.9% or Gluc 5% taken from a 500-mL infusion bag and mix thoroughly to dissolve.
2. Withdraw the required dose (ensuring the entire vial contents are transferred) and add to the 500-mL bag, e.g. 5 × 40-mg vials added to 500 mL NaCl 0.9% gives a solution containing 400 micrograms/mL. Mix well.
3. The solution should be clear and colourless. Inspect visually for particulate matter or discoloration prior to administration and discard if present.
4. Give by IV infusion at a rate of 8 mg/hour, i.e. 20 mL/hour of a 400 micrograms/mL solution. Prepare a fresh infusion bag every 24 hours.

## Technical information

| | |
|---|---|
| Incompatible with | Lorazepam, midazolam, vancomycin. |
| Compatible with | **Flush**: NaCl 0.9%<br>**Solutions**: NaCl 0.9%, Gluc 5%. Some generic brands state that only Gluc 5% may be used as a diluent but all preparations are similarly formulated.<br>**Y-site**: No information but likely to be unstable. |
| pH | 8.8–10 |
| Sodium content | Negligible |
| Storage | Store below 25°C in original packaging. |
| Stability after preparation | From a microbiological point of view, should be used immediately; however:<br>• Reconstituted vials may be stored at room temperature and used within 4 hours.<br>• Prepared infusions may be infused (at room temperature) within 24 hours. |

## Monitoring

| Measure | Frequency | Rationale |
|---|---|---|
| Signs of infection | Throughout treatment | • Use of antisecretory drugs may ↑risk of infections such as community acquired pneumonia, salmonella, campylobacter and *Clostridium difficile*-associated disease. |
| LFTs | Periodically | • Altered LFTs and hepatitis have been reported. |
| Renal function | | • Acute interstitial nephritis has been reported with PPIs.<br>• ↓Na has been reported with PPIs. |
| Vitamin B$_{12}$ | | • In long-term therapy, malabsorption of vitamin B$_{12}$ has been reported. |

## Additional information

| | |
|---|---|
| Common and serious undesirable effects | *Immediate:* Hypersensitivity reactions including anaphylaxis and bronchospasm have been reported very rarely.<br>*Injection/infusion-related:* Local: Administration-site reactions, particularly with prolonged infusion.<br>*Other:*<br>• Common: Nausea, vomiting, abdominal pain, flatulence, diarrhoea, constipation, headache, dry mouth, peripheral oedema, dizziness, sleep disturbances, fatigue, paraesthesia, arthralgia, myalgia, rash, and pruritus.<br>• Rare: Taste disturbance, stomatitis, ↑liver enzymes, hepatitis, jaundice, fever, depression, hallucinations, confusion, gynaecomastia, interstitial nephritis, ↓Na, blood disorders (including leucopenia, leucocytosis, pancytopenia and thrombocytopenia), visual disturbances, sweating, photosensitivity, alopecia, Stevens-Johnson syndrome, and toxic epidermal necrolysis. |
| Pharmacokinetics | Approximate plasma half-life is 0.5–3 hours. The IV infusion produces an immediate decrease in intragastric acidity and a mean decrease over 24 hours of approximately 90%. |
| Significant interactions | • Tipranavir may ↓omeprazole levels or effect.<br>• Omeprazole may ↑levels or effect of the following drugs (or ↑side-effects): cilostazol (avoid combination), coumarins (monitor INR), raltegravir (avoid combination).<br>• Omeprazole may ↓levels or effect of the following drugs: atazanavir (avoid combination), clopidogrel (avoid combination), nelfinavir (avoid combination).<br>• Omeprazole may affect the following tests:<br>Antisecretory drug therapy may cause a false-negative urea breath test.<br>May give false positive tetrahydrocannabinol (THC) urine screening test results. |
| Action in case of overdose | Stop administration and give supportive therapy as appropriate. |

| | |
|---|---|
| Risk rating: **AMBER** | Score = 4<br>Moderate-risk product: Risk-reduction strategies are recommended. |

This assessment is based on the full range of preparation and administration options described in the monograph. These may not all be applicable in some clinical situations.

### Reference

1. Hasselgren G *et al.* Optimization of acid suppression for patients with peptic ulcer bleeding: an intragastric pH-metry study with omeprazole. *Eur J Gastroenterol Hepatol* 1998; 10: 601–606.

### Bibliography

SPC Losec IV injection 40 mg, AstraZeneca UK (accessed 28 March 2010).

# Ondansetron

**2 mg/mL solution in 2-mL and 4-mL ampoules**

* Ondansetron hydrochloride is a 5-HT$_3$ antagonist with antiemetic activity.
* It is used in the management of nausea and vomiting associated with cytotoxic chemotherapy and radiotherapy and in postoperative nausea and vomiting (PONV).
* Co-administration of dexamethasone may ↑efficacy of ondansetron.
* Doses given by injection are expressed as ondansetron hydrochloride.

## Pre-treatment checks

* Caution with cardiac rhythm or conduction problems, check whether the patient is being treated with any antiarrhythmic, beta-blocker or any medication that may prolong the QT interval – IV ondansetron may cause transient ECG changes.
* Caution if there are any signs of subacute intestinal obstruction – ondansetron can ↑large-bowel transit time.

*Biochemical and other tests (not all are necessary in an emergency situation)*

LFTs

## Dose

**Chemotherapy and radiotherapy:** usually 8 mg by IM or IV injection immediately before treatment. Further doses are given by IM or IV injection, or by continuous IV infusion, depending on the emetogenic potential of the cytotoxic regimen.

**Prevention of PONV:** 4 mg by IM or IV injection at induction of anaesthesia.

**Treatment of PONV:** a single dose of 4 mg by IM or IV injection.

**Dose in hepatic impairment:** in moderate to severe hepatic impairment the total daily dose should not exceed 8 mg.

## Intramuscular injection

*Preparation and administration*

1. Withdraw the required dose.
2. Give by IM injection.

## Intravenous injection

*Preparation and administration*

1. Withdraw the required dose.
2. The solution should be clear and colourless. Inspect visually for particulate matter or discoloration prior to administration and discard if present.
3. Give by IV injection over at least 30 seconds and preferably over 2–5 minutes.

## Intermittent intravenous infusion

*Preparation and administration*

1. Withdraw the required dose and add to 50–100 mL of NaCl 0.9% or Gluc 5%.
2. The solution should be clear and colourless. Inspect visually for particulate matter or discoloration prior to administration and discard if present.
3. Give by IV infusion over at least 15 minutes.

## Continuous intravenous infusion

*Preparation and administration*

1. Withdraw the required dose and add to a suitable volume of compatible infusion fluid. Mix well.
2. The solution should be clear and colourless. Inspect visually for particulate matter or discoloration prior to administration and discard if present.
3. Give by IV infusion for up to 24 hours.

## Technical information

| | |
|---|---|
| Incompatible with | Sodium bicarbonate.<br>Aciclovir, aminophylline, amphotericin, ampicillin, furosemide, ganciclovir, lorazepam, meropenem, methylprednisolone sodium succinate, micafungin. |
| Compatible with | **Flush**: NaCl 0.9%<br>**Solutions**: NaCl 0.9%, Gluc 5% (both with added KCl), Ringer's, Hartmann's<br>**Y-site**: Amikacin, aztreonam, cefotaxime, ceftazidime, cefuroxime, cisatracurium, clindamycin, dexamethasone, dopamine, fluconazole, gentamicin, hydrocortisone sodium succinate, imipenem with cilastatin, linezolid, magnesium sulphate, piperacillin with tazobactam, ranitidine, remifentanil, ticarcillin with clavulanate, vancomycin |
| pH | 3.3-4 |
| Sodium content | Negligible |
| Storage | Store below 25°C in original packaging. |
| Stability after preparation | From a microbiological point of view, should be used immediately; however, prepared infusions may be stored at 2-8°C and infused (at room temperature) within 24 hours. |

## Monitoring

| Measure | Frequency | Rationale |
|---|---|---|
| Dizziness during IV infusion | During infusion period | • May be avoided or resolved by increasing infusion period |
| Clinical improvement | Periodically | • To ensure that treatment is effective. |
| IV injection site | | • Injection-site reactions have occurred. |

## Additional information

| | |
|---|---|
| Common and serious undesirable effects | *Injection/infusion-related*: Local: Injection-site reactions are common.<br>*Other*: Headache, constipation, sensation of warmth or flushing. |
| Pharmacokinetics | Elimination half-life is approximately 3 hours. |
| Significant interactions | • The following may ↓ondansetron levels or effect: carbamazepine, phenytoin, rifampicin.<br>• Ondansetron may ↑levels or effect (or ↑side-effects) of QT-prolonging drugs (may result in additional QT prolongation).<br>• Ondansetron may ↓levels or effect of tramadol (higher doses of tramadol required, which also increase its emetogenicity). |
| Action in case of overdose | Stop administration and give supportive therapy as appropriate. |

| Risk rating: **GREEN** | Score = 1 Lower-risk product: Risk-reduction strategies should be considered. |

This assessment is based on the full range of preparation and administration options described in the monograph. These may not all be applicable in some clinical situations.

## Bibliography

SPC Zofran Injection, Flexi-Amp injection (accessed 21 January 2010).
SPC Ondansetron 2 mg/mL injection, Hospira UK (accessed 21 January 2010).
SPC Ondansetron 2 mg/mL solution for injection, Wockhardt UK Ltd (accessed 21 January 2010).

# Oxycodone hydrochloride

**10 mg/mL solution in 1-mL and 2-mL ampoules**
**50 mg/mL solution in 1-mL ampoules**

* Oxycodone hydrochloride is a potent opioid analgesic. It is roughly twice as potent as morphine for a given dose and route.
* It is used parenterally for the treatment of moderate to severe pain, particularly in palliative care.

## Pre-treatment checks

* Do not use in acute respiratory depression, where there is a risk of paralytic ileus, in ↑intracranial pressure and in head injury, in comatose patients; in acute abdomen; delayed gastric emptying; chronic constipation; cor pulmonale; acute porphyria.
* Caution in ↓BP, shock, convulsive disorders, supraventricular tachycardias, atrial flutter, chronic obstructive pulmonary disease and acute asthma attack, obstructive or inflammatory bowel diseases, biliary tract diseases, alcoholism, prostatic hyperplasia, myasthenia gravis, hypothyroidism (reduce dose), adrenocortical insufficiency (reduce dose).
* Caution in toxic psychosis and pancreatitis.
* Ensure resuscitation equipment and naloxone are available especially for IV administration.

*Biochemical and other tests (not all are necessary in an emergency situation)*

| | |
|---|---|
| Blood pressure and pulse | Pain score |
| Bodyweight (certain indications) | Renal function: U, Cr, CrCl (or eGFR) |
| LFTs | Respiratory rate |

## Dose

Note: Doses above those stated must not be given to opioid-naive patients.

**Moderate to severe pain:** initially 1–10 mg by IV injection or 5 mg by SC injection every 4 hours when required. Halve the dose in elderly or frail patients. The initial dose is dependent on previous opioid exposure – see below.

**Approximate equivalents for patients switched from oral to parenteral dosing**

5 mg orally every 4 hours (or 30 mg daily as oral modified release) is equivalent to
* 2.5 mg by SC injection every 4 hours (total 15 mg daily)
* 2.5 mg by IV injection every 4 hours (total 15 mg daily)
* 15 mg by IV or SC infusion over 24 hours

Alternatively, give 2 mg/hour by IV infusion and adjust dose according to requirements.

**Patient-controlled analgesia:** the usual setting for the PCA device is to deliver a 0.03 mg/kg bolus with a minimum 5-minute lock-out period.

**Dose in renal impairment:** reduce the dose if creatinine clearance < 10 mL/minute.

**Dose in hepatic impairment:** reduce dose or avoid (may precipitate coma).

## Subcutaneous injection

*Preparation and administration*

Check that you have selected the correct strength of ampoule. High-strength ampoules are available for use in PCA and palliative care. These are not suitable for use in acute situations.

1. Withdraw the required dose.
2. Give by SC injection.
3. Close monitoring of respiratory rate and consciousness recommended for 30 minutes in patients receiving initial dose, especially elderly patients or those of low bodyweight.

## Intravenous injection

*Preparation and administration*

Check that you have selected the correct strength of ampoule. High-strength ampoules are available for use in PCA and palliative care. These are not suitable for use in acute situations.

1. Withdraw the required dose and dilute with NaCl 0.9% or Gluc 5% to give a solution containing 1 mg/mL.
2. The solution should be clear and colourless. Inspect visually for particulate matter or discoloration prior to administration and discard if present.
3. Give by slow IV injection over a minimum of 2 minutes.
4. Close monitoring of respiratory rate and consciousness recommended for 30 minutes in patients receiving initial dose, especially elderly patients or those of low bodyweight.

## Intravenous infusion

*Preparation and administration*

1. Withdraw the required dose and add to a suitable volume of NaCl 0.9% or Gluc 5% to give a solution containing 1 mg/mL.
2. The solution should be clear and colourless. Inspect visually for particulate matter or discoloration prior to administration and discard if present.
3. Give by IV infusion at the desired rate via a volumetric infusion device or syringe pump. Adjust the dose to clinical response.

## Patient-controlled analgesia[1]

*Preparation and administration*

Strength used may vary depending on local policies.

1. Make 50 mg oxycodone up to 50 mL with NaCl 0.9% or Gluc 5% in a PCA syringe to give a solution containing 1 mg/mL.
2. The solution should be clear and colourless. Inspect visually for particulate matter or discoloration prior to administration and discard if present.
3. The usual setting for the PCA device is to deliver a 0.03 mg/kg bolus with a minimum 5-minute lock-out period. Lower doses are used in patients with severe renal impairment.

## Technical information

| | |
|---|---|
| Incompatible with | No information |
| Compatible with | **Flush**: NaCl 0.9%<br>**Solutions**: Gluc 5%, NaCl 0.9%, WFI<br>**Y-site**: No information |
| pH | 4.5 to 5.5 |
| Sodium content | Negligible |
| Storage | Store below 25°C in original packaging. Controlled Drug.<br>After opening, use immediately and discard unused portion. |
| Stability after preparation | From a microbiological point of view, should be used immediately; however, prepared infusions may be stored at 2–8°C and infused (at room temperature) within 24 hours. |

## Monitoring

Close monitoring of respiratory rate and consciousness recommended for 30 minutes in patients receiving initial dose, especially elderly patients or those of low bodyweight.

| Measure | Frequency | Rationale |
|---|---|---|
| Pain | At regular intervals | • To ensure therapeutic response. |
| Blood pressure, pulse and respiratory rate | | • ↓BP, ↓pulse, ↑pulse, palpitations and respiratory depression with ↓oxygen saturation can occur. |
| Sedation | | • May cause sedation. |
| Monitor for side-effects and toxicity | | • May cause side-effects such as nausea and constipation, which may need treating. |

## Additional information

| | |
|---|---|
| Common and serious undesirable effects | *Immediate:* Anaphylaxis has rarely been reported, bronchospasm.<br>*Other:* Nausea and vomiting (particularly initially), constipation, dry mouth, urticaria, pruritus, biliary spasm, ↑ or ↓pulse, hallucinations, euphoria, drowsiness.<br>At higher doses: ↓BP, sedation, respiratory depression, muscle rigidity. |
| Pharmacokinetics | Elimination half-life is 2-4 hours. |
| Significant interactions | • The following may ↑oxycodone levels or effect (or ↑side-effects): antihistamines-sedating (↑sedation), MAOIs (avoid combination and for 2 weeks after stopping MAOI), moclobemide.<br>• Oxycodone may ↑levels or effect (or ↑side-effects) of sodium oxybate (avoid combination). |
| Action in case of overdose | *Symptoms to watch for:* ↑sedation, respiratory depression.<br>*Antidote:* Naloxone (see the Naloxone monograph). Stop administration and give supportive therapy as appropriate. |
| Counselling | May cause drowsiness which may affect the ability to perform skilled tasks; if affected, do not drive or operate machinery, avoid alcoholic drink (the effects of alcohol are enhanced).<br>If you are pregnant or breast feeding inform your doctor.<br>Inform the patient of possible side-effects: see above. |

| | |
|---|---|
| Risk rating: **AMBER** | Score = 3<br>Moderate-risk product: Risk-reduction strategies are recommended. |

This assessment is based on the full range of preparation and administration options described in the monograph. These may not all be applicable in some clinical situations.

## Reference

1. Walder B *et al.* Efficacy and safety of patient controlled opioid analgesia for acute postoperative pain. *Acta Anaesthesiol Scand* 2001; 45: 795–804.

## Bibliography

SPCs OxyNorm 10 mg/mL and 50 mg/mL solution for injection or infusion (accessed 13 July 2009).

# Pabrinex Intramuscular High Potency Injection

**No. 1 (5-mL) and No. 2 (2-mL) ampoules**

*Each No. 1 ampoule (5 mL) contains:*

**Thiamine 250 mg, riboflavin (as phosphate sodium) 4 mg, pyridoxine 50 mg**

*Each No. 2 ampoule (2 mL) contains:*

**Ascorbic acid 500 mg, nicotinamide BP 160 mg**

* Pabrinex ampoules are given in pairs and each pair of Pabrinex ampoules provides high potency B complex vitamins and vitamin C.
* Pabrinex is used to reverse severe depletion or malabsorption of these vitamins, particularly in alcoholism, after acute infections, postoperatively and in psychiatric states.

---

**MHRA/CHM advice (September 2007)**

Although potentially serious allergic adverse reactions may rarely occur during, or shortly after, parenteral administration, the CHM has recommended that:

* This should not preclude the use of parenteral thiamine in patients where this route of administration is required, particularly in patients at risk of Wernicke-Korsakoff syndrome where treatment with thiamine is essential.
* Facilities for treating anaphylaxis (including resuscitation facilities) should be available when parenteral thiamine is administered.

---

## Pre-treatment checks

* Repeated injections may give rise to anaphylactic shock. Mild allergic reactions such as sneezing or mild asthma are warning signs that further injections may give rise to anaphylactic shock.
* In thiamine deficiency ↑carbohydrate load including the use of high-strength parenteral glucose solutions may ↑thiamine requirements and worsen symptoms.

## Dose

Pabrinex injection is also available in an IV form which **must not** be given IM. Ensure the correct preparation has been selected before administration.

The contents of ampoules No. 1 and No. 2 (total 7 mL) combine to form the dose.

**Standard dose:** 7 mL twice daily for up to 7 days.

## Intramuscular injection

*Preparation and administration*

1. Make up the total dose by mixing the contents of ampoules Nos. 1 and 2 in a syringe (total 7 mL).
2. Give by slow IM injection high into the gluteal muscle, 5 cm below the iliac crest. Rotate injection sites for subsequent injections.

## Technical information

| | |
|---|---|
| Incompatible with | Not relevant |
| Compatible with | Not relevant |
| pH | No relevant |
| Sodium content | Negligible |
| Excipients | Contains benzyl alcohol. |
| Storage | Store at 2-8°C in original packaging. Do not freeze. |
| Stability after preparation | Mixed ampoules should be used immediately after mixing. |

## Monitoring

| Measure | Frequency | Rationale |
|---|---|---|
| Hypersensitivity reactions | During and for one hour after administration | • Thiamine injections may give rise to anaphylactic shock and less severe hypersensitivity reactions such as mild asthma or sneezing. |
| Fluid balance | Regularly during treatment | • Dehydration increases the likelihood of renal oxalate calculi formation with high dose ascorbic acid therapy. |
| Ability to urinate | Daily | • High-dose ascorbic acid can cause renal oxalate calculi. |

## Additional information

| | |
|---|---|
| Common and serious undesirable effects | *Immediate:* Repeated injections of high concentrations of thiamine may cause anaphylactic shock. Mild allergic reactions, e.g. sneezing or wheeze are a warning that further injections may give rise to anaphylactic shock. *Other:* Occasionally ↓BP and mild paraesthesia is seen following continued high doses of thiamine. Large doses of ascorbic acid have resulted in haemolysis in patients with glucose-6-phosphate dehydrogenase (G6PD) deficiency. |
| Pharmacokinetics | Thiamine, riboflavin, pyridoxine, nicotinamide and ascorbic acid are widely distributed in the body tissues. Higher doses in excess of the body's needs are rapidly eliminated unchanged in the urine. |
| Significant interactions | • Use of high-strength parenteral glucose solutions may ↑thiamine requirements and worsen symptoms. <br> • Pabrinex Intramuscular High Potency Injection may affect the following tests: <br> ascorbic acid is a strong reducing agent and interferes with a number of laboratory tests based on oxidation reduction reactions. |
| Action in case of overdose | Stop treatment and give supportive therapy as appropriate. |

| Risk rating: **GREEN** | Score = 1 |
| --- | --- |
| | Lower-risk product: Risk-reduction strategies should be considered. |

This assessment is based on the full range of preparation and administration options described in the monograph. These may not all be applicable in some clinical situations.

## Bibliography

SPC Pabrinex IM HP (accessed 21 October 2008).
SPC Ascorbic Acid Injection BPC UCB Pharma (accessed 20 October 2008).

# Pabrinex Intravenous High Potency Injection

**No. 1 and No. 2 ampoules each containing 5 mL**

*Each No. 1 ampoule contains per 5 mL:*

**Thiamine 250 mg, riboflavin (as phosphate sodium) 4 mg, pyridoxine 50 mg**

*Each No. 2 ampoule contains per 5 mL:*

**Ascorbic acid 500 mg, nicotinamide BP 160 mg, anhydrous glucose BP 1g**

* Pabrinex ampoules are given in pairs and each pair of Pabrinex ampoules provides high potency B complex vitamins and vitamin C.
* Pabrinex is used to reverse severe depletion or malabsorption of these vitamins, particularly in alcoholism, after acute infections, postoperatively, in psychiatric states and in prevention of refeeding syndrome.
* The IV form is also used to maintain levels of vitamins B and C in patients on chronic intermittent haemodialysis.

### MHRA/CHM advice (September 2007)

Although potentially serious allergic adverse reactions may rarely occur during, or shortly after, parenteral administration, the CHM has recommended that:

* This should not preclude the use of parenteral thiamine in patients where this route of administration is required, particularly in patients at risk of Wernicke–Korsakoff syndrome where treatment with thiamine is essential.
* IV administration should be by infusion over 30 minutes.
* Facilities for treating anaphylaxis (including resuscitation facilities) should be available when parenteral thiamine is administered.

## Pre-treatment checks

* Repeated injections may give rise to anaphylactic shock. Mild allergic reactions such as sneezing or mild asthma are warning signs that further injections may give rise to anaphylactic shock.

- In thiamine deficiency ↑carbohydrate load including the use of high-strength parenteral glucose solutions may ↑thiamine requirements and worsen symptoms.

## Dose

Pabrinex injection is also available in an IM form which **must not** be given IV. Ensure the correct preparation has been selected before administration.

Equal volumes of the contents of ampoules No. 1 and No. 2 combine to form the dose.

**Coma or delirium from alcohol, narcotics or barbiturates; collapse following continuous narcosis:** give 20–30 mL of the mixed ampoules by IV infusion every 8 hours.

**Psychosis following narcosis or ECT; toxicity from acute infections:** give 10 mL of the mixed ampoules by IV infusion twice daily for up to 7 days.

**Haemodialysis:** give 10 mL of the mixed ampoules by IV infusion every 2 weeks at the completion of dialysis.

**Prevention of refeeding syndrome in susceptible individuals (unlicensed):** 10 mL of the mixed ampoules has been given by IV infusion twice daily for 10 days.

## Intravenous infusion

*Preparation and administration*

1. Make up the total dose by mixing equal volumes of ampoules Nos. 1 and 2 in a syringe.
2. Add to 100 mL of NaCl 0.9% or Gluc 5%.
3. Give by IV infusion over 30 minutes.

## Technical information

| | |
|---|---|
| Incompatible with | Sodium bicarbonate.<br>Aminophylline, chloramphenicol sodium succinate, erythromycin, doxapram, propofol. |
| Compatible with | **Flush**: NaCl 0.9%<br>**Solutions**: NaCl 0.9%, Gluc 5%, Gluc-NaCl<br>**Y-site**: No Information |
| pH | 4.9 (mixed) |
| Sodium content | 2.95 mmol per pair of ampoules |
| Storage | Store below 25°C in original packaging. |
| Stability after preparation | Mixed ampoules should be used immediately.<br>From a microbiological point of view, prepared infusions should be used immediately; however, they may be stored at 2-8°C for 4 hours. Do not freeze. |

## Monitoring

| Measure | Frequency | Rationale |
|---|---|---|
| Hypersensitivity reactions | During and for 1 hour after administration | • Thiamine injections may give rise to anaphylactic shock and less severe hypersensitivity reactions such as mild asthma or sneezing. |

*(continued)*

## Monitoring *(continued)*

| Measure | Frequency | Rationale |
|---|---|---|
| Fluid balance | Regularly during treatment | • Dehydration increases the likelihood of renal oxalate calculus formation with high-dose ascorbic acid therapy. |
| Ability to urinate | Daily | • High-dose ascorbic acid can cause renal oxalate calculi. |

## Additional information

| | |
|---|---|
| Common and serious undesirable effects | *Immediate:* Repeated injections of high concentrations of thiamine may cause anaphylactic shock. Mild allergic reactions, e.g. sneezing or wheezing, are a warning that further injections may give rise to anaphylactic shock.<br>*Other:* Occasionally ↓BP and mild paraesthesia are seen following continued high doses of thiamine. Large doses of ascorbic acid have resulted in haemolysis in patients with G6PD deficiency. |
| Pharmacokinetics | Thiamine, riboflavin, pyridoxine, nicotinamide and ascorbic acid are widely distributed in the body tissues. Doses in excess of the body's needs are rapidly eliminated unchanged in the urine. |
| Significant interactions | • Use of high-strength parenteral glucose solutions may ↑thiamine requirements and worsen symptoms.<br>• Pabrinex Intravenous High Potency Injection may affect the following tests: ascorbic acid is a strong reducing agent and interferes with a number of laboratory tests based on oxidation-reduction reactions. |
| Action in case of overdose | Stop treatment and give supportive therapy as appropriate. |

| Risk rating: **AMBER** | Score = 3<br>Moderate-risk product: Risk-reduction strategies are recommended. |
|---|---|

This assessment is based on the full range of preparation and administration options described in the monograph. These may not all be applicable in some clinical situations.

## Bibliography

SPC Pabrinex IV HP (accessed 21 October 2008).
SPC Ascorbic Acid Injection BPC UCB Pharma (accessed 20 October 2008).

# Palifermin

**6.25-mg dry powder vials**

* Palifermin is a human keratinocyte growth factor (KGF) produced by recombinant DNA technology in *Escherichia coli*.
* It is used to reduce the incidence and duration of severe oral mucositis in patients with haematological neoplasms undergoing myeloablative chemotherapy, before stem cell transplantation.

## Pre-treatment checks

Do not use if there is known hypersensitivity to palifermin or any *E. coli*-derived proteins and avoid in breast feeding.

*Biochemical and other tests*

Bodyweight

## Dose

In all cases be guided by the oncology team responsible for treating the patient.

**Standard dose:** 60 micrograms/kg daily on three consecutive days (*doses 1 to 3*) before and three consecutive days after myeloablative chemotherapy (doses 4 to 6).

*Doses 1 to 3* are given on the three consecutive days prior to myeloablative chemotherapy, with the third dose administered 24–48 hours before chemotherapy.

*Doses 4 to 6* are given on the three consecutive days after myeloablative chemotherapy with the first of these (dose 4) administered after, but on the same day as, stem cell infusion and at least 4 days after dose 3.

## Intravenous injection

*Preparation and administration*

1. Slowly inject 1.2 mL WFI into the vial.
2. Swirl the contents gently to dissolve (usually takes less than 5 minutes) but do not shake vigorously. This produces a solution containing 5 mg/mL.
3. The solution should be clear and colourless. Inspect visually for particulate matter or discoloration prior to administration and discard if present.
4. Withdraw the required dose.
5. Give by IV injection. If heparin is being used to maintain the IV line, NaCl 0.9% should be used to flush the line prior to and after administration of palifermin. Palifermin should **not** be filtered during preparation or administration.

## Technical information

| Incompatible with | Heparin sodium |
|---|---|
| Compatible with | **Flush**: NaCl 0.9%<br>**Solutions**: NaCl 0.9%<br>**Y-site**: No information but likely to be unstable |
| pH | 6.5 |

*(continued)*

## Technical information (continued)

| | |
|---|---|
| Sodium content | Nil |
| Storage | Store at 2-8°C in original packaging. Do not freeze. |
| Displacement value | Negligible |
| Stability after preparation | From a microbiological point of view, should be used immediately; however, reconstituted vials may be stored at 2-8°C for 24 hours (only stable for a maximum of 1 hour at room temperature). |

## Monitoring

Nothing specific. Palifermin can sometimes cause ↑lipase and amylase levels with or without symptoms of abdominal pain or backache thought to be salivary in origin and non-serious.

## Additional information

| | |
|---|---|
| Common and serious undesirable effects | Skin rash, pruritus, erythema, an increase in the thickness in the mouth or tongue, change in colour of the mouth or tongue, oedema, pain, fever, arthralgia and altered taste. |
| Pharmacokinetics | Elimination half-life is 4.5 hours. |
| Significant interactions | No significant interactions. |
| Action in case of overdose | *Antidote:* No known antidote; stop administration and give supportive therapy as appropriate. |
| Counselling | Discuss likely side-effects and their usual transient nature (most often start a few days after the first three injections and can last about a week). |

| Risk rating: **AMBER** | Score = 3<br>Moderate-risk product: Risk-reduction strategies are recommended. |
|---|---|

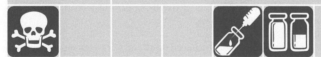

This assessment is based on the full range of preparation and administration options described in the monograph. These may not all be applicable in some clinical situations.

## Bibliography

SPC Kepivance 6.25 mg powder for solution for injection (accessed 2 April 2009).

# Palonosetron

### 50 micrograms/mL solution 5-mL ampoules

* Palonosetron hydrochloride is a 5-HT$_3$ antagonist with antiemetic activity.
* It is used in the prevention of nausea and vomiting associated with moderate and highly emetogenic cytotoxic chemotherapy.
* Co-administration of a corticosteroid may ↑efficacy of palonosetron.
* Doses are expressed in terms of the base:
  Palonosetron 250 micrograms ≅ 281 micrograms palonosetron hydrochloride.

### Pre-treatment checks

* Caution in patients receiving drugs that may ↑QT interval or patients who have or may develop prolongation of the QT interval.
* Caution in history of constipation or intestinal obstruction – may ↑large bowel transit time.

*Biochemical and other tests*

Electrolytes: serum K

### Dose

**Standard dose**: 250 micrograms by IV injection 30 minutes before the start of chemotherapy. Do not repeat the dose within 7 days.

### Intravenous injection

*Preparation and administration*

1. Withdraw the required dose.
2. The solution should be clear and colourless. Inspect visually for particulate matter or discoloration prior to administration and discard if present.
3. Give by IV injection over 30 seconds.

## Technical information

| | |
|---|---|
| Incompatible with | Methylprednisolone sodium succinate |
| Compatible with | **Flush**: NaCl 0.9%<br>**Solutions**: NaCl 0.9%, Gluc 5%, Gluc-NaCl<br>**Y-site**: Dexamethasone, lorazepam, midazolam |
| pH | 4.5–5.5 |
| Sodium content | Negligible |
| Storage | Store below 30°C in original packaging. |

## Monitoring

| Measure | Frequency | Rationale |
|---|---|---|
| Improvement in nausea/vomiting | Post chemotherapy | • To ensure that treatment is effective. |
| Serum K | Periodically | • Can sometimes cause ↑K. |

## Additional information

| | |
|---|---|
| Common and serious undesirable effects | *Injection/infusion-related:* Local: Injection-site reactions are very rare. *Other:* Headache, dizziness, constipation, diarrhoea. Rarely non-sustained ↑pulse, ↑K, anxiety, sensation of warmth or flushing. |
| Pharmacokinetics | Elimination half-life is about 40 hours. |
| Significant interactions | None reported. |
| Action in case of overdose | Stop administration and give supportive therapy as appropriate. |

Risk rating: **GREEN**   Score = 0
Lower-risk product: Risk-reduction strategies should be considered.

This assessment is based on the full range of preparation and administration options described in the monograph. These may not all be applicable in some clinical situations.

### Bibliography

SPC Aloxi (accessed 29 December 2009).

# Pamidronate disodium (disodium pamidronate)

**15-mg, 30-mg, 90-mg dry powder vials with either 5 mL or 10 mL solvent (Aredia)**
**15 mg/mL solution in 1-mL, 2-mL, 4-mL and 6-mL ampoules**
**3 mg/mL solution in 5-mL, 10-mL, 20-mL and 30-mL vials**

* Pamidronate disodium is an aminobisphosphonate with properties similar to other bisphosphonates. It inhibits bone resorption, but appears to have less effect on bone mineralisation.
* It is used to treat conditions characterised by increased osteoclast activity: tumour-induced ↑Ca; osteolytic lesions and bone pain in patients with bone metastases associated with breast cancer or multiple myeloma; Paget disease (of bone).
* Not all products are licensed for all indications; individual products vary in their specifications for suitable dilutions and rates of administration.
* Doses are expressed as pamidronate disodium.

### Pre-treatment checks

* Do not give to patients already receiving other bisphosphonates.
* Do not give in renal impairment when CrCl (or eGFR) < 30 mL/minute unless life-threatening tumour-induced ↑Ca where the benefit outweighs risk.

- Osteonecrosis of the jaw can occur: consider dental examination and preventive dentistry prior to *planned* treatment in patients with risk factors (e.g. cancer, chemotherapy, radiotherapy, corticosteroids, poor oral hygiene). Avoid invasive dental procedures during treatment if possible.
- Give cautiously to patients who have had previous thyroid surgery (increased risk of ↓Ca).
- Contraindicated in pregnancy. Women of child-bearing potential should take contraceptive precautions during *planned* treatment.
- Unless being used for ↑Ca, prescribe oral calcium and vitamin D supplements in those at risk of deficiency (e.g. through malabsorption or lack of exposure to sunlight) and in patients with Paget disease to minimise ↓Ca.
- Hydrate the patient adequately before, during and after infusions. Calcium level may return to normal simply by rehydration of the patient. Recheck Ca before commencing infusion.

*Biochemical and other tests*

Electrolytes: serum Na, K, Ca, PO$_4$, Mg
Renal function: U, Cr, CrCl (or eGFR)

## Dose

**Tumour-induced hypercalcaemia (TIH):** the total dose is dependent on initial serum Ca (see Table P1 below – dose ranges are valid for both 'uncorrected' and 'corrected' Ca). Give the total dose either as a single infusion or as multiple smaller infusions over 2–4 consecutive days, with a maximum dose per treatment course of 90 mg.

**Table P1** Pamidronate dosing regimen in TIH

| Initial serum calcium ('corrected' or 'uncorrected') | | Recommended total dose (mg) |
|---|---|---|
| mmol/L | mg/dL | |
| <3.0 | <12.0 | 15-30 |
| 3.0-3.5 | 12.0-14.0 | 30-60 |
| 3.5-4.0 | 14.0-16.0 | 60-90 |
| >4.0 | >16.0 | 90 |

**Dose in renal impairment for TIH:** adjusted according to creatinine clearance:[1]
- CrCl ≥10 mL/minute: dose as in normal renal function.
- CrCl <10 mL/minute: Ca >4.0 mg/dL, dose at 60 mg; Ca <4.0 mg/dL, dose at 30 mg.

**Osteolytic lesions and bone pain in multiple myeloma:** 90 mg every 4 weeks.
**Osteolytic lesions and bone pain in bone metastases associated with breast cancer:** 90 mg every 4 weeks (or may also be given 3-weekly to coincide with chemotherapy).
**Paget disease of bone:** give the course either as:
- 30 mg weekly for 6 consecutive weeks (total dose 180 mg).
- An initial dose of 30 mg (to minimise first-dose side-effects), followed by three doses of 60 mg every other week (total dose of 210 mg).

Increase the dose according to disease severity, to a maximum total dose of 360 mg (in divided doses of 60 mg). Repeat the course every 6 months until disease remission, or if relapse occurs.

## Intermittent intravenous infusion

- Pamidronate disodium is incompatible with Hartmann's and Ringer's (contain Ca).
- The patient must be adequately hydrated using NaCl 0.9% before dosing for ↑Ca.
- Infusion into a relatively large vein minimises patient discomfort.

*Preparation and administration*

1. For dry powder vials: reconstitute with the solvent supplied. Dissolve vial contents completely before withdrawing the dose. Concentration is 15 mg/5 mL, 30 mg/10 mL or 90 mg/10 mL depending on vial size.
2. For all presentations: withdraw the required dose.
3. Add each dose of 30 mg to a minimum of 100 mL NaCl 0.9%; add each dose of 60–90 mg to a minimum of 250 mL NaCl 0.9%.
4. The solution should be clear and colourless. Inspect visually for particulate matter or discoloration prior to administration and discard if present.
5. Give by IV infusion into a relatively large vein (to minimise local reactions) at a maximum rate of 60 mg/hour (1 mg/minute). In impaired renal function give at a maximum rate of 20 mg/hour.

## Technical information

| | |
|---|---|
| Incompatible with | Pamidronate disodium is incompatible with Hartmann's and Ringer's (contain Ca). |
| Compatible with | **Flush**: NaCl 0.9%<br>**Solutions**: NaCl 0.9%, Gluc 5%<br>**Y-site**: No information |
| pH | 6-7 |
| Sodium content | Negligible |
| Storage | Store below 25°C in original packaging. |
| Displacement value | Negligible (Aredia) |
| Stability after preparation | From a microbiological point of view, should be used immediately; however, prepared infusions may be stored at 2-8°C and infused (at room temperature) within 24 hours. |

## Monitoring

| Measure | Frequency | Rationale |
|---|---|---|
| Hypersensitivity reactions | During and just after infusion | • Anaphylactic reactions, bronchospasm, dyspnoea, angioedema have occasionally been reported. |
| Fluid balance | Frequently during therapy | • Hydration ↑Ca diuresis.<br>• Hydration reduces decline in renal function and decreases formation of calcium renal calculi. |

*(continued)*

## Monitoring (continued)

| Measure | Frequency | Rationale |
|---------|-----------|-----------|
| U&Es, CrCl (or eGFR) | Prior to each dose; periodically post dose | • Enables the infusion to be given at the correct rate.<br>• If renal function declines during therapy, withhold further treatment until renal function returns to within 10% of the baseline value.<br>• ↑K, ↓K, ↑Na have been reported. |
| Serum Ca, PO$_4$, Mg | | • A significant fall in serum Ca is usually seen 24-48 hours after administration, with normalisation within 3-7 days. If normocalcaemia is not achieved within this time, a further dose may be given.<br>• The duration of the response varies. Treatment can be repeated whenever ↑Ca recurs but may become less effective as the number of treatments increase.<br>• Stop treatment if ↓Ca develops.<br>• PO$_4$ and Ca share common control systems. Disruption to Ca metabolism affects PO$_4$ levels.<br>• ↓Mg occurs commonly during treatment. |

## Additional information

| | |
|---|---|
| Common and serious undesirable effects | *Immediate:* Angioedema and bronchospasm have been reported.<br>*Injection/infusion-related:* Injection-site reactions have been observed. Care should be taken to avoid extravasation or inadvertent intra-arterial administration.<br>*Other:* Renal dysfunction, haematuria, asymptomatic and symptomatic ↓Ca (paraesthesia, tetany), pruritus, urticaria, exfoliative dermatitis, fever and influenza-like symptoms, malaise, rigors, fatigue and flushes (usually resolve spontaneously), eye disorders (uveitis, scleritis, conjunctivitis), jaw osteonecrosis (see above). |
| Pharmacokinetics | The apparent elimination half-life in plasma is about 0.8 hour. |
| Significant interactions | None. |
| Action in case of overdose | *Symptoms to watch for:* Clinically significant ↓Ca (paraesthesia, tetany, ↓BP).<br>*Antidote:* Calcium gluconate infusion.<br>Stop administration and give supportive therapy as appropriate. Monitor Ca, PO$_4$, Mg, K. |
| Counselling | Patients should be warned against driving or operating machinery after treatment with pamidronate as somnolence or dizziness may occur for up to 24 hours.<br>Maintain oral fluid intake during the post-infusion hours.<br>Inform of symptoms of ↓Ca (e.g. paraesthesia, tetany, muscle cramps, confusion).<br>Advise of the importance of taking calcium and vitamin D supplements as prescribed where these are indicated.<br>Report any ocular discomfort/loss of visual acuity or injection-site reactions.<br>Advise patients with risk factors for osteonecrosis of the jaw (see Pre-treatment checks) not to undergo invasive dental procedures during treatment. |

Risk rating: **AMBER**    Score = 4
Moderate-risk product: Risk-reduction strategies are recommended.

     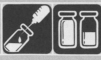

This assessment is based on the full range of preparation and administration options described in the monograph. These may not all be applicable in some clinical situations.

## Reference

1. Ashley C, Currie A, eds. *The Renal Drug Handbook*, 3rd edn. Oxford: Radcliffe Medical Press, 2009.

## Bibliography

SPC AREDIA dry powder 15 mg, 30 mg and 90 mg (accessed 10 February 2009).

SPC Disodium pamidronate 15 mg/ml concentrate for solution for infusion, Wockhardt UK Ltd (accessed 10 February 2009).

SPC Pamidronate disodium 3 mg/mL, 6 mg/mL, 9 mg/mL sterile concentrate, Hospira UK Ltd (accessed 10 February 2009).

SPC Medac Disodium pamidronate 3 mg/ml, sterile concentrate (accessed 10 February 2009).

# Pantoprazole

### 40-mg dry powder vials

• Pantoprazole sodium is a proton pump inhibitor (PPI).
• It may be used IV when the oral route is temporarily unavailable, to treat conditions where inhibition of gastric acid secretion may be beneficial: treatment and prevention of gastric and duodenal ulcers, gastro-oesophageal reflux disease (GORD) and Zollinger–Ellison syndrome.
• Doses are expressed in terms of pantoprazole:
  Pantoprazole 40 mg ≅ 45.1 mg pantoprazole sodium.

## Pre-treatment checks

• Zinc supplementation should be considered during IV therapy in patients prone to zinc deficiency – the preparation contains edetate disodium, which is a potent metal ion chelator.
• Caution also when used concomitantly with other IV preparations containing edetate disodium.

*Biochemical tests*

LFTs

## Dose

**Duodenal ulcer, gastric ulcer, and gastro-oesophageal reflux:** 40 mg daily.

**Zollinger–Ellison syndrome (and other hypersecretory conditions):** initially 80 mg (160 mg if rapid acid control is required) then 80 mg once daily, adjusted according to response; give daily doses above 80 mg in two divided doses.

**Dose in hepatic impairment:** in severe impairment, the daily dose should be reduced to 20 mg.

## Intravenous injection

*Preparation and administration*

1. Reconstitute each 40-mg vial with 10 mL NaCl 0.9% to make a 4 mg/mL solution.
2. Withdraw the required dose.
3. The solution should be clear and colourless. Inspect visually for particulate matter or discoloration prior to administration. Discard if present.
4. Give by IV injection over 2 minutes.

## Intravenous infusion

*Preparation and administration*

1. Reconstitute each 40-mg vial with 10 mL NaCl 0.9% to make a 4 mg/mL solution.
2. Withdraw the required dose and add to 100 mL of compatible infusion fluid (NaCl 0.9% or Gluc 5%).
3. The solution should be clear and colourless. Inspect visually for particulate matter or discoloration prior to administration. Discard if present.
4. Give by IV infusion over 15 minutes.

## Technical information

| | |
|---|---|
| Incompatible with | Mannitol, sodium bicarbonate.<br>Aciclovir, adrenaline (epinephrine), amikacin, amiodarone, amphotericin, calcium gluconate, cefotaxime, ceftazidime, cefuroxime, ciprofloxacin, clindamycin phosphate, co-trimoxazole, dexamethasone, diazepam, digoxin, dobutamine, dopamine, esmolol, fentanyl, fluconazole, furosemide, gentamicin, glyceryl trinitrate, heparin sodium, hydralazine, hydrocortisone sodium succinate, insulin (soluble), labetalol, magnesium sulfate, meropenem, methylprednisolone sodium succinate, metoclopramide, metronidazole, midazolam, naloxone, noradrenaline (norepinephrine), octreotide, phenytoin sodium, piperacillin with tazobactam, propofol, tobramycin, vecuronium bromide, verapamil. |
| Compatible with | **Flush**: NaCl 0.9%<br>**Solutions**: NaCl 0.9%, Gluc 5%, Hartmann's<br>**Y-site**: Aminophylline, ampicillin, benzylpenicillin, ceftriaxone, ticarcillin with clavulanate, vancomycin, vasopressin |
| pH | 9-10.5 |
| Sodium content | Negligible |
| Storage | Store below 25°C in original packaging. |
| Stability after preparation | From a microbiological point of view, should be used immediately; however:<br>• Reconstituted vials may be stored at 2-8°C for 12 hours.<br>• Prepared infusions may be stored at 2-8°C and infused (at room temperature) within 12 hours. |

## Monitoring

| Measure | Frequency | Rationale |
|---|---|---|
| Signs of infection | Throughout treatment | • Use of anti-secretory drugs may ↑risk of infections such as community-acquired pneumonia, *Salmonella*, *Campylobacter* and *Clostridium difficile*-associated disease. |
| LFTs | Periodically | • Altered LFTs and hepatitis have been reported rarely.<br>• If this occurs, stop treatment. |
| Renal function | | • Acute interstitial nephritis has been reported with PPI's.<br>• ↓Na has been reported with PPIs. |
| Serum vitamin B₁₂ | | • In long-term therapy malabsorption of vitamin $B_{12}$ has been reported. |

## Additional information

| | |
|---|---|
| Common and serious undesirable effects | *Common:* GI disturbances (including nausea, vomiting, abdominal pain, flatulence, diarrhoea, constipation), and headache.<br>*Rare:* Peripheral oedema, paraesthesia, arthralgia, myalgia, rash, and pruritus, ↑liver enzymes, hepatitis, jaundice, hypersensitivity reactions (including anaphylaxis, bronchospasm), hallucinations, confusion, gynaecomastia, interstitial nephritis, ↓Na, blood disorders (including leucopenia, leucocytosis, pancytopenia, thrombocytopenia), visual disturbances, alopecia, Stevens-Johnson syndrome, toxic epidermal necrolysis. |
| Pharmacokinetics | Elimination half-life is about 1–2 hours but may be prolonged (up to 10 hours) in poor metabolisers and patients with liver impairment. |
| Significant interactions | • Pantoprazole may ↓levels or effect of atazanavir (avoid combination).<br>• Pantoprazole may affect the following tests:<br>Antisecretory drug therapy may cause a false-negative urea breath test.<br>May give false-positive tetrahydrocannabinol (THC) urine screening test results. |
| Action in case of overdose | Stop administration and give supportive therapy as appropriate. Pantoprazole is extensively plasma protein bound and is therefore not readily dialysable. |

| | |
|---|---|
| Risk rating: **GREEN** | Score = 1<br>Lower-risk product: Risk-reduction strategies should be considered. |

This assessment is based on the full range of preparation and administration options described in the monograph. These may not all be applicable in some clinical situations.

## Bibliography

SPC Protium i.v. powder for solution for injection (accessed 26 June 2009).

# Papaveretum

**15.4 mg/mL solution in 1-mL ampoules**

This preparation must not be confused with papaverine.

* Papaveretum is a mixture of opium alkaloids and in the UK contains the hydrochlorides of morphine, codeine, and papaverine. In the past it additionally contained noscapine but this was removed from the UK formulation in 1993; it may still be contained in this product in other countries.
* It is licensed for premedication, enhancement of anaesthesia, postoperative analgesia and for severe chronic pain.
* Doses are expressed as papaveretum:
  Papaveretum 15.4 mg ≅ 10 mg anhydrous morphine.

## Pre-treatment checks

* Do not use in acute respiratory depression, where there is a risk of paralytic ileus, in ↑intracranial pressure and in head injury, in comatose patients, in heart failure secondary to chronic lung disease and phaeochromocytoma.
* Caution in ↓BP, shock, convulsive disorders, supraventricular tachycardias, atrial flutter, chronic obstructive pulmonary disease and acute asthma attack, obstructive or inflammatory bowel diseases, biliary tract diseases, alcoholism, prostatic hyperplasia, myasthenia gravis, hypothyroidism (reduce dose), adrenocortical insufficiency (reduce dose).
* Caution in elderly patients or those of low bodyweight.
* Ensure that resuscitation equipment and naloxone are available, especially for IV administration.

*Biochemical and other tests (not all are necessary in an emergency situation)*

| | |
|---|---|
| Blood pressure and pulse | Renal function: U, Cr, CrCl (or eGFR) |
| LFTs | Respiratory rate |
| Pain score | |

## Dose

The CSM has advised (in 1993) that to avoid confusion the figures 7.7 mg or 15.4 mg should be used for prescribing purposes.

**Standard dose:** 7.7–15.4 mg by IM or SC injection every 4 hours if necessary (elderly patients initially 7.7 mg) If given by IV injection the dose should be reduced to 25–50% of the corresponding IM or SC dose.
**Pre-operative medication:** 7.7–15.4 mg by IM or SC injection.
**Dose in renal impairment:** reduce the dose or avoid (especially if severe).
**Dose in hepatic impairment:** reduce the dose or avoid.

## Intramuscular injection (preferred route)

*Preparation and administration*

1. Withdraw the required dose.
2. Give by IM injection.
3. Close monitoring of respiratory rate and consciousness is recommended for 30 minutes in patients receiving an initial dose, especially elderly patients or those of low bodyweight.

## Subcutaneous injection

*Preparation and administration*

1. Withdraw the required dose.
2. Give by SC injection.
3. Close monitoring of respiratory rate and consciousness is recommended for 30 minutes in patients receiving an initial dose, especially elderly patients or those of low bodyweight.

## Intravenous injection

*Preparation and administration*

1. Withdraw the required dose. It may be diluted to 10 mL with NaCl 0.9% or Gluc 5% to facilitate slow administration.
2. The solution should be clear and colourless. Inspect visually for particulate matter or discoloration prior to administration and discard if present.
3. Give by slow IV injection over 2–3 minutes.
4. Close monitoring of respiratory rate and consciousness is recommended for 30 minutes in patients receiving an initial dose, especially elderly patients or those of low bodyweight.

## Technical information

| | |
|---|---|
| Incompatible with | Flucloxacillin, furosemide. |
| Compatible with | **Flush**: NaCl 0.9%<br>**Solutions**: NaCl 0.9%, Gluc 5%<br>**Y-site**: No information |
| pH | 3.7–4.7 |
| Sodium content | Negligible |
| Excipients | Contains sulfites (may cause hypersensitivity reactions). |
| Storage | Store below 25°C in original packaging. Do not freeze. Controlled Drug. |

## Monitoring

Close monitoring of respiratory rate and consciousness is recommended for 30 minutes in patients receiving an initial dose, especially elderly patients or those of low bodyweight.

| Measure | Frequency | Rationale |
|---|---|---|
| Pain | At regular intervals | • To ensure therapeutic response. |
| Blood pressure, pulse and respiratory rate | | • ↓BP, ↓pulse, ↑pulse, palpitations and respiratory depression with ↓oxygen saturation can occur. |
| Sedation | At regular intervals | • Can cause sedation. |
| Monitor for side-effects and toxicity | | • Can cause side-effects such as itching and nausea and vomiting and constipation, which may need treating. |

## Additional information

| | |
|---|---|
| Common and serious undesirable effects | *Common:* Nausea and vomiting (particularly initially), constipation, dry mouth, urticaria, pruritus, biliary spasm, ↑ or ↓pulse, hallucinations, euphoria, drowsiness.<br>*At higher doses:* ↓BP, sedation, respiratory depression, muscle rigidity. |
| Pharmacokinetics | Elimination half-life of morphine is about 2 hours; 2.4-6.7 hours for morphine-3-glucuronide (active metabolite); 2.5-4 hours for codeine; about 100 minutes for papaverine. |
| Significant interactions | • The following may ↑papaveretum levels or effect (or ↑side-effects): antihistamines-sedating (↑sedation), MAOIs (avoid combination and for 2 weeks after stopping MAOI), moclobemide.<br>• Papaveretum may ↑levels or effect (or ↑side-effects) of sodium oxybate (avoid combination). |
| Action in case of overdose | *Symptoms to watch for:* ↑Sedation, respiratory depression.<br>*Antidote:* Naloxone (see the Naloxone monograph) Stop administration and give supportive therapy as appropriate. |
| Counselling | If the patient is pregnant or breast feeding she should inform her doctor. Inform the patient of possible side-effects: see above.<br>May cause drowsiness and dizziness that may affect the ability to perform skilled tasks; if affected do not drive or operate machinery. To help avoid dizziness, get up slowly from a sitting or lying position.<br>Drink plenty of fluids to help avoid constipation and use a laxative if required. |

| | |
|---|---|
| Risk rating: **GREEN** | Score = 2<br>Lower-risk product: Risk-reduction strategies should be considered. |

This assessment is based on the full range of preparation and administration options described in the monograph. These may not all be applicable in some clinical situations.

## Bibliography

SPC Martindale Pharmaceuticals Papaveretum Injection BP 15.4 mg/mL (received 26 February 2009).

# Papaveretum with hyoscine hydrobromide

**Solution in 1-mL ampoules (≡ papaveretum 15.4 mg/mL with hyoscine hydrobromide 400 micrograms/mL)**

This preparation must not be confused with papaverine.

* Papaveretum is a mixture of opium alkaloids and in the UK contains the hydrochlorides of morphine, codeine, and papaverine. In the past it additionally contained noscapine but this was removed from the UK formulation in 1993; it may still be contained in this product in other countries.
* Hyoscine hydrobromide is a tertiary amine with antimuscarinic activity which reduces secretions during surgery.
* The preparation is licensed for premedication.
* Papaveretum 15.4 mg ≅ 10 mg anhydrous morphine.
* Doses below are quoted in millilitres of the combined product.

## Pre-treatment checks

* Do not use in acute respiratory depression, where there is a risk of paralytic ileus, in ↑intracranial pressure and in head injury, in comatose patients, in heart failure secondary to chronic lung disease and phaeochromocytoma.
* Caution in ↓BP, shock, convulsive disorders, supraventricular tachycardias, atrial flutter, chronic obstructive pulmonary disease and acute asthma attack, obstructive or inflammatory bowel diseases, biliary tract diseases, alcoholism, prostatic hyperplasia, myasthenia gravis, hypothyroidism (reduce dose), adrenocortical insufficiency (reduce dose).
* Caution in elderly patients or those of low bodyweight.
* Ensure that resuscitation equipment and naloxone are available, especially for IV administration.

*Biochemical and other tests (not all are necessary in an emergency situation)*

Blood pressure and pulse
LFTs

Renal function: U, Cr, CrCl (or eGFR)
Respiratory rate

## Dose

**Preoperative medication:** 0.5–1 mL as a single dose by IM or SC injection 45–60 minutes before anaesthesia (use 0.5 mL in elderly patients or those of low bodyweight and frail).
**Dose in renal impairment:** avoid if CrCl <20 mL/minute.
**Dose in hepatic impairment:** reduce dose or avoid (may precipitate coma).

## Intramuscular injection (preferred route)

*Preparation and administration*

1. Withdraw the required dose.
2. Give by IM injection.
3. Close monitoring of respiratory rate and consciousness is recommended for 30 minutes in patients receiving an initial dose, especially elderly patients or those of low bodyweight.

## Subcutaneous injection

*Preparation and administration*

1. Withdraw the required dose.
2. Give by SC injection.
3. Close monitoring of respiratory rate and consciousness is recommended for 30 minutes in patients receiving an initial dose, especially elderly patients or those of low bodyweight.

## Technical information

| | |
|---|---|
| Incompatible with | Not relevant |
| Compatible with | Not relevant |
| pH | 2.5-4.0 |
| Sodium content | Negligible |
| Excipients | Contains sulfites (may cause hypersensitivity reactions). |
| Storage | Store below 25°C in original packaging. Do not freeze. Controlled Drug. |

## Monitoring

Close monitoring of respiratory rate and consciousness is recommended for 30 minutes in patients receiving an initial dose, especially elderly patients or those of low bodyweight.

| Measure | Frequency | Rationale |
|---|---|---|
| Pain | At regular intervals | • To ensure therapeutic response. |
| Blood pressure, pulse and respiratory rate | | • ↓BP, ↓pulse, ↑pulse, palpitations and respiratory depression with ↓oxygen saturation can occur. |
| Sedation | | • Can cause sedation. |
| Monitor for side-effects and toxicity | | • Can cause side-effects such as itching and nausea and vomiting and constipation, which may need treating. |

## Additional information

| | |
|---|---|
| Common and serious undesirable effects | *Common:* Nausea and vomiting (particularly initially), constipation, dry mouth, urticaria, pruritus, biliary spasm, ↑ or ↓pulse, hallucinations, euphoria, drowsiness, blurred vision, difficulty with micturition.<br>*At higher doses:* ↓BP, sedation, respiratory depression, muscle rigidity. |
| Pharmacokinetics | Elimination half-life of morphine is about 2 hours; 2.4-6.7 hours for morphine-3-glucuronide (active metabolite); 2.5-4 hours for codeine; about 100 minutes for papaveretum; about 8 hours for hyoscine hydrobromide. |

*(continued)*

## Additional information (*continued*)

| | |
|---|---|
| Significant interactions | • The following may ↑papaveretum levels or effect (or ↑side-effects): antihistamines-sedating (↑sedation), MAOIs (avoid combination and for 2 weeks after stopping MAOI), moclobemide.<br>• Papaveretum may ↑levels or effect (or ↑side-effects) of sodium oxybate (avoid combination). |
| Action in case of overdose | *Symptoms to watch for (papaveretum):* ↑Sedation, respiratory depression.<br>*Antidote (papaveretum):* Naloxone (see the Naloxone monograph). Stop administration and give supportive therapy as appropriate. |
| Counselling | If the patient is pregnant or breast feeding she should inform her doctor. Inform the patient of possible side-effects: see above.<br>May cause drowsiness and dizziness that may affect the ability to perform skilled tasks; if affected do not drive or operate machinery. To help avoid dizziness, get up slowly from a sitting or lying position.<br>Drink plenty of fluids to help avoid constipation and use a laxative if required. |

| Risk rating: **GREEN** | Score = 2<br>Lower-risk product: Risk-reduction strategies should be considered. |
|---|---|

This assessment is based on the full range of preparation and administration options described in the monograph. These may not all be applicable in some clinical situations.

## Bibliography

SPC Martindale Pharmaceuticals, Papaveretum and hyoscine injection 15.4 mg and 400 micrograms/mL (received 26 February 2009).

# Paracetamol (acetaminophen)

**10 mg/mL solution in 50-mL and 100-mL vials**
• Paracetamol has analgesic and antipyretic activity and some anti-inflammatory activity.
• It is used IV for the short-term treatment of moderate pain and pyrexia when administration by other routes is not possible or appropriate.
• It provides onset of pain relief within 5–10 minutes and exerts its antipyretic effect within 30 minutes.

## Pre-treatment checks

• Avoid in severe hepatic impairment.
• Caution in non-severe hepatic impairment, renal impairment, alcoholism, chronic malnutrition due to low hepatic glutathione reserves and dehydration.

*Biochemical and other tests*

LFTs

Renal function: U, Cr, CrCl (or eGFR)

## Dose

**Adult ≥50 kg:** 1 g every 4–6 hours when required. Maximum 4 g in any 24-hour period.

**Adult <50 kg:** 15 mg/kg (1.5 mL/kg) every 4–6 hours when required. Maximum 60 mg/kg daily (without exceeding 3 g in any 24-hour period).

**Dose in renal impairment:** adjusted according to CrCl:

*   CrCl < 30 mL/minute: normal adult dose but increase dose interval to a minimum of 6 hours.

**Dose in hepatic impairment:** in adults with hepatocellular insufficiency, chronic alcoholism, chronic malnutrition (low reserves of hepatic glutathione) or dehydration, the maximum daily dose must not exceed 3 g.

## Intermittent intravenous infusion

*Preparation and administration*

1.  Select the appropriate dose.
2.  The infusion is pre-prepared for use. It should be clear and slightly yellowish. Inspect visually for particulate matter or discoloration prior to administration and discard if present.
3.  Give by IV infusion over 15 minutes.

## Technical information

| Incompatible with | No information |
|---|---|
| Compatible with | **Flush**: NaCl 0.9%<br>**Solutions**: NaCl 0.9%, Gluc 5%<br>**Y-site**: No information |
| pH | 5.5 |
| Sodium content | Negligible |
| Storage | Store below 30°C. Do not refrigerate or freeze. |

## Monitoring

| Measure | Frequency | Rationale |
|---|---|---|
| Infusion reactions | Throughout infusion | • May cause irritation at site of infusion. |
| Body temperature | At regular intervals | • To ensure therapeutic response. |
| Pain | | |
| Renal function | Periodically if prolonged usage | • Changes in renal function may require a dose frequency adjustment. |
| LFTs | | • If hepatic function deteriorates may require cessation. |

## Additional information

| | |
|---|---|
| Common and serious undesirable effects | *Immediate:* Anaphylaxis and other hypersensitivity reactions have been rarely reported.<br>*Other:* ↓BP, ↑LFTs; rarely rashes, thrombocytopenia, leucopenia, neutropenia. |
| Pharmacokinetics | Elimination half-life is 2.7 hours. |
| Significant interactions | No significant interactions known. |
| Action in case of overdose | See Acetylcysteine monograph. |
| Counselling | Avoid other paracetamol-containing products. |

| | |
|---|---|
| Risk rating: **GREEN** | Score = 0<br>Lower-risk product: Risk-reduction strategies should be considered. |

This assessment is based on the full range of preparation and administration options described in the monograph. These may not all be applicable in some clinical situations.

## Bibliography

SPC Perfalgan 10 mg/mL solution for infusion (accessed 25 January 2010).

# Parathyroid hormone (human recombinant parathyroid hormone)

**1.61 mg powder plus solvent in dual-chamber cartridge for use in Preotact pen**

- Parathyroid hormone (PTH) is secreted by the parathyroid gland and maintains normal concentrations of ionised Ca in extracellular fluid. It increases renal reabsorption of Ca and decreases $PO_4$ excretion. It also promotes the conversion of vitamin D to its active metabolite, which increases Ca absorption from the GI tract.
- PTH acts on bone to accelerate the release of Ca and $PO_4$ into the extracellular fluid: ↓Ca stimulates PTH secretion, whereas ↑Ca has an inhibitory effect. 1,25-Dihydroxycholecalciferol can also suppress PTH secretion.
- Therapeutically, PTH is used for the treatment of osteoporosis in postmenopausal women at high risk of fractures.

## Pre-treatment checks

- PTH is for use in postmenopausal women, there is no data available for other patient groups.
- Do not use in hypercalcaemia, other disturbances of calcium–phosphate metabolism or if bone-specific Alk Phos is raised.
- Do not use in patients with metabolic bone disease such as hyperparathyroidism and Paget disease.
- Do not use in patients who have received radiation therapy to the skeleton.
- May be used in mild to moderate hepatic impairment (Child–Pugh 7–9). Do not use in severe hepatic impairment.
- Prescribe oral calcium and vitamin D supplements if dietary intake is inadequate.

*Biochemical and other tests*

Electrolytes: serum Ca, $PO_4$, Mg
LFTs
Renal function: U, Cr, CrCl (or eGFR)

## Dose

**Standard dose:** 100 micrograms once daily by SC injection for up to 24 months.
Each dual-chamber cartridge provides 14 doses of 100 micrograms. All patients should receive training in the use of the pen and a user manual is provided with each pen.
**Dose in renal impairment:** do not give if CrCl < 30 mL/minute.

## Subcutaneous injection

*Preparation and administration*

1. Refer to the Preotact user manual for full details of reconstitution and administration.
2. The solution should be clear and colourless. Inspect visually and discard cartridge if solution is cloudy, coloured or contains particles.
3. Give the dose by SC injection, taking care to rotate injection sites.

## Technical information

| | |
|---|---|
| Incompatible with | Not relevant |
| Compatible with | Not relevant |
| pH | Not relevant |
| Sodium content | Negligible |
| Excipients | Contains metacresol which may cause hypersensitivity reactions. |
| Storage | Store below 25°C in original packaging. Do not freeze. |
| Stability after preparation | *Mixed solution in cartridge:*<br>Store between 2–8°C for up to 28 days. Do not freeze.<br>May be stored at room temperature (<25°C) for up to 7 days of the 28-day use period if necessary.<br>The mixed cartridge must not be removed from the pen whilst in use.<br>Do not shake at any point as this may denature the active substance. |

## Monitoring

| Measure | Frequency | Rationale |
|---|---|---|
| Serum Ca, PO₄ | On initiation, and at months 1, 3 and 6 of treatment (further monitoring is not necessary if stable at this point) | • Can cause ↑Ca. Take samples at least 20 hours after the most recent dose.<br>• PO₄ and Ca share common control systems. Disruption to Ca metabolism affects PO₄ levels.<br>• If serum Ca is elevated:<br>  • Stop calcium and vitamin D supplements.<br>  • Change dosing to 100 micrograms on alternate days.<br>  • If persistently raised, stop PTH treatment and monitor Ca. |

## Additional information

| | |
|---|---|
| Common and serious undesirable effects | *Immediate:* Hypersensitivity reactions have been reported (possibly preservative related).<br>*Injection-related:* Local: Erythema at injection sites.<br>*Other:* Transient ↑Ca (in both serum and urine), nausea (occasionally with vomiting), diarrhoea, constipation, headache. |
| Pharmacokinetics | SC PTH produces peak plasma concentrations 1-2 hours after injection. Average half-life is about 1.5 hours and absolute bioavailability is about 55%. Serum Ca concentrations reach a maximum at 6-8 hours post dose and normally return to baseline by 20-24 hours after each dose. |
| Significant interactions | No significant interactions. |
| Action in case of overdose | In severe ↑Ca give supportive therapy as appropriate. |
| Counselling | Training in the preparation, use and storage of the pen and rotation of injection sites.<br>Report symptoms of ↑Ca: persistent constipation or diarrhoea, constant headache, vertigo, loss of appetite, polyuria, thirst, sweating.<br>Advise of the need for further blood tests. |

| Risk rating: **GREEN** | Score = 2<br>Lower-risk product: Risk-reduction strategies should be considered. |
|---|---|

This assessment is based on the full range of preparation and administration options described in the monograph. These may not all be applicable in some clinical situations.

## Bibliography

SPC Preotact (accessed 27 February 2009).

# Parecoxib

**20-mg and 40-mg dry powder vials with solvent (NaCl 0.9%)**

* Parecoxib sodium is a selective COX-2 inhibitor.
* It is used for the short-term management of acute postoperative pain.
* Doses are expressed in terms of the base:
  Parecoxib 40 mg ≡ 42.4 mg parecoxib sodium.

## Pre-treatment checks

Avoid in patients with a history of severe allergic drug reactions to aspirin or NSAIDs (including COX-2 inhibitors), active peptic ulceration or GI bleeding, inflammatory bowel disease, congestive heart failure, post coronary artery bypass graft, severe hepatic failure (Child–Pugh score >10 or serum albumin <25 g/L).

*Biochemical and other tests*

Blood pressure
Electrolytes: serum Na, K

LFTs
Renal function: U, Cr, CrCl (or eGFR)

## Dose

**Postoperative pain:** 40 mg by IV or IM injection, then 20–40 mg every 6–12 hours as required. Maximum daily dose is 80 mg. There is limited experience of treating for more than 3 days.

**Dose in renal impairment:** adjusted according to creatinine clearance:[1]

* CrCl >30–50 mL/minute: dose as in normal renal function; use with caution.
* CrCl 10–30 mL/minute: dose as in normal renal function; avoid if possible.
* CrCl <10 mL/minute: dose as in normal renal function but avoid unless on dialysis.

## Intravenous injection

*Preparation and administration*

1. Reconstitute each 20-mg vial with 1 mL solvent (use 2 mL for each 40-mg vial).
2. Gently swirl the vial to dissolve the powder to give a solution containing 20 mg/mL.
3. The solution should be clear and colourless. Inspect visually for particulate matter or discoloration prior to administration and discard if present.
4. Withdraw the required dose.
5. Give by rapid IV injection.

## Intramuscular injection

*Preparation and administration*

1. Reconstitute each 20-mg vial with 1 mL solvent (use 2 mL for each 40-mg vial).
2. Gently swirl the vial to dissolve the powder to give a solution containing 20 mg/mL.
3. Withdraw the required dose.
4. Give by deep IM injection

## Technical information

| | |
|---|---|
| Incompatible with | Parecoxib is incompatible with Hartmann's; reconstitution with WFI is not recommended (the resultant solution is not isotonic). |
| Compatible with | **Flush**: NaCl 0.9%<br>**Solutions**: NaCl 0.9%, Gluc 5%, Gluc-NaCl (may be used to reconstitute vials)<br>**Y-site**: No information |
| pH | 7.5-8.5 (reconstituted) |
| Sodium content | Negligible |
| Storage | Store below 30°C in original packaging.<br>Vials are single use only - discard the unused portion. |
| Stability after preparation | From a microbiological point of view, should be used immediately; however, reconstituted vials are stable for 24 hours at 25°C. |

## Monitoring

| Measure | Frequency | Rationale |
|---|---|---|
| Pain relief | Post injection | • To ensure that treatment is effective. |
| Blood pressure | Periodically | • May cause ↑BP or ↓BP. |
| Skin | | • Check for any rash or other reaction. |
| U&Es, Cr, LFTs and FBC | | • If on long-term treatment. |

## Additional information

| | |
|---|---|
| Common and serious undesirable effects | *Immediate*: Anaphylaxis and other hypersensitivity reactions may occur.<br>*Other*: Postoperative anaemia, ↓K, agitation, insomnia, hypo-aesthesia, ↑ or ↓BP, respiratory insufficiency, pharyngitis, dyspepsia, flatulence, pruritus, back pain, oliguria, peripheral oedema. |
| Pharmacokinetics | Elimination half-life is approximately 8 hours. |
| Significant interactions | • The following may ↑risk of bleeding with parecoxib: antidepressants-SSRIs, aspirin, dabigatran, erlotinib, ketorolac, NSAIDs, venlafaxine.<br>• Parecoxib may ↑levels or effect of the following drugs (or ↑side-effects): ciclosporin (↑risk of nephrotoxicity), coumarin anticoagulants (monitor INR), lithium (monitor levels), methotrexate (↑toxicity, avoid combination), phenindione (monitor INR), phenytoin (monitor levels), quinolones (↑risk of seizures), sulfonylureas. |
| Action in case of overdose | *Antidote*: No known antidote; stop administration and give supportive therapy as appropriate. |
| Counselling | Advise the patient to report skin reactions. |

| Risk rating: **GREEN** | Score = 1<br>Lower-risk product: Risk-reduction strategies should be considered. |
| --- | --- |

This assessment is based on the full range of preparation and administration options described in the monograph. These may not all be applicable in some clinical situations.

## Reference

1. Ashley C, Currie A, eds. *The Renal Drug Handbook*, 3rd edn. Oxford: Radcliffe Medical Press, 2009.

## Bibliography

SPC Dynastat (accessed 14 February 2010).

# Paricalcitol

### 5 micrograms/mL solution in 1-mL and 2-mL ampoules

* Paricalcitol is an analogue of calcitriol, the active form of vitamin D. It is reported to have less effect on Ca and $PO_4$ concentrations while retaining the suppressive effect on parathyroid hormone (PTH).
* It is indicated for the prevention and treatment of secondary hyperparathyroidism in patients with chronic renal failure undergoing haemodialysis. Paricalcitol may also be given orally for this indication.

## Pre-treatment checks

Do not give to patients with hypercalcaemia, including hypercalcaemia of malignancy.

*Biochemical and other tests*

Baseline PTH level (measured in either picomol/L or pg/mL)
Electrolytes: serum Ca (corrected), $PO_4$

Liver function: Alk Phos
Renal function: U, Cr, CrCl (or eGFR)

## Dose

**Initial dose:** calculated using baseline intact PTH levels (formula depends on reported PTH units):

$$\text{Initial dose (micrograms)} = \frac{\text{Baseline intact PTH level (picomol/L)}}{8}$$

$$\text{Initial dose (micrograms)} = \frac{\text{Baseline intact PTH level (picograms/mL)}}{80}$$

Give the dose no more frequently than every other day at any time during dialysis. The maximum dose used in clinical studies was as high as 40 micrograms.

*Titration dose*

- The currently accepted target range for PTH levels in end-stage renal failure subjects undergoing dialysis is no more than 1.5–3 times the non-uremic ULN, i.e. 15.9–31.8 picomol/L (150–300 picograms/mL) for intact PTH.
- Close monitoring and individual dose titration are necessary to adjust treatment.
- If the patient is hypercalcaemic or (corrected Ca × PTH level) > 5.2 mmol²/L² (65 mg²/dL²), reduce the dose or stop treatment until these parameters have returned to normal values.
- At this point, paricalcitol may be restarted at a lower dose.
- The dose may need to be decreased as the PTH levels reduce in response to therapy.
- Table P2 gives further guidance on how to adjust the dose.

**Table P2**  Suggested paricalcitol dosing guidelines (dose adjustments at 2–4 week intervals)

| Intact PTH level relative to baseline | Paricalcitol dose adjustment |
|---|---|
| Same or increased | Increase by 2–4 micrograms |
| Decreased by <30% | |
| Decreased by 30–60% | Continue with current dose |
| Decreased >60% | Decrease by 2–4 micrograms |
| Intact PTH <15.9 picomol/L (150 picograms/mL) | |

## Via haemodialysis access

*Preparation and administration*

1. Withdraw the required dose.
2. The solution should be clear and colourless. Inspect visually for particulate matter or discoloration prior to administration.
3. Give by IV injection via haemodialysis access before, during or after haemodialysis sessions.

| Technical information | |
|---|---|
| Incompatible with | *Haemodialysis access:* heparin sodium (give through a different injection port because the propylene glycol component of paricalcitol injection neutralises the effect of heparin). |
| Compatible with | **Flush**: WFI<br>**Solutions**: not relevant<br>**Y-site**: not relevant |
| pH | Not relevant |
| Sodium content | Nil |

*(continued)*

## Technical information (continued)

| | |
|---|---|
| Excipients | Contains ethanol (may interact with metronidazole, possible religious objections).<br>Contains propylene glycol (adverse effects seen in ↓renal function, may interact with disulfiram and metronidazole). |
| Storage | Store below 25°C in original packaging but do not refrigerate. Use immediately after opening. |

## Monitoring

| Measure | Frequency | Rationale |
|---|---|---|
| Serum intact PTH | Every 2–4 weeks during dosage adjustment; every 3 months once stable | • Necessary for dosage adjustment.<br>• See Table P2 for dose adjustment guidance. |
| Ca (corrected) and PO$_4$ | Every 2–4 weeks during dosage adjustment; at least every month once stable | • ↑Ca and ↑PO$_4$ can occur during treatment with paricalcitol. This is dependent on the level of PTH oversuppression and can be minimised by proper dose titration.<br>• Plasma PO$_4$ should be controlled during therapy to reduce the risk of ectopic calcification. |
| Alk Phos | Monthly | • A fall in Alk Phos levels often precedes ↑Ca. |
| Ophthalmological examination | Periodically | • To check for ectopic calcification. |

## Additional information

| | |
|---|---|
| Common and serious undesirable effects | *Injection-related:* Local: Rarely injection-site pain.<br>*Other:* ↑Ca (persistent constipation or diarrhoea, constant headache, vertigo, loss of appetite, polyuria, thirst, sweating), pruritus, taste disturbance, headache. |
| Pharmacokinetics | The mean half-life in patients with chronic renal failure requiring haemodialysis is about 15 hours. No accumulation of paricalcitol was observed with multiple dosing. |
| Significant interactions | Injectable preparation contains ethanol and propylene glycol: may interact with disulfiram and metronidazole. |
| Action in case of overdose | Stop treatment if ↑Ca develops until plasma Ca levels return to normal.<br>In severe ↑Ca give supportive therapy as appropriate.<br>Restart treatment at a lower dose if appropriate. |
| Counselling | Advise patients to report symptoms of ↑Ca: persistent constipation or diarrhoea, constant headache, vertigo, loss of appetite, polyuria, thirst, sweating.<br>Advise of the need for further blood tests. |

Risk rating: **GREEN**    Score = 2
Lower-risk product: Risk-reduction strategies should be considered.

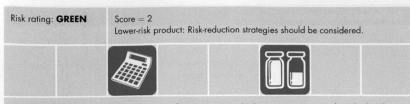

This assessment is based on the full range of preparation and administration options described in the monograph. These may not all be applicable in some clinical situations.

## Bibliography

SPC Zemplar 5 microgram/ml solution for injection (accessed 25 January 2009).

# Pegfilgrastim

**10 mg/mL (expressed as filgrastim) solution in pre-filled syringe: 6 mg/0.6 mL**

* Pegfilgrastim is pegylated recombinant methionyl human granulocyte colony-stimulating factor (G-CSF), produced using r-DNA technology in *E. coli*. It acts primarily on neutrophil precursors to increase neutrophil levels and has a more sustained action than filgrastim.
* It is used to treat or prevent neutropenia in patients receiving myelosuppressive cancer chemotherapy (except in chronic myeloid leukaemia and myelodysplastic syndromes),
* Doses are expressed as milligrams of filgrastim.

## Pre-treatment checks

* Contraindicated in chronic myeloid leukaemia, secondary acute myeloid leukaemia, and myelodysplastic syndromes.
* Caution recommended in acute myeloid leukaemia.
* Check recent pulmonary history (recent history of pulmonary infiltrates or pneumonia ↑risk of pulmonary adverse events).
* Confirm whether women of child-bearing potential are pregnant or breast feeding (contraindicated unless benefit outweighs risk, at discretion of clinician).
* Ensure patient is adequately hydrated.
* Ensure patient not allergic to latex (needle sheath of the pre-filled syringe contains natural dry rubber).

*Biochemical and other tests*

FBC

## Dose

**Standard dose:** 6 mg given by SC injection for each chemotherapy cycle starting approximately 24 hours after cytotoxic chemotherapy.

## Subcutaneous injection

*Preparation and administration*

1. The pre-filled syringe should not be shaken as this may inactivate pegfilgrastim.
2. Give by SC injection.

## Technical information

| | |
|---|---|
| Incompatible with | Not relevant |
| Compatible with | Not relevant |
| pH | Not relevant |
| Sodium content | Negligible |
| Storage | Store at 2-8°C in original packaging (accidental freezing for < 24 hours does not affect stability).<br>May be stored at room temperature for up to 72 hours. |

## Monitoring

| Measure | Frequency | Rationale |
|---|---|---|
| Signs of respiratory distress (cough, dyspnoea) | Throughout course of treatment | • May be initial signs of ARDS; discontinue at the discretion of the clinician. |
| Body temperature | Throughout course of treatment | • Pyrexia may indicate ARDS or febrile neutropenia<br>• Discontinue at the discretion of the clinician. |
| Neutrophil count | As regularly as clinically indicated, minimum once each cycle before chemotherapy administration | • ↑Neutrophil count may be preliminary sign of ARDS in association with radiological evidence of pulmonary infiltrations.<br>• Discontinue at the discretion of the clinician. |
| Platelet count | As regularly as clinically indicated, minimum once each cycle before chemotherapy administration | • Thrombocytopenia may occur. |
| Haematocrit | | • Anaemia may occur. |
| WBC count | | • White blood cell counts of ≥100 000 cells/mm³ (≥100 × 10⁹/L) have been reported in rare cases. This is usually transient, occurring within 48 hours of administration. |
| Bone pain | Ongoing | • Relatively common adverse effect due to ↑haemopoietic activity - usually transient.<br>• Usually controlled with standard analgesia. |
| Spleen size (by physical examination/ ultrasound) | If indicated, potentially at each cycle | • Splenomegaly is common, and usually asymptomatic.<br>• Splenic rupture has been reported (consider if patient complains of left upper abdominal pain or shoulder tip pain). |

## Additional information

| | |
|---|---|
| Common and serious undesirable effects | *Immediate:* Anaphylaxis has been reported rarely.<br>*Injection-related:* Local: Injection-site reactions.<br>*Other:*<br>• Common: GI disturbances, anorexia, headache, asthenia, fever, musculoskeletal pain, bone pain, rash, alopecia, thrombocytopenia, and leucocytosis. Less commonly chest pain can occur.<br>• Rare: Pulmonary side-effects, particularly interstitial pneumonia. Splenic rupture. |
| Pharmacokinetics | Elimination half-life is 15-80 hours (neutrophil-mediated clearance, so serum concentrations decline in accordance with neutrophil recovery). |
| Significant interactions | • Lithium may ↑pegfilgrastim effect (or ↑side-effects): potential ↑neutrophil release – more frequent monitoring of neutrophil counts is recommended.<br>• Fluorouracil may ↓pegfilgrastim effect: neutropenia possibly exacerbated. |
| Action in case of overdose | No experience in humans. |
| Counselling | Recognition of sensitivity reactions or signs of infection; importance of regular monitoring of FBC; importance of female patients informing clinicians of plans to become pregnant or to breast feed; provision of full patient information leaflet for self-administration purposes. |

| Risk rating: **GREEN** | Score = 1<br>Lower-risk product: Risk-reduction strategies should be considered. |
|---|---|

This assessment is based on the full range of preparation and administration options described in the monograph. These may not all be applicable in some clinical situations.

## Bibliography

SPC Neulasta, Amgen (accessed 5 June 2009).

# Pegvisomant

### 10-mg, 15-mg, 20-mg dry powder vials plus solvent

• Pegvisomant is a genetically modified analogue of human growth hormone and is a highly selective growth hormone receptor antagonist.
• It is licensed for the treatment of acromegaly in patients who have had an inadequate response to surgery and/or radiation therapy and in whom an appropriate medical treatment with somato-statin analogues did not normalise IGF-I concentrations or was not tolerated.

## Pre-treatment checks

- The vial stopper contains natural rubber latex which may cause latex-sensitivity reactions in susceptible individuals.
- Avoid in pregnancy and breast feeding (insufficient information). Reduction in IGF-I concentration may potentially ↑fertility in female patients. Women of child-bearing potential should take contraceptive precautions.
- The safety and effectiveness of pegvisomant in patients with renal or hepatic insufficiency has not been established and no dosing recommendations are available.
- Initiate and titrate doses only under the supervision of a physician experienced in the treatment of acromegaly.

*Biochemical and other tests*

Liver function: AST; ALT; bilirubin
Renal function: U, Cr, CrCl (or eGFR)
Serum IGF-I concentrations (the use of commercially available growth hormone assays is not appropriate – see Interactions below)

## Dose

**Loading dose:** 80 mg by SC injection.
**Maintenance dose:** the dose is then adjusted (based on serum IGF-I concentration) every 4–6 weeks in increments (or decrements) of 5 mg/day to a suitable maintenance dose (maximum 30 mg daily).

## Subcutaneous injection

*Preparation and administration*

1. Add 1 mL solvent to dry powder vial.
2. Gently dissolve the powder with a slow, swirling motion. Do not shake vigorously, as this might cause denaturation of the active ingredient. After reconstitution, vials contain 10 mg/mL, 15 mg/mL or 20 mg/mL dependent on vial size.
3. Discard the product if the resulting solution is cloudy or contains particulate matter.
4. Give by SC injection into the upper arm, upper thigh, abdomen or buttocks. Rotate injection sites daily to prevent lipohypertrophy.

## Technical information

| | |
|---|---|
| Incompatible with | Not relevant |
| Compatible with | Not relevant |
| pH | Not relevant |
| Sodium content | Negligible |
| Storage | Store at 2-8°C in original packaging. Do not freeze. |
| Displacement value | Negligible |
| Stability after reconstitution | Use the prepared solution immediately. |

## Monitoring

| Measure | Frequency | Rationale |
|---------|-----------|-----------|
| Serum IGF-I levels | Every 4–6 weeks | • Enables dose adjustments to be made (see Dose above). |
| ALT, AST, bilirubin | Every 4–6 weeks for the first 6 months of treatment and periodically thereafter | • Rule out evidence of obstructive biliary tract disease in patients with elevations of ALT and AST.<br>• Monitor ALT and AST at any time in patients exhibiting symptoms suggestive of hepatitis.<br>• Stop therapy if signs of liver disease persist. Tests should normalise following discontinuation. |
| Tumour growth | Assess each time the patient is reviewed | • Growth hormone-secreting pituitary tumours may sometimes expand, causing serious complications (for example, visual field defects). Treatment with pegvisomant does not halt this.<br>• Periodic imaging scans of the sella turcica may facilitate monitoring. |

## Additional information

| | |
|---|---|
| Common and serious undesirable effects | *Injection-related:* Local: erythema, soreness, bruising, bleeding, hypertrophy, lipohypertrophy.<br>*Other:* ↑Liver enzymes, chronic hepatitis, diarrhoea, constipation, nausea, vomiting, abdominal distension, dyspepsia, headache, dizziness, drowsiness, tremor, sweating, pruritus, rash, arthralgia, hunger, weight gain, hyperglycaemia, ↑cholesterol, ↑BP, sleep disturbances, influenza-like syndrome, fatigue, arthralgia. |
| Pharmacokinetics | Absorption of pegvisomant following SC administration is slow and prolonged, and peak serum concentrations are not generally attained for 33–77 hours. Half-life ranges from 74–172 hours. |
| Significant interactions | Cross-reaction with commercially available growth hormone assays. These assays should not be used to monitor pegvisomant therapy. |
| Action in case of overdose | Discontinue until IGF-I levels return to within or above the normal range. |
| Counselling | Instructions for proper storage, preparation, and injection technique.<br>Importance of regular monitoring of IGF-I levels.<br>Importance of reporting signs or symptoms of possible liver dysfunction (e.g. jaundice, dark urine, light stools, loss of appetite, nausea, fatigue, abdominal pain).<br>For patients with diabetes mellitus; close monitoring of blood glucose levels.<br>Stress the importance for women of informing clinicians if they are, or plan to become, pregnant or plan to breast feed. |

| Risk rating: **GREEN** | Score = 2<br>Lower-risk product: Risk-reduction strategies should be considered |
|---|---|

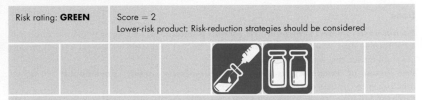

This assessment is based on the full range of preparation and administration options described in the monograph. These may not all be applicable in some clinical situations.

## Bibliography

SPC Somavert (accessed 3 February 2009).

# Pentamidine isetionate (pentamidine isethionate)

### 300-mg dry powder vials

- Pentamidine isetionate is an antiprotozoal agent.
- It is used in the treatment of the early stages of African trypanosomiasis (especially *Trypanosoma brucei gambiense* infections), in some forms of leishmaniasis, and in the treatment and prophylaxis of pneumocystis pneumonia.
- The injection is also licensed for use by nebulisation in the treatment of pneumocystis pneumonia (a ready-made solution for nebulisation also exists).
- Doses are expressed in terms of the base:
  Pentamidine 1 mg ≅ 1.74 mg pentamidine isetionate.

Pentamidine isetionate is toxic and personnel must be adequately protected during handling and administration – consult product literature.

## Pre-treatment checks

- Caution in ↓K, ↓Mg, coronary heart disease, ↓pulse (<50 bpm), history of ventricular arrhythmias, concomitant use with other drugs which prolong QT-interval, ↑BP or ↓BP, pancreatitis, hyperglycaemia or hypoglycaemia, leucopenia, thrombocytopenia or anaemia.
- Ensure that appropriate equipment for maintenance of an adequate airway, other supportive measures and agents (e.g. IV fluids, vasopressor agents) for the management of severe ↓BP are readily available.

*Biochemical and other tests*

Blood pressure
Bodyweight
ECG
Electrolytes: serum K, Ca, Mg

Fasting blood glucose
FBC
LFTs
Renal function: U Cr, CrCl (or eGFR)

## Dose

*Pneumocystis jiroveci (Pneumocystis carinii)* **pneumonia:** 4 mg/kg by IV infusion once daily for at least 14 days. Alternatively give 600 mg via nebuliser once daily for 3 weeks (consult product literature for suitable equipment to be used).

**Prevention of** *Pneumocystis jiroveci (Pneumocystis carinii)* **pneumonia:** 300 mg via nebuliser every 4 weeks or 150 mg every 2 weeks.

**Visceral leishmaniasis:** 3–4 mg/kg by IM injection on alternate days to a maximum of 10 injections. A repeat course may be necessary.

**Cutaneous leishmaniasis:** 3–4 mg/kg by IM injection once or twice weekly until the condition resolves.

**Trypanosomiasis:** 4 mg/kg by IM injection or IV infusion once daily or on alternate days for 7–10 doses.

**Dose in renal impairment:** adjusted according to creatinine clearance:[1]

- CrCl >20–50 mL/minute: dose as in normal renal function.
- CrCl 10–20 mL/minute: dose as in normal renal function.
- CrCl <10 mL/minute: where IV infusion is required, dependent on the severity of the infection, 4 mg/kg/day IV for 7 days then on alternate days to complete a minimum 14 doses *or* 4 mg/kg on alternate days to complete a minimum 14 doses.

## Intramuscular injection

See Special handling below.

*Preparation*

1. Reconstitute a vial with 3 mL WFI to give 300 mg/mL.
2. Withdraw the require dose and discard any remainder in accordance with local protocol.

*Administration*

1. Administer with patient lying down (see Monitoring).
2. Give by deep IM injection into the buttock using the Z-track technique. Rotate injection sites for subsequent injections.

## Intravenous infusion

See Special handling below.

*Preparation*

1. Determine the required dose then reconstitute each vial with a volume of WFI or Gluc 5% to produce a concentration of pentamidine that will give a concentration suitable for delivering this dose, i.e.

| Volume of diluent added | 3 mL | 4 mL | 5 mL |
|---|---|---|---|
| Approximate concentration of pentamidine | 100 mg/mL | 75 mg/mL | 60 mg/mL |

2. Withdraw the required dose and dilute in 50–250 mL NaCl 0.9% or Gluc 5% and discard any remaining vial contents in accordance with local protocol.

*Administration*

1. The patient should be lying down (see Monitoring).
2. Give by slow IV infusion over 60–120 minutes.

## Nebulisation

Consult product literature for detailed guidance on administration and protection of bystanders.

## Technical information

| | |
|---|---|
| Incompatible with | Do not mix with other drugs during infusion. |
| Compatible with | **Flush**: NaCl 0.9%<br>**Solutions**: NaCl 0.9%, Gluc 5%, WFI<br>**Y-site**: No information but likely to be unstable |
| pH | 4.09–5.4 |
| Sodium content | Negligible |
| Storage | Store below 30°C in original packaging. |
| Stability after preparation | Reconstituted vials should be used immediately (risk of precipitation particularly if refrigerated).<br>From a microbiological point of view, it should be used immediately; however, prepared infusions may be stored at 2–8°C and infused (at room temperature) within 24 hours. |
| Displacement volume | 0.15 mL/300 mg |
| Special handling | The manufacturer recommends that initial reconstitution should take place in a fume cupboard, although in practice this may not be feasible.<br>All ward-based preparation should be done in a manner that reduces risk, i.e. wear a face mask and visor alongside normal glove and apron practices in a well-ventilated treatment room, with the door closed and a sign outside indicating no entry during the preparation.<br>Consult product literature when giving via nebuliser. |

## Monitoring

| Measure | Frequency | Rationale |
|---|---|---|
| Blood pressure | During administration and regularly thereafter | • Life-threatening ↓BP may occur.<br>• Measurement should continue until therapy has concluded. |
| ECG | Regularly | • Can prolong the QT interval and life-threatening arrhythmias may occur.<br>• If the QTc interval exceeds 500 milliseconds, consider continuous cardiac monitoring. |
| Renal function, serum K and urinalysis | Daily during therapy | • ↑Cr may require a dose adjustment.<br>• Acute renal failure and severe ↑K may occur. |
| FBC | | • Severe leucopenia and thrombocytopenia may occur. |

*(continued)*

## Monitoring (continued)

| Measure | Frequency | Rationale |
|---------|-----------|-----------|
| Fasting blood glucose | Daily during therapy and regularly thereafter | • Life-threatening hypoglycaemia may occur.<br>• Hyperglycaemia and diabetes mellitus (with or without preceding hypoglycaemia) may occur up to several months after cessation of therapy. |
| Serum Mg | Twice weekly | • ↓Mg may occur. |
| Serum Ca | Weekly | • Severe ↓Ca may occur. |
| LFTs | At least weekly | • If baseline measurements are normal and remain so during therapy, test weekly.<br>• If baseline is elevated or if LFTs increase during therapy, continue monitoring weekly unless the patient is on other hepatotoxic agents, in which case monitor every 3-5 days. |

## Additional information

| | |
|---|---|
| Common and serious undesirable effects | *Injection/infusion-related:* Local: Pain, induration, abscess formation and muscle necrosis.<br>*Other:* Severe reactions, sometimes fatal, due to ↓BP, hypoglycaemia, pancreatitis, and arrhythmias; also leucopenia, thrombocytopenia, acute renal failure, ↓Ca.<br>*On inhalation:* Bronchoconstriction (may be prevented by prior use of bronchodilators), cough, and shortness of breath. |
| Pharmacokinetics | Elimination half-life is 6 hours after IV infusion; 9 hours after IM injection. |
| Significant drug interactions | • Pentamidine may ↑risk of ventricular arrhythmias with the following drugs: amiodarone (avoid combination), amisulpride (avoid combination), antidepressants-tricyclic, droperidol (avoid combination), erythromycin-parenteral, ivabradine, moxifloxacin (avoid combination), phenothiazines. |
| Overdose | No specific antidote; treatment is symptomatic - see Monitoring above. |

| Risk rating: **AMBER** | Score = 4<br>Moderate-risk product: Risk-reduction strategies are recommended. |
|---|---|

This assessment is based on the full range of preparation and administration options described in the monograph. These may not all be applicable in some clinical situations.

## Reference

1. Ashley C, Currie A, eds. *The Renal Drug Handbook*, 3rd edn. Oxford: Radcliffe Medical Press, 2009.

## Bibliography

SPC Pentacarinat 300 mg (accessed 16 February 2009).

# Pentazocine

**30 mg/mL solution 1-mL and 2-mL ampoules**

* Pentazocine lactate has both opioid agonist and antagonist properties. If used in combination with other opioids it may precipitate withdrawal symptoms including the re-emergence of pain.
* It is used for the treatment of moderate to severe pain.
* Parenteral doses are expressed in terms of the base:
  Pentazocine 100 mg ≡ 131.6 mg pentazocine lactate.

## Pre-treatment checks

* Do not use in patients dependent on opioids (can precipitate withdrawal), in heart failure secondary to chronic lung disease and in acute porphyria.
* Caution in pancreatitis, arterial or pulmonary hypertension, cardiac arrhythmias, myocardial infarction, phaeochromocytoma.
* Caution in renal and hepatic impairment.

*Biochemical tests*

LFTs
Renal function: U, Cr, CrCl (or eGFR)

## Dose

**Moderate to severe pain:** 30–60 mg by IM or SC injection or 30 mg by IV injection every 3–4 hours when required to a maximum total daily dose of 360 mg. Individual doses should not exceed 1 mg/kg SC or IM, or 500 micrograms/kg IV.
**Dose in renal impairment:** reduce dose or avoid.
**Dose in hepatic impairment:** reduce dose or avoid.

## Intramuscular injection (preferred to SC route if repeated doses are to be given)

*Preparation and administration*

1. Withdraw the required dose.
2. Give by IM injection. Rotate injection sites for subsequent injections.
3. Close monitoring of respiratory rate and consciousness is recommended for 30 minutes in patients receiving an initial dose, especially elderly patients or those of low bodyweight.

## Intravenous injection

*Preparation and administration*

1. Withdraw the required dose.
2. The solution should be clear and colourless. Inspect visually for particulate matter or discoloration prior to administration and discard if present.
3. Give by IV injection over 3–5 minutes. It may be diluted to 10 mL with NaCl 0.9% to facilitate slow administration.
4. Close monitoring of respiratory rate and consciousness is recommended for 30 minutes in patients receiving an initial dose, especially elderly patients or those of low bodyweight.

## Subcutaneous injection (only use if other routes are not available — risk of tissue damage)

*Preparation and administration*

1. Withdraw the required dose.
2. Give by SC injection.
3. Close monitoring of respiratory rate and consciousness is recommended for 30 minutes in patients receiving an initial dose, especially elderly patients or those of low bodyweight.

## Technical information

| | |
|---|---|
| Incompatible with | Sodium bicarbonate.<br>Aminophylline, diazepam. |
| Compatible with | **Flush**: NaCl 0.9%<br>**Solutions**: NaCl 0.9%, Gluc 5%, Hartmann's, Ringer's (all with added KCl)<br>**Y-site**: Hydrocortisone sodium succinate |
| pH | 4-5 |
| Sodium content | Negligible |
| Storage | Store below 25°C in original packaging. Controlled Drug. |

## Monitoring

Close monitoring of respiratory rate and consciousness is recommended for 30 minutes in patients receiving an initial dose, especially elderly patients or those of low bodyweight.

| Measure | Frequency | Rationale |
|---|---|---|
| Pain | At regular intervals | • To ensure therapeutic response. |
| Blood pressure, pulse and respiratory rate | | • ↓ or ↑BP, ↓ or ↑pulse, palpitations and respiratory depression can occur. |
| Sedation | | • May cause sedation. |
| Monitor for side-effects and toxicity | | • Consider appropriate treatment if itching or constipation occurs. |
| Injection site | | • Can cause ulceration of subcutaneous tissues. |

## Additional information

| | |
|---|---|
| Common and serious undesirable effects | *Immediate:* Anaphylaxis and other hypersensitivity reactions have been reported.<br>*Injection/infusion-related:* Local: Stinging.<br>*Other:* Nausea and vomiting (particularly initially), constipation, dry mouth, urticaria, pruritus, biliary spasm, ↑ or ↓pulse, hallucinations, euphoria, drowsiness. At higher doses: ↓BP, sedation, respiratory depression, muscle rigidity. |
| Pharmacokinetics | Elimination half-life is 2-5 hours. |

*(continued)*

| **Additional information** (continued) | |
|---|---|
| Significant interactions | • The following may ↑pentazocine levels or effect (or ↑side-effects): antihistamines-sedating (↑sedation), MAOIs (avoid combination and for 2 weeks after stopping MAOI), moclobemide.<br>• Pentazocine may ↑levels or effect (or ↑side-effects) of sodium oxybate (avoid combination). |
| Action in case of overdose | *Symptoms to watch for:* ↑Sedation, respiratory depression.<br>*Antidote:* Naloxone (see the Naloxone monograph), but may only partially reverse toxicity.<br>Stop administration and give supportive therapy as appropriate. |
| Counselling | As for other opioids (e.g. see the Dihydrocodeine monograph).<br>Avoid abrupt withdrawal after prolonged exposure; withdrawal symptoms may be atypical and problematic. |

| Risk rating: **GREEN** | Score = 2<br>Lower-risk product: Risk-reduction strategies should be considered. |
|---|---|

This assessment is based on the full range of preparation and administration options described in the monograph. These may not all be applicable in some clinical situations.

## Bibliography

SPC Fortral injection 30 mg/mL (accessed 19 January 2009).

# Pethidine hydrochloride (meperidine hydrochloride)

**50 mg/mL solution in 1-mL and 2-mL ampoules**

* Pethidine hydrochloride is an opioid analgesic.
* It is used to treat moderate to severe acute pain including labour pain. It is also used as a preoperative medication and as an adjunct to anaesthesia.
* Pethidine is less potent and has a shorter duration of action than morphine but is also less constipating. It has ↓effect on smooth muscle and biliary pressure compared with morphine, and therefore may be considered a better analgesic for biliary colic and pancreatitis.

## Pre-treatment checks

* Do not use in acute respiratory depression, where there is a risk of paralytic ileus, in ↑intracranial pressure and in head injury, in comatose patients and phaeochromocytoma.
* Caution in ↓BP, shock, convulsive disorders, supraventricular tachycardias, atrial flutter, chronic obstructive pulmonary disease and acute asthma attack, obstructive or inflammatory bowel

diseases, biliary tract diseases, alcoholism, prostatic hyperplasia, myasthenia gravis, hypothyroidism (reduce dose), adrenocortical insufficiency (reduce dose).
* Caution in elderly patients or those of low bodyweight – use lower doses; the initial dose should not exceed 25 mg.
* Ensure that resuscitation equipment and naloxone are available, especially for IV administration.

*Biochemical and other tests (not all are necessary in an emergency situation)*

Blood pressure and pulse
LFTs
Pain score

Renal function: U, Cr, CrCl (or eGFR)
Respiratory rate

## Dose

Pethidine is no longer considered suitable for the management of chronic pain because of its short duration of action and ↑risk of seizures due to the accumulation of its toxic metabolite norpethidine.

**Acute pain:** 25–100 mg by IM or SC injection or 25–50 mg by slow IV injection repeated after 4 hours if required.
**Obstetric pain:** 50–100 mg by IM or SC injection once contractions are at regular intervals, repeated as required up to a maximum 400 mg in 24 hours.
**Premedication:** 25–100 mg by IM injection 1 hour before procedure.
**Dose in renal impairment:** adjusted according to creatinine clearance,[1]
* CrCl >20 mL/minute: normal adult dose.
* CrCl 10–20 mL/minute: increase dosing interval to 6-hourly and ↓dose by 25%.
* CrCl <10 mL/minute: avoid if possible. If not, increase dosing interval to 8-hourly and ↓dose by 50%.

**Dose in hepatic impairment:** reduce dose or avoid.

## Intramuscular injection (preferred to SC route for repeated doses but absorption is variable)

*Preparation and administration*

1. Withdraw the required dose.
2. Ensure that the patient is sitting or lying down.
3. Give by IM injection into a large muscle such as the gluteus or the lateral aspect of the thigh; take care to avoid nerve trunks.
4. Close monitoring of respiratory rate and consciousness is recommended for 30 minutes in patients receiving an initial dose, especially elderly patients or those of low bodyweight.

## Subcutaneous injection (may be irritant if repeated doses are given)

*Preparation and administration*

1. Withdraw the required dose.
2. Ensure that the patient is sitting or lying down.
3. Give by SC injection.
4. Close monitoring of respiratory rate and consciousness is recommended for 30 minutes in patients receiving an initial dose, especially elderly patients or those of low bodyweight.

## Intravenous injection (↑incidence of adverse effects)

*Preparation and administration*

1. Withdraw the required dose and dilute to 10 mg/mL using WFI, NaCl 0.9% or Gluc 5%.
2. The solution should be clear and colourless. Inspect visually for particulate matter or discoloration prior to administration and discard if present.

3. Ensure that the patient is lying down.
4. Give by slow IV injection over a minimum of 2–3 minutes.
5. Close monitoring of respiratory rate and consciousness is recommended for 30 minutes in patients receiving an initial dose, especially elderly patients or those of low bodyweight.

## Technical information

| | |
|---|---|
| Incompatible with | Sodium bicarbonate.<br>Aciclovir, aminophylline, amphotericin, flucloxacillin, furosemide, heparin sodium, imipenem with cilastatin, micafungin, pantoprazole, phenytoin sodium. |
| Compatible with | **Flush**: NaCl 0.9%<br>**Solutions**: NaCl 0.9%, Gluc 5%, Gluc-NaCl, Hartmann's, Ringer's (all with added KCl)<br>**Y-site**: Amikacin, ampicillin, atenolol, aztreonam, benzylpenicillin, bumetanide, cefotaxime, ceftazidime, ceftriaxone, cefuroxime, chloramphenicol sodium succinate, cisatracurium, clindamycin, co-trimoxazole, dexamethasone, digoxin, dobutamine, dopamine, erythromycin, fluconazole, gentamicin, granisetron, hydrocortisone sodium succinate, labetalol, linezolid, magnesium sulfate, methylprednisolone sodium succinate, metoclopramide, metronidazole, ondansetron, oxytocin, piperacillin with tazobactam, promethazine (in-syringe compatible), propofol, ranitidine, remifentanil, ticarcillin with clavulanate, tobramycin, vancomycin, verapamil |
| pH | 3.5–6 |
| Sodium content | Negligible |
| Storage | Store below 25°C in original packaging. Controlled Drug. |

## Monitoring

Close monitoring of respiratory rate and consciousness is recommended for 30 minutes in patients receiving an initial dose, especially elderly patients or those of low bodyweight.

| Measure | Frequency | Rationale |
|---|---|---|
| Pain score | At regular intervals | • To ensure therapeutic response. |
| Blood pressure, pulse and respiratory rate | | • ↓BP, ↓pulse, ↑pulse, palpitations and respiratory depression with ↓oxygen saturation can occur. |
| Sedation | | • Can cause sedation and CNS depression. |
| Monitor for side-effects and toxicity | | • Itching, nausea and constipation may occur, requiring treatment.<br>• Pruritus can occur with PCA and epidural pethidine. It is not an allergic reaction - it can be eased with low-dose naloxone infusion.<br>• Accumulation of the metabolite, norethidine, can result in agitation, irritability, nervousness, twitches, tremors, myoclonus or seizures. |

## Additional information

| | |
|---|---|
| Common and serious undesirable effects | *Injection/infusion-related:* Local: Injection-site reactions.<br>*Common:* Nausea and vomiting (particularly initially), constipation, dry mouth, urticaria, pruritus, biliary spasm, ↑ or ↓pulse, hallucinations, euphoria, drowsiness.<br>*At higher doses:* ↓BP, sedation, respiratory depression, muscle rigidity. |
| Pharmacokinetics | Elimination half-life is 3 to 6 hours. The onset of analgesia is around 10 minutes; the duration of action is around 2-4 hours following SC or IM administration. The metabolite norpethidine has a half-life up to about 20 hours and may accumulate. |
| Significant interactions | • The following may ↑pethidine levels or effect (or ↑side-effects): antihistamines-sedating (↑sedation), MAOIs (avoid combination and for 2 weeks after stopping MAOI), moclobemide (avoid combination), rasagiline (avoid combination and for 2 weeks after stopping rasagiline), ritonavir (accumulation of toxic pethidine metabolite – avoid combination), selegiline (avoid combination).<br>• Pethidine may ↑levels or effect (or ↑side-effects) of sodium oxybate (avoid combination). |
| Action in case of overdose | *Symptoms to watch for:* ↑Sedation, respiratory depression. Accumulation of the toxic metabolite norpethidine can cause tremors, twitching and seizures.<br>*Antidote:* Naloxone (see the Naloxone monograph). Stop administration and give supportive therapy as appropriate. |
| Counselling | May cause drowsiness that may affect the ability to perform skilled tasks; if affected do not drive or operate machinery, avoid alcoholic drink (the effects of alcohol are enhanced).<br>Inform the patient of possible side-effects: See above.<br>Drink plenty of fluids to help avoid constipation. |

| Risk rating: **GREEN** | Score = 2<br>Lower-risk product: Risk-reduction strategies should be considered. |
|---|---|

This assessment is based on the full range of preparation and administration options described in the monograph. These may not all be applicable in some clinical situations.

## Reference

1. Ashley C, Currie A, eds. *The Renal Drug Handbook*, 3rd edn. Oxford: Radcliffe Medical Press, 2009.

## Bibliography

SPC Pethidine, Goldshield (accessed 31 December 2009).

# Phenobarbital sodium (phenobarbitone sodium)

**200 mg/mL solution in 1-mL ampoules (other strengths may be available)**
* Phenobarbital sodium is a long-acting barbiturate.
* It is sometimes used as an antiepileptic for the treatment of tonic-clonic and partial seizures. To prevent rebound seizures in patients maintained on the drug, withdrawal should be gradual.
* The use of parenteral therapy may have a place in patients normally maintained on phenobarbital when the oral route is temporarily unavailable.
* It may also used parenterally for the treatment of status epilepticus after other methods have failed.

## Pre-treatment checks

* Avoid in severe respiratory depression, acute porphyria and severe hepatic impairment.
* Caution in elderly patients or those of low bodyweight, senile patients, debilitated patients, history of drug or alcohol abuse, renal impairment.

*Biochemical and other tests (not all are necessary in an emergency situation)*

| | |
|---|---|
| Blood pressure and pulse | Pregnancy test (when appropriate) |
| FBC | Renal function: U, Cr, CrCl (or eGFR) |
| LFTs | |

## Dose

**Patients previously established on oral therapy:** oral therapy has good bioavailability and therefore parenteral replacement doses should be close to the previous oral dose (e.g. between 75% and 100% of the oral dose) with the same dose frequency, preferably by IV route. Review for signs of toxicity if parenteral therapy is prolonged.

**Status epilepticus:** 10 mg/kg by IV injection up to maximum 1 g. Up to 30 minutes may be required for maximum effect – allow sufficient time for the therapeutic effect to develop before giving additional doses. Do not use in patients who have recently received oral phenobarbital or primidone.

**Dose in renal impairment:** if CrCl <10 mL/minute reduce the dose by 25–50% avoiding large single doses.[1]

**Dose in hepatic impairment:** reduce dose and avoid if severe.

## Intravenous injection

*Preparation and administration*

1. Withdraw the required dose and dilute each 1 mL of injection to 10 mL with WFI.
2. The solution should be clear and colourless. Inspect visually for particulate matter or discoloration prior to administration and discard if present.
3. Give by IV injection at a rate of not more than 100 mg/minute. Care must be taken to avoid inadvertent intra-arterial injection as this may cause spasm, severe pain and tissue damage. Stop injection if patches of discoloured skin or a white hand with cyanosed skin are seen, or if the patient complains of pain.

## Intramuscular injection

Avoid this route if possible; absorption is likely to be delayed from IM sites, and injection-site reactions are likely.

*Preparation and administration*

1. Withdraw the required dose. May be further diluted with WFI if required.
2. Give by deep IM injection into a large muscle.

## Technical information

| | |
|---|---|
| Incompatible with | Amphotericin, atracurium, benzylpenicillin, clindamycin, noradrenaline (norepinephrine). |
| Compatible with | **Flush**: NaCl 0.9%<br>**Solutions**: NaCl 0.9%, Gluc 5%, Hartmann's, Ringer's, WFI (for dilution)<br>**Y-site**: Fentanyl, fosphenytoin sodium, linezolid, meropenem, propofol |
| pH | 8.5–10.5 |
| Sodium content | Negligible |
| Excipients | May contain propylene glycol (adverse effects seen in ↓renal function, may interact with disulfiram and metronidazole). |
| Storage | Store below 30°C in original packaging. Controlled Drug. |

## Monitoring

| Measure | Frequency | Rationale |
|---|---|---|
| Seizure duration and frequency | Throughout treatment | • To assess therapeutic response. |
| Sedation score | | • May cause drowsiness mental depression and confusion and severe sedation at higher doses. |
| Blood pressure | | • May cause ↓BP. |
| Heart rate | | • May cause ↑pulse and at higher doses cardiovascular depression. |
| Respiratory rate | | • May cause respiratory depression. |
| Injection site | Throughout administration and then periodically | • Inadvertent intra-arterial injection can cause spasm and severe pain.<br>• Local reactions varying in severity from transient pain to gangrene may occur.<br>• Stop injection if the patient complains of pain or if patches of discoloured skin or a white hand with cyanosed skin develop.<br>• SC injection can cause tissue necrosis. |
| Therapeutic levels | If required or if toxicity suspected | • The plasma-phenobarbital concentration for optimum response is 15–40 mg/L (60–180 micromol/L).<br>• Sampling time is just before a dose (trough) and should be after at least 5 half-lives. |

## Additional information

| | |
|---|---|
| Common and serious undesirable effects | *Injection-related:* Too rapid administration: Hypotension, shock, respiratory depression, apnoea, bronchospasm.<br>*Local:* Extravasation can cause tissue necrosis. Pain on IM dosing. SC administration is not recommended due to risk of necrosis.<br>*Other:* Sedation, impaired cognition, headache, dizziness, depression, hypotension, respiratory depression. Rarely blood dyscrasias, Stevens-Johnson syndrome, toxic epidermal necrolysis, allergic skin reactions, suicidal ideation.<br>*Chronic use:* Chronic use of phenobarbital leads to physical dependence on the substance. Withdrawal effects include anxiety, ↑heart rate, sweating, confusion, seizures and death (very rarely). |
| Pharmacokinetics | Elimination half-life is 75-120 hours. |
| Significant interactions | • The following may ↓phenobarbital levels or effect: antidepressants tricyclic (↓seizure threshold), antidepressants-tricyclic, related (↓seizure threshold), antipsychotics (↓seizure threshold), St John's wort (avoid combination).<br>• Phenobarbital may ↑levels or effect (or ↑side-effects) of sodium oxybate (avoid combination).<br>• Phenobarbital may ↓levels or effect of the following drugs: aripiprazole (↑dose required), calcium channel blockers, chloramphenicol, ciclosporin, corticosteroids, coumarins (monitor INR), eplerenone (avoid combination), indinavir, lopinavir, mianserin, nelfinavir, oestrogens (↓contraceptive effect), posaconazole, progestogens (↓contraceptive effect), saquinavir, tacrolimus, telithromycin (avoid combination and for 2 weeks after phenobarbital), voriconazole (avoid combination). |
| Action in case of overdose | *Symptoms to watch for:* Drowsiness, coma, ↓BP, hypothermia, respiratory and cardiovascular depression.<br>*Antidote:* No known antidote but charcoal haemoperfusion may be effective.<br>Stop administration and give supportive therapy as appropriate |

| Risk rating: **GREEN** | Score = 2<br>Lower-risk product: Risk-reduction strategies should be considered. |
|---|---|

This assessment is based on the full range of preparation and administration options described in the monograph. These may not all be applicable in some clinical situations.

## Reference

1. Ashley C, Currie A, eds. *The Renal Drug Handbook*, 3rd edn. Oxford: Radcliffe Medical Press, 2009.

## Bibliography

SPC Phenobarbital Sodium Injection BP 200 mg/mL, Martindale Pharmaceuticals (accessed 17 March 2009).

# Phenoxybenzamine hydrochloride

**50 mg/mL solution in 2-mL ampoules**

* Phenoxybenzamine hydrochloride is a powerful alpha-adrenoceptor blocker with a prolonged duration of action.
* It is used in the management of phaeochromocytoma to control the hypertension associated with excessive catecholamine release.
* It is also licensed for use as an adjunct in the treatment of severe shock not responding to conventional therapy in the presence of an adequate circulatory blood volume.

## Pre-treatment checks

* Avoid if there is a history of cerebrovascular accident and during the recovery period after myocardial infarction (usually 3–4 weeks); and in acute porphyria.
* Do not use in hypovolaemia in patient with severe shock.
* Caution in elderly patients or those of low bodyweight; congestive heart failure; severe heart disease; renal impairment and in those in whom a fall in BP and/or ↑pulse is undesirable.
* Take care not to cause extravasation (irritant to muscle tissues).
* Intensive care facilities and facilities for rapid infusion of IV fluid should be available.
* Phenoxybenzamine is carcinogenic in rats and should only be used after very careful consideration of the risks, in patients where alternative treatment is inappropriate.

*Biochemical and other tests (not all are necessary in an emergency situation)*

Blood pressure
Bodyweight
Renal function: U, Cr, CrCl (or eGFR)

## Dose

Intensive monitoring is required: phenoxybenzamine should only be given in a critical care facility.

**Phaeochromocytoma**: initially 1 mg/kg by IV infusion in 200 mL NaCl 0.9% over 2 hours. Dose may be titrated as necessary. No more than one dose should be given in any 24-hour period.
**Shock**: 1 mg/kg by IV infusion in 200–500 mL NaCl 0.9% over not less than 2 hours. No more than one dose should be given in any 24-hour period.

## Intermittent intravenous infusion

See Special handling below.

*Preparation and administration*

1. Withdraw the required dose and add to the appropriate volume of NaCl 0.9% as described above.
2. The solution should be clear and almost colourless. Inspect visually for particulate matter or discoloration prior to administration and discard if present.
3. Patient should be recumbent and BP must be checked every few minutes during infusion.
4. Give by IV infusion into a large vein via a volumetric infusion device over at least 2 hours (and a maximum of 4 hours).

## Technical information

| | |
|---|---|
| Incompatible with | No information |
| Compatible with | **Flush**: NaCl 0.9%.<br>**Solutions**: NaCl 0.9%<br>**Y-site**: No information but unlikely to be stable |
| pH | 2.5–3.1 |
| Sodium content | Nil |
| Storage | Store below 25°C in original packaging. |
| Excipients | Contains ethanol (may interact with metronidazole; possible religious objections).<br>Contains propylene glycol (adverse effects seen in ↓renal function; may interact with disulfiram and metronidazole). |
| Special handling | Wear gloves to reduce risk of contact sensitisation. |
| Stability after preparation | Use prepared infusions immediately. The entire infusion must be complete within 4 hours of preparation. |

## Monitoring

| Measure | Frequency | Rationale |
|---|---|---|
| Blood pressure | Continuously during treatment | • The infusion should be slowed or stopped if there is a precipitous fall in BP.<br>• There may be an idiosyncratic profound ↓BP within few minutes of starting infusion.<br>• If BP drops and subsequently has been stabilised by the administration of appropriate fluids, the infusion may be restarted under close supervision. |

## Additional information

| | |
|---|---|
| Common and serious undesirable effects | *Infusion-related:*<br>• Too rapid administration: Convulsions have been reported.<br>• Local: Extravasation may cause tissue damage.<br>*Other:* Idiosyncratic profound ↓BP within a few minutes of starting infusion; ↓sweating, dry mouth, postural ↓BP with dizziness and marked compensatory ↑pulse, drowsiness, nasal congestion, miosis. |
| Pharmacokinetics | Elimination half-life is 24 hours. A single large dose may cause alpha-blockade for 3 days or more. |
| Significant interactions | • The following may ↑hypotensive effect of phenoxybenzamine: adrenaline, anaesthetics-general, beta-blockers, calcium channel blockers, diuretics, moxisylyte, sildenafil.<br>• Phenoxybenzamine may ↓levels or effect of noradrenaline (hypertensive effects abolished).<br>• Injectable preparation contains ethanol and propylene glycol: may interact with disulfiram and metronidazole. |

*(continued)*

| **Additional information** (*continued*) | |
|---|---|
| Action in case of overdose | *Symptoms to watch for:* Severe ↓BP.<br>*Antidote:* There is no specific antidote. Plasma expanders may be used and the 'head down' position adopted. Adrenaline should not be used as stimulation of beta-receptors will further ↓BP (noradrenaline is of little value when alpha-adrenergic receptors are blocked). If BP has been stabilised by the administration of appropriate fluids, the infusion may be restarted under close supervision. |

| Risk rating: **AMBER** | Score = 3<br>Moderate-risk product: Risk-reduction strategies are recommended. |
|---|---|

This assessment is based on the full range of preparation and administration options described in the monograph. These may not all be applicable in some clinical situations.

## Bibliography

SPC Dibenyline injection concentrate (accessed 21 August 2009).

# Phentolamine mesilate

### 10 mg/mL solution in 1-mL ampoules

* Phentolamine mesilate is an alpha-adrenoceptor blocker that produces vasodilatation, ↑cardiac output and has a positive inotropic effect. It reportedly has little effect on the BP of patients with essential hypertension.
* It is used in the diagnosis of phaeochromocytoma, and also to treat hypertensive episodes due to phaeochromocytoma, e.g. during surgery.
* It may also be used (unlicensed) in erectile dysfunction and extravasation of noradrenaline (norepinephrine).

### Pre-treatment checks

* Do not use in ↓BP, history of MI, coronary insufficiency, angina, or other evidence of coronary artery disease.
* Caution if a history of peptic ulcer – may cause exacerbation.
* For diagnosis of phaeochromocytoma: antihypertensive drugs are withheld until BP returns to the untreated, hypertensive level; sedatives, analgesics and all other medications except those that might be deemed essential are withheld for at least 24 hours, and preferably 48–72 hours, prior to the test. The test is **not** performed on a patient who is normotensive.

*Biochemical and other tests*

Blood pressure: in diagnosis of phaeochromocytoma the patient must be kept at rest and lying down throughout the test preferably in a quiet, darkened room. The injection should be delayed until BP is stabilised, i.e. BP is taken every 10 minutes for at least 30 minutes.
Electrolytes: serum K

## Dose

**Management of hypertensive episodes in patients with phaeochromocytoma** (e.g. peri-surgery): 2–5 mg by IV injection repeated as necessary. Use a lower dose in elderly patients or those of low bodyweight in case of undiagnosed coronary insufficiency.

**Diagnosis of phaeochromocytoma**: 5 mg by IV or IM injection. See product literature for full details of test procedure and interpretation.

**Serious hypertensive conditions associated with excess circulating catecholamines (unlicensed)**: 2–5 mg by IV injection repeated as necessary. Use a lower dose in elderly patients or those of low bodyweight in case of undiagnosed coronary insufficiency.

**Extravasation of noradrenaline (unlicensed)**: infiltrate the affected area with 5–10 mg phentolamine diluted to 10–15 mL with NaCl 0.9%. This has been shown to be effective in treating dermal necrosis and sloughing if given within 12 hours of extravasation.

**Prevention of dermal necrosis during infusion of noradrenaline (unlicensed)**: 10 mg (1 mL) phentolamine has been added to each 1 L of noradrenaline infusion.

## Intravenous injection

*Preparation and administration*

1. Withdraw the required dose.
2. The solution should be clear and colourless to pale yellow. Inspect visually for particulate matter or discoloration prior to administration.
3. Give by rapid IV injection.

## Intramuscular injection

*Preparation and administration*

1. Withdraw the required dose.
2. Give by IM injection.

| Technical information | |
|---|---|
| Incompatible with | No information |
| Compatible with | **Flush**: NaCl 0.9%<br>**Solutions**: NaCl 0.9%<br>**Y-site**: No information |
| pH | 3–6.5 |
| Sodium content | Negligible |
| Excipients | Contains sulfites (may cause hypersensitivity reactions). |
| Storage | Store at 2–8°C in original packaging. Do not freeze. |
| Stability after preparation | Use prepared infusions immediately. |

## Monitoring

| Measure | Frequency | Rationale |
|---------|-----------|-----------|
| ECG/heart rate | Continuously | • ↑Pulse and arrhythmias may be precipitated. |
| Blood pressure | | • Response to therapy.<br>• May cause serious ↓BP with attendant risk of MI or CVA. |
| Respiratory function | Throughout treatment | • Risk of bronchospasm in asthmatics. |

## Additional information

| | |
|---|---|
| Common and serious undesirable effects | *Immediate:* Bronchospasm or shock especially in asthma due to sulfite content.<br>*Injection-related:* Local: Pain on injection into the corpus cavernosum; induration and fibrosis may occur with repeated use. Priapism.<br>*Other:* ↑Pulse, arrhythmias and ↓BP, flushing, sweating and apprehension. |
| Pharmacokinetics | Serum half-life is approximately 19 minutes. |
| Significant interactions | • The following may ↑hypotensive effect of phentolamine: adrenaline (severe ↑pulse), anaesthetics-general, beta-blockers, calcium channel blockers, diuretics, moxisylyte, sildenafil. |
| Action in case of overdose | *Symptoms to watch for:* Severe ↓BP.<br>*Antidote:* The drug has a short duration of action; the patient should remain recumbent and fluids and electrolytes may be required. Noradrenaline may be used cautiously to overcome alpha blockade but adrenaline must be avoided. |
| Counselling | Patients should report wheezing or shortness of breath. |

| Risk rating: **GREEN** | Score = 2<br>Lower-risk product. Risk-reduction strategies should be considered. |
|---|---|

This assessment is based on the full range of preparation and administration options described in the monograph. These may not all be applicable in some clinical situations.

## Bibliography

SPC Rogitine ampoules 10 mg (accessed 26 June 2009).

# Phenylephrine hydrochloride

**10 mg/mL solution in 1-mL ampoules**

- Phenylephrine hydrochloride is a sympathomimetic with mainly alpha-adrenergic activity.
- It is licensed for the treatment of hypotensive states, e.g. circulatory failure, during spinal anaesthesia or drug-induced ↓BP.
- It has also been used to treat priapism (unlicensed).

## Pre-treatment checks

- Avoid in severe ↑BP and hyperthyroidism.
- Do not give with MAOIs, or within 14 days of ceasing such treatment.
- Caution in patients with pre-existing cardiovascular disease such as ischaemic heart disease, arrhythmias, occlusive vascular disease including arteriosclerosis, ↑BP or aneurysms. Anginal pain may be precipitated in patients with angina pectoris.
- Caution in patients with diabetes mellitus or closed-angle glaucoma.

*Biochemical and other tests (not all are necessary in an emergency situation)*

Blood pressure
TFTs

## Dose

The route of administration should be determined by the needs of the individual patient; patients who are in shock may require IV administration to ensure absorption of the drug.

**By SC or IM injection:** 2–5 mg, with further doses of 1–10 mg if necessary according to response.

**By slow IV injection:** 100–500 micrograms, repeated as necessary after a minimum of 15 minutes.

**By IV infusion:** initially at a rate of up to 180 micrograms/minute, reduced according to response to 30–60 micrograms/minute.

## Subcutaneous injection

*Preparation and administration*

1. Withdraw the required dose.
2. Give by SC injection.

## Intramuscular injection

*Preparation and administration*

1. Withdraw the required dose.
2. Give by IM injection.

## Intravenous injection

*Preparation and administration*

The initial dilution of this injection produces more than the required dose. Adjust the volume before administration.

1. Withdraw 0.1 mL (1 mg) and dilute to 1 mL with WFI.
2. Cap the syringe and mix well to give a solution containing 1 mg/mL (1000 micrograms/mL).
3. Expel the excess solution from the syringe so that the prescribed dose remains.

*(continued)*

4. The solution should be clear and colourless. Inspect visually for particulate matter or discoloration prior to administration and discard if present.
5. Give by slow IV injection over 3–5 minutes.

## Continuous intravenous infusion

*Preparation and administration*

1. Withdraw 10 mg (1 mL) and add to 500 mL NaCl 0.9% or Gluc 5%.
2. Mix well to give a solution containing 20 micrograms/mL.
3. The solution should be clear and colourless. Inspect visually for particulate matter or discoloration prior to administration and discard if present.
4. Give by IV infusion via a volumetric infusion device at an initial rate of 180 micrograms/minute (540 mL/hour). Adjust the rate to clinical response: usually 30–60 micrograms/minute (90–180 mL/hour).

## Technical information

| | |
|---|---|
| Incompatible with | Furosemide, phenytoin sodium, propofol. |
| Compatible with | **Flush**: NaCl 0.9%, Gluc 5%<br>**Solutions**: NaCl 0.9%, Gluc 5% (with added KCl)<br>**Y-site**: Cisatracurium, micafungin, remifentanil, sodium bicarbonate, vasopressin |
| pH | 3–6.5 |
| Sodium content | Negligible |
| Storage | Store at 2–25°C in original packaging. |
| Stability after preparation | From a microbiological point of view, prepared infusions should be used immediately; however, they are known to be stable at room temperature for up to 24 hours. |

## Monitoring

| Measure | Frequency | Rationale |
|---|---|---|
| Blood pressure | Frequently throughout infusion and for short time after stopping treatment | • Continue therapy until adequate BP and tissue perfusion are maintained.<br>• When IV infusions are discontinued, the infusion rate should be slowed gradually and abrupt withdrawal avoided.<br>• Observe carefully so that therapy may be resumed if the BP falls too rapidly.<br>• Pressor therapy should not be reinstated until the systolic BP falls to 70-80 mmHg.<br>• In some patients, additional IV fluids may be necessary before phenylephrine can be discontinued. |

## Additional information

| | |
|---|---|
| Common and serious undesirable effects | ↑BP, headache, arrhythmias, peripheral ischaemia, ↑pulse or reflex ↓pulse. |
| Pharmacokinetics | Elimination half-life is 2-3 hours. When injected SC or IM, phenylephrine takes 10-15 minutes to act and effects last for up to 1 or 2 hours respectively. IV injections are effective for up to about 20 minutes. |
| Significant interactions | • The following may ↑phenylephrine levels or effect (or ↑side-effects): MAOIs (risk of hypertensive crisis), moclobemide (risk of hypertensive crisis), rasagiline (avoid combination).<br>• Phenylephrine may ↓levels or effect of guanethidine (↓hypotensive effect). |
| Action in case of overdose | No known antidote. Treatment should consist of symptomatic and supportive measures.<br>The hypertensive effects may be treated with an alpha-adrenoceptor blocking drug, e.g. phentolamine (see the Phentolamine monograph). |

| | |
|---|---|
| Risk rating: **AMBER** | Score = 4<br>Moderate-risk product: Risk-reduction strategies are recommended. |

This assessment is based on the full range of preparation and administration options described in the monograph. These may not all be applicable in some clinical situations.

### Bibliography

SPC Phenylephrine Injection BP 10 mg/mL, Sovereign Medical (accessed 21 August 2009).

# Phenytoin sodium

### 50 mg/mL solution in 5-mL ampoules

- Phenytoin sodium is a hydantoin antiepileptic agent believed to act by preventing the spread of seizure activity, rather than by raising seizure threshold.
- It is used parenterally in the management of status epilepticus and for prophylactic control of seizures in neurosurgery or following serious head injury.
- Phenytoin therapy should not be withdrawn abruptly as this may precipitate seizures and status epilepticus: may be used parenterally in patients normally maintained on phenytoin when the oral route is temporarily unavailable.
- Phenytoin sodium is also licensed for use in cardiac arrhythmias, but this use is now obsolete.
- Injection doses are expressed in terms of phenytoin sodium.

## Pre-treatment checks

* Ensure that resuscitation facilities are available.
* Avoid in acute porphyria.
* Caution in ↓BP, ↓pulse, heart failure, previous myocardial infarction, sinoatrial block, second- and third-degree heart block and Stokes-Adams syndrome.

*Biochemical and other tests (not all are necessary in an emergency situation)*

| | |
|---|---|
| Blood pressure | FBC |
| Bodyweight | LFTs including albumin |
| ECG | Pregnancy test |

## Dose

**Status epilepticus:**

* *Loading dose* (in patients not maintained on oral phenytoin): 18 mg/kg, by slow IV injection or infusion. Blood levels may be checked 2 hours after giving the loading dose to ensure that they are in the correct range.
* *Maintenance dose:* Up to 100 mg every 6–8 hours. Adjust maintenance dose according to plasma levels.

**Maintenance in patients temporarily unable to take oral therapy:** the maintenance dose may be given as a single daily infusion, or in divided doses (see information below)

---

**For existing epilepsy patients switched from oral maintenance to parenteral dosing**

* Capsules (containing phenytoin sodium) 100 mg ≡ 100 mg phenytoin sodium IV.
* Suspension (containing phenytoin base) 90 mg ≅ 100 mg phenytoin sodium IV.
* Maintenance therapy by the IM route is not recommended as absorption is slow and erratic. However, if use of the IM route is deemed essential, the manufacturers advise increasing the usual oral dose by 50%. The IM route is not usually used for longer than 1 week. When oral therapy is resumed, reduce usual oral dosage by 50% for the same amount of time the patient was receiving IM therapy. This may ↓risk of accumulation as residual phenytoin is released from IM injection sites.
* Phenytoin exhibits non-linear pharmacokinetics (minor dose changes can have a significant effect on phenytoin levels) – always monitor levels closely when route is changed.

---

**Intramuscular dosing:** not advised – see notes above.
**Dose in hepatic impairment:** a reduced maintenance dose may be adequate to control seizures. Monitor levels closely.

## Intravenous injection

*Preparation and administration*

1. Withdraw the required dose.
2. The solution should be clear and colourless to faintly yellow. Inspect visually for particulate matter or discoloration prior to administration and discard if present.
3. Flush with NaCl 0.9% before administration.
4. Give by slow IV injection into a large vein (using a syringe pump if necessary) at a maximum rate of 25 mg/minute (to avoid ↓BP). The rate of administration may be further reduced in higher-risk patients to 5–10 mg/minute (e.g. elderly patients or those of low bodyweight and those with heart disease).
5. After administration, flush with NaCl 0.9% to reduce the risk of irritation (phenytoin is highly alkaline).

## Intermittent intravenous infusion

Phenytoin sodium is incompatible with Gluc 5%, Gluc-NaCl, Hartmann's, Ringer's.
Stability is limited in NaCl 0.9% (precipitates may form).
ECG monitoring during IV administration is strongly advised: risk of serious arrhythmias.

*Preparation and administration*

1. Doses may be given as undiluted injection via syringe pump because this reduces the likelihood of precipitation that is seen when using dilutions in NaCl 0.9%. This practice is commonplace though unlicensed.
2. Alternatively, withdraw the required dose and add to 50–100 mL of NaCl 0.9% (maximum concentration 10 mg/mL).
3. The solution should be clear and colourless to faintly yellow. Inspect visually for particulate matter or discoloration prior to administration and discard if present.
4. Flush the line with NaCl 0.9% before administration.
5. Give by IV infusion into a large vein (via a 0.22–0.50-micron in-line filter if using diluted solution) using a volumetric infusion device. The rate of infusion should be no more than 25 mg/minute (to avoid ↓BP). The rate of administration may be further reduced in higher-risk patients to 5–10 mg/minute (e.g. elderly patients or those of low bodyweight and those with heart disease).
6. Throughout the infusion inspect for particulate matter and discoloration.
7. After administration, flush with NaCl 0.9% to reduce risk of irritation.

## Intramuscular injection (not recommended)

Maintenance therapy by the IM route is not recommended as absorption is slow and erratic (see information above).

*Preparation and administration*

1. Withdraw the required dose.
2. Give by deep IM injection. SC injection should be avoided because of the risk of tissue necrosis.

## Technical information

| | |
|---|---|
| Incompatible with | Phenytoin sodium is incompatible with Gluc 5%, Gluc-NaCl, Hartmann's, Ringer's.<br>Precipitation is likely if phenytoin sodium is mixed with other drugs. Flush lines well before and after administration of phenytoin to avoid contact with other drugs. |
| Compatible with | **Flush**: NaCl 0.9%<br>**Solutions**: NaCl 0.9% (but precipitates may form; use of a 0.22–0.50-micron in-line filter is essential if the injection solution is diluted for infusion)<br>**Y-site**: Not recommended, precipitates may form with all drugs and solutions |
| pH | 12 |
| Sodium content | 1.1 mmol/5 mL |
| Excipients | Ethanol (may interact with metronidazole, possible religious objections).<br>Propylene glycol (adverse effects seen in ↓renal function, may interact with disulfiram and metronidazole). |

*(continued)*

## Technical information (continued)

| | |
|---|---|
| Storage | Store below 25°C in original packaging. Do not refrigerate or freeze. The solution may develop a faint yellow colour; this does not affect the potency. |
| Stability after preparation | Use prepared dilutions in NaCl 0.9% immediately. Do not refrigerate or freeze. Complete the infusion within one hour of preparation. |

## Monitoring

| Measure | Frequency | Rationale |
|---|---|---|
| ECG and blood pressure | During IV administration | • There is a risk of serious arrhythmias and ↓BP. |
| Seizures | Continuously | • For therapeutic effect. |
| Blood glucose | Frequently | • May ↑blood glucose concentration.<br>• Adjust the dosage of insulin or oral antidiabetic drugs if required. |
| Phenytoin serum levels | Twice weekly while on IV (more frequently if needed). At steady state to ensure in therapeutic window (after 5-7 half lives). If dosage adjustments are required. If toxicity suspected | • Therapeutic total plasma phenytoin level for optimum response in epilepsy is 10-20 mg/L (40-80 micromol/L); unbound plasma phenytoin level is 1-2 mg/L (4-8 micromol/L). |
| LFTs including albumin | Periodically | • Albumin levels should also be measured to indicate whether protein binding is affected. If albumin is low, free phenytoin levels will be high even if total plasma-phenytoin levels are in range.<br>• Liver dysfunction sometimes occurs. |
| FBC | | • Thrombocytopenia, leucopenia, neutropenia, agranulocytosis, pancytopenia and aplastic anaemia have all been reported. |
| Pregnancy test | If pregnancy suspected | • May cause blood clotting abnormalities and congenital malformations in the neonate. |

## Additional information

| | |
|---|---|
| Common and serious undesirable effects | *Injection/infusion-related:*<br>• Too rapid administration: Arrhythmias, ↓pulse, heart block, vasodilation, ↓BP, cardiovascular collapse, asystole, impaired respiratory function and respiratory arrest.<br>• Local: Injection-site reaction or pain. Inadvertent SC, intra-arterial or perivascular injection may cause severe local tissue damage due to the high pH.<br>*Other:* Nausea, vomiting, constipation, anorexia, insomnia, transient nervousness, tremor, paraesthesia, dizziness, headache, peripheral neuropathy, dyskinesia, rash, megaloblastic anaemia, leucopenia, thrombocytopenia, aplastic anaemia, hepatotoxicity, lymphadenopathy, polyarteritis nodosa, lupus erythematosus, Stevens-Johnson syndrome, toxic epidermal necrolysis, pneumonitis, interstitial nephritis. |

*(continued)*

## Additional information (*continued*)

| | |
|---|---|
| Pharmacokinetics | Elimination half-life is 13–46 hours. The half-life may increase if the metabolism pathway becomes saturated - risk of toxicity.<br>Phenytoin is highly protein bound (about 90% and mainly to albumin). |
| Significant interactions | • The following may ↑phenytoin levels or effect (or ↑side-effects): amiodarone, azapropazone (avoid combination), chloramphenicol (monitor), cimetidine, co-trimoxazole, diltiazem, disulfiram (monitor levels), esomeprazole, ethosuximide, fluconazole-multiple dosing (monitor levels), fluoxetine, fluvoxamine, indinavir, isoniazid, metronidazole-systemic, miconazole, NSAIDs-systemic, sulfinpyrazone, topiramate, trimethoprim, voriconazole (monitor levels).<br>• The following may ↓phenytoin levels or effect: antipsychotics (↓seizure threshold), mefloquine, pyrimethamine, rifabutin, rifampicin, theophylline, SSRIs (↓seizure threshold), St John's wort, tricyclic antidepressants (↓seizure threshold).<br>• Phenytoin may ↑levels or effect (or ↑side-effects) of coumarins.<br>• Phenytoin may ↓levels or effect of the following drugs: aripiprazole, ciclosporin, corticosteroids, coumarins, diltiazem, eplerenone (avoid combination), ethosuximide, imatinib (avoid combination), indinavir, itraconazole (avoid combination), ketoconazole, lapatinib (avoid combination), mianserin, nifedipine, theophylline, oestrogens (↓contraceptive effect), posaconazole, progestogens (↓contraceptive effect), telithromycin (avoid combination), topiramate, voriconazole (↑dose needed), tricyclic antidepressants.<br>• Injectable preparation contains ethanol and propylene glycol: may interact with disulfiram and metronidazole. |
| Action in case of overdose | *Symptoms to watch for:* ↑ or ↓pulse, asystole, respiratory or circulatory depression, cardiac arrest, syncope, ↓Ca, metabolic acidosis and death.<br>*Antidote:* No known antidote but haemodialysis may be used, as about 10% of phenytoin is not protein bound.<br>Stop administration and give supportive therapy as appropriate. Phenytoin plasma levels should be checked as soon as possible. |
| Counselling | Women who have been relying on the combined contraceptive pill should be advised to take additional precautions. |

| | |
|---|---|
| Risk rating: **AMBER** | Score = 5<br>Moderate-risk product: Risk-reduction strategies are recommended. |

This assessment is based on the full range of preparation and administration options described in the monograph. These may not all be applicable in some clinical situations.

## Bibliography

SPC Phenytoin Injection BP, Hospira UK Ltd (accessed 21 April 2008).

SPC Phenytoin 250mg/5ml solution for injection, Beacon Pharmaceuticals (accessed 21 April 2008).

SPC Epanutin Ready Mixed Parenteral, Pfizer Ltd (accessed 21 April 2008).

SPC Pro-Epanutin concentrate for infusion/solution for injection, Pfizer Ltd (accessed 10 October 2008).

# Phosphates

### Solution in 500-mL Polyfusor infusion container

* Phosphorus plays an important part in the structure of bones and teeth and, as adenosine triphosphate, is crucial in the transfer of cellular energy.
* Normal range for plasma phosphate: 0.8–1.44 mmol/L.
* Phosphate infusions are used to treat hypophosphataemia due to inadequate intake, refeeding syndrome, or ↑phosphate losses.

| Phosphates solution 500 mL contains: | 50 mmol phosphate |
| --- | --- |
| | 81 mmol sodium |
| | 9.5 mmol potassium |

## Pre-treatment checks

* Avoid in ↑$PO_4$, ↑K, ↑Na, ↓Ca or over-hydration.
* Caution in patients with cardiac disease, ↑BP, peripheral or pulmonary oedema, renal impairment and pre-eclampsia.
* Care with patients on potassium-sparing diuretics.

*Biochemical and other tests (not all are necessary in an emergency situation)*

| | |
| --- | --- |
| Acid–base balance | Electrolytes: serum K, Na, Ca, $PO_4$ |
| Blood pressure | Fluid balance |
| Bodyweight | Renal function: U, Cr, CrCl (or eGFR) |
| ECG | |

## Dose

The doses below are as advised by the manufacturer; however, IV phosphates are associated with serious adverse effects if hypophosphataemia is over-corrected.
Some authorities advise giving no more than 9 mmol (90 mL) phosphate over 12 hours (7.5 mL/hour) unless given within a critical care facility.

**Moderate hypophosphataemia:** 0.1–0.2 mmol/kg ($\equiv$ 1–2 mL/kg) by IV infusion over 6–12 hours.
**Severe hypophosphataemia:** 0.2–0.5 mmol/kg ($\equiv$ 2–5 mL/kg) by IV infusion over 6–24 hours up to a maximum of 50 mmol (500 mL) per infusion. Repeat as necessary over subsequent days in response to phosphate levels.
**Dose in renal impairment:** reduce the dose in elderly patients or those of low bodyweight with renal impairment.
**Dose in hepatic impairment:** no information available.

## Intermittent intravenous infusion

*Preparation and administration*

1. The infusion is pre-prepared for use. It should be clear and colourless. Inspect visually for particulate matter or discoloration prior to administration and discard if present.
2. Give by IV infusion over 12 hours at a maximum rate of 7.5 mL/hour (see warning above) unless given within a critical care facility.

## Technical information

| | |
|---|---|
| Incompatible with | Calcium chloride, calcium gluconate, magnesium sulfate - may precipitate. |
| Compatible with | **Flush**: NaCl 0.9 %<br>**Solutions**: No information<br>**Y-site**: No information |
| pH | 7-7.7 |
| Sodium content | 81 mmol/500 mL |
| Storage | Store at 2-25°C. |

## Monitoring

| Measure | Frequency | Rationale |
|---|---|---|
| Serum PO$_4$ | Periodically | • To ensure that treatment is effective. |
| Serum K | | • May cause ↑K - monitor closely. |
| Serum Ca | | • May cause ↓Ca - monitor closely. |
| Serum Na | | • May cause ↑Na - monitor closely. |
| ECG | | • To check for any problems caused by ↑K. |
| Acid-base balance | | • To ensure that treatment is effective. |
| Fluid balance | | • To check hydration status. |

## Additional information

| | |
|---|---|
| Common and serious undesirable effects | *Infusion-related:* Local: Pain and phlebitis at injection site. |
| Pharmacokinetics | Not relevant |
| Significant interactions | None known |
| Action in case of overdose | *Symptoms to watch for:* ↑PO$_4$, ↑K, ↑Na, ↓Ca, tetany.<br>Stop administration and give supportive therapy as appropriate. |

| | |
|---|---|
| Risk rating: **AMBER** | Score = 3<br>Moderate-risk product: Risk-reduction strategies are recommended. |

This assessment is based on the full range of preparation and administration options described in the monograph. These may not all be applicable in some clinical situations.

**Bibliography**

SPC Phosphates Polyfusor (accessed 14 October 2009).

# Phytomenadione (vitamin K₁, phytonadione)

**10 mg/mL solution (mixed micelles vehicle) in 0.2-mL and 1-mL ampoules**

This monograph refers to the mixed micelles formulation available in the UK.
Information given does not apply to formulations containing polyoxyl castor oil, which can cause severe hypersensitivity reactions if given IV.

* Vitamin K is an essential cofactor in the hepatic synthesis of prothrombin (factor II) and other blood clotting factors (factors VII, IX, and X, and proteins C and S). It has a role in the function of proteins such as osteocalcin that are important for bone development.
* Phytomenadione is a naturally occurring vitamin K substance used to reverse ↑INR and haemorrhage caused by warfarin. It can be used IV or the injectable preparation can be given orally for this indication.
* Phytomenadione may be used to reverse ↑INR and haemorrhage caused by phenindione therapy. It may also be used to reverse acenocoumarol (nicoumalone) but may have a lesser effect. It is not effective as a heparin antidote (see the Protamine sulfate monograph).
* Phytomenadione is also indicated in the treatment of haemorrhage or threatened haemorrhage associated with a low blood level of prothrombin or factor VII.

## Pre-treatment checks

Time to onset of action is a minimum of 1–2 hours if given IV, irrespective of dose, and 6–10 hours if given orally. If a faster response is needed, prothrombin complex concentrate (factors II, VII, IX, and X) 30–50 units/kg or (if no concentrate available) fresh frozen plasma 15 mL/kg should also given.

*Biochemical and other tests*

LFTs
Prothrombin time or INR

## Dose

Parenterally, for the mixed micelles formulation the IV route is preferred (see caution above) because absorption is irregular if given IM, and there is a risk of haematoma formation. SC delivery is reported to be less effective in treating over-anticoagulation.

**As an antidote to warfarin (or other 4-hydroxycoumarin):**
* *Major bleeding:* stop warfarin; give phytomenadione 5–10 mg by slow IV injection.
* Larger doses of up to 40 mg in 24 hours have been given but this can cause considerable delay when anticoagulant therapy is planned. If anticoagulation is needed following overdosage of phytomenadione, heparin may be used.

- *INR >8.0, no bleeding or minor bleeding:* stop warfarin, restart when INR <5.0; if there are other risk factors for bleeding, give phytomenadione 500 micrograms by slow IV injection or 5 mg orally (for partial reversal of anticoagulation give smaller oral doses of phytomenadione, e.g. 0.5–2.5 mg orally); repeat the dose of phytomenadione if INR is still too high after 24 hours.
- *INR <8.0:* stop warfarin, restart when INR<5.0; phytomenadione is unnecessary unless there is bleeding (in which case investigate the possibility of underlying pathology).

**To reverse raised INR associated with liver impairment:** give 10 mg IV and monitor INR to assess the need for further doses; if using the oral route, water-soluble menadiol sodium phosphate is more effective.

## Intravenous injection

*Preparation and administration*

1. Withdraw the required dose.
2. The solution should be clear to slightly opalescent and pale yellow. Inspect visually for particulate matter or discoloration prior to administration.
3. Give by IV injection over 3–5 minutes.

## Intermittent intravenous infusion

*Preparation and administration*

1. Withdraw the required dose and add to 50 mL Gluc 5%.
2. The solution should be clear to slightly opalescent and pale yellow. Inspect visually for particulate matter or discoloration prior to administration.
3. Give by IV infusion over 15–30 minutes.

## Oral use (use unlicensed in adults)

Konakion MM and Konakion MM Paediatric are identical formulations[1]: either preparation may be used.

*Preparation and administration*

1. Withdraw the required dose using an oral syringe.
2. Place the dose directly into the patient's mouth.

| Technical information | |
|---|---|
| Incompatible with | No information |
| Compatible with | **Flush**: Gluc 5%, NaCl 0.9% <br>**Solutions**: Gluc 5% <br>**Y-site**: No information |
| pH | 5–7.5 |
| Sodium content | Negligible |
| Storage | Store below 25°C in original packaging. Do not use if the solution is turbid. |
| Stability after preparation | Use prepared infusions immediately. |

## Monitoring

| Measure | Frequency | Rationale |
|---------|-----------|-----------|
| INR | Minimum 3 hours after IV dose, otherwise daily | • INR should have fallen in response to the dose; if the response has been inadequate, the dose may be repeated.<br>• Monitor INR daily until <5, at which point warfarin may be reintroduced if appropriate. |

## Additional information

| | |
|---|---|
| Common and serious undesirable effects | *Immediate:* Hypersensitivity reactions have been reported rarely. An anaphylaxis-like reaction (facial flushing, sweating, chest constriction, dyspnoea, cyanosis, cardiovascular collapse) has previously been associated with IV use of polyethoxylated castor oil formulations, which are no longer available in the UK.<br>*Injection/infusion-related:* Local: Very rarely phlebitis (IV use), injection-site reactions (IM use).<br>*Other:* Various adverse cutaneous reactions, e.g. pruritic, erythematous, eczematous plaques may occur up to 2 weeks after a dose. Treat symptomatically. |
| Pharmacokinetics | Blood coagulation factors increase in 1-2 hours following IV dosing and about 6-10 hours after oral dosing. |
| Significant interactions | Orlistat may ↓phytomenadione levels or effect: ↓GI absorption of fat-soluble vitamins such as phytomenadione. |
| Action in case of overdose | Hypervitaminosis of vitamin $K_1$ is unknown in adults although it has been reported in neonates and infants. |
| Counselling | Report any itchy or red skin rashes occurring within 2 weeks of a dose. |

| Risk rating: **GREEN** | Score = 1<br>Lower-risk product: Risk-reduction strategies should be considered. |
|---|---|

This assessment is based on the full range of preparation and administration options described in the monograph. These may not all be applicable in some clinical situations.

## Reference

1. Communication with Roche Products Ltd, 18 May 2009.

## Bibliography

SPC Konakion MM (accessed 8 September 2009).

Toxbase. Acenocoumarol and Phenindione monographs. www.toxbase.org (accessed 20 April 2009).

# Piperacillin with tazobactam

### 2.25-g and 4.5-g dry powder vials

- Piperacillin is a ureidopenicillin. It is given in combination with the beta-lactamase inhibitor tazobactam to widen its spectrum of action.
- The combined preparation is used in the treatment of severe infections including neutropenic sepsis, peritonitis and septicaemia.
- Doses of piperacillin are expressed in terms of the base:
  Piperacillin 1 g ≡ 1.04 g piperacillin sodium.
- Piperacillin with tazobactam doses are expressed below as the combined mg of the two constituents:
  Piperacillin with tazobactam 4.5 g ≡ piperacillin 4 g with tazobactam 500 mg.

---

**MHRA advice (January 2009)**

Generic piperacillin/tazobactam products have different compatibilities with other medicines compared with Tazocin, raising a risk of serious medication errors.
Generic piperacillin/tazobactam must not be mixed or co-administered with any aminoglycoside, and must not be reconstituted or diluted with Hartmann's solution.

---

## Pre-treatment checks

- Check for history of allergy/hypersensitivity to any beta-lactam drug or beta-lactamase inhibitors.
- Patients to be treated for gonorrhoea should be evaluated for syphilis (it may mask or delay the symptoms of incubating syphilis).

*Biochemical and other tests (not all are necessary in an emergency situation)*

Electrolytes: serum K
FBC

LFTs
Renal function: U, Cr, CrCl (or eGFR)

## Dose

**Standard dose:** 2.25–4.5 g every 6–8 hours, usually 4.5 g every 8 hours.
**Neutropenic sepsis** (in combination with an aminoglycoside, but see above): 4.5 g every 6 hours.
Neutropenic patients with signs of infection (e.g. fever) should receive immediate empirical antibiotic therapy before laboratory results are available.
**Dose in renal impairment:** adjusted according to creatinine clearance:[1]

- CrCl >20–50 mL/minute: dose as in normal renal function.
- CrCl 10–20 mL/minute: 4.5 g every 8–12 hours, or 2.25 g every 6 hours.
- CrCl <10 mL/minute: 4.5 g every 12 hours, or 2.25 g every 8 hours.

## Intravenous injection

*Preparation and administration*

---

If used in combination with an aminoglycoside (e.g. amikacin, gentamicin, tobramycin), preferably administer at a different site. If this is not possible then flush the line thoroughly with a compatible solution between drugs.

1. Reconstitute each 2.25-g vial with 10 mL WFI or NaCl 0.9% (each 4.5-g vial requires 20 mL) and swirl until dissolved. This may take up to 10 minutes depending on brand.
2. The solution should be clear and colourless. Inspect visually for particulate matter or discoloration prior to administration and discard if present (it is not uncommon with this preparation to find small particles of the bung to be forced into the ampoule).
3. Give by IV injection over at least 3–5 minutes.

## Intravenous infusion

*Preparation and administration*

If used in combination with an aminoglycoside (e.g. amikacin, gentamicin, tobramycin), preferably administer at a different site. If this is not possible then flush the line thoroughly with a compatible solution between drugs.

NB: some manufacturers' vials may be 'docked' for reconstitution with a 'minibag plus'.

1. Reconstitute each 2.25-g vial with 10 mL WFI or NaCl 0.9% (each 4.5-g vial requires 20 mL) and swirl until dissolved. This may take up to 10 minutes depending on brand.
2. Add to 50–100 mL of compatible infusion fluid (usually NaCl 0.9%).
3. The solution should be clear and colourless. Inspect visually for particulate matter or discoloration prior to administration and discard if present (it is not uncommon with this preparation to find small particles of the bung that have been forced into the vial).
4. Give by IV infusion over 20–30 minutes.

## Technical information

| | |
|---|---|
| Incompatible with | Piperacillin with tazobactam is incompatible with Hartmann's. Sodium bicarbonate. Amikacin, amiodarone, amphotericin, chlorpromazine, cisatracurium, dobutamine, drotrecogin alfa (activated), ganciclovir, gentamicin, tobramycin, vancomycin. |
| Compatible with | **Flush**: NaCl 0.9% <br> **Solutions**: NaCl 0.9%, Gluc 5%, WFI <br> **Y-site**: Brands vary |
| pH | 5.7 |
| Sodium content | 5.6 mmol/2.25 g; 11.2 mmol/4.5 g |
| Storage | Store below 25°C in original packaging. |
| Displacement value | 1.6 mL for every 2.25 g; 3.2 mL for every 4.5 g |
| Stability after preparation | From a microbiological point of view, should be used immediately; however: <br> • Reconstituted vials may be stored at 2–8°C for 24 hours. <br> • Prepared infusions may be stored at 2–8°C and infused (at room temperature) within 24 hours. |

## Monitoring

| Measure | Frequency | Rationale |
|---|---|---|
| Temperature | Minimum daily | • For clinical signs of fever resolution. |
| Signs of hypersensitivity reaction | Throughout treatment | • Occurs occasionally and fatalities have occurred. The antibiotic must be stopped. |
| LFTs | Periodically | • Occasional mild ↑ALT, AST, bilirubin and Alk Phos occur.<br>• Dosage adjustments in patients with hepatic impairment are not considered necessary. |
| Renal function and serum K | | • A dose adjustment may be necessary if renal function changes.<br>• ↓K may occur especially if other potential hypokalaemic agents are present. |
| FBC | Periodically (especially if duration >21 days) | • Anaemia, leucopenia, neutropenia and thrombocytopenia occasionally occur.<br>• WCC will also show signs of the infection resolving. |
| Prothrombin time | If indicated | • Bleeding abnormalities have occurred (rarely). If manifest, the antibiotic should be discontinued and appropriate therapy commenced. |
| Development of diarrhoea | Throughout and up to 2 months after treatment | • Development of severe, persistent diarrhoea may be suggestive of *Clostridium difficile*-associated diarrhoea and colitis (pseudomembranous colitis). Discontinue drug and treat. Do not use drugs that inhibit peristalsis. |

## Additional information

| | |
|---|---|
| Common and serious undesirable effects | *Immediate:* Anaphylaxis and other hypersensitivity reactions have been reported.<br>*Injection/infusion-related:* Local: Injection-site reaction.<br>*Other:* Diarrhoea, nausea, vomiting. |
| Pharmacokinetics | Elimination half-life is 0.7–1.2 hours. |
| Significant interactions | No significant interactions known. |
| Action in case of overdose | *Antidote:* No know antidote but haemodialysis may be effective.<br>Stop administration and give supportive therapy as appropriate. |

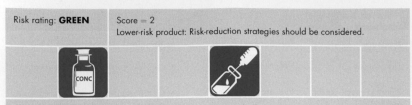

Risk rating: **GREEN**

Score = 2
Lower-risk product: Risk-reduction strategies should be considered.

This assessment is based on the full range of preparation and administration options described in the monograph. These may not all be applicable in some clinical situations.

### Reference

1. Ashley C, Currie A, eds. *The Renal Drug Handbook*, 3rd edn. Oxford: Radcliffe Medical Press, 2009.

### Bibliography

SPC Tazocin 2 g/0.25 g and 4g/0.5 g powder for solution for injection or infusion (accessed 2 April 2009).
SPC Piperacillin/Tazobactam 2 g/0.25 g powder for solution for injection or infusion, Hospira UK Ltd (accessed 2 April 2009).

# Pipotiazine palmitate (pipothiazine palmitate)

**50 mg/mL oily solution in 1-mL and 2-mL ampoules**

* Pipotiazine palmitate is a phenothiazine antipsychotic with a wide range of actions. It is a dopamine inhibitor; it has antiemetic activity; it has muscle relaxant properties; and it inhibits the heat-regulating centre.
* It is used as a long-acting depot injection in the treatment of schizophrenia and other psychoses.

### Pre-treatment checks

* Do not use in comatose states, including alcohol, barbiturate, or opiate poisoning.
* Do not use if there is severe renal or hepatic impairment, in phaeochromocytoma, or in patients with marked cerebral atherosclerosis or severe cardiac insufficiency.
* Caution in epilepsy, Parkinson disease, liver disease, renal failure, cardiac disease, depression, myasthenia gravis, prostatic hypertrophy, narrow-angle glaucoma, hypothyroidism, hyperthyroidism, severe respiratory disease or if there are risk factors for stroke.
* Concomitant administration with other antipsychotics should be avoided.

*Biochemical and other tests*

| | |
|---|---|
| Blood pressure | FBC |
| Bodyweight | LFTs |
| ECG | Renal function |

### Dose

**Test dose:** 25 mg by IM injection to assess tolerability. Reduce dose to 5–10 mg if patient is elderly.
**Maintenance dose:** 25–50 mg to be administered at least 4–7 days after test dose; the usual dose range is 50–100 mg every 4 weeks. Some patients may require up to 200 mg every 4 weeks.

## Intramuscular injection

*Preparation and administration*

1. Withdraw the required dose.
2. Give by deep IM injection into the gluteal muscle. Volumes >2 mL should be distributed between two injection sites. Rotate injection sites for subsequent injections.

## Technical information

| | |
|---|---|
| Incompatible with | Not relevant |
| Compatible with | Not relevant |
| pH | Not relevant - oily injection |
| Sodium content | Nil |
| Storage | Store below 25°C and protect from light. |

## Monitoring

| Measure | Frequency | Rationale |
|---|---|---|
| Therapeutic improvement | Periodically | • To ensure that treatment is effective. |
| EPSEs | During dose adjustment and every 3 months | • Causes extrapyramidal symptoms, e.g. dystonias. |
| Renal function | At least annually | • As part of regular health check. |
| LFTs | | |
| Blood pressure | | |
| Glucose | | |
| Lipids (including cholesterol, HDL, LDL and triglycerides) | | |
| Weight and obesity | | • As part of regular health check.<br>• May cause weight gain.<br>• Obesity measured by waist:hip ratio or waist circumference. |
| ECG | Annually | • Can increase QT interval. |
| Prolactin | See rationale | • If symptoms of hyperprolactinaemia develop. |

## Additional information

| | |
|---|---|
| Common and serious undesirable effects | Drowsiness and sedation are more common at start of treatment and at high doses. EPSE. <br><br> Other reported side-effects include orthostatic dizziness, weight gain, hyperprolactinaemia, ↑pulse, ↓BP, abnormalities of visual accommodation, urinary incontinence and frequency, convulsions. <br><br> Rare cases of QT prolongation, ventricular arrhythmias - ventricular fibrillation, ventricular tachycardia, torsade de pointes and sudden unexplained death have been reported. Blood dyscrasias. |
| Pharmacokinetics | Rate-limiting half-life is 14-21 days. |
| Significant interactions | • The following may ↑pipotiazine levels or effect (or ↑side-effects): anaesthetics-general (↑risk of ↓BP), antidepressants-tricyclic, artemether with lumefantrine (avoid combination), ritonavir, sibutramine (avoid combination). <br> • Pipotiazine may ↓levels or effect of levodopa. <br> • Pipotiazine may ↑risk of ventricular arrhythmias with the following drugs: amiodarone (avoid combination), antidepressants-tricyclic, atomoxetine, disopyramide, droperidol (avoid combination), methadone, moxifloxacin (avoid combination), pentamidine isetionate, pimozide (avoid combination), sotalol. <br> • Pipotiazine ↓convulsive threshold and may ↓effect of the following drugs: barbiturates, carbamazepine, ethosuximide, oxcarbazepine, phenytoin, primidone, valproate. |
| Action in case of overdose | Treat EPSE with anticholinergic antiparkinsonian drugs. <br> If agitation or convulsions occur, treat with benzodiazepines. <br> If the patient is in shock, treatment with metaraminol or noradrenaline may be appropriate. <br> Adrenaline must not be given (may further ↓BP). |
| Counselling | Advise patients not to drink alcohol especially at the beginning of treatment. <br> May impair alertness so do not drive or operate machinery until susceptibility is known. |

| Risk rating: **GREEN** | Score = 2 <br> Lower-risk product: Risk-reduction strategies should be considered. |
|---|---|

This assessment is based on the full range of preparation and administration options described in the monograph. These may not all be applicable in some clinical situations.

## Bibliography

SPC Piportil (accessed 7 January 2010).

Bazire S. *Psychotropic Drug Directory* 2010. Aberdeen: HealthComm UK Ltd, 2010.

NICE (2009) *Clinical Guideline 82: Core interventions in the treatment and management of schizophrenia in primary and secondary care (update)*. London: National Institute for Health and Clinical Excellence. http://guidance.nice.org.uk/CG82 (accessed 1 October 2009).

# Piroxicam

**20 mg/mL solution 1-mL ampoules**
* Piroxicam is a non-steroidal anti-inflammatory drug (NSAID).
* It is licensed for symptomatic relief of osteoarthritis, rheumatoid arthritis or ankylosing spondylitis.

### CHMP advice (June 2007)

* The maximum dose of piroxicam should be 20 mg per day.
* It should only be initiated by physicians experienced in treating inflammatory or degenerative rheumatic diseases.
* Piroxicam should not be used as first line treatment and should not be used for acute, painful and inflammatory conditions.

## Pre-treatment checks

* Avoid in active peptic ulceration, history of recurrent ulceration, severe heart failure, asthma induced by aspirin or other NSAIDs, nasal polyps, angioedema or urticaria.
* Caution in elderly patients or those of low bodyweight, and in renal and hepatic impairment.
* Consider prescribing a gastro-protective agent.

*Biochemical and other tests*

Blood pressure
FBC

LFTs
Renal function: U, Cr, CrCl (or eGFR)

## Dose

**Standard dose:** 20 mg daily.
**Dose in renal impairment:** avoid if possible.

## Intramuscular injection

*Preparation and administration*

1. Withdraw the required dose.
2. Give by deep IM injection into the upper outer quadrant of the buttock.

| Technical information | |
|---|---|
| Incompatible with | Not relevant |
| Compatible with | Not relevant |
| pH | Not relevant |
| Sodium content | Negligible |

*(continued)*

## Technical information (*continued*)

| | |
|---|---|
| Excipients | Contains benzyl alcohol.<br>Contains ethanol (may interact with metronidazole, possible religious objections).<br>Contains propylene glycol (adverse effects seen in ↓renal function, may interact with disulfiram and metronidazole). |
| Storage | Store below 25°C in original packaging. |

## Monitoring

| Measure | Frequency | Rationale |
|---|---|---|
| Blood pressure | Periodically | • May cause ↑BP. |
| Skin reactions | | • Has been associated with serious skin reactions. |
| Renal function | 6- to 12-monthly if on long-term therapy | • Although rare can cause interstitial nephritis, glomerulitis, papillary necrosis and the nephrotic syndrome. |
| FBC | | • Can cause GI bleeds leading to ↓Hb etc. |
| LFTs | | • If hepatic function deteriorates may need to discontinue therapy. |

## Additional information

| | |
|---|---|
| Common and serious undesirable effects | *Immediate:* Anaphylaxis and other hypersensitivity reactions have rarely been reported.<br>*Injection-related:* Local: Temporary pain on injection.<br>*Other:* GI side-effects, skin reactions, oedema, ↑BP, cardiac failure. |
| Pharmacokinetics | Elimination half-life is 50 hours. |
| Significant interactions | • The following may ↑risk of bleeding with piroxicam: antidepressants-SSRIs, aspirin, dabigatran, erlotinib, ketorolac, NSAIDs, venlafaxine.<br>• Piroxicam may ↑levels or effect of the following drugs (or ↑side-effects): ciclosporin (↑risk of nephrotoxicity), coumarin anticoagulants (monitor INR), lithium (monitor levels), methotrexate (↑toxicity, avoid combination), phenindione (monitor INR), phenytoin (monitor levels), quinolones (↑risk of seizures), ritonavir (avoid combination), sulfonylureas.<br>• Injectable preparation contains ethanol and propylene glycol: may interact with disulfiram and metronidazole. |
| Action in case of overdose | *Antidote:* No known antidote; haemodialysis is unlikely to be effective.<br>Stop administration and give supportive therapy as appropriate. |

| Risk rating: **GREEN** | Score = 1<br>Lower-risk product: Risk-reduction strategies should be considered. |
|---|---|

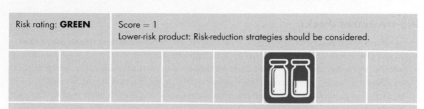

This assessment is based on the full range of preparation and administration options described in the monograph. These may not all be applicable in some clinical situations.

## Bibliography

SPC Feldene (accessed 16 October 2008).

# Potassium chloride

**20 mmol (1.5 g)/L in NaCl 0.9%, Gluc 5%, or Gluc-NaCl solution in 500-mL and 1-L infusion containers**
**40 mmol (3 g)/L in NaCl 0.9%, Gluc 5%, or Gluc-NaCl solution in 500-mL and 1-L infusion containers**
*Concentrated solutions (restricted use):*
**20 or 40 mmol in 100-mL NaCl 0.9% infusion bags**
**20 mmol/10 mL (1.5 g/10 mL; 15%) ampoules – other strengths may be available**

* Potassium is the major intracellular electrolyte.
* Normal range for serum potassium: 3.5–5.0 mmol/L.
* Potassium is given IV as the initial treatment for the correction of severe ↓K (<2.5 mmol/L) and for treatment and prevention of ↓K where the oral route is unavailable.
* Pre-prepared solutions containing up to 40 mmol/L KCl are considered safe for routine use in general clinical areas; more concentrated solutions should only be used in critical care with intensive monitoring because of the risk of arrhythmias and asystole.
* Potassium chloride 3 g = 20 mmol of $K^+$ and $Cl^-$.

---

### The UK NPSA Patient Safety Alert (Oct 2002)

Potassium chloride concentrate solution can be fatal if given inappropriately, therefore:
* Commercially prepared ready to use dilute solutions containing potassium chloride should be used wherever possible.
* If a suitable solution is not available commercially, dilutions should be made in the hospital pharmacy wherever possible.
* Storage of concentrated potassium chloride solutions should be restricted to pharmacy departments and to those critical care areas where concentrated solutions are needed for urgent use.
* Receipt and use of these solutions should be recorded in a similar way to Controlled Drugs and stocks should be kept in a separate locked cupboard away from commonly used diluting solutions.
* Potassium chloride concentrate solution should not be transferred between clinical areas.

## Pre-treatment checks

* Potassium chloride concentrate must not be injected undiluted as **instant death may occur**.
* Do not give in cases of ↑K, ↑Cl or if CrCl <10 mL/minute.
* Caution in cardiac disease or conditions predisposing to ↑K such as renal or adrenocortical insufficiency, acute dehydration, and extensive tissue destruction as occurs with severe burns and in patients who are receiving potassium-sparing diuretics or other medications that may ↑K.
* In cases of renal insufficiency due to severe dehydration, excretory function should be restored by correction of the fluid deficit in order to ensure adequate urinary excretion of potassium before its parenteral administration.
* Initial potassium replacement therapy should not involve glucose infusions, because glucose may further decrease serum K.

*Biochemical and other tests (not all are necessary in an emergency situation)*

ECG
Electrolytes: serum K, Cl
Renal function: U, Cr, CrCl (or eGFR)

## Dose

**Treatment of hypokalaemia:** the dose is dependent upon the biochemistry and clinical condition of the patient.

**Mild to moderate ↓K (K > 2.5 mmol/L):** oral KCl supplements are usually adequate. If the oral route is temporarily unavailable, a single dose of 20–40 mmol by IV infusion over 6–8 hours may be sufficient to treat acute deficiency.

**Severe ↓K (K < 2.5 mmol/L):** 20–40 mmol (as a 40 mmol/L solution) by IV infusion at a maximum rate of 20 mmol/hour (10 mmol/hour is the usual maximum in a general ward area) governed by the clinical status and hydration of the patient. Repeat as necessary according to biochemistry results.

More concentrated solutions may be given in a critical care area with ECG monitoring, particularly where fluid overload is problematic.

NB: There is a high risk of asystole if the administration rate reaches 40 mmol/hour.

**Prevention of hypokalaemia where the oral route is unavailable:** average adult requirement is considered to be approximately 1 mmol/kg/day by IV infusion although this may rise to 2–3 mmol/kg/day where there are large losses such as those from drains, fistulae, etc.

## Continuous intravenous infusion

*Preparation and administration*

Check that you have selected the correct strength of KCl-containing infusion fluid.
Owing to the risk of thrombophlebitis, solutions containing >30 mmol/L should be given via the largest vein available.

1. The infusion is pre-prepared for use*. It should be clear and colourless. Inspect visually for particulate matter or discoloration prior to administration and discard if present.
2. Give by IV infusion via a volumetric infusion device at a maximum rate of 10–20 mmol/hour (10 mmol/hour is the usual maximum in a general ward area) unless the patient is being treated under specialist supervision in a critical care area. Owing to the risk of thrombophlebitis, solutions containing >30 mmol/L should be given via the largest vein available.
3. Discard any unused portion. Do not reconnect partially used infusion containers.

\*_Important_: If a pre-prepared infusion is not available at the required strength, and it is necessary to add concentrated KCl to an infusion fluid:

- Additions must never be made to an infusion container that has already been connected to a giving set.
- After the correct quantity of KCl has been added mix thoroughly by squeezing and inverting the bag at least 10 times.
- KCl is particularly prone to a 'layering' effect when added without adequate mixing: a concentrated layer of KCl will form at the bottom of the bag, which may cause the patient to receive an inadvertent bolus.

## Technical information

| | |
|---|---|
| Incompatible with | The following drugs are incompatible with potassium chloride-containing solutions (however this list is not be exhaustive, check individual drug monographs): amoxicillin, amphotericin, dantrolene, diazepam emulsion, enoximone, methylprednisolone sodium succinate, phenytoin sodium. |
| Compatible with | **Flush**: NaCl 0.9% **Solutions**: NaCl 0.9%, Gluc 5%, Gluc-NaCl, Hartmann's, Ringer's **Y-site**: See individual drug monographs |
| pH | 3.5–6.5 |
| Sodium content | Depends on diluent infusion fluid used – see relevant entries. |
| Storage | Store below 25°C. See the UK NPSA Patient Safety Alert information above concerning appropriate storage. |

## Monitoring

| Measure | Frequency | Rationale |
|---|---|---|
| Serum K | Throughout treatment | • Measured at regular intervals to avoid the development of ↑K, especially in patients with renal impairment. • The aim of potassium replacement therapy is to elevate the plasma concentration to within the normal range. |
| ECG monitoring (when infusion rate exceeds 20 mmol/hour) | | • ECG changes are an important indicator of K toxicity and include tall, peaked T waves, depression of the ST segment, disappearance of the P wave, prolongation of the QT interval, and widening and slurring of the QRS complex. |
| Clinical symptoms | | • Symptoms indicating toxicity related to ↑K include paraesthesia of the extremities, muscle weakness, paralysis, ↓BP, cardiac arrhythmias, heart block, cardiac arrest, and confusion. |

_(continued)_

## Monitoring (*continued*)

| Measure | Frequency | Rationale |
|---------|-----------|-----------|
| Renal function | Throughout treatment | • ↑K is more likely to occur in patients with impaired renal function.<br>• Use of KCl should be avoided where possible if CrCl <10 mL/minute. |
| Acid-base balance | | • Potassium deficiency can be evaluated by acid-base status. |

## Additional information

| | |
|---|---|
| Common and serious undesirable effects | *Infusion-related:*<br>• Too rapid administration: Life threatening ↑K.<br>• Local: Pain and thrombophlebitis may occur during IV administration of solutions containing >30 mmol/L. Extravasation may cause tissue damage.<br>*Other:* ↑K especially in patients with renal impairment. |
| Pharmacokinetics | Not applicable |
| Significant interactions | • The following may ↑K levels:<br>  ACE inhibitors, aliskiren, amiloride, angiotensin II receptor antagonists, ciclosporin, eplerenone, spironolactone, tacrolimus, triamterene, K supplements, K-containing salt substitutes for flavouring food, e.g. Lo-Salt.<br>• Glucose infusions may ↓K (in patients with ↓K). |
| Action in case of overdose | *Symptoms to watch for:* Extremely high serum K concentrations (8-11 mmol/L) may cause death from cardiac depression, arrhythmias or arrest.<br>*Antidote:* Emergency treatment is needed if serum potassium concentration is >6.5 mmol/L. Give calcium gluconate to stabilise the myocardium and insulin/glucose to lower serum K rapidly. Salbutamol has also been used but its use is controversial. See relevant entries. Review all potassium-retaining medication. |

| | |
|---|---|
| Risk rating: **RED** | Scoring system not suitable for this substance.<br>*Caution:* Extreme risk posed by inappropriate IV administration. |

This assessment is based on the full range of preparation and administration options described in the monograph. These may not all be applicable in some clinical situations.

## Bibliography

SPC Sterile Potassium Chloride Concentrate 15%, Hameln Pharmaceuticals Ltd (accessed 18 September 2009).

SPC Sterile Potassium Chloride Concentrate 20%, Hameln Pharmaceuticals Ltd (accessed 18 September 2009).

SPC Sterile Potassium Chloride Concentrate BP 15% w/v, 1.5 g in 10 mL, Goldshield plc (accessed 18 September 2009).

# Pralidoxime

**1-g dry powder vial (from designated centres)**

- Pralidoxime chloride is a cholinesterase reactivator.
- It is used (unlicensed) as an adjunct to atropine in the treatment of poisoning due to organophosphorus chemicals.
- It is available from designated centres – in the UK see Toxbase at www.toxbase.org for this list.

## Pre-treatment checks

- Do not use in the treatment of poisoning due to phosphorus, inorganic phosphates or organophosphates not having anticholinesterase activity.
- Use with caution in myasthenia gravis as it may cause a myasthenic crisis.
- Morphine, theophylline, aminophylline, and suxamethonium are contraindicated in organophosphorus poisoning. Avoid tranquillisers such as reserpine or phenothiazines.
- Pralidoxime should be administered within 36 hours after termination of exposure to the organophosphate. However, if the poison was ingested, exposure will continue for some time owing to the slow absorption from the lower bowel.
- If the skin has been exposed, clothing should be removed and the hair and skin washed thoroughly with sodium bicarbonate, alcohol or a washing-up liquid solution as soon as possible.
- Use with caution in renal impairment.

*Biochemical and other tests (not all are necessary in an emergency situation)*

| | |
|---|---|
| Blood pressure and pulse | will aid diagnosis and help monitor progress, but do not wait for results before initiating treatment. |
| Bodyweight | |
| Red blood cell, plasma cholinesterase and urinary paranitrophenol (if exposed to parathion) | |
| | Renal function: U, Cr, CrCl (or eGFR) |

## Dose

It is essential to consult a poisons information service, e.g. Toxbase at www.toxbase.org (password or registration required) for full details of the management of organophosphorus poisoning.

*Organophosphorus poisoning (unlicensed)[1]*

**Loading dose:** 30 mg/kg by IV infusion over 20 minutes. In patients weighing 60–80 kg this dose can be rounded up or down to 2 g.

**Subsequent dose:** 8 mg/kg/hour by IV infusion. In patients weighing 60–80 kg this can be rounded up or down to 0.5 g/hour. Usual maximum dose is 12 g in 24 hours. Continue treatment until the patient has not required atropine treatment for at least 12 hours; treatment may be required for several days.

**Fluid restriction:** if pulmonary oedema is present, the loading dose may be given by IV injection.

**Dose in renal impairment:** pralidoxime is renally excreted therefore dose reduction is probably required, particularly for prolonged infusions, but little information available.

## Intravenous infusion (loading dose)

*Preparation and administration*

1. Reconstitute each 1-g vial with 20 mL WFI.
2. Withdraw required dose and add to 100 mL NaCl 0.9%.

*(continued)*

3. The solution should be clear and colourless. Inspect visually for particulate matter or discoloration prior to administration and discard if present.
4. Give by IV infusion over 20 minutes.

## Continuous intravenous infusion (subsequent dosing)

*Preparation and administration*

1. The aim is to produce a solution containing 1–2% pralidoxime in NaCl 0.9% (e.g. 10 g could be made up to 500 mL).
2. Withdraw 20 mL for each vial to be used from an infusion bag containing the desired final volume of NaCl 0.9% and discard.
3. Reconstitute each 1-g vial with 20 mL WFI.
4. Withdraw required total dose and add to the prepared infusion bag to give a solution containing 1–2% pralidoxime. Mix well.
5. The solution should be clear and colourless. Inspect visually for particulate matter or discoloration prior to administration and discard if present.
6. Give by IV infusion using a volumetric infusion device at the required rate (see Dose above).
7. Prepare a fresh infusion bag at least every 24 hours.

## Intravenous injection (loading dose if IV infusion is not possible)

*Preparation and administration*

1. Reconstitute each 1-g vial with 20 mL WFI.
2. Withdraw the required dose.
3. The solution should be clear and colourless. Inspect visually for particulate matter or discoloration prior to administration and discard if present.
4. Give by slow IV injection over 5–10 minutes.

## Technical information

| Incompatible with | No information |
|---|---|
| Compatible with | **Flush**: NaCl 0.9%<br>**Solutions**: NaCl 0.9%<br>**Y-site**: No information |
| pH | 3.5-4.5 |
| Sodium content | Negligible |
| Storage | Store at 20-25°C in original packaging. |
| Displacement value | Negligible |
| Stability after preparation | Use prepared infusions immediately. |

## Monitoring

| Measure | Frequency | Rationale |
|---|---|---|
| ECG | During treatment and periodically after | • In severe cases of poisoning heart block may occur. |

*(continued)*

## Monitoring (continued)

| Measure | Frequency | Rationale |
|---|---|---|
| RBC, plasma cholinesterase, urinary paranitrophenol | Periodically | • For signs of clinical improvement, patients should be closely observed for at least 24 hours after resolution of symptoms.<br>• If poison was ingested symptoms may re-occur as the effects of pralidoxime wear off. Repeat doses may be required. |
| Blood pressure | | • May cause ↑BP. |
| Pulse | | • May cause ↑pulse. |

## Additional information

| | |
|---|---|
| Common and serious undesirable effects | *Injection/infusion-related:*<br>• Too rapid administration: ↑Pulse, laryngospasm and muscle rigidity.<br>• Local. Pain at injection site 40–60 minutes after IM administration.<br>*Other:* Drowsiness, dizziness, visual disturbances, nausea, ↑pulse, headache, hyperventilation and muscle rigidity. |
| Pharmacokinetics | As an adjunct to atropine and it should improve muscle tone within 30 minutes. Elimination half-life is 1–3 hours. |
| Significant interactions | No significant interactions. |
| Action in case of overdose | *Symptoms to watch for:* It can be difficult to distinguish the side-effects due to drug from those due to poison, but the following may occur: dizziness, blurred vision, diplopia, headache, impaired accommodation, ↑pulse.<br>*Antidote:* No specific antidote. Review benefits and risks of continued treatment. |

| Risk rating: **AMBER** | Score – 5<br>Moderate-risk product: Risk-reduction strategies are recommended. |
|---|---|

This assessment is based on the full range of preparation and administration options described in the monograph. These may not all be applicable in some clinical situations.

## Reference

1. Toxbase. www.toxbase.org (accessed 23 April 2010).

## Bibliography

SPC Protopam (accessed 25 November 2008).

# Prednisolone acetate

**25 mg/mL aqueous suspension in 1-mL ampoules**
* Prednisolone acetate is a corticosteroid with mainly glucocorticoid activity.
* It is used in the treatment of conditions for which systemic corticosteroid therapy is indicated (except adrenal-deficiency states). Deep IM injections have a depot effect, allowing dosing once or twice weekly.
* It may also be given by intra-articular or intrasynovial injection for various inflammatory conditions.
* Doses for injection are expressed in terms of prednisolone acetate.

## Pre-treatment checks

* Avoid where systemic infection is present (unless specific therapy given).
* Avoid live virus vaccines in those receiving immunosuppressive doses.
* May activate or exacerbate amoebiasis or strongyloidiasis (exclude before initiating a corticosteroid in those at risk or with suggestive symptoms). Fungal or viral ocular infections may also be exacerbated.
* Caution in patients predisposed to psychiatric reactions, including those who have previously suffered corticosteroid-induced psychosis, or who have a personal or family history of psychiatric disorders.
* Do not inject directly into tendons.

*Intra-articular:*
* Do not inject into unstable joints.
* Do not give in the presence of active infection in or near joints.

## Dose

**Intramuscular:** 25–100 mg once or twice weekly, adjusted according to patient response.
**Intra-articular or intrasynovial:** 5–25 mg according to size of joint; not more than three joints should be treated on any one day; where appropriate it may be repeated when relapse occurs.

## Intramuscular injection

*Preparation and administration*

* Withdraw the required dose.
* Give by IM injection.

## Intra-articular or intrasynovial injection

*Preparation and administration*

1. Withdraw the required dose.
2. Inject into the affected area. Treatment failure after intra-articular injection is most frequently the result of failure to enter the joint space.

| Technical information | |
|---|---|
| Incompatible with | Not relevant |
| Compatible with | Not relevant |
| pH | Not relevant |
| Sodium content | Negligible |

*(continued)*

## Technical information (continued)

| | |
|---|---|
| Excipients | Contains benzyl alcohol. |
| Storage | Store at 15-25°C in original packaging. |

## Monitoring (dependent on dose and site of injection)

| Measure | Frequency | Rationale |
|---|---|---|
| Serum Na, K, Ca | Throughout systemic treatment | • May cause fluid and electrolyte disturbances. |
| Withdrawal symptoms and signs | During withdrawal and after stopping systemic treatment | • During prolonged therapy with corticosteroids, adrenal atrophy develops and can persist for years after stopping. Abrupt withdrawal after a prolonged period can lead to acute adrenal insufficiency, ↓BP or death.<br>• The UK CSM has recommended that gradual withdrawal of systemic corticosteroids should be considered in patients whose disease is unlikely to relapse. Full details can be found in the BNF. |
| Signs of infection | During systemic treatment | • Prolonged courses ↑susceptibility to infections and severity of infections. Serious infections may reach an advanced stage before being recognised. |
| Signs of chickenpox | | • Unless they have had chickenpox, patients receiving corticosteroids for purposes other than replacement should be regarded as being at risk of severe chickenpox.<br>• Confirmed chickenpox requires urgent treatment; corticosteroids should not be stopped and the dosage may need to be increased. |
| Exposure to measles | | • Patients should be advised to take particular care to avoid exposure to measles and to seek immediate medical advice if exposure occurs.<br>• Prophylaxis with IM normal immunoglobulin may be needed. |
| Symptoms of septic arthritis | Following intra-articular injection | • A marked increase in pain accompanied by local swelling, further restriction of joint motion, fever, and malaise are suggestive of septic arthritis. |

## Additional information

| | |
|---|---|
| Common and serious undesirable effects | *Immediate:* Anaphylaxis and other hypersensitivity reactions have been reported.<br>*Short-term use:* Undesirable effects which may result from short-term use (minimise by using the lowest effective dose for the shortest time): ↑BP, Na and water retention, ↓K, ↓Ca, ↑blood glucose, peptic ulceration and perforation, psychiatric reactions, ↑susceptibility to infection, muscle weakness, tendon rupture, insomnia, ↑intracranial pressure, ↓seizure threshold, impaired healing.<br>*Long-term use:* For undesirable effects resulting from long-term corticosteroid use refer to the BNF. |

*(continued)*

## Additional information (*continued*)

| | |
|---|---|
| Pharmacokinetics | Elimination half-life is 2-4 hours (biological half-life will be longer). |
| Significant interactions | • The following may ↓corticosteroid levels or effect: barbiturates, carbamazepine, phenytoin, primidone, rifabutin, rifampicin.<br>• Corticosteroids may ↑levels or effect of the following drugs (or ↑side-effects): anticoagulants (monitor INR), methotrexate (↑risk of blood dyscrasias).<br>• If using amphotericin IV monitor fluid balance and K level closely.<br>• Corticosteroids may ↓levels or effect of vaccines (↓immunological response, ↑risk of infection with live vaccines). |
| Action in case of overdose | Give supportive therapy as appropriate. Following chronic overdose the possibility of adrenal suppression should be considered. |
| Counselling | Patients should be specifically warned to avoid over-use of joints in which symptomatic benefit has been obtained.<br>Patients on long-term corticosteroid treatment should read and carry a Steroid Treatment Card. |

| Risk rating: **GREEN** | Score = 2<br>Lower-risk product: Risk-reduction strategies should be considered. |
|---|---|

This assessment is based on the full range of preparation and administration options described in the monograph. These may not all be applicable in some clinical situations.

### Bibliography

SPC Deltastab injection (accessed 16 January 2010).

# Prochlorperazine (chlormeprazine, prochlorpemazine)

### 12.5 mg/mL solution in 1-mL ampoules

* Prochlorperazine mesilate is a phenothiazine antipsychotic with a wide range of actions. It is a dopamine inhibitor; it has antiemetic activity; it has muscle relaxant properties; and it inhibits the heat-regulating centre.
* It is used in the treatment of nausea and vomiting and in schizophrenia and acute mania.
* Doses below are expressed in terms of prochlorperazine mesilate.

### Pre-treatment checks

* Do not use in comatose states, CNS depression, and phaeochromocytoma.

- Caution in renal or hepatic impairment, Parkinson disease, hypothyroidism, cardiac failure, myasthenia gravis, prostate hypertrophy, history of narrow-angle glaucoma or agranulocytosis.
- Use with caution in patients with risk factors for stroke.
- Concomitant treatment with other antipsychotics should be avoided.
- Monitor patients with epilepsy or a history of seizures closely because prochlorperazine may lower the seizure threshold.

*Biochemical and other tests (not all are necessary in an emergency situation)*

ECG – to rule out any risk factors
LFTs
Renal function: U, Cr, CrCl (or eGFR) – start with small doses in severe renal impairment as increased cerebral sensitivity

## Dose

**Nausea and vomiting:** 12.5 mg by deep IM injection followed by oral medication 6 hours later if required.
**Schizophrenia and other psychotic disorders:** 12.5–25 mg two or three times a day by deep IM injection until oral treatment can be initiated.
**Dose in renal impairment:** reduce dose if CrCl <10 mL/minute.
**Dose in hepatic impairment:** reduce dose or avoid.

## Intramuscular injection

See Special handling below.

*Preparation and administration*

1. Withdraw the required dose.
2. Give by deep IM injection into a large muscle such as the gluteal muscle.

## Technical information

| Incompatible with | Not relevant |
|---|---|
| Compatible with | Not relevant |
| pH[1] | 5.5–6.5 |
| Sodium content | Negligible |
| Excipients | Contains sulfites (may cause hypersensitivity reactions) |
| Storage | Store below 25°C in original packaging. Do not use discoloured solutions. |
| Special handling | Handle solutions with care to avoid risk of contact sensitisation. |

## Monitoring

| Measure | Frequency | Rationale |
|---|---|---|
| Blood pressure | Post injection | • May cause ↓BP particularly after IM injection. |

*(continued)*

## Monitoring (*continued*)

| Measure | Frequency | Rationale |
|---|---|---|
| Therapeutic improvement | Periodically | • Reduction in nausea and vomiting or improvement in symptoms of schizophrenia or mania. |
| FBC | | • In long-term use there is a risk of agranulocytosis. |
| ECG | | • In long-term use there may be ECG changes. |
| LFTs | | • Can precipitate coma if used in hepatic impairment.<br>• Phenothiazines are hepatotoxic. |

## Additional information

| | |
|---|---|
| Common and serious undesirable effects | ↓BP, ↓sweating, photosensitivity, constipation, xerostomia, EPSEs, blurred vision, nasal congestion. |
| Pharmacokinetics | Elimination half-life is approximately 7 hours. |
| Significant drug interactions | • The following may ↑prochlorperazine levels or effect (or ↑side-effects): anaesthetics-general (↑risk of ↓BP), antidepressants-tricyclic, artemether with lumefantrine (avoid combination), ritonavir, sibutramine (avoid combination).<br>• Prochlorperazine may ↓levels or effect of levodopa.<br>• Prochlorperazine may ↑risk of ventricular arrhythmias with the following drugs:<br>amiodarone (avoid combination), antidepressants-tricyclic, atomoxetine, disopyramide, droperidol (avoid combination), methadone, moxifloxacin (avoid combination), pentamidine isetionate, pimozide (avoid combination), sotalol.<br>• Prochlorperazine ↓convulsive threshold and may ↓effect of the following drugs: barbiturates, carbamazepine, ethosuximide, oxcarbazepine, phenytoin, primidone, valproate. |
| Overdose | Treatment is supportive and symptomatic.<br>Severe dystonic reactions may be treated with 5-10 mg procyclidine.<br>Convulsions may be treated with IV diazepam.<br>Neuroleptic malignant syndrome should be treated with cooling. Dantrolene sodium may be used.<br>Do not give adrenaline. |
| Counselling | Patients on long-term prochlorperazine should avoid exposure to direct sunlight as they may develop photosensitisation. |

| | |
|---|---|
| Risk rating: **GREEN** | Score = 1<br>Lower-risk product: Risk-reduction strategies should be considered. |

This assessment is based on the full range of preparation and administration options described in the monograph. These may not all be applicable in some clinical situations.

## Reference

1. Personal communiqué from Sanofi Aventis, 09 June 20009.

## Bibliography

SPC Stemetil (accessed 11 July 2008).

# Procyclidine hydrochloride

**5 mg/mL solution in 2-mL ampoules**

* Procyclidine hydrochloride is an antimuscarinic drug.
* It is used parenterally to treat drug-induced acute dystonic reactions and extrapyramidal symptoms.

## Pre-treatment checks

* Avoid in individuals with untreated urinary retention, closed-angle glaucoma and GI obstruction.
* Caution in cardiovascular disease, ↑BP, psychotic disorders, prostatic hypertrophy and pyrexia.

## Dose

**Standard dose:** 5–10 mg by IV or IM injection, repeated after 20 minutes if necessary. Maximum daily dose 20 mg. Use the lower end of the dosage range in elderly patients or those of low bodyweight. The IV route should be effective within 5–10 minutes; occasionally patients may require up to 30 minutes for full effect.

## Intravenous injection

*Preparation and administration*

1. Withdraw the required dose.
2. The solution should be clear and colourless. Inspect visually for particulate matter or discoloration prior to administration and discard if present.
3. Give by IV injection.

## Intramuscular injection

*Preparation and administration*

1. Withdraw the required dose.
2. Give by IM injection.

| Technical information | |
|---|---|
| Incompatible with | No information |
| Compatible with | **Flush**: NaCl 0.9%<br>**Solutions**: NaCl 0.9%<br>**Y-site**: No information |
| pH | 3.9–4.5 |

*(continued)*

## Technical information (continued)

| | |
|---|---|
| Sodium content | Nil |
| Storage | Store below 25°C in original packaging. |

## Monitoring

| Measure | Frequency | Rationale |
|---|---|---|
| Observe extrapyramidal movements, rigidity, tremor, gait disturbances | For acute dystonias: the first 20–30 minutes. For Parkinson's disease: daily until maintenance dose achieved. | • To ensure that treatment is effective.<br>• To establish maintenance dose. |

## Additional information

| | |
|---|---|
| Common and serious undesirable effects | *Common:* Constipation, nausea, dry mouth, blurred vision, urinary retention. |
| Pharmacokinetics | Elimination half-life is approximately 12 hours. |
| Significant interactions | No significant interactions known. |
| Action in case of overdose | *Symptoms to watch for:* Agitation, restlessness and severe sleeplessness lasting 24 hours or more. Visual and auditory hallucinations have been reported. ↑Pulse has also been reported.<br>*Antidote:* Stop administration and give supportive therapy as appropriate. Active measures such as the use of cholinergic agents or haemodialysis are unlikely to be of value. |

| | |
|---|---|
| Risk rating: **GREEN** | Score = 1<br>Lower-risk product: Risk-reduction strategies should be considered. |

This assessment is based on the full range of preparation and administration options described in the monograph. These may not all be applicable in some clinical situations.

## Bibliography

SPC Kemadrin injection (10 April 2007 version).

# Progesterone

**50 mg/mL oily solution in 1-mL and 2-mL ampoules**

* Progesterone is a natural hormone that acts on the endometrium.
* It may be given by IM injection to treat dysfunctional uterine bleeding.
* It is also licensed (but no longer recommended) for the maintenance of early pregnancy following recurrent miscarriages due to inadequate luteal phase, or following in-vitro fertilisation or gamete intrafallopian transfer.

## Pre-treatment checks

* Avoid in undiagnosed vaginal bleeding, missed or incomplete abortion, mammary or genital tract carcinoma, thrombophlebitis, cerebral haemorrhage, severe hepatic dysfunction.
* Caution in patients with conditions that might be affected by fluid retention, e.g. ↑BP, cardiac disease or with a history of depression, diabetes, mild–moderate hepatic impairment, acute intermittent porphyria, migraine or photosensitivity.
* Progesterone may ↓glucose tolerance and patients with diabetes should be closely monitored.

*Biochemical and other tests (not all are necessary in an emergency situation)*

Blood pressure
LFTs

## Dose

**Dysfunctional uterine bleeding:** 5–10 mg daily by IM injection for 5–10 days until 2 days before anticipated onset of menstruation.

## Intramuscular injection

*Preparation and administration*

1. Withdraw the required dose.
2. Give by deep IM injection into the buttock.

| Technical information | |
|---|---|
| Incompatible with | Not relevant |
| Compatible with | Not relevant |
| pH | Not relevant - oily injection |
| Sodium content | Nil |
| Excipients | Contains benzyl alcohol. |
| Storage | Store at 15-25°C in original packaging. |

## Monitoring

| Measure | Frequency | Rationale |
|---|---|---|
| Uterine bleeding | Periodically | • For signs of clinical improvement. |
| Pregnancy | | • To ensure that treatment is effective. |
| Blood glucose | | • May ↓glucose tolerance. |
| Visual disturbances | On presentation | • If unexplained, sudden or gradual, partial or complete loss of vision, proptosis or diplopia, papilloedema, retinal vascular lesions or migraine occur, the drug should be discontinued and appropriate diagnostic and therapeutic measures instituted. |

## Additional information

| | |
|---|---|
| Common and serious undesirable effects | *Injection-related:* Local: pain and swelling at the injection site.<br>*Other:* Menstrual disturbances, breast changes, oedema, weight gain, nausea, headache, dizziness, sleep disturbances, depression, alopecia, hirsutism, jaundice, acne. |
| Pharmacokinetics | The IM injection is rapidly absorbed and provides depot therapy. |
| Significant interactions | • Progesterone may ↑levels or effect of the following drugs (or ↑side-effects): ciclosporin (monitor levels), coumarin anticoagulants (monitor INR).<br>• Progesterone may ↓levels or effect of the following drugs: coumarin anticoagulants (monitor INR), lamotrigine, phenindione (monitor INR). |
| Action in case of overdose | Observe and if required symptomatic and supportive measures should be provided. |

| Risk rating: **GREEN** | Score = 1<br>Lower-risk product: Risk-reduction strategies should be considered. |
|---|---|

This assessment is based on the full range of preparation and administration options described in the monograph. These may not all be applicable in some clinical situations.

## Bibliography

SPC Gestone (accessed 29 September 2009).

# Promethazine hydrochloride

**25 mg/mL solution in 1-mL and 2-mL ampoules**

* Promethazine hydrochloride is a phenothiazine derivative. It acts as a sedating antihistamine with significant sedative, antimuscarinic, and some serotonin-antagonist properties.
* It is used for the symptomatic treatment of allergic conditions of the upper respiratory tract and skin including allergic rhinitis, urticaria and anaphylactic reactions to drugs and foreign proteins.
* It may be given IV as an adjunct in the emergency treatment of anaphylactic shock.
* It may also be used pre- and postoperatively in surgery and obstetrics for its sedative effects and for the relief of apprehension; it is often given with pethidine hydrochloride.

## Pre-treatment checks

* Avoid in patients taking monoamine oxidase inhibitors up to 14 days previously because of ⏐risk of extrapyramidal side-effects.
* Use with caution in asthma, bronchitis or bronchiectasis as it may thicken secretions.
* Use with care in narrow-angle glaucoma, prostatic hypertrophy, urinary retention and pyloro-duodenal obstruction because of its antimuscarinic effects.
* Use with care in epilepsy as it may lower the convulsive threshold.
* Promethazine is thought to be safe in acute porphyria.

*Biochemical and other tests (not all are necessary in an emergency situation)*

LFTs

## Dose

**Standard dose:** 25–50 mg by deep IM injection. If used for pre-medication, give 1 hour prior to surgery.

**Adjunctive treatment of anaphylactic shock:** 25–50 mg by slow IV injection (maximum 100 mg).

**Dose in hepatic impairment:** avoid in severe liver disease, may precipitate coma and is hepatotoxic.

## Intramuscular injection (preferred route)

*Preparation and administration*

1. Withdraw the required dose.
2. Give by deep IM injection. Take care to avoid inadvertent SC injection (can cause local necrosis).

## Intravenous injection

*Preparation and administration*

1. Withdraw the required dose and dilute each 1 mL of injection to 10 mL with WFI.
2. The solution should be clear and colourless. Inspect visually for particulate matter or discoloration prior to administration and discard if present.
3. Give by slow IV injection at a maximum rate of 25 mg/minute.
4. Take care to avoid extravasation or inadvertent intra-arterial injection (can cause necrosis and peripheral gangrene). If a patient complains of pain during IV injection, stop immediately.

## Technical information

| | |
|---|---|
| Incompatible with | Amphotericin, foscarnet, heparin sodium, hydrocortisone sodium succinate, piperacillin with tazobactam, potassium chloride. |
| Compatible with | **Flush**: NaCl 0.9%<br>**Solutions**: WFI, NaCl 0.9%, Gluc 5%, Gluc-NaCl, Hartmann's, Ringer's<br>**Y-site**: Aztreonam, ciprofloxacin, cisatracurium, fluconazole, granisetron, metoclopramide, ondansetron, pethidine (in-syringe compatible), remifentanil |
| pH | 4-5.5 |
| Sodium content | Negligible |
| Excipients | Contains sulfites (may cause allergic reactions). |
| Storage | Store below 30°C in original packaging. Discard if discoloured or contains a precipitate. |
| Stability after preparation | Use prepared dilutions immediately. |

## Monitoring

| Measure | Frequency | Rationale |
|---|---|---|
| Pain at injection site | During administration | • Extravasation or inadvertent intra-arterial injection may cause necrosis and peripheral gangrene.<br>• Inadvertent SC injection may cause local necrosis.<br>• Stop injection immediately. |
| Blood pressure and pulse | | • May cause ↓BP and ↑pulse. |
| Hypersensitivity reactions | During and for 1 hour after administration | • Rash, pruritus and anaphylaxis have been reported.<br>• These may be a reaction to the preservatives in the injection rather than to the drug itself. |

## Additional information

| | |
|---|---|
| Common and serious undesirable effects | *Immediate:* Anaphylaxis and other hypersensitivity reactions have been reported very rarely.<br>*Other:* Drowsiness, dizziness, restlessness, headaches, nightmares, tiredness, disorientation, blurred vision, dry mouth, urinary retention, rash, pruritus. |
| Pharmacokinetics | After IM dosing, peak plasma concentrations are seen after 2-3 hours. Elimination half-lives of 5-14 hours have been reported. |
| Significant interactions | • Promethazine may ↑side-effects of the following drugs: MAOIs (↑risk of EPSE; avoid within 14 days), opioid analgesics (↑sedation). |

*(continued)*

## Additional information (*continued*)

| | |
|---|---|
| Action in case of overdose | *Symptoms to watch for:* ↑Drowsiness.<br>*Antidote:* No known antidote; stop administration and give supportive therapy as appropriate. |
| Counselling | May cause drowsiness; if affected do not drive or operate machinery. Do not drink alcohol for a few hours after injection. |

| | |
|---|---|
| Risk rating: **GREEN** | Score = 1<br>Lower-risk product: Risk-reduction strategies should be considered. |

This assessment is based on the full range of preparation and administration options described in the monograph. These may not all be applicable in some clinical situations.

## Bibliography

SPC Phenergan (accessed 24 January 2009).

# Propranolol hydrochloride

**1 mg/mL solution in 1-mL ampoules**

* Propranolol hydrochloride is a non-cardioselective beta-adrenoceptor blocker.
* It is used IV for the emergency treatment of cardiac dysrhythmias and thyrotoxic crisis.

## Pre-treatment checks

* Treatment should be avoided in sick sinus syndrome, ↓BP, heart block greater than first degree, ↓pulse (<45–50 bpm), cardiogenic shock, overt heart failure and asthma.
* Caution in patients with a history of wheezing or peripheral circulatory conditions.
* Caution in elderly patients or those of low bodyweight.

## Dose

**Standard dose:** 1 mg by IV injection which may be repeated at 2-minute intervals if necessary until a response is observed, or to a maximum dose of 10 mg in conscious patients or 5 mg in patients under anaesthesia.

## Intravenous injection

*Preparation and administration*

1. Withdraw the required dose.
2. The solution should be clear and colourless. Inspect visually for particulate matter or discoloration prior to administration and discard if present.
3. Give by IV injection over 1 minute.

## Technical information

| | |
|---|---|
| Incompatible with | Amphotericin, pantoprazole. |
| Compatible with | **Flush**: NaCl 0.9%<br>**Solutions**: NaCl 0.9%, Gluc 5%, Gluc-NaCl, Hartmann's (all including added KCl)<br>**Y-site**: Alteplase, dobutamine, hydrocortisone sodium succinate, linezolid, propofol |
| pH | 2.8-4 |
| Sodium content | Nil |
| Storage | Store below 30°C in original packaging. |

## Monitoring

| Measure | Frequency | Rationale |
|---|---|---|
| Heart rate | Continuously | • Consider withholding therapy if pulse drops to 50–55 bpm or lower.<br>• Excessive ↓pulse can be countered with IV atropine sulfate in doses of 600 micrograms repeated every 3-5 minutes up to a maximum of 2.4 mg. |
| Blood pressure | | • Stop dosing if ↓BP occurs that requires corrective measures. |
| Respiratory function or oxygen saturation in at-risk individuals | After initial dosing | • May cause bronchoconstriction in susceptible individuals, e.g. patients with history of bronchospasm or respiratory disease. |
| Injection site | For 24 hours after dosing | • Extravasation may cause tissue damage. |

## Additional information

| | |
|---|---|
| Common and serious undesirable effects | ↓Pulse, cold extremities, fatigue.<br>Bronchospasm may occur in patients with asthma or other respiratory disease. |
| Elimination half-life | Approximately 2 hours. |
| Significant drug interactions | • The following may ↑propranolol levels or effect (or ↑side-effects): adrenaline (risk of severe ↑BP and ↓pulse), alpha-blockers (severe ↓BP), amiodarone (risk of ↓pulse and AV block), antiarrhythmics (risk of myocardial depression), chlorpromazine, clonidine (↑risk of withdrawal ↑BP), diltiazem (risk of ↓pulse and AV block), dobutamine (risk of severe ↑BP and ↓pulse), flecainide (risk of myocardial depression and ↓pulse), moxisylyte (severe ↓BP), nifedipine (severe ↓BP and heart failure), noradrenaline (risk of severe ↑BP and ↓pulse), verapamil (risk of asystole and severe ↓BP).<br>• Propranolol may ↑levels or effect of the following drugs (or ↑side-effects): bupivacaine, chlorpromazine, lidocaine. |

*(continued)*

| Additional information | (continued) |
|---|---|
| Overdose | *Symptoms to watch for:* ↓Pulse, ↓BP, acute cardiac insufficiency and bronchospasm. *Antidote:* Stop administration and give supportive therapy as appropriate (may include atropine, bronchodilators, glucagon, dopamine – see relevant entries). |
| Counselling | Patients may experience fatigue and cold extremities during therapy, and should report wheezing. |

| Risk rating: **GREEN** | Score = 1 |
|---|---|
| | Lower-risk product: Risk-reduction strategies should be considered. |

This assessment is based on the full range of preparation and administration options described in the monograph. These may not all be applicable in some clinical situations.

## Bibliography

SPC Inderal injection (accessed 17 September 2009).

# Protamine sulfate (protamine sulphate)

**10 mg/mL solution in 5-mL and 10-mL ampoules**

* Protamine sulfate is composed of a mixture of the sulfates of basic peptides prepared from the sperm or mature testes of suitable species of fish, usually *Clupeidae* or *Salmonidae*.
* It combines with heparin to form a stable inactive complex. It can therefore be used to treat haemorrhage resulting from severe heparin overdosage, both for unfractionated heparins (UFH) or low-molecular-weight heparins (LMWH).

## Pre-treatment checks

* Use with caution in patients with known sensitivity to fish, in vasectomised or infertile males, and in patients who have received previous protamine sulfate therapy or protamine insulin due to ↑risk of allergic reactions (see Counselling).
* Identification of type of heparin, route used and dose given.

*Biochemical and other tests (not all are necessary in an emergency situation)*

APTT or ACT

## Dose

Dose is dependent on the amount and type of heparin to be neutralised, route of administration and the time that has elapsed since it was last given (heparin is continuously being excreted). Excessive doses of protamine sulfate can have an anticoagulant effect.

Protamine sulfate 1 mg can be expected to inhibit the effects of:

* Heparin (mucous) 100 units (UFH)
* Heparin (lung) 80 units (UFH)
* Bemiparin sodium 71 units (LMWH), i.e. 1.4 mg protamine sulfate for every 100 units
* Dalteparin sodium 100 units (LMWH)
* Enoxaparin sodium 1 mg (LMWH)
* Tinzaparin sodium 100 units (LMWH)

**Neutralisation of UFH given by IV injection:** by slow IV injection give 1 mg protamine sulfate for each 100 units of heparin (mucous) up to a maximum of 50 mg. Reduce the dose if more than 15 minutes have elapsed since IV injection of heparin; e.g. if 30–60 minutes have elapsed give 0.5–0.75 mg/100 units; if 2 hours or more have elapsed give 0.25–0.375 mg/100 units.

**Neutralisation of UFH given by IV infusion:** stop the infusion and give 25–50 mg protamine sulfate by slow IV injection. Maximum dose is 50 mg.

**Neutralisation of UFH given by SC injection:** give a total dose of 1 mg/100 units of heparin (mucous) as follows: initially with 25–50 mg by slow IV injection, then the remainder by IV infusion over 8–16 hours. Total maximum dose is 50 mg.

**Neutralisation of LMWH:** according to the dose equivalents stated above, give the required dose (up to a maximum of 50 mg) as an intermittent or continuous IV infusion. The anti-Factor Xa activity of LMWHs may not be completely reversed by protamine and may persist for up to 24 hours after administration.

## Intravenous injection

*Preparation and administration*

1. Withdraw the required dose.
2. The solution should be clear and colourless. Inspect visually for particulate matter or discoloration prior to administration and discard if present.
3. Give by IV injection over about 10 minutes at a maximum rate of 5 mg/minute.

## Intermittent or continuous intravenous infusion

*Preparation and administration*

1. Withdraw the required dose and add to a convenient volume of NaCl 0.9% or Gluc 5%. Mix well.
2. The solution should be clear and colourless. Inspect visually for particulate matter or discoloration prior to administration and discard if present.
3. Give by IV infusion via a volumetric infusion device. Rate depends on indication.

## Technical information

| | |
|---|---|
| Incompatible with | Cephalosporins, penicillins. |
| Compatible with | **Flush**: NaCl 0.9%<br>**Solutions**: NaCl 0.9%, Gluc 5%<br>**Y-site**: No information |
| pH | 2.5–3.5 |
| Sodium content | Negligible |
| Storage | Store at 15–25°C. Do not refrigerate. |
| Stability after preparation | Use prepared infusions immediately. |

## Monitoring

| Measure | Frequency | Rationale |
|---------|-----------|-----------|
| APTT or ACT | 5-15 minutes after administration; then after 2-8 hours | • For signs of clinical improvement.<br>• Further doses may be needed as protamine is cleared more rapidly from the blood than heparin, especially LMWH. |
| Bleeding | Up to 5 hours after protamine administration | • If insufficient protamine is given, a heparin rebound occurs within 5 hours of neutralisation; this may be associated with clinical bleeding. |

## Additional information

| | |
|---|---|
| Common and serious undesirable effects | *Immediate:* Anaphylaxis has been reported rarely.<br>*Other:* Sudden ↓BP, ↓pulse, pulmonary and systemic ↑BP, dyspnoea, transitory flushing and a feeling of warmth, back pain, nausea and vomiting, lassitude. |
| Pharmacokinetics | Elimination half-life is 7.4 minutes. |
| Significant interactions | Protamine may affect fluorescence methods of estimating plasma catecholamines. |
| Action in case of overdose | Monitor coagulation tests, respiratory ventilation and symptomatic treatment. If bleeding is a problem, fresh frozen plasma or fresh whole blood should be given |
| Counselling | Caution in fish sensitivity and in vasectomised men.<br>During vasectomy, antibodies develop against natural nucleoproteins (a component of human sperm cells) in 22-33% of patients. These antibodies have been shown to cross-react with medicinal protamines, which are extracted commercially from the testes of salmon and certain other fish.[1] |

| Risk rating: **AMBER** | Score = 4<br>Moderate risk product: Risk-reduction strategies are recommended. |
|---|---|

This assessment is based on the full range of preparation and administration options described in the monograph. These may not all be applicable in some clinical situations.

## Reference

1. Watson RA *et al.* Allergic reaction to protamine: a late complication of elective vasectomy? *Urology* 1983; 22(5): 493–495.

## Bibliography

SPC Prosulf 10 mg/mL solution for injection (accessed 23 August 2009).
SPC Protamine Sulphate Injection BP (UCB Pharma Ltd) (accessed 23 August 2009).
SPC Protamine Sulphate Injection BP 1%, Sovereign Medical (accessed 23 August 2009).

# Protirelin (thyrotrophin-releasing hormone, TRH, TRF)

**100 micrograms/mL solution in 2-mL ampoules**

- Protirelin is a hypothalamic releasing hormone that stimulates the release of thyrotrophin (thyroid-stimulating hormone, TSH) from the anterior pituitary.
- It is licensed for the diagnosis of mild hyperthyroidism or hypothyroidism, but its use has been largely superseded by immunoassays for TSH.
- It may be used to assess hypothalamic and pituitary function and TSH reserve by the interpretation of the various thyroid hormone levels pre and post dose.

## Pre-treatment checks

- Protirelin may have an effect on smooth muscle; closely monitor patients with asthma or other types of obstructive airways disease.
- Give cautiously to patients with myocardial ischaemia and severe hypopituitarism.

*Biochemical and other tests*

Thyroid function: baseline TSH assay (and other thyroid hormones if appropriate) immediately prior to dose

## Dose

**Standard adult dose:** 200 micrograms.

## Intravenous injection

*Preparation and administration*

1. Take blood sample immediately prior to the dose.
2. Withdraw the required dose.
3. Give by IV injection over 30 seconds.
4. Take a blood sample exactly 20 minutes after the injection for peak thyroid hormone assay and, if necessary, a further sample at exactly 60 minutes after injection to detect a delayed thyroid hormone response.

| Technical information | |
|---|---|
| Incompatible with | Not relevant |
| Compatible with | **Flush**: NaCl 0.9%<br>**Solutions**: Not relevant<br>**Y-site**: Not relevant |
| pH | 4.5-6.5 |
| Sodium content | Nil |
| Storage | Store below 30°C in original packaging. |

## Monitoring

| Measure | Frequency | Rationale |
| --- | --- | --- |
| Thyroid function | Immediately before administration, 20 (and possibly 60) minutes after | • See detail in Administration above. |
| Blood pressure and pulse | For 15 minutes after administration | • BP changes may occur; the patient should be lying down when receiving the drug and for 15 minutes afterwards. |

## Additional information

| | |
| --- | --- |
| Common and serious undesirable effects | Following rapid IV injection most side-effects are mild and transient: nausea, desire to micturate, flushing, slight dizziness, peculiar taste, ↑ or ↓BP, ↑pulse. Protirelin also has prolactin-releasing activity and may cause breast enlargement and milk leakage in breast-feeding women. |
| Pharmacokinetics | TSH disappears rapidly from the plasma after IV injection. Over 90% is removed within 20 minutes with a half-life of about 5.3 minutes. About 5.5% of the dose is excreted in the urine, mostly within 30 minutes. |
| Significant interactions | • The following may ↑protirelin levels or effect (or ↑side-effects): amiodarone, metoclopramide, oestrogens (in men), theophylline, thyroid hormones (overtreatment).<br>• The following may ↓protirelin levels or effect: bromocriptine, carbamazepine, corticosteroids, levodopa, lithium, phenothiazines, salicylates, thyroid hormones (pharmacological doses). |
| Action in case of overdose | No symptoms of overdosage have been noted in patients receiving up to 1 mg IV. |

| Risk rating: **GREEN** | Score = 0<br>Lower-risk product. Risk-reduction strategies should be considered. |
| --- | --- |

This assessment is based on the full range of preparation and administration options described in the monograph. These may not all be applicable in some clinical situations.

## Bibliography

SPC Protirelin ampoules (Cambridge Laboratories), Alliance Pharmaceuticals (accessed 9 February 2009).

# Quinine dihydrochloride

**300 mg/mL solution in 1-mL and 2-mL ampoules**

* Quinine is an alkaloid originally obtained from the bark of the cinchona tree. It is the levorotatory isomer of quinidine.
* Quinine dihydrochloride (unlicensed product) is given by slow IV infusion in the treatment of falciparum malaria if the patient is seriously ill or unable to take oral therapy.
* Quinine doses are expressed as the salt; the dihydrochloride and sulphate (but not the bisulphate) contain about the same amounts of quinine base.

## Pre-treatment checks

* Do not give if there is known hypersensitivity to quinine, quinidine or mefloquine.
* Contraindicated in haemoglobinuria, myasthenia gravis, optic neuritis, tinnitus and in patients with a prolonged QT interval.
* Caution in cardiac disease (including atrial fibrillation, conduction defects, heart block) and G6PD deficiency.
* Omit the loading dose if the patient has received quinine or mefloquine during the previous 24 hours.

*Biochemical and other tests*

Blood glucose concentration
Blood pressure
Bodyweight
Electrolytes: serum Na, K

FBC
LFTs (accumulation may occur with hepatitis)
Pulse
Renal function: U, Cr, CrCl (or eGFR)

## Dose

Quinine should not be given by direct IV injection as this is now considered too hazardous.

*WHO recommended regimen for severe or complicated falciparum malaria*

**Initial loading dose:** 20 mg/kg (up to a maximum of 1.4 g) with maintenance infusions starting 8 hours after the start of the first infusion. Higher doses have been given in the critical care environment. A loading dose should **not be given** if the patient has received quinine or mefloquine during the previous 24 hours.
**Maintenance dose:** 10 mg/kg (up to a maximum of 700 mg) by IV infusion every 8 hours. If parenteral therapy is required for more than 48 hours, the maintenance dose should be reduced to 5–7 mg/kg. A switch to oral therapy should be made as soon as possible.
**Dose in renal impairment:** adjusted according to creatinine clearance:[1]

* CrCl >20–50 mL/minute: 5–7 mg/kg every 8 hours.
* CrCl 10–20 mL/minute: 5–7 mg/kg every 8–12 hours.
* CrCl <10 mL/minute: 5–7 mg/kg every 24 hours.

## Intravenous infusion (preferred route)

*Preparation and administration*

1. Withdraw the required dose and add to 250 mL NaCl 0.9% or Gluc 5%.
2. The solution should be clear and colourless to very pale straw in colour. Inspect visually for particulate matter or discoloration prior to administration and discard if present.
3. Give by slow IV infusion over 4 hours via a volumetric infusion device, taking care to avoid extravasation.

## Intramuscular injection (very irritant, use only if no alternative – efficacy not proven; dose as IV)

*Preparation and administration*

1. Withdraw half the required dose and further dilute with NaCl 0.9% to give a solution containing 60–100 mg/mL (i.e. dilute each 1 mL to 3–5 mL).
2. Withdraw the other half of the dose and dilute in the same way.
3. Give each half dose by IM injection into the anterior thigh (not the buttock). Rotate injection sites for subsequent injections.

## Technical information

| | |
|---|---|
| Incompatible with | No information |
| Compatible with | **Flush**: NaCl 0.9%<br>**Solutions**: Gluc 5%, NaCl 0.9%<br>**Y site**: No information |
| pH | 2.0-3.0 |
| Sodium content | Nil |
| Storage | Store below 25°C in original packaging. |
| Stability after preparation | Use prepared infusions immediately. |

## Monitoring

| Measure | Frequency | Rationale |
|---|---|---|
| Signs of cardiotoxicity (including blood pressure and heart rate) | See Rationale | • Monitor BP and pulse every 15 minutes for the first hour, then hourly during infusion.<br>• Monitor ECG during infusion, especially in elderly patients.<br>• Symptoms of cardiotoxicity include conduction disturbances, arrhythmias, anginal symptoms and ↓BP.<br>• In overdose this can lead to cardiac arrest and circulatory failure. |
| Blood glucose concentration | Every 4 hours during infusion | • Hypoglycaemia is a common adverse effect and may also manifest as a complication in falciparum malaria.<br>• Increase monitoring frequency if diminished consciousness or convulsions occur. |
| Renal function and serum K | Periodically | • Renal failure occurs rarely.<br>• ↓K may also occur. |
| FBC | | • Thrombocytopenia and other haematological effects may occur.<br>• Haemolytic anaemia has been reported when given to patients with G6PD. |
| Signs of visual disturbances | Throughout treatment | • Can cause retinal and optic nerve damage.<br>• May be indicative of overdose, e.g. blurred or double vision or loss of vision. |

## Additional information

| | |
|---|---|
| Common and serious undesirable effects | A cluster of symptoms referred to as 'cinchonism' (i.e. tinnitus, headache, hot and flushed skin, nausea, abdominal pain, rashes, confusion and visual disturbances including temporary blindness).<br>Cardiovascular effects; hypersensitivity reactions including angioedema; hypoglycaemia; blood disorders (including thrombocytopenia and intravascular coagulation); acute renal failure; photosensitivity. |
| Pharmacokinetics | Elimination half-life is 11 hours. |
| Significant interactions | • Quinine may ↑risk of ventricular arrhythmias with the following drugs (avoid combined use):<br>amiodarone, artemether/lumefantrine, droperidol, moxifloxacin, pimozide.<br>• Quinine may ↑levels or effect of the following drugs (or ↑side-effects): digoxin, flecainide, mefloquine (↑risk of convulsions but combined use may be necessary in severe cases). |
| Action in case of overdose | Quinine is very toxic in overdose and there are no effective antidotes.<br>It is essential to consult a Poisons Information Service, e.g. Toxbase at www.toxbase.org (password or registration required) for information on how to manage overdose. |
| Counselling | Once switched to oral therapy, if symptoms of hypoglycaemia occur (e.g. light-headedness, dizziness, fainting, seizure, sweating, confusion, shakiness, anxiety or weakness) consume fruit juice or a snack and contact the clinician. |

| Risk rating: **AMBER** | Score = 5<br>Moderate-risk product: Risk-reduction strategies are recommended. |
|---|---|

This assessment is based on the full range of preparation and administration options described in the monograph. These may not all be applicable in some clinical situations.

## Reference

1. Ashley C, Currie A, eds. *The Renal Drug Handbook*, 3rd edn. Oxford: Radcliffe Medical Press, 2009.

# Quinupristin with dalfopristin

**500-mg dry powder vials**

- Quinupristin and dalfopristin (both as mesilate salts) are semi-synthetic streptogramin antibacterials and are used in the ratio 3:7. They each have bacteriostatic activity and in combination usually act synergistically to produce bactericidal activity.
- The combination is used against a range of Gram-positive and some Gram-negative organisms, but is reserved for the treatment of serious infections with multidrug-resistant Gram-positive bacteria, such as MRSA and vancomycin-resistant *Enterococcus faecium*.
- Quinupristin with dalfopristin doses are expressed as the combined mass (mg) of the two constituents:
  Quinupristin with dalfopristin 500 mg ≡ quinupristin 150 mg with dalfopristin 350 mg.

## Pre-treatment checks

- Do not give if there is known hypersensitivity to quinupristin, dalfopristin, or other streptogramins.
- Caution if predisposed to cardiac arrhythmias (including congenital QT syndrome, concomitant use of drugs that prolong QT interval, cardiac hypertrophy, dilated cardiomyopathy, ↓K, ↓Mg, ↓pulse).

*Biochemical and other tests (not all are necessary in an emergency situation)*

Bodyweight
LFTs

## Dose

**Standard dose:** 7.5 mg/kg every 8 hours for 7 days in skin and soft-tissue infections; for 10 days in hospital-acquired pneumonia; duration of treatment in *E. faecium* infection is dependent on clinical response. The product is licensed for 12-hourly dosing for skin and soft-tissue infections.
**Dose in hepatic impairment:** 5 mg/kg (if 7.5 mg/kg is not tolerated) in moderate hepatic impairment. Avoid in severe hepatic impairment. Do not use if plasma bilirubin is >3 times ULN.

## Intermittent intravenous infusion

*Preparation and administration*

> Give via central venous catheter.
> In an emergency the first dose may be diluted in 250 mL Gluc 5% and given over 60 minutes via a peripheral line, but this is very likely to cause venous irritation.
> Quinupristin with dalfopristin is incompatible with NaCl 0.9%.

1. Reconstitute each 500-mg vial with 5 mL WFI or Gluc 5%, gently swirling vial without shaking to dissolve the powder, to give a solution containing 100 mg/mL.
2. Allow to stand for at least 2 minutes until foam disappears and the solution is clear.
3. Within 30 minutes of reconstitution withdraw the required dose and add to 100 mL Gluc 5%.
4. The solution should be clear and colourless to yellow. Inspect visually for particulate matter or discoloration prior to administration and discard if present.
5. Flush the line with Gluc 5% before commencing infusion.
6. Give by IV infusion over 60 minutes via a central venous catheter.
7. Flush the line again with Gluc 5% at the end of the infusion.

## Technical information

| | |
|---|---|
| Incompatible with | Quinupristin with dalfopristin is incompatible with NaCl 0.9%. |
| Compatible with | **Flush**: Gluc 5%.<br>**Solutions**: Gluc 5%, WFI<br>**Y-site** (but only if prepared in Gluc 5%): Aztreonam, metoclopramide, potassium chloride |
| pH | 4.3-5.0 |
| Sodium content | 16 mmol/500 mg |
| Storage | Store at 2-8°C in original packaging. |
| Displacement value | Negligible |
| Stability after preparation | From a microbiological point of view, should be used immediately; however:<br>• Reconstituted vials must be further diluted within 30 minutes.<br>• Prepared infusions may be stored at 2-8°C and infused (at room temperature) within 24 hours. |

## Monitoring

| Measure | Frequency | Rationale |
|---|---|---|
| LFTs | Periodically | • If plasma-bilirubin concentration rises to >3 times ULN, discontinue use. |
| FBC | | • Eosinophilia, anaemia, leucopenia, and neutropenia are common. |
| Signs of supra-infection or superinfection | Throughout treatment | • May result in the overgrowth of non-susceptible organisms - appropriate therapy should be commenced; treatment may need to be interrupted. |
| Development of diarrhoea | Throughout and up to 2 months after treatment | • Development of severe, persistent diarrhoea may be suggestive of *Clostridium difficile*-associated diarrhoea and colitis (pseudomembranous colitis). If needed, discontinue drug and treat. Do not use drugs that inhibit peristalsis. |

## Additional information

| | |
|---|---|
| Common and serious undesirable effects | *Injection/infusion-related:* Local: injection-site reactions on peripheral venous administration.<br>*Other:* Nausea, vomiting, diarrhoea, headache, arthralgia, myalgia, asthenia, rash, pruritus, anaemia, leucopenia, eosinophilia, ↑urea and creatinine. |
| Pharmacokinetics | Elimination half-life is about 1 hour for both drugs. |

*(continued)*

## Additional information (*continued*)

| | |
|---|---|
| Significant interactions | • Quinupristin with dalfopristin may ↑risk of ventricular arrhythmias with:<br>disopyramide, lidocaine.<br>• Quinupristin with dalfopristin may ↑levels of the following drugs (or ↑side-effects):<br>ciclosporin (monitor levels), ergotamine (avoid combination), methysergide (avoid combination), midazolam, nifedipine, tacrolimus (monitor levels). |
| Action in case of overdose | No specific antidote; observe carefully and give supportive treatment. Not removed by peritoneal dialysis or haemodialysis. |

| Risk rating: **AMBER** | Score = 5<br>Moderate-risk product: Risk-reduction strategies are recommended. |
|---|---|

This assessment is based on the full range of preparation and administration options described in the monograph. These may not all be applicable in some clinical situations.

## Bibliography

SPC Synercid IV (accessed 2 April 2009).

# Ranitidine

**25 mg/mL solution in 2-mL ampoules**
- Ranitidine hydrochloride is a histamine $H_2$-receptor antagonist that rapidly inhibits both basal and stimulated gastric acid secretion and reduces pepsin output.
- It is used where inhibition of gastric acid secretion may be beneficial: the treatment of duodenal and benign gastric ulceration, stress ulceration, pathological hypersecretory states such as the Zollinger–Ellison syndrome and in patients at risk of acid aspiration during general anaesthesia or childbirth.
- Doses are expressed in terms of the base:
  Ranitidine 50 mg $\cong$ 56 mg of ranitidine hydrochloride.

## Pre-treatment checks
- Avoid in patients with a history of porphyria.
- $H_2$-receptor antagonists may mask symptoms of gastric cancer and particular care is required in those whose symptoms change and in those who are middle-aged or older.

*Biochemical and other tests*

Bodyweight
Renal function: U, Cr, CrCl (or eGFR)

## Dose

**Standard dose:** 50 mg by IV injection, IV infusion or IM injection, repeated every 6–8 hours if necessary.
**Continuous infusion:** for the prophylaxis of upper GI haemorrhage from stress ulceration in seriously ill patients, initially 50 mg by IV injection followed by 125–250 micrograms/kg/hour by IV infusion.
**Patients at risk of acid aspiration:** 50 mg by IV or IM injection 45–60 minutes before induction of general anaesthesia.
**Dose in renal impairment:** adjusted according to creatinine clearance:
- CrCl >50 mL/minute: dose as in normal renal function.
- CrCl <50 mL/minute: reduce individual doses to 25 mg.

## Intramuscular injection

*Preparation and administration*

1. Withdraw the required dose.
2. Give by deep IM injection into a large muscle such as the gluteus or lateral aspect of the thigh.

## Intravenous injection

*Preparation and administration*

1. Withdraw the required dose and dilute to 20 mL with NaCl 0.9%.
2. Give by IV injection over 2–5 minutes.

## Intermittent intravenous infusion

*Preparation and administration*

1. Withdraw the required dose and add to a suitable volume of compatible infusion fluid (e.g. 100 mL NaCl 0.9%).
2. Give by IV infusion at a rate of 25 mg/hour.

## Continuous intravenous infusion

*Preparation and administration*

1. Withdraw the required dose and add to a suitable volume of compatible infusion fluid. Mix well.
2. Give by IV infusion at a rate of 125–250 micrograms/kg/hour.

## Technical information

| | |
|---|---|
| Incompatible with | Amphotericin, drotrecogin alfa (activated), insulin (soluble). |
| Compatible with | **Flush**: NaCl 0.9%<br>**Solutions**: NaCl 0.9%, Gluc 5%, Gluc-NaCl, Hartmann's<br>**Y-site**: Aciclovir, adrenaline (epinephrine), aminophylline, atracurium, aztreonam, ceftazidime, ciprofloxacin, cisatracurium, clarithromycin, dobutamine, dopamine, esmolol, fentanyl, fluconazole, foscarnet, furosemide, glyceryl trinitrate, granisetron, labetalol, linezolid, midazolam, norepinephrine (norepinephrine), ondansetron, piperacillin with tazobactam, propofol, remifentanil, sodium bicarbonate, vecuronium |
| pH | 6.7-7.3 |
| Sodium content | Negligible |
| Storage | Store below 25°C, in original packaging. |
| Stability after preparation | From a microbiological point of view, should be used immediately; however, prepared infusions may be stored at 2-8°C and infused (at room temperature) within 24 hours. |

## Monitoring

| Measure | Frequency | Rationale |
|---|---|---|
| Renal function | Periodically | • A decline in renal function may require a dose reduction.<br>• Interstitial nephritis has rarely been observed. |
| LFTs | | • Altered LFTs, reversible liver damage and (rarely) cases of hepatitis have been reported. |
| FBC | | • Agranulocytosis, leucopenia, pancytopenia, thrombocytopenia and aplastic anaemia have been reported rarely. |
| Signs of infection | Throughout treatment | • Use of antisecretory drugs may ↑risk of infections such as community-acquired pneumonia, *Salmonella*, *Campylobacter* and *Clostridium difficile*-associated disease. |

## Additional information

| | |
|---|---|
| Common and serious undesirable effects | *Injection/infusion-related:* Too rapid administration: ↓pulse reported rarely.<br>*Other:* Rarely hepatotoxicity, acute pancreatitis, AV block, hallucinations particularly in elderly or very ill patients, hypersensitivity reactions, interstitial nephritis. |
| Pharmacokinetics | Elimination half-life is 2-3 hours. |
| Significant drug interactions | • Ranitidine may ↓levels or effect of tolazoline.<br>• Ranitidine may cause a false-negative urea breath test when testing for *H. pylori* infection - the test should not be performed for at least 2 weeks after stopping therapy. |
| Overdose | No particular problems expected. Stop administration and give supportive therapy as appropriate. |

| Risk rating: **GREEN** | Score = 1<br>Lower-risk product: Risk-reduction strategies should be considered. |
|---|---|

This assessment is based on the full range of preparation and administration options described in the monograph. These may not all be applicable in some clinical situations.

## Bibliography

SPC Ranitidine 50 mg/2 mL solution for injection and infusion, Beacon Pharmaceuticals (accessed 28 March 2010).

# Rasburicase

**1.5-mg and 7.5-mg dry powder vials with solvent**
• Rasburicase is a recombinant form of urate oxidase.
• It is used in the treatment and prophylaxis of acute hyperuricaemia, in order to prevent acute renal failure, in patients with haematological malignancy at risk of rapid tumour lysis at the start of chemotherapy.

## Pre-treatment checks

Do not administer to patients with G6PD or other cellular metabolic disorders known to cause haemolytic anaemia.

*Biochemical and other tests*

Bodyweight

## Dose

**Standard dose:** 200 micrograms/kg/day for up to 7 days depending upon plasma uric acid levels and clinical judgement.

### Intermittent intravenous infusion

*Preparation and administration*

1. Reconstitute each 1.5-mg vial with 1 mL supplied solvent (use 5 mL for each 7.5-mg vial). Swirl very gently (do not shake) to give a solution containing 1.5 mg/mL.
2. Withdraw the required dose (more than one vial may be required) and add to 50 mL NaCl 0.9%.
3. The solution should be clear and colourless. Inspect visually for particulate matter or discoloration prior to administration and discard if present.
4. Give by IV infusion over 30 minutes through a different line to that used for chemotherapy treatment. If this is not possible, flush the line with at least 15 mL of NaCl 0.9% before and after the rasburicase infusion. Do not use a filter for the infusion.

## Technical information

| | |
|---|---|
| Incompatible with | Likely to be incompatible with Gluc 5%. |
| Compatible with | **Flush**: NaCl 0.9% <br> **Solutions**: NaCl 0.9% <br> **Y-site**: No information |
| pH[1] | 8 |
| Sodium content | Negligible |
| Storage | Store at 2–8°C in original packaging. Do not freeze. |
| Displacement value | Negligible |
| Stability after preparation | From a microbiological point of view, should be used immediately; however: <br> • Reconstituted vials may be stored at 2–8°C for 24 hours. <br> • Prepared infusions may be stored at 2–8°C and infused (at room temperature) within 24 hours. |

## Monitoring

| Measure | Frequency | Rationale |
|---|---|---|
| Allergic reactions | Following administration | • If severe hypersensitivity reactions occur, stop treatment immediately. |
| Plasma uric acid levels | Periodically | • To ensure that treatment is effective. <br> • Collect the blood sample into a pre-chilled tube containing heparin and immerse in ice/water bath. <br> • Keep plasma sample in ice/water bath and analyse for uric acid within 4 hours (a centrifuge pre-cooled to 4°C must be used). |
| Creatinine and U&Es | | • To check for signs of tumour lysis syndrome. |

## Additional information

| | |
|---|---|
| Common and serious undesirable effects | *Immediate:* Anaphylaxis has been reported rarely. <br> *Other:* Fever. |
| Pharmacokinetics | Elimination half-life is about 18 hours. |
| Significant interactions | • Rasburicase degrades uric acid *in vitro*. Samples taken for plasma uric acid assessment must be handled in a precise way – see Monitoring above. |
| Action in case of overdose | *Symptoms to watch for:* Monitor for haemolysis. <br> *Antidote:* No known antidote; stop administration and give supportive therapy as appropriate. |

| | |
|---|---|
| Risk rating: **AMBER** | Score = 4 <br> Moderate-risk product. Risk-reduction strategies are recommended. |

This assessment is based on the full range of preparation and administration options described in the monograph. These may not all be applicable in some clinical situations.

### Reference

1. Personal communiqué from Sanofi Aventis, 9 June 2009.

### Bibliography

SPC Fasturtec (accessed 26 November 2008).

# Reteplase

**10-units dry powder vials with 10 mL WFI in pre-filled syringe**

• Reteplase is a recombinant plasminogen activator with some fibrin specificity. It has thrombolytic activity.
• It is licensed for the dissolution of clots in STEMI.
• Reteplase doses are expressed in units specific to reteplase that are not directly comparable with units of other thrombolytic agents.

## Pre-treatment checks

• Contraindicated in recent haemorrhage, trauma, or surgery (including dental extraction), coagulation defects, bleeding diatheses, aortic dissection, aneurysm, coma, history of cerebrovascular disease especially recent events or with any residual disability, recent symptoms of possible peptic ulceration, heavy vaginal bleeding, severe ↑BP, active pulmonary disease with cavitation, acute pancreatitis, pericarditis, bacterial endocarditis, severe liver disease, and oesophageal varices.

- Do not use in ↓glycaemia, ↑glycaemia.
- Use with caution if there is a risk of bleeding including that from venepuncture or invasive procedures.
- Caution in external chest compression, pregnancy, elderly patients, ↑BP, conditions in which thrombolysis might give rise to embolic complications such as enlarged left atrium with atrial fibrillation (risk of dissolution of clot and subsequent embolisation), and recent or concurrent use of drugs that ↑risk of bleeding.
- Heparin and aspirin should be administered before and after reteplase to reduce the risk of re-thrombosis.

*Biochemical and other tests (not all are necessary in an emergency situation)*

APTT ratio if heparin is to be used                                    LFTs
Blood pressure and pulse – do not give if systolic BP >160

## Dose

**Acute MI (initiated within 12 hours of onset of symptoms):** 10 units by IV injection as soon as possible after the onset of symptoms. Repeat the dose once after 30 minutes.
**Concomitant therapy with aspirin:** 300 mg prior to thrombolysis, followed by 75–150 mg once daily at least until discharge.
**Concomitant therapy with unfractionated heparin:** 5000 units given by IV injection prior to reteplase therapy followed by an infusion of 1000 units/hour starting after the second reteplase dose. Heparin should be given for at least 24 hours, preferably for 48–72 hours with the aim of keeping APTT ratio at 1.5–2.
**Central venous catheter occlusion (unlicensed):** a dose of 0.4 units has been used, repeated after 2 hours if necessary. See below for administration method.
**Dose in renal impairment:** use with caution if CrCl <10 mL/minute.
**Dose in hepatic impairment:** do not give in severe disease.

## Intravenous injection

*Preparation*

1. Remove the protective flip-cap from the vial and clean the rubber closure with an alcohol wipe.
2. Open the package containing the reconstitution spike; remove both protective caps from this.
3. Insert the spike through the rubber closure into the vial of reteplase.
4. Take the 10-mL syringe out of the package. Remove the tip cap from the syringe. Connect the syringe to the reconstitution spike and transfer the 10 mL of solvent into the vial.
5. With the reconstitution spike and syringe still attached to the vial, swirl the vial gently to dissolve the injection powder. Do not shake.
6. Withdraw 10 mL of the solution back into the syringe. A small amount of solution may remain in the vial owing to overfill. Disconnect the syringe from the reconstitution spike.
7. The solution should be clear and colourless. Inspect visually for particulate matter or discoloration prior to administration and discard if present.

*Administration*

1. Check the compatibility of the syringe with the IV access device. If necessary an adaptor may be used.
2. Give by slow IV injection over a maximum of 2 minutes.

## Catheter lock (unlicensed)

*Preparation and administration*

1. Prepare as steps 1–5 above.
2. Withdraw 0.4 mL into a second empty syringe and dilute to the catheter volume with WFI.
3. Aspirate the catheter.
4. Inject the reteplase solution into the catheter.
5. Allow to dwell for at least 30 minutes, then aspirate.

## Technical information

| | |
|---|---|
| Incompatible with | Bivalirudin, heparin sodium. |
| Compatible with | Flush: NaCl 0.9%<br>Solutions: NaCl 0.9%, Gluc 5%<br>Y-site: No information but unlikely to be stable |
| pH | 5.7–6.3 |
| Sodium content | Negligible |
| Excipients | Contains tranexamic acid. |
| Storage | Store below 25°C in original packaging. |
| Displacement value | Negligible |
| Stability after preparation | From a microbiological point of view, should be used immediately; however, reconstituted vials may be stored at 2–8°C and used within 8 hours. |

## Monitoring in treatment of myocardial infarction

| Measure | Frequency | Rationale |
|---|---|---|
| Heart rate | Continuously | • ↓Pulse may result from reperfusion. |
| ECG | | • Arrhythmias may result from reperfusion. |
| Blood pressure | | • ↓BP may occur. Raise the legs and slow or stop infusion temporarily. |

## Additional information

| | |
|---|---|
| Common and serious undesirable effects | *Immediate:* Anaphylaxis and other hypersensitivity reactions have been reported rarely.<br>*Injection-related:* Local: Burning sensation or haemorrhage at the injection site.<br>*Other:* Bleeding, ↓BP, ↑or ↓pulse, coronary artery reperfusion events, e.g. rhythm disorders. |
| Pharmacokinetics | Biphasic elimination with terminal half-life of 1.6 hours. |
| Significant interactions | • The following may ↑risk of haemorrhage with reteplase: anticoagulants, heparins, antiplatelet agents, e.g. aspirin, clopidogrel, dipyridamole, GP IIb/IIIa inhibitors. |
| Action in case of overdose | *Symptoms to watch for:* severe bleeding.<br>*Antidote:* No specific antidote. Stop administration and give supportive therapy as appropriate, including fresh frozen plasma, fresh blood and tranexamic acid if necessary. |
| Counselling | Report bleeding events. |

| Risk rating: **GREEN** | Score = 2<br>Lower-risk product. Risk-reduction strategies should be considered. |
| --- | --- |

This assessment is based on the full range of preparation and administration options described in the monograph. These may not all be applicable in some clinical situations.

## Bibliography

SPC Rapilysin 10 U (accessed 31 March 2010).

# Rifampicin (rifampin)

### 600-mg dry powder vials with solvent

* Rifampicin belongs to the rifamycin group of antimycobacterials.
* It is used in the treatment of various infections due to mycobacteria and other susceptible organisms and is usually given with other antibacterials to prevent the emergence of resistant organisms.
* Rifampicin is well absorbed from the GI tract following oral dosing, so the IV route should be used only when the oral route is unavailable.

## Pre-treatment checks

* Do not give if there is known hypersensitivity to rifamycins or in jaundice.
* Contraindicated if given concomitantly with saquinavir/ritonavir combination.
* Caution in acute porphyria, pregnancy and breast feeding.

*Biochemical and other tests*

Bodyweight

Electrolytes: serum Na, K

FBC

LFTs

Renal function: U, Cr

Sputum cultures and chest X-ray if tuberculosis suspected

U&Es

## Dose

Rifampicin must not be given by the IM or SC route (local irritation and inflammation can occur).

**Tuberculosis:** 600 mg daily in combination with other antibacterials.

**Brucellosis, Legionnaires' disease, endocarditis and serious staphylococcal infections:** 300–600 mg every 12 hours in combination with other antibacterials (may also be given as 150–300 mg every 6 hours).

**Multibacillary leprosy:** 600 mg monthly for adults (or 450 mg if <35 kg) in combination with clofazimine and dapsone. Treatment is continued for 12 months.

**Paucibacillary leprosy:** 600 mg monthly for adults (or 450 mg if <35 kg) in combination with dapsone. Treatment is continued for 6 months.

**Dose in hepatic impairment:** the total daily dose should not exceed 8 mg/kg.

## Intermittent intravenous infusion

*Preparation and administration*

1. Reconstitute each 600-mg vial with the solvent provided. Swirl gently until fully dissolved to give a solution containing 60 mg/mL.
2. Withdraw the required dose and add to 500 mL Gluc 5% (preferred) or other compatible infusion fluid.
3. The solution should be clear and red to reddish brown in colour. Inspect visually for particulate matter or discoloration prior to administration and discard if present.
4. Give by IV infusion over 2–3 hours taking care to avoid extravasation. If local irritation or inflammation occurs at the infusion site, the infusion should be discontinued and restarted at another site.

**Fluid restriction (unlicensed):** 300–600 mg may be added to 100 mL Gluc 5% (preferred) or NaCl 0.9% and given by IV infusion over 2–3 hours.

## Technical information

| | |
|---|---|
| Incompatible with | Do not mix with other drugs during infusion. |
| Compatible with | **Flush**: NaCl 0.9%<br>**Solutions**: Gluc 5%, NaCl 0.9%<br>**Y-site**: No information but likely to be unstable |
| pH | 8–8.8 |
| Sodium content | Negligible |
| Storage | Store below 25°C in original packaging. |
| Displacement value | Not relevant |
| Stability after preparation | From a microbiological point of view, should be used immediately; however:<br>• Reconstituted vials may be stored at room temperature for 6 hours.<br>• Prepared infusions should be used immediately (precipitation may occurs beyond 3–4 hours). |

## Monitoring

| Measure | Frequency | Rationale |
|---|---|---|
| LFTs | See Rationale | • In patients with normal LFTs at start of therapy, recheck only if there is fever, vomiting or jaundice or if the condition deteriorates.<br>• In patients with pre-existing hepatic impairment monitor LFTs (especially AST and ALT) weekly for 2 weeks then every 2–4 weeks.<br>• If signs of hepatocellular damage occur, withdraw rifampicin.<br>• If rifampicin is re-introduced after liver function has returned to normal, LFTs should be monitored daily. |

*(continued)*

## Monitoring *(continued)*

| Measure | Frequency | Rationale |
|---------|-----------|-----------|
| Renal function | Throughout treatment | • If renal failure occurs rifampicin should be stopped and never restarted. |
| FBC | Periodically in prolonged treatment | • If thrombocytopenia purpura or anaemia occurs rifampicin should be stopped and never restarted. |
| Development of diarrhoea | Throughout and up to 3 weeks after treatment | • Development of severe, persistent diarrhoea may be suggestive of *Clostridium difficile*-associated diarrhoea and colitis (pseudomembranous colitis). Consider discontinuing drug. Treat the other infection. Do not use drugs that inhibit peristalsis. |

## Additional information

| | |
|---|---|
| Common and serious undesirable effects | *Infusion-related:* Local: Thrombophlebitis reported if infusion used for prolonged period.<br>*Other:* Anorexia, nausea, vomiting, diarrhoea, headache, drowsiness, altered LFTs, flushing, urticaria, rashes. |
| Pharmacokinetics | Elimination half-life is 2-3 hours. |
| Significant interactions | • Avoid combination of rifampicin with the following (rifabutin may be an alternative in some cases):<br>atanazavir, atovaquone, bosentan, darunavir, dasatinib, eplerenone, fosamprenavir, imatinib, indinavir, lapatinib, lopinavir, mefloquine, nelfinavir, nevirapine, nilotinib, ranolazine, saquinavir, sirolimus, telithromycin, temsirolimus, tipranavir, voriconazole.<br>• Ketoconazole may ↓rifampicin levels or effect.<br>• Rifampicin may ↓levels or effect of the following drugs: aripiprazole, chlorpropamide, ciclosporin (monitor levels), corticosteroids, coumarin anticoagulants (monitor INR), diltiazem, disopyramide, fluconazole, haloperidol, isradipine, itraconazole, ketoconazole, lamotrigine, maraviroc, mycophenolate, nicardipine, nifedipine, nimodipine, oestrogens (↓contraceptive effect), posaconazole, propafenone, raltegravir, rosiglitazone, tacrolimus, terbinafine, tolbutamide, verapamil. |
| Action in case of overdose | No specific antidote. Management should be symptomatic. |
| Counselling | Warn patient that orange-reddish discoloration of the urine, faeces, sweat, saliva, sputum and tears may occur, and soft contact lenses may be permanently stained. Explain how to recognise signs of liver disorder, and advise to discontinue treatment and seek immediate medical attention if symptoms such as persistent nausea, vomiting, malaise or jaundice develop.<br>Women taking the combined contraceptive pill should be should be advised to use an alternative method. |

| Risk rating: **AMBER** | Score = 3<br>Moderate-risk product: Risk-reduction strategies are recommended. |
| --- | --- |

This assessment is based on the full range of preparation and administration options described in the monograph. These may not all be applicable in some clinical situations.

## Bibliography

SPC Rifadin for infusion 600 mg (accessed 2 April 2009).

# Risperidone long-acting injection

### 25-mg, 37.5-mg and 50-mg dry powder vials with solvent

- Risperidone is a benzisoxazole atypical antipsychotic, reported to be an antagonist at dopamine, serotonin, adrenergic, and histamine receptors.
- As a long-acting depot injection it is used in the maintenance treatment of schizophrenia in patients already stabilised on oral antipsychotics.

## Pre-treatment checks

Patients with no history of risperidone use should be given oral risperidone for several days to assess tolerability.

*Biochemical and other tests*

| | |
| --- | --- |
| Blood pressure | LFTs |
| Bodyweight | Prolactin |
| ECG | Renal function |

## Dose

> After administration, initially <1% risperidone will be released, followed by a lag time of 3 weeks before the main release of risperidone occurs. When initiating treatment with risperidone depot injection, oral risperidone (or the patient's previous antipsychotic if not risperidone) should also be provided for the first 3 weeks after the first injection.

**Patients not stabilised on risperidone or patients stabilised on up to 4 mg oral risperidone daily for at least 2 weeks:** initiate therapy at 25 mg by IM injection every 2 weeks.
**Patients stabilised more than 4 mg oral risperidone daily for at least 2 weeks:** initiate therapy at 37.5 mg by IM injection every 2 weeks.
**Maintenance therapy:** increase the dose if necessary at intervals of at least 4 weeks in steps of 12.5 mg up to a maximum of 50 mg every 2 weeks.

## Intramuscular injection

*Preparation and administration*

1. The pack should be removed from the refrigerator and allowed to come to room temperature before reconstitution.
2. Follow the manufacturer's instructions to reconstitute the vial with the diluent provided to give a thick, milky suspension containing 25 mg/2 mL, 37.5 mg/2 mL or 50 mg/2 mL depending on vial size.
3. The entire contents of the suspension in the vial should be drawn up.
4. Shake the syringe vigorously to re-suspend the microspheres and give the dose by deep IM injection into the gluteal or deltoid muscle. For gluteal administration use a 50-mm needle and alternate injections between the buttocks; for deltoid administration use a 25-mm needle and alternate between the arms

## Technical information

| Incompatible with | Not relevant |
|---|---|
| Compatible with | Not relevant |
| pH | 6.7-7.3 |
| Sodium content | Negligible |
| Storage | Store at 2-8°C. If refrigeration is not available the product may be stored below 25°C for up to 7 days prior to administration |
| Stability after preparation | From a microbiological point of view, should be used immediately; however, reconstituted suspension may be stored at 25°C for up to 6 hours. Shake the syringe vigorously to re-suspend the microspheres before administration. |

## Monitoring

| Measure | Frequency | Rationale |
|---|---|---|
| Therapeutic effect | During dose adjustment and periodically | • To ensure reduction/elimination of psychotic symptoms. |
| EPSEs | During dose adjustment and every 3 months | • Causes extrapyramidal symptoms, e.g. dystonias. |
| Renal function and LFTs | At least annually | • To check renal and hepatic function as part of regular health check. |
| Glucose | | • May cause hyperglycaemia. |
| Blood pressure | | • May cause ↓BP. |
| Weight gain and obesity | | • As part of regular health check.<br>• May cause weight gain.<br>• Obesity measured by waist : hip ratio or waist circumference. |
| Lipids (including cholesterol, HDL, LDL and triglycerides) | | • As part of regular health check. |

*(continued)*

## Monitoring (continued)

| Measure | Frequency | Rationale |
|---------|-----------|-----------|
| Prolactin | See rationale | • If symptoms of hyperprolactinaemia develop. |

## Additional information

| | |
|---|---|
| Common and serious undesirable effects | Weight gain, depression, fatigue and extrapyramidal symptoms. |
| Pharmacokinetics | See under Dose above: half-life is 3-6 days. |
| Significant drug interactions | • The following may ↑risperidone levels or effect (or ↑side-effects): anaesthetics-general (↑risk of ↓BP), antidepressants-tricyclic, artemether with lumefantrine (avoid combination), clozapine (avoid combination – depot preparation cannot be withdrawn quickly if neutropenia occurs), ritonavir, sibutramine (avoid combination).<br>• Risperidone may ↓levels or effect of levodopa.<br>• Risperidone may ↑risk of ventricular arrhythmias with the following drugs: antiarrhythmics, antidepressants-tricyclic, atomoxetine, methadone.<br>• Risperidone ↓convulsive threshold and may ↓effect of the following drugs: barbiturates, carbamazepine, ethosuximide, oxcarbazepine, phenytoin, primidone, valproate. |
| Action in case of overdose | Treat EPSE with anticholinergic antiparkinsonian drugs.<br>If agitation or convulsions occur, treat with benzodiazepines.<br>If the patient is in shock, treatment with metaraminol or noradrenaline may be appropriate.<br>Adrenaline **must not** be given (may further ↓BP). |
| Counselling | Advise patients not to drink alcohol especially at the beginning of treatment. May impair alertness so do not drive or operate machinery until susceptibility is known. |

| Risk rating: **AMBER** | Score = 3<br>Moderate-risk product: Risk-reduction strategies are recommended. |
|---|---|

This assessment is based on the full range of preparation and administration options described in the monograph. These may not all be applicable in some clinical situations.

## Bibliography

NICE (2009). *Clinical Guideline 82: Core interventions in the treatment and management of schizophrenia in primary and secondary care (update)*. London: National Institute for Health and Clinical Excellence. http://guidance.nice.org.uk/CG82 (accessed 1 October 2009).

SPC Risperdal Consta (accessed 27 August 2008).

# Rituximab

**10 mg/mL solution in 10-mL and 50-mL vials**

* Rituximab is a genetically engineered chimeric monoclonal antibody that binds specifically to the CD20 antigen.
* It is used with methotrexate in adults with severe active rheumatoid arthritis who have had an inadequate response to DMARDs including anti-TNF agents.
* It is also licensed for use in non-Hodgkin lymphoma and chronic lymphocytic leukaemia (see specialist literature for dosing details).

## Pre-treatment checks

* Caution in patients with a history of cardiovascular disease because exacerbation of angina, arrhythmia, and heart failure have been reported.
* Patients should be premedicated with paracetamol (acetaminophen) and an antihistamine.
* Screen for the presence of active or severe infection; screen for hepatitis B virus (HBV) in high-risk patients.
* Ensure full resuscitation facilities are immediately available throughout the administration period.

*Biochemical and other tests*

Blood pressure
FBC
Possibly bodyweight and height

## Dose

**Rheumatoid arthritis:** 1 g by IV infusion followed 2 weeks later by a second dose of 1 g.

* Give methylprednisolone 100 mg by IV injection 30 minutes prior to rituximab to ↓severity of acute infusion reactions.
* If a repeat course of treatment is considered, it should be given after a minimum interval of 16 weeks.

## Intravenous infusion through a dedicated line

*Preparation and administration*

Preparation should take place in a CIVAS unit.
Administer only in an environment where full resuscitation facilities are immediately available.

1. The solution should be clear and colourless. Inspect visually for particulate matter or discoloration prior to administration and discard if present.
2. Give by IV infusion.
   * *For the first infusion:* initially administer at 50 mg/hour increased in 50 mg/hour increments every 30 minutes to a maximum of 400 mg/hour.
   * *For subsequent infusions:* initially administer at 100 mg/hour increased in 100 mg/hour increments at 30-minute intervals to a maximum of 400 mg/hour.

## Technical information

| | |
|---|---|
| Incompatible with | No information but do not mix with any other drug. |
| Compatible with | **Flush**: NaCl 0.9%<br>**Solutions**: NaCl 0.9%, Gluc 5%<br>**Y-site**: No information but likely to be unstable |
| pH | 6.2-6.8 |
| Sodium content | 2.4 mmol/10 mL |
| Storage | Store at 2-8°C in original packaging. |
| Special handling | Prepare in a CIVAS unit. |
| Stability after preparation | As recommended by the CIVAS unit. |

## Monitoring

| Measure | Frequency | Rationale |
|---|---|---|
| Observe for symptoms of cytokine release syndrome: severe dyspnoea (with bronchospasm and hypoxia), fever, chills, rigors, urticaria and angioedema | During infusion | • May occur within 30-120 minutes of starting the first infusion - immediately stop infusion and institute aggressive symptomatic treatment.<br>• The infusion should not be restarted until complete resolution of all symptoms. Recommence initially at no more than one-half the previous rate.<br>• If severe adverse reactions occur a second time, a decision to stop the treatment should be considered. |
| Observe for mild infusion-related reactions: fevers, chills rigors | | • ↓Infusion rate usually resolves these symptoms. May be increased when symptoms improve.<br>• If required, treat symptomatically with an antipyretic, antihistamine, and if necessary oxygen, IV NaCl, bronchodilators and glucocorticoids. |
| Blood pressure | | • ↓BP may occur during infusion.<br>• Consider withholding antihypertensive drugs 12 hours prior to infusion. |
| Respiratory function | | • In patients with pre-existing pulmonary conditions or in whom adverse pulmonary events have occurred at previous infusions. |

*(continued)*

## Monitoring (continued)

| Measure | Frequency | Rationale |
|---|---|---|
| Signs of infection | Post infusion | • Rituximab is immunosuppressive and any infections should be treated promptly. |
| FBC | According to local policy | • Thrombocytopenia, neutropenia and anaemia have been reported. These may persist for a considerable time following discontinuation of rituximab. |
| Signs of HBV infection and LFTs | During and for several months post treatment | • Carriers of HBV are at high risk of active HBV infection or hepatitis. |

## Additional information

| | |
|---|---|
| Common and serious undesirable effects | *Immediate:* Transient ↓BP occurs frequently during infusion and antihypertensives may need to be withheld for 12 hours before infusion. *Infusion-related:* Occur predominantly during the first infusion and include cytokine release syndrome (see Monitoring above), fever and chills, nausea and vomiting, allergic reactions (such as rash, pruritus, angiooedema, bronchospasm and dyspnoea), flushing and tumour pain. *Other:* Exacerbation of angina, arrhythmia, and heart failure. |
| Pharmacokinetics | Elimination half-life is 31.5-152.6 hours (mean 76 hours) after the first infusion; 83.9-407 hours (mean 205 hours) after the fourth infusion. |
| Significant interactions | None known. |
| Action in case of overdose | There is no specific antidote and treatment should be symptomatic. |
| Counselling | Any vaccination schedule should be completed at least 4 weeks prior to the first treatment. |

| Risk rating: **AMBER** | Score = 4 Moderate-risk product: Risk-reduction strategies are recommended. |
|---|---|

This assessment is based on the full range of preparation and administration options described in the monograph. These may not all be applicable in some clinical situations.

## Bibliography

SPC Mabthera 100 mg and 500 mg concentrate for solution for infusion (accessed 4 March 2010).

# Salbutamol (albuterol)

**500 micrograms/mL solution in 1-mL ampoules; 1 mg/mL solution in 5-mL ampoules**
* Salbutamol sulfate is a direct-acting sympathomimetic with mainly beta-adrenergic activity and a selective action on beta$_2$ receptors.
* It can be given by various parenteral routes in the management of severe bronchospasm and by IV infusion to delay uncomplicated premature labour.
* It has been used (unlicensed) to treat ↑K but this use is controversial.
* Doses are expressed in terms of the base:
Salbutamol 1 mg ≅ 1.2 mg salbutamol sulfate.

## Pre-treatment checks

* Avoid use in patients with underlying severe heart disease, e.g. ischaemic heart disease, arrhythmia or severe heart failure.
* Use with caution in thyrotoxicosis.
* In asthma, use should be combined with oxygen and corticosteroid therapy.
* Hypoglycaemic therapy in diabetes may require review.

*Biochemical and other tests (not all are necessary in an emergency situation)*

| | |
|---|---|
| Blood glucose | Bodyweight |
| Blood pressure and pulse (in the USA an ECG is sometimes performed in addition) | Electrolytes: serum K |
| | Respiratory function: ABGs, pulse oximetry |

## Dose

**Severe bronchospasm:**
* By IV infusion, initially 5 micrograms/minute, adjusted according to response and heart rate; usually in range 3–20 micrograms/minute, or more if necessary.
* Alternatively, give 250 micrograms (4 micrograms/kg) by slow IV injection (repeated if necessary) or 500 micrograms (8 micrograms/kg bodyweight) by SC or IM injection repeated every 4 hours as required.

**Premature labour:** glucose is the preferred diluent and use of a syringe pump is the preferred means of administration (↑risk of maternal pulmonary oedema if saline or large volumes of fluid are used).
* Initially 10 micrograms/minute given by IV infusion, increasing the rate at 10-minute intervals until there is diminution in strength, frequency or duration of contractions.
* The infusion rate may then be increased slowly until contractions cease.
* The infusion is maintained at this level for one hour and then gradually decreased over several hours.
* Infusion rates providing 10–45 micrograms/minute are generally adequate to control uterine contractions.
* After stopping the infusion, treatment may be continued by giving salbutamol 4 mg orally 3–4 times daily, bearing in mind that risk to the mother increases after 48 hours of treatment.

**Hyperkalaemia (unlicensed):** 500 micrograms by slow IV injection has been used, repeated after 2 hours if necessary. However, this use is controversial as it is reportedly no more effective than 10–20 mg nebulised salbutamol and may be more likely to cause cardiac arrhythmias. If effective, ↓K levels are seen in 30 minutes and the effect may last for up to 2 hours.[1]

## Continuous intravenous infusion via a syringe pump

*Preparation of a 200 micrograms/mL solution*

1. Using the 5 mg/5 mL strength, withdraw 10 mg (10 mL).
2. Make up to 50 mL in a syringe pump with NaCl 0.9% or Gluc 5% (Gluc 5% is the preferred diluent in premature labour).
3. Cap the syringe and mix well to give a solution containing 200 micrograms/mL.
4. The solution should be clear and colourless or faintly straw-coloured. Inspect visually for particulate matter or discoloration prior to administration and discard if present.

*Administration*

Give by IV infusion at the required rate, adjusting the dose according to response and heart rate.

## Continuous intravenous infusion (large volume infusion)

*Preparation of a 20 micrograms/mL solution*

1. Withdraw 10 mL from a 500-mL bag of NaCl 0.9% or Gluc 5% and discard.
2. Using the 5 mg/5 mL strength of salbutamol, withdraw 10 mg (10 mL) and add to the prepared infusion bag to give a solution containing 20 micrograms/mL. Mix well.
3. The solution should be clear and colourless or faintly straw-coloured. Inspect visually for particulate matter or discoloration prior to administration and discard if present.

*Administration*

Give by IV infusion at the required rate via a volumetric infusion device, adjusting the dose according to response and heart rate.

## Intravenous injection

*Preparation and administration*

1. Using the 500 micrograms/mL strength, withdraw 250 micrograms (0.5 mL).
2. Dilute to 5 mL with WFI to give a solution containing 50 micrograms/mL.
3. The solution should be clear and colourless or faintly straw-coloured. Inspect visually for particulate matter or discoloration prior to administration and discard if present.
4. Give by slow IV injection over 3–5 minutes.

## Subcutaneous injection

*Preparation and administration*

1. Using the 500 micrograms/mL strength, withdraw the required dose.
2. Give by SC injection.

## Intramuscular injection

*Preparation and administration*

1. Using the 500 micrograms/mL strength, withdraw the required dose.
2. Give by IM injection.

| Technical information | |
|---|---|
| Incompatible with | Aminophylline, pantoprazole. |
| Compatible with | **Flush**: NaCl 0.9%<br>**Solutions**: Gluc 5% (preferred diluent in premature labour), NaCl 0.9%, Gluc-NaCl<br>**Y-site**: No information |

*(continued)*

## Technical information (*continued*)

| | |
|---|---|
| pH | 3.5 |
| Sodium content | Negligible |
| Storage | Store below 30°C in original packaging. |
| Stability after preparation | From a microbiological point of view, should be used immediately; however, it may be stored at 2-8°C and infused (at room temperature) within 24 hours. |

## Monitoring

| Measure | Frequency | Rationale |
|---|---|---|
| Respiratory function | Frequently during treatment | • For signs of clinical improvement. |
| Blood pressure and pulse | | • May cause ↑pulse, ↓BP and myocardial ischaemia. |
| Serum K | | • May cause ↓K. |
| Blood glucose | | • May ↑blood glucose levels. |

## Additional information

| | |
|---|---|
| Common and serious undesirable effects | *Immediate:* Hypersensitivity reactions including angioedema, urticaria, bronchospasm, ↓BP and collapse have rarely been reported.<br>*Other:* ↑Pulse, palpitations, arrhythmias, peripheral vasodilation, ↓BP, myocardial ischaemia and collapse, ↓K, fine tremor, nervous tension, headache, muscle cramps. May ↑blood glucose levels. |
| Pharmacokinetics | IV salbutamol has a half-life of 4-6 hours and is cleared partly renally and partly by metabolism to an inactive metabolite that is also excreted primarily in the urine. |
| Significant interactions | • Beta-blockers (including eye drops) may ↓salbutamol levels or effect.<br>• Salbutamol may ↑ effect (or ↑side-effects) of methyldopa (profound ↓BP with IV salbutamol). |
| Action in case of overdose | *Symptoms to watch for:* ↑Pulse, tremor, ↓K, lactic acidosis.<br>*Antidote:* The preferred antidote is a cardioselective beta-blocker, but use it with caution in patients with a history of bronchospasm. Give supportive therapy as appropriate. |
| Counselling | Advise that shaking and a feeling of anxiety are common side-effects.<br>Report palpitations or ↑ heart rate. |

| | |
|---|---|
| Risk rating: **AMBER** | Score = 5<br>Moderate-risk product: Risk-reduction strategies are recommended. |

This assessment is based on the full range of preparation and administration options described in the monograph. These may not all be applicable in some clinical situations.

## Reference

1. CREST (2006).). *Guidelines for the treatment of hyperkalaemia in adults*. www.crestni.org.uk/publications/hyperkalaemia-booklet.pdf (accessed 28 April 2008).

## Bibliography

SPC Ventolin injection 500 mcg (accessed 13 May 2010).
SPC Ventolin solution for IV infusion (accessed 13 May 2010).

# Selenium

### 50 micrograms/mL solution in 2-mL and 10-mL ampoules

* Selenium is an essential trace element that acts as a co-factor in various enzymes in the human body.
* Sodium selenite pentahydrate injection is used when there is proven selenium deficiency that cannot be remedied from food sources.
* Doses are expressed as selenium:
  Selenium 100 micrograms ≡ 333 micrograms sodium selenite pentahydrate.

## Pre-treatment checks

Avoid in selenosis.

## Dose

**Standard dose:** 100–200 micrograms daily by IM or IV injection increased to a maximum of 500 micrograms daily if required.
**Dose in renal and hepatic impairment:** no information available.

## Intravenous injection

*Preparation and administration*

1. Withdraw the required dose.
2. The solution should be clear and colourless. Inspect visually for particulate matter or discoloration prior to administration and discard if present.
3. Give by IV injection.

## Intramuscular injection

*Preparation and administration*

1. Withdraw the required dose.
2. Give by IM injection.

## Technical information

| | |
|---|---|
| Incompatible with | A precipitate forms if the pH falls below 7 and if the solution is mixed with reducing substances, e.g. ascorbic acid. |
| Compatible with | **Flush**: NaCl 0.9%<br>**Solutions**: NaCl 0.9%<br>**Y-site**: No information |

*(continued)*

## Technical information (*continued*)

| | |
|---|---|
| pH | No information |
| Sodium content | Negligible |
| Storage | Store below 25°C in original packaging. |

## Monitoring

| Measure | Frequency | Rationale |
|---|---|---|
| Selenium level | Periodically | • For signs of clinical improvement.<br>• In the UK the plasma reference range is 70–130 micrograms/L. |

## Additional information

| | |
|---|---|
| Common and serious undesirable effects | None known |
| Pharmacokinetics | Elimination is dependent on the selenium status of the body. It occurs in three phases, with the half-lives being 0.7–1.2 days in the first phase, 7–11 days in the second phase and 96–144 days in the third phase. |
| Significant interactions | No significant interactions. |
| Action in case of overdose | *Symptoms to watch for:* Odour of garlic on the breath, tiredness, nausea, diarrhoea and abdominal pain. Chronic overdose can affect growth of nails and hair and may lead to peripheral polyneuropathy.<br>*Antidote:* Forced diuresis or the administration of high doses of ascorbic acid may be of use. In the case of an extreme overdose (1000–10 000 times the normal dose) dialysis may help. |

| | |
|---|---|
| Risk rating: **GREEN** | Score = 1<br>Lower-risk product: Risk-reduction strategies should be considered. |

This assessment is based on the full range of preparation and administration options described in the monograph. These may not all be applicable in some clinical situations.

## Bibliography

SPC Selenase solution for injection (50 micrograms/mL) (accessed 30 September 2009).

# Sodium aurothiomalate

**20 mg/mL solution in 0.5-mL (10-mg) ampoules; 100 mg/mL solution in 0.5-mL (50-mg) ampoules**

Sodium aurothiomalate should be used under specialist supervision only.

* Sodium aurothiomalate is gold-containing compound with anti-inflammatory activity.
* It is used as a DMARD in the management of active progressive rheumatoid arthritis and juvenile idiopathic arthritis.

## Pre-treatment checks

Do not use in pregnancy, or severe renal or hepatic disease, a history of blood disorders, exfoliative dermatitis, systemic lupus erythematosus, necrotising enterocolitis, pulmonary fibrosis or porphyria.

*Biochemical and other tests*

Follow any local guidelines.

| | |
|---|---|
| FBC | Signs of abnormal bruising or severe sore throat |
| LFTs | Skin examination |
| Pulmonary function | Urinalysis |
| Renal function: U, Cr | |

## Dose

**Test dose:** 10 mg by IM injection in first week to assess tolerability.

**Maintenance dose:** after the test dose give 50 mg weekly by IM injection until there is evidence of remission. Benefit is not expected until 300–500 mg has been given. The dose frequency may then be reduced to every 2 weeks until full remission occurs and then further reduced on specialist advice. If there is no evidence of improvement after a total dose of 1 g has been given, and if there are no signs of gold toxicity, then 100 mg may be given every week for 6 weeks. Discontinue if there is no evidence of remission.

## Intramuscular injection

*Preparation and administration*

1. Withdraw the required dose.
2. Inspect visually and do not use if the solution has darkened (i.e. more than pale yellow).
3. The patient should be lying down.
4. Give by deep IM injection preferably into the gluteal muscle. Gently massage the area after administration. Rotate injection sites for subsequent injections.

| Technical information | |
|---|---|
| Incompatible with | Not relevant |
| Compatible with | Not relevant |
| pH | Not relevant |

*(continued)*

## Technical information (continued)

| | |
|---|---|
| Sodium content | Negligible |
| Storage | Store below 25°C in original packaging. |

## Monitoring

| Measure | Frequency | Rationale |
|---|---|---|
| FBC (including total and differential white cell and platelet counts) | Prior to each injection | • Blood dyscrasias may occur.<br>• If WBC <35 000-40 000 cells/mm$^3$ (<3.5-4.0 × 10$^9$/L) or neutrophils <20 000 cells/mm$^3$ (<2.0 × 10$^9$/L) or platelets <50 000 cells/mm$^3$ (<50 × 10$^9$/L), withhold therapy until discussed with the specialist team.<br>• Check for signs of abnormal bruising or a sore throat. |
| Urine albumin | | • The presence of albumin is an indication of developing toxicity.<br>• If 2+ proteinuria, withhold therapy until discussed with the specialist team. |
| Skin inspection | | • Rashes often occur after 2-6 months of treatment and may necessitate stopping treatment.<br>• If a rash (usually itchy) or oral ulceration presents, withhold therapy until discussed with the specialist team. |
| Medical observation | For a period of 30 minutes after injection | • Anaphylactoid reactions have been reported. |
| CRP and ESR | Periodically | • To track disease progression and therapeutic effect. |
| U&Es, LFTs | | • Changes in renal or hepatic function may require discontinuation of therapy (contraindicated in severe renal and hepatic impairment). |
| Chest radiograph | Annually | • Pulmonary fibrosis very rarely occurs. |

## Additional information

| | |
|---|---|
| Common and serious undesirable effects | *Immediate:* Anaphylaxis and other hypersensitivity reactions have been reported.<br>*Other:* Severe reactions (occasionally fatal) in up to 5% of patients; mouth ulcers, skin reactions, proteinuria, blood disorders, irreversible pigmentation in sun-exposed areas. |
| Pharmacokinetics | Elimination half-life is 5-6 days; this can increase with multiple doses and gold may be found in the urine for up to 12 months owing to its presence in deep body compartments. |
| Significant drug interactions | Sodium aurothiomalate may ↑levels or effect (or ↑side-effects) of ACE inhibitors (↑risk of severe anaphylactoid reaction). |

*(continued)*

| **Additional information** (*continued*) | |
|---|---|
| Overdose | *Symptoms to watch for:* Pruritus, blood dyscrasias.<br>*Antidote:* Dimercaprol or penicillamine may be used to enhance gold excretion. Pruritus may be treated symptomatically with antihistamines. Give other supportive therapy as appropriate. |
| Counselling | The patient is to tell the doctor immediately if sore throat, fever, infection, non-specific illnesses, unexplained bleeding and bruising, purpura, mouth ulcers, metallic taste or rashes develop. Signs of breathlessness or cough should also be reported. |

| Risk rating: **GREEN** | Score = 2<br>Lower-risk product. Risk-reduction strategies should be considered |
|---|---|

This assessment is based on the full range of preparation and administration options described in the monograph. These may not all be applicable in some clinical situations.

## Bibliography

SPC Myocrisin (accessed 2 December 2008).

# Sodium bicarbonate

**1.26% solution in 500-mL and 1000-mL infusion containers**
**4.2% solution in 10-mL pre-filled syringes and 500-mL infusion containers**
**8.4% solution in 10-mL and 50-mL pre-filled syringes and 200-mL infusion containers**

* Sodium bicarbonate is a buffer that breaks down to water and $CO_2$ after combining with hydrogen ions. It is reabsorbed by the kidney following glomerular filtration and this action is balanced by the excretion of hydrogen ions to maintain the systemic pH.
* Normal range for serum bicarbonate: 20–30 mmol/L.
* It is sometimes used IV to ↑serum bicarbonate, buffer excess hydrogen ion concentration and ↑blood pH, thus correcting metabolic acidosis.
* Sodium bicarbonate 1 g ≡ 12 mmol of Na and $HCO_3$.
* Table S1 shows the electrolyte content of different strengths and volumes of solution.

## Pre-treatment checks

* Do not use in renal failure, metabolic or respiratory alkalosis, ↑BP, oedema, congestive heart failure, hypoventilation, a history of urinary calculi, and co-existent ↓K, ↓Ca, ↓Cl or ↑Na.
* Whenever respiratory acidosis is concomitant with metabolic acidosis, both pulmonary ventilation and perfusion must be adequately supported to remove excess $CO_2$.
* Caution should also be used in patients receiving corticosteroids and in geriatric or postoperative patients.

**Table S1** Electrolyte content of various strengths and volumes of sodium bicarbonate solutions

| Strength: | 1.26% | 1.26% | 4.2% | 4.2% | 8.4% | 8.4% | 8.4% |
|---|---|---|---|---|---|---|---|
| Volume: | 500 mL | 1000 mL | 10 mL | 500 mL | 10 mL | 50 mL | 200 mL |
| Sodium (mmol) | 75 | 150 | 5 | 250 | 10 | 50 | 200 |
| Bicarbonate (mmol) | 75 | 150 | 5 | 250 | 10 | 50 | 200 |

*Biochemical tests (not all are necessary in every situation)*

Acid–base balance

Electrolytes: serum Na, K, Ca, Cl

LFTs

Renal function: U, Cr, CrCl (or eGFR)

## Dose

**Correction of metabolic acidosis:**

- *Mild metabolic acidosis associated with dehydration:* manage initially with appropriate fluid replacement. Acidosis usually improves as tissue and renal perfusion improve.
- *Severe metabolic acidosis (pH <7.1):* the advice of a senior doctor should be sought before proceeding – use is controversial. An appropriate volume of sodium bicarbonate 1.26% may be given by IV infusion over 3–4 hours according to body base deficit. The rate may be increased in 'life-threatening' conditions, e.g. 50 mmol may be given over 1 hour in severe DKA. Plasma pH, electrolytes (particularly K) and $pCO_2$ must be closely monitored and over-correction avoided. Allow natural compensatory mechanisms to make the final approach to normal acid–base balance.

**Correction of acidosis during advanced cardiac life support:** routine use is not recommended. Give sodium bicarbonate 50 mmol (as 50 mL 8.4%) by IV injection if cardiac arrest is associated with ↑K or tricyclic antidepressant overdose. Repeat the dose according to the clinical condition of the patient and the results of repeated blood gas analysis.[1]

## Intravenous injection

*Preparation and administration*

Concentrations >1.26% should be given via a central line except in emergencies.
Sodium bicarbonate solution is incompatible with Hartmann's and Ringer's solutions.

1. Either assemble a pre-filled syringe according to the manufacturer's instructions or withdraw the required dose from an infusion container.
2. The solution should be clear and colourless. Inspect visually for particulate matter or discoloration prior to administration and discard if present.
3. Give by slow IV injection. Concentrations >1.26% should be given via a central line (see Osmolarity below) except in emergency situations.

## Intravenous infusion

*Preparation and administration*

Concentrations >1.26% should be given via a central line.
Sodium bicarbonate solution is incompatible with Hartmann's and Ringer's solutions.

1. The infusion is pre-prepared for use. It should be clear and colourless. Inspect visually for particulate matter or discoloration prior to administration and discard if present.
2. Give by IV infusion via a volumetric infusion device at the required rate. Concentrations >1.26% should be given via a central line (see Osmolarity below) except in emergency situations.
3. Discard any unused portion. Do not reconnect partially used infusion containers.

## Technical information

| | |
|---|---|
| Incompatible with | Hartmann's, Ringers.<br>Amiodarone, amphotericin, anidulafungin, calcium chloride, calcium folinate, calcium gluconate, ciprofloxacin, magnesium sulfate, midazolam, ondansetron, phosphate, verapamil. |
| Compatible with | **Flush**: NaCl 0.9%<br>**Solutions**: NaCl 0.9%, Gluc 5%, Gluc-NaCl<br>**Y-site**: Aciclovir, aztreonam, bivalirudin, ceftriaxone, dexamethasone, granisetron, linezolid, mesna, methylprednisolone sodium succinate, piperacillin with tazobactam, potassium chloride, remifentanil, vancomycin |
| pH | 7-8.5 |
| Electrolyte content | See Table S1 above. |
| Osmolarity<br>(plasma osmolality = 280-300 mOsmol/L)[2] | Sodium bicarbonate 1.26% ≅ 300 mOsmol/L.<br>Sodium bicarbonate 4.2% ≅ 1000 mOsmol/L.<br>Sodium bicarbonate 8.4% ≅ 2000 mOsmol/L. |
| Storage | Store below 25°C. Do not freeze. |

## Monitoring

| Measure | Frequency | Rationale |
|---|---|---|
| Arterial blood gas analyses | Regularly throughout treatment | • To minimise the possibility of overdosage and resultant alkalosis. |
| Serum electrolytes | | • Replacement of Ca, Cl, and K may be of particular importance if alkalosis occurs.<br>• Too rapid correction of Na can lead to severe neurological adverse effects.<br>• Excessive IV administration of Na may result in ↓K. |
| Fluid balance | | • Retention of excess Na can lead to the accumulation of extracellular fluid and may result in pulmonary and peripheral oedema and their consequent effects. |
| Acid-base balance | | • Frequent monitoring of acid-base balance is essential.<br>• Bicarbonate-induced metabolic alkalosis can occur with excessive administration of bicarbonate-containing compounds.<br>• Na is associated with chloride and bicarbonate in the regulation of acid-base balance. |

### Additional information

| | |
|---|---|
| Common and serious undesirable effects | *Infusion-related:* Local: Extravasation may cause tissue damage.<br>*Other:* Alkalosis, ↑Na, ↓K (especially in patients with impaired renal function). |
| Pharmacokinetics | Not applicable |
| Significant interactions | No significant interactions in emergency use. |
| Action in case of overdose | *Symptoms to watch for:* Metabolic alkalosis, compensatory hyperventilation, ↑Na, severe ↓K, hyperirritability, tetany.<br>*Antidote:* Stop administration and give supportive therapy as appropriate. |

| | |
|---|---|
| Risk rating: **AMBER** | Score = 3<br>Moderate-risk product: Risk-reduction strategies are recommended. |

This assessment is based on the full range of preparation and administration options described in the monograph. These may not all be applicable in some clinical situations.

### References

1. Resuscitation Council (UK) (2005). *Resuscitation Guidelines 2005*. London: Resuscitation Council (UK). www.resus.org.uk/pages/mediMain.htm (accessed 7 May 2010).
2. Longmore M *et al.*, eds. *Oxford Handbook of Clinical Medicine*, 6th edn. Oxford: Oxford University Press, 2004.

### Bibliography

SPC Sodium Bicarbonate Injection BP Minijet 8.4%, International Medication Systems (accessed 7 May 2010).

SPC Sodium Bicarbonate Injection BP Minijet 4.2%, International Medication Systems (accessed 7 May 2010).

# Sodium chloride

**0.9% solution in ampoules, vials and infusion containers of various volumes**
**0.45%, 1.8%, 2.7% and 5% solution in 500-mL infusion containers**
**30% solution in 10-mL ampoules**

* Sodium is the major extracellular electrolyte and its role and metabolism are closely related to the body's water balance.
* Sodium chloride in water forms a crystalloid intravenous fluid. The 0.9% solution is commonly called normal saline or physiological saline because it is isotonic with plasma, but prescriptions should always specify strength as a percentage.

- Normal range for serum sodium: 135–145 mmol/L.
- NaCl 0.9% is used to replenish extracellular fluid and is also widely used as a vehicle or diluent for the administration of compatible parenteral drugs.
- NaCl 1.8% may sometimes be used cautiously to correct ↓Na; other strengths may be added to parenteral nutrition regimens to provide Na supplementation.
- NaCl 0.9% and NaCl 0.45% may also be given (unlicensed) by SC infusion (hypodermoclysis).
- Sodium chloride 1 g ≡ 17.1 mmol of Na and Cl.
- Sodium chloride 2.54 g ≡ 1 g sodium.
- Table S2 shows the electrolyte content of different strengths and volumes of solution.

**Table S2**  Electrolyte content of various volumes and strengths of NaCl solutions

| Strength: | 0.9% | 0.9% | 0.9% | 0.9% | 0.9% | 0.9% | 1.8% |
|---|---|---|---|---|---|---|---|
| **Volume:** | **10 mL** | **50 mL** | **100 mL** | **250 mL** | **500 mL** | **1000 mL** | **500 mL** |
| Sodium (mmol) | 1.5 | 7.5 | 15 | 37.5 | 75 | 150 | 150 |
| Chloride (mmol) | 1.5 | 7.5 | 15 | 37.5 | 75 | 150 | 150 |

## Pre-treatment checks

- Caution in patients with ↑BP, heart failure, peripheral or pulmonary oedema, renal impairment, liver cirrhosis, pre-eclampsia, toxaemia of pregnancy or other conditions associated with Na retention.
- Caution should also be used in patients receiving corticosteroids and in elderly or postoperative patients.

*Biochemical tests (not all are necessary in every situation)*

Acid–base balance

Electrolytes: serum Na, K

## Dose

**Treatment or prevention of fluid depletion:** dose is dependent upon the age, weight, biochemistry and clinical condition of the patient. Normal fluid requirements are generally about 40 mL/kg/ 24 hours. The use of colloid solutions should be considered where plasma expansion is required due to ↑losses.

**Hyponatraemia:** therapy is guided by the rate of development and degree of ↓Na, accompanying symptoms, the state of water balance, and taking into account the underlying cause.

- Mild asymptomatic ↓Na: does not usually require specific therapy.
- Chronic mild to moderate ↓Na due to, e.g. salt-losing bowel or renal disease: give oral NaCl supplements whilst ensuring adequate fluid intake.
- Chronic dilutional ↓Na, which is often asymptomatic, can be managed by correcting the underlying cause. Fluid restriction may be necessary, particularly in the short term, and drugs interfering with the action of ADH should be stopped if possible.
- Severe acute (or chronic) ↓Na may require the use of NaCl 0.9% by IV infusion (which is effectively hypertonic in these circumstances). In very severe ↓Na, cautious use of NaCl 1.8% may be necessary. The deficit should be corrected slowly to avoid the risk of osmotic demyelination syndrome:

rise in serum Na should be no more than 10 mmol/L in 24 hours. The aim is to render the patient asymptomatic (serum Na 120–130 mmol/L). Loop diuretics, e.g. furosemide are often also given, especially if fluid overload is likely to be a problem. Hypertonic solutions should be used with caution as over-rapid correction may have severe neurological adverse effects.

**Hypernatraemia:** hypernatraemia is usually due to water loss in excess of Na loss. Treatment should correct the underlying cause and usually involves water replacement: simply drinking water may be sufficient in some patients. In more severe conditions, Gluc 5% may be given by slow IV infusion. Alternatively, if volume depletion is severe, NaCl 0.9% may be given by IV infusion (as it is relatively hypotonic).

## Intravenous infusion

*Preparation and administration*

1. The infusion is pre-prepared for use. It should be clear and colourless. Inspect visually for particulate matter or discoloration prior to administration and discard if present.
2. Give by IV infusion at the required rate.
3. Discard any unused portion. Do not reconnect partially used infusion containers.

| Technical information | |
|---|---|
| Incompatible with | The following drugs are incompatible with sodium chloride solutions (however this list is not exhaustive, check individual drug monographs): amiodarone, amphotericin, dantrolene, diazepam emulsion, filgrastim, mycophenolate, quinupristin with dalfopristin. |
| Compatible with | **Flush**: Not relevant<br>**Y-site**: See individual drug monographs |
| pH | 4.5-7 |
| Electrolyte content | See Table S2 above. |
| Storage | Store below 25°C. |

| Monitoring | | |
|---|---|---|
| **Measure** | **Frequency** | **Rationale** |
| Serum Na | Periodically during treatment (at least daily in some situations) | • Too rapid correction can lead to severe neurological adverse effects. |
| Serum K | | • Excessive IV administration of NaCl may result in ↓K. |
| Acid-base balance | | • Sodium is associated with chloride and bicarbonate in the regulation of acid-base balance. |
| Fluid accumulation | | • Retention of excess sodium can lead to the accumulation of extracellular fluid and may result in pulmonary and peripheral oedema and their consequent effects. |

## Additional information

| | |
|---|---|
| Common and serious undesirable effects | Fluid overload may cause peripheral and pulmonary oedema particularly in cardiac failure and renal impairment.<br>↑Na (following excessive use of hypertonic NaCl) may cause dehydration of the brain leading to somnolence, confusion, convulsions, coma, respiratory failure and death.<br>Excessive Cl infusion (particularly during prolonged IV fluid replacement) causes bicarbonate loss resulting in hyperchloraemic acidosis. |
| Pharmacokinetics | Not applicable. |
| Significant interactions | No significant interactions. |
| Action in case of overdose | Stop administration and give supportive therapy as appropriate. |

| Risk rating: **GREEN** | Score = 1<br>Lower-risk product: Risk-reduction strategies should be considered. |
|---|---|

This assessment is based on the full range of preparation and administration options described in the monograph. These may not all be applicable in some clinical situations.

### Bibliography

SPC Sodium Chloride Injection BP 0.9% w/v, Hameln Pharmaceuticals Ltd (accessed 07 May 2010).
SPC Sodium chloride 0.45%, 0.9%. www.baxterhealthcare.co.uk (accessed 07 May 2010).

# Sodium fusidate (fusidate sodium)

**500-mg dry powder vials with buffered solvent**
- Sodium fusidate is a steroidal antibacterial with a bacteriostatic or bactericidal activity.
- It is used mainly against Gram-positive bacteria, particularly in susceptible staphylococcal infections. It is usually given in combination with other antibacterials to prevent the emergence of resistance.
- Doses are expressed in terms of sodium fusidate:
  Sodium fusidate 500 mg ≡ 480 mg fusidic acid.

## Pre-treatment checks

*Biochemical tests*

Bodyweight
FBC
LFTs

## Dose

Sodium fusidate must not be given by IM or SC injection as this causes local tissue necrosis.

**Adults 50 kg or more**: 500 mg three times daily.
**Adults less than 50 kg**: 6–7 mg/kg three times daily (equivalent to 6–7 mL/kg of the final infusion solution).

## Intermittent intravenous infusion

*Preparation and administration*

Infusion via a central venous line is preferred (risk of vasospasm); if use of a peripheral line is essential use a large vein and infuse over a longer period (see below).

1. Reconstitute a 500-mg vial with 10 mL of the solvent provided and add the entire contents of the vial to 500 mL of compatible infusion fluid (usually NaCl 0.9%)
2. Mix well to give a solution containing approximately 1 mg/mL.
3. The solution should be clear and colourless. Inspect visually for particulate matter or discoloration prior to administration and discard if present. If opalescence develops, the solution must be discarded.
4. Give by IV infusion via a central venous line (preferred) over at least 2 hours. If a peripheral vein is used (must be a wide-bore vein with a good blood flow), give by IV infusion over at least 6 hours as there is a risk of vasospasm, thrombophlebitis and haemolysis if it is given too rapidly.

## Technical information

| Incompatible with | Unstable in solutions of pH < 7.4 |
|---|---|
| Compatible with | **Flush**: NaCl 0.9%<br>**Solutions**: NaCl 0.9%, Gluc 5%, Hartmann's (with added KCl)<br>**Y-Site**: No information |
| pH | 7.4–7.6 |
| Electrolyte content | Sodium: 3.1 mmol/500 mg; phosphate: 1.1 mmol/500 mg (reconstituted) |
| Storage | Store below 25°C in original packaging.<br>Single use only – discard the unused portion. |
| Displacement value | Negligible |
| Stability after preparation | From a microbiological point of view, should be used immediately; however, it may be stored at room temperature and infused within 24 hours. |

## Monitoring

| Measure | Frequency | Rationale |
|---|---|---|
| LFTs | Periodically in prolonged use | • Use with caution in liver dysfunction and biliary disease.<br>• If jaundice occurs, normal liver function and bilirubin level usually return when treatment is stopped |
| FBC | | • Abnormalities in white and red blood cells and platelets have been reported. |

## Additional information

| | |
|---|---|
| Common and serious undesirable effects | *Infusion-related:*<br>• Too rapid administration: Reversible jaundice.<br>• Local: Vasospasm, thrombophlebitis.<br>*Other:* Nausea, vomiting, reversible jaundice, especially after high dosage (withdraw therapy if persistent). |
| Pharmacokinetics | Elimination half-life is 10–15 hours. |
| Significant interactions | • Ritonavir may ↑sodium fusidate levels or ↑side-effects (avoid combination).<br>• Sodium fusidate may ↑levels or effect of the following drugs (or ↑side-effects): ritonavir (avoid combination), simvastatin (↑risk of myopathy). |
| Action in case of overdose | *Antidote:* No known antidote and sodium fusidate is not removed by haemodialysis.<br>Stop administration and give supportive therapy as appropriate. |

| | |
|---|---|
| Risk rating: **AMBER** | Score = 4<br>Moderate-risk product: Risk-reduction strategies are recommended. |

This assessment is based on the full range of preparation and administration options described in the monograph. These may not all be applicable in some clinical situations.

## Bibliography

SPC Sodium Fusidate 500 mg for intravenous infusion, Leo Laboratories Ltd (accessed 2 April 2009).

# Sodium nitrite

**300 mg/10 mL solution in vials**

• Sodium nitrite is used with sodium thiosulfate in the treatment of cyanide poisoning.
• Sodium nitrite produces methaemoglobinaemia and it is thought that cyanide ions combine with the methaemoglobin to produce cyanmethaemoglobin, thus protecting cytochrome oxidase from the cyanide ions; however, other mechanisms may have a significant role. As the cyanmethaemoglobin slowly dissociates, the cyanide is converted to relatively non-toxic thiocyanate and is excreted in the urine.
• Sodium thiosulfate provides an additional source of sulfur for this reaction and this accelerates the process.

## Pre-treatment checks

• Do not give sodium nitrite to asymptomatic patients who have been exposed to cyanide.
• Do not give sodium nitrite to symptomatic patients if dicobalt edetate is available.

- It is important to be aware if any cyanide antidote therapy has been given in the pre-hospital setting as repeat doses of some antidotes can cause serious side-effects.
- Use with caution in patients with acquired or congenital methaemoglobinaemia, as sodium nitrite will exacerbate this condition.
- Patients with G6PD are theoretically at great risk from sodium nitrite therapy because of the likelihood of haemolysis, although no such cases have been reported.

## Doses of cyanide poisoning antidotes (see relevant entries)[1]

It is essential to consult a poisons information service, e.g. Toxbase at www.toxbase.org (password or registration required) for full details of the management of cyanide toxicity.

**Mild poisoning (nausea, dizziness, drowsiness, hyperventilation, anxiety):**
- Observe.
- Give 12.5 g sodium thiosulfate (50 mL of 25% or 25 mL of 50% solution) IV over 10 minutes.

**Moderate poisoning (reduced conscious level, vomiting, convulsions, ↓BP):** as well as other supportive measures:

*If dicobalt edetate is available:*
- Give 300 mg (20 mL) of 1.5% dicobalt edetate solution IV over 1 minute.
- Follow immediately with 50 mL Gluc 50%.

*If dicobalt edetate is not available:*
- Give 12.5 g sodium thiosulfate (50 mL of 25% or 25 mL of 50% solution) IV over 10 minutes.

**Severe poisoning (coma, fixed dilated pupils, cardiovascular collapse, respiratory failure, cyanosis):**

*If dicobalt edetate is available:*
As well as other supportive measures:
- Give 300 mg (20 mL) of 1.5% dicobalt edetate solution IV over 1 minute.
- Follow immediately with 50 mL Gluc 50%.
- If there is only a partial response to dicobalt edetate 300 mg, or the patient relapses after recovery, give a further dose of dicobalt edetate 300 mg. If a second dose of dicobalt edetate is given there is ↑risk of cobalt toxicity but only if the diagnosis is not cyanide poisoning.

*If dicobalt edetate is not available:*
As well as other supportive measures:
- Give 300 mg (10 mL) of 3% sodium nitrite solution IV over 5–20 minutes.
- Follow with 12.5 g sodium thiosulfate (50 mL of 25% or 25 mL of 50% solution) IV over 10 minutes.
- A further dose of sodium thiosulfate 12.5 g IV over 10 minutes may then be given.
- A second dose of sodium nitrite should **not** be given because of the risk of excessive methaemoglobinaemia.

## Intravenous injection

*Preparation and administration*

1. Withdraw the required dose.
2. The solution should be clear and colourless. Inspect visually for particulate matter or discoloration prior to administration.
3. Give by IV injection over 5–20 minutes monitoring the patient for adverse effects.
4. Give sodium thiosulfate as above.
5. The sodium nitrite dose should **not** be repeated.

## Technical information

| | |
|---|---|
| Incompatible with | Hydroxocobalamin |
| Compatible with | Not relevant |
| pH | No information |
| Sodium content | Contains sodium, but not relevant in an emergency situation. |
| Storage | Store below 25°C in original packaging. |

## Monitoring

| Measure | Frequency | Rationale |
|---|---|---|
| Blood pressure | During treatment | • ↓BP may result if given too rapidly. |
| Methaemoglobin concentration | | • Sodium nitrite produces methaemoglobinaemia. Methaemoglobin concentration should not exceed 40%. |

## Additional information

| | |
|---|---|
| Common and serious undesirable effects | Flushing and headache due to vasodilatation, nausea and vomiting, abdominal pain, dizziness, cyanosis, tachypnoea, dyspnoea, syncope, ↓BP and ↑pulse. |
| Pharmacokinetics | After IV administration the time to peak effect of sodium nitrite is 30–70 minutes. An injection of 1 mg/kg sodium nitrite produces a peak methaemoglobin concentration of approximately 6%. |
| Significant interactions | No information. |
| Action in case of overdose | Give intensive supportive therapy as appropriate. Methylthioninium chloride (methylene blue, an antidote for nitrite toxicity) should **not** be given if sodium nitrite has been used to treat cyanide poisoning since cyanide may be displaced. |

| Risk rating: **GREEN** | Score = 1<br>Lower-risk product: Risk-reduction strategies should be considered. |
|---|---|

This assessment is based on the full range of preparation and administration options described in the monograph. These may not all be applicable in some clinical situations.

### Reference

1. Toxbase. www.toxbase.org (accessed 1 May 2010).

### Bibliography

SPC Sodium nitrite. www.phebra.com.au (accessed 21 January 2009).

# Sodium nitroprusside

### 50-mg dry powder vials

* Sodium nitroprusside is a short-acting peripheral arteriolar and venous vasodilator that lowers peripheral resistance and ↓arterial blood pressure.
* It is used in the management of hypertensive emergencies, for controlled hypotension in anaesthesia, and in acute or chronic heart failure.
* It is no longer marketed in the UK but is available from 'special-order' manufacturers or specialist importing companies.
* Treatment should be restricted to no more than 72 hours if possible to avoid toxicity.

## Pre-treatment checks

* Do not use in compensatory hypertension such as arteriovenous bypass or coarctation of aorta.
* Use with caution, if at all, in patients with hepatic impairment, and in patients with low plasma cobalamin concentrations or Leber's optic atrophy.
* Caution in patients with impaired renal or pulmonary function and with particular caution in patients with impaired cerebrovascular circulation or ischaemic heart disease.

*Biochemical and other tests*

Blood pressure
Bodyweight (in certain indications)

## Dose (no longer licensed in UK; doses specified are previously licensed doses)

**Hypertensive emergencies**: 0.5–1.5 microgram/kg/minute, increasing in steps of 500 nanograms/kg/minute every 5 minutes to 0.5–8 microgram/kg/minute (use lower doses if the patient is already receiving other antihypertensives); stop if response is unsatisfactory with the maximum dose after 10 minutes. Treatment with an oral antihypertensive should be introduced as soon as possible.

**Controlled hypotension in surgery**: up to 1.5 micrograms/kg/minute.

**Cardiac failure**: 10–15 micrograms/minute, increasing by 10–15 micrograms/minute every 5–10 minutes as necessary; usual range 10–200 micrograms/minute (maximum 4 micrograms/kg/minute), normally for a maximum of 3 days.

**Calculation of infusion rate:** NB: cardiac failure doses above are **not** given per kg bodyweight.

$$\text{Infusion rate (mL/hour)} = \frac{\text{Bodyweight (kg)} \times \text{rate required (micrograms/kg/minute)} \times 60}{\text{Concentration of solution (micrograms/mL)}}$$

## Continuous intravenous infusion (large volume infusion)

*Preparation and administration*

The infusion and giving set must be protected from light.
Any strong discoloration (bright orange, dark brown or blue) indicates serious degradation in the presence of light and these solutions should be discarded.

1. Reconstitute each vial with 5 mL of the supplied solvent (use Gluc 5% if solvent is not supplied) and shake gently to dissolve to produce a solution containing 10 mg/mL.
2. Withdraw 50 mg (5 mL) and add to 250, 500 or 1000 mL Gluc 5% infusion and mix well. The resulting solution will contain 200 micrograms/mL, 100 micrograms/mL or 50 micrograms/mL respectively.
3. The solution should be clear and may vary in colour from light brown, brownish-pink, light orange or straw. Inspect visually for particulate matter or discoloration prior to administration and discard if present. Any strong discoloration (bright orange, dark brown or blue) indicates serious degradation in the presence of light and these solutions should be discarded.
4. Wrap the prepared infusion immediately in foil (which may be provided) or other light-occlusive material, and do the same with the infusion set once attached.
5. Give by IV infusion via a volumetric infusion device at a rate appropriate for the indication. Continue to protect from light. Monitor the colour of the infusion periodically during administration and discard if discoloration has occurred.
6. Prepare a fresh infusion at least every 24 hours if required.
7. Treatment should not be stopped abruptly; taper off over 30 minutes to avoid rebound effects.

## Continuous intravenous infusion via a syringe pump

*Preparation and administration*

The infusion and giving set must be protected from light.
Any strong discoloration (bright orange, dark brown or blue) indicates serious degradation in the presence of light and these solutions should be discarded.

1. Reconstitute each vial with 5 mL supplied solvent (use Gluc 5% if solvent is not supplied) and shake gently to dissolve to produce a solution containing 10 mg/mL.
2. Withdraw 50 mg (5 mL) and make up to 50 mL in a syringe pump with Gluc 5%.
3. Mix well to give a solution containing 1 mg/mL.
4. The solution should be clear and may vary in colour from light brown, brownish-pink, light orange or straw. Inspect visually for particulate matter or discoloration prior to administration and discard if present. Any strong discoloration (bright orange, dark brown or blue) indicates serious degradation in the presence of light and these solutions should be discarded.
5. Wrap the prepared syringe immediately in foil (which may be provided) or other light-occlusive material, and do the same with the infusion set once attached.
6. Give by IV infusion at a rate appropriate for the indication. Continue to protect from light. Monitor the colour of the infusion periodically during administration and discard if discoloration has occurred.
7. Prepare a fresh syringe at least every 24 hours if required.
8. Treatment should not be stopped abruptly; taper off over 30 minutes to avoid rebound effects.

## Technical information

| Incompatible with | Amiodarone, cisatracurium, dobutamine, drotrecogin alfa (activated). |
|---|---|
| Compatible with | **Flush**: NaCl 0.9%<br>**Solutions**: Gluc 5%, NaCl 0.9% (manufacturer specifies Gluc 5% but known to be stable in NaCl 0.9%)<br>**Y-site**: Atracurium, dopamine, esmolol, furosemide, glyceryl trinitrate, labetalol, lidocaine, magnesium sulfate, micafungin, midazolam, midazolam, noradrenaline (norepinephrine) |
| pH | 3.5–6 in Gluc 5% |

*(continued)*

## Technical information (*continued*)

| | |
|---|---|
| Sodium content | Negligible |
| Storage | Store at 15-30°C in original packaging. Protect from light. |
| Displacement volume | Negligible |
| Stability after reconstitution | Use prepared infusions immediately. Solutions adequately protected from light are stable for up to 24 hours.<br>Any strong discoloration (bright orange, dark brown or blue) indicates serious photodegradation and these solutions should be discarded. |

## Monitoring

| Measure | Frequency | Rationale |
|---|---|---|
| Blood pressure | Continuously | • Response to therapy.<br>• The average dose required to maintain BP 30-40% below the pre-treatment diastolic BP is 3 micrograms/kg per minute and the usual dose range is 0.5-6 micrograms/kg per minute. |
| Infusion site | Every 30 minutes | • Extravasation must be avoided. |
| Blood cyanide concentration | After high dose or renal/hepatic impairment or treatment >3 days | • Blood concentration of cyanide should not exceed 1 microgram/mL and the serum concentration should not exceed 80 nanograms/mL. |
| Blood thiocyanate concentration | | • Should not exceed 100 micrograms/mL although toxicity may be apparent at lower thiocyanate concentrations. |
| Blood pH | Daily | • Cyanide toxicity includes acidosis. |

## Additional information

| | |
|---|---|
| Common and serious undesirable effects | *Infusion-related:*<br>• Too rapid administration: Headache, dizziness, nausea, retching, abdominal pain, ↑perspiration, palpitations, anxiety, retrosternal discomfort.<br>• Local: Acute transient phlebitis.<br>*Other:* Side-effects caused by ↑plasma concentration of the cyanide metabolite include ↑pulse, sweating, hyperventilation, arrhythmias, marked metabolic acidosis. |
| Pharmacokinetics | The drug is rapidly eliminated; when infusion is stopped blood pressure returns to pre-treatment levels within 1-10 minutes. |
| Significant drug interactions | • Other hypotensive agents may ↑sodium nitroprusside effect. |
| Overdose | ↓BP responds rapidly to dose reduction or cessation. If cyanide or thiocyanate toxicity occur, expert advice should be sought. |
| Counselling | Ask the patient to report infusion-site reactions. |

| Risk rating: **RED** | Score = 7 |
| --- | --- |
| | High-risk product. Risk-reduction strategies are required to minimise these risks. |

This assessment is based on the full range of preparation and administration options described in the monograph. These may not all be applicable in some clinical situations.

## Bibliography

SPC Sodium Nitroprussiat Fides package insert [undated]. Fides Ecopharma S.A.

# Sodium stibogluconate

**100 mg/mL solution in 100-mL vials**
* Sodium stibogluconate is a pentavalent antimony compound.
* It is used as first-line treatment for all forms of leishmaniasis except *Leishmania aethiopica* infections.
* Doses are expressed as pentavalent antimony:
  Sodium stibogluconate injection contains pentavalent antimony 100 mg/mL.

## Pre-treatment checks

* Do not give if a serious reaction was experienced to the previous dose.
* Caution in patients with cardiovascular disease, a history of ventricular arrhythmias or other risk factors that predispose towards QT prolongation.
* Caution in existing infections, e.g. pneumonia should be actively treated concomitantly.

*Biochemical and other tests*

ECG (if unavailable the risks and benefits of therapy will need to be assessed)
LFTs
Renal function: not to be given in moderate to severe renal impairment. Unfortunately the degree of renal impairment at which the drug should not be given (or should be given at a reduced dose) is poorly defined and no precise data is available based on creatinine clearance.

## Dose

**Visceral leishmaniasis:** 20 mg (0.2 mL)/kg up to a maximum of 850 mg (8.5 mL) by IM or IV injection daily for a minimum period of 20 days. Patients should be examined for evidence of relapse after 2 and 6 months and in Africa again after 12 months.

Expert advice should be sought for dosing information in other forms of leishmaniasis as treatment regimens vary by species and geographical source of infection.

**Dose in renal impairment:** avoid in 'significant' renal impairment.

## Intramuscular injection (preferred route)

*Preparation and administration*

1. Withdraw the required dose into a syringe immediately before administration through a filter of 5 microns or less (if the volume exceeds 10 mL the dose should be split between two sites[1]).
2. Remove the filter and give by deep IM injection into the buttock or thigh. Rotate injection sites for subsequent injections.

## Intravenous injection

*Preparation and administration*

1. Withdraw the required dose into a syringe immediately before administration through a filter of 5 microns or less.
2. Remove the filter and replace with a fine needle, which may help to avoid thrombophlebitis.
3. Give by slow IV injection over at least 5 minutes.

## Technical information

| | |
|---|---|
| Incompatible with | No information but do not mix with any other drug. |
| Compatible with | **Flush**: WFI<br>**Solutions**: WFI<br>**Y-site**: No information but likely to be unstable |
| pH | 5.0–5.6 |
| Sodium content | Approximately 0.5 mmol/mL |
| Storage | Store below 25°C in original packaging. Do not freeze.<br>*In use*: The manufacturer states that the vial contents should not be used more than 1 month after removing the first dose. |

## Monitoring

| Measure | Frequency | Rationale |
|---|---|---|
| Coughing, vomiting or substernal pain | During administration | • The presence of these symptoms during administration may indicate serious adverse effects and therapy should be discontinued immediately. |
| ECG | | • If clinically significant prolongation of QTc interval occurs, therapy should be discontinued.<br>• ↓Pulse and arrhythmias are signs of antimony intoxication. |
| Renal function | Periodically | • If renal function deteriorates therapy may need to be stopped. Renal impairment may lead to high antimony plasma levels and increased renal and cardiotoxicity.[2] |
| LFTs | | • Mild, transient ↑LFTs may occur.<br>• Antimony may be deposited in the liver and visceral leishmaniasis may cause abnormal LFTs. |

## Additional information

| | |
|---|---|
| Common and serious undesirable effects | *Injection/infusion-related:* Local: Pain and thrombosis on IV administration, IM injection also painful.<br>*Other:* Anorexia, vomiting, nausea, malaise, arthralgia and myalgia, headache, lethargy, and pancreatitis. |
| Pharmacokinetics | The elimination half-life of the initial phase is about 1.7 hours and that of the slow terminal phase is about 33 hours. |
| Significant drug interactions | • Sodium stibogluconate may ↑side-effects of the following drugs:<br>    Caution with drugs which prolong the QT interval, e.g. amiodarone, sotalol. |
| Action in case of overdose | *Antidote:* Dimercaprol has been reported to be effective as a chelating agent in the treatment of intoxication with antimony compounds (see the Dimercaprol monograph). |

| | |
|---|---|
| Risk rating: **AMBER** | Score = 3<br>Moderate-risk product: Risk-reduction strategies are recommended. |

This assessment is based on the full range of preparation and administration options described in the monograph. These may not all be applicable in some clinical situations.

### References

1. World Health Organization (1988). *WHO Essential Medicines Library*. Geneva: WHO. http://apps. who.int/emlib/Default.aspx?Language=EN (accessed 17 February 2009).
2. Dollery C, ed. *Therapeutic Drugs*, 2nd edn, vol.2. Edinburgh: Churchill Livingstone, 1999. S64–S67.

# Sodium thiosulfate (sodium thiosulphate, disodium thiosulfate)

**2.5 g/10 mL (25%) or 5 g/10 mL (50%) solution in ampoules**

* Sodium thiosulfate is used in the treatment of cyanide poisoning. It acts as a sulfur-donating substrate for the enzyme rhodanese, which catalyses the conversion of cyanide to relatively non-toxic thiocyanate, and thus accelerates the detoxification of cyanide.
* It may be effective alone in less severe cases of cyanide poisoning, but it may be used with dicobalt edetate or sodium nitrite in more severe poisoning (see below).

## Pre-treatment checks

* It is important to be aware whether any cyanide antidote therapy has been given in the pre-hospital setting as repeat doses of some antidotes can cause serious side-effects.

## Doses of cyanide poisoning antidotes (see relevant entries)[1]

It is essential to consult a poisons information service, e.g. Toxbase at www.toxbase.org (password or registration required) for full details of the management of cyanide toxicity.

**Mild poisoning (nausea, dizziness, drowsiness, hyperventilation, anxiety):**
* Observe.
* Give 12.5 g sodium thiosulfate (50 mL of 25% or 25 mL of 50% solution) IV over 10 minutes.

**Moderate poisoning (reduced conscious level, vomiting, convulsions, ↓BP):** as well as other supportive measures:
*If dicobalt edetate is available:*
* Give 300 mg (20 mL) of 1.5% dicobalt edetate solution IV over 1 minute.
* Follow immediately with 50 mL Gluc 50%.

*If dicobalt edetate is not available:*
* Give 12.5 g sodium thiosulfate (50 mL of 25% or 25 mL of 50% solution) IV over 10 minutes.

**Severe poisoning (coma, fixed dilated pupils, cardiovascular collapse, respiratory failure, cyanosis):**
*If dicobalt edetate is available:*
As well as other supportive measures:
* Give 300 mg (20 mL) of 1.5% dicobalt edetate solution IV over 1 minute.
* Follow immediately with 50 mL Gluc 50%.
* If there is only a partial response to dicobalt edetate 300 mg, or the patient relapses after recovery, give a further dose of dicobalt edetate 300 mg. If a second dose of dicobalt edetate is given, there is ↑risk of cobalt toxicity but only if the diagnosis is not cyanide poisoning.

*If dicobalt edetate is not available:*
As well as other supportive measures:
* Give 300 mg (10 mL) of 3% sodium nitrite solution IV over 5–20 minutes.
* Follow with 12.5 g sodium thiosulfate (50 mL of 25% or 25 mL of 50% solution) IV over 10 minutes.
* A further dose of sodium thiosulfate 12.5 g IV over 10 minutes may then be given.
* A second dose of sodium nitrite should **not** be given because of the risk of excessive methaemoglobinaemia.

## Intravenous injection

*Preparation and administration*

1. Give sodium nitrite first if appropriate (see above).
2. Withdraw the required dose.
3. Give by IV injection over about 10 minutes.

| Technical information | |
|---|---|
| Incompatible with | Hydroxocobalamin |
| Compatible with | Not relevant |
| pH | 7–9 |
| Sodium content | Contains sodium, but not relevant in an emergency situation. |
| Storage | Store below 25°C in original packaging. |

## Monitoring

| Measure | Frequency | Rationale |
|---|---|---|
| Blood pressure | During treatment | May cause ↓BP. |

## Additional information

| | |
|---|---|
| Common and serious undesirable effects | ↓BP may be seen following rapid IV infusion of very large doses; this should be self-limiting and transient. Care should be taken to avoid extravasation. |
| Pharmacokinetics | After IV injection sodium thiosulfate is distributed throughout the extracellular fluid and primarily rapidly excreted unchanged in the urine. Plasma elimination half-life is reported to be about 80 minutes. |
| Significant interactions | No information available. |
| Action in case of overdose | Treat unresolved ↓BP symptomatically. |

| Risk rating: **GREEN** | Score = 1 Lower-risk product: Risk-reduction strategies should be considered. |
|---|---|

This assessment is based on the full range of preparation and administration options described in the monograph. These may not all be applicable in some clinical situations.

### Reference

1. Toxbase. www.toxbase.org (accessed 1 May 2010).

# Sodium valproate (valproate sodium)

**100 mg/mL solution in 3-mL and 10-mL ampoules (Episenta)**
**400-mg dry powder vials with 4 mL WFI (Epilim)**

- Sodium valproate is an antiepileptic drug.
- It is used to treat all forms of epilepsy as monotherapy or as an adjunct to other antiepileptic agents.
- It is usually used parenterally in patients normally maintained on sodium valproate when the oral route is temporarily unavailable.

## Pre-treatment checks

* Do not give if there is active liver disease or family history of severe hepatic dysfunction, and in acute porphyria.
* Caution in SLE.
* Use extreme caution in pregnancy (may cause congenital malformations).

*Biochemical and other tests (not all are necessary in an emergency situation)*

FBC – ensure there is no excess potential for bleeding
LFTs

Pregnancy test – where appropriate
Renal function: U, Cr, CrCl (or eGFR)

## Dose

> For existing epilepsy patients switched from oral maintenance to parenteral dosing:
> * No adjustment of dose or frequency is necessary.

**Patients previously established on oral therapy:** doses are given by IV injection or infusion at the same dose and frequency as previous oral therapy.

**Initiation of treatment in patients temporarily unable to tolerate oral therapy:** 400–800 mg (up to 10 mg/kg) by slow IV injection, followed by intermittent IV infusion. Increase dose gradually up to a maximum of 2.5 g daily.

**Dosage in hepatic impairment**: avoid if possible.

### Intermittent intravenous infusion

*Preparation and administration*

1. If used, reconstitute dry powder vials with 3.8 mL WFI (provided) to give a solution containing 100 mg/mL (if the full 4 mL of diluent is used then the resultant solution contains 95 mg/mL).
2. Add the required dose to at least 50 mL of compatible infusion fluid (usually 100 mL NaCl 0.9%).
3. The solution should be clear and colourless. Inspect visually for particulate matter or discoloration prior to administration and discard if present.
4. Give by IV infusion over 60 minutes via volumetric infusion device at a maximum rate of 20 mg/minute.

### Intravenous injection

*Preparation and administration*

1. If used, reconstitute dry powder vials with 3.8 mL WFI (provided) to give a solution containing 100 mg/mL (if the full 4 mL of diluent is used then the resultant solution contains 95 mg/mL).
2. Withdraw the required dose. It may be further diluted with NaCl 0.9% or Gluc 5% to facilitate slow administration.
3. The solution should be clear and colourless. Inspect visually for particulate matter or discoloration prior to administration and discard if present.
4. Give by IV injection over 3–5 minutes.

| Technical information | |
| --- | --- |
| Incompatible with | No information |
| Compatible with | **Flush**: NaCl 0.9%<br>**Solutions**: NaCl 0.9%, Gluc 5%<br>**Y-site**: Ceftazidime |

*(continued)*

## Technical information (*continued*)

| | |
|---|---|
| pH | 7.6 |
| Sodium content | 0.6 mmol/100 mg |
| Storage | Store below 30°C in original packaging. Do not freeze. |
| Displacement value | 400 mg displaces approximately 0.2 mL (Epilim). |
| Stability after preparation | Use reconstituted vials immediately. From a microbiological point of view, prepared infusions should be used immediately; however, they may be stored at 2–8°C and infused (at room temperature) within 24 hours. |

## Monitoring

| Measure | Frequency | Rationale |
|---|---|---|
| Seizure frequency and severity | Throughout treatment | • Monitor for reduction in the frequency and severity to ensure therapeutic effect. |
| Bodyweight | Throughout therapy | • ↑Appetite and weight gain are common. |
| LFTs | Periodically during first 6 months | • Liver toxicity may occur during therapy, particularly during the first 6 months of therapy.<br>• Patients most at risk, e.g. those with organic brain damage or metabolic disorder, prior history of liver disease will require closer monitoring.<br>• Transient elevations often occur that do not require cessation of therapy.<br>• If prothrombin time is abnormally prolonged or if there are clinical symptoms of liver toxicity, therapy should be stopped (see below). |
| Symptoms of liver dysfunction | Throughout therapy and particularly during first 6 months | • Symptoms often occur before alterations to LFTs and include: nausea and vomiting (may be persistent), abdominal pain, ↓appetite, haematomas, epistaxis, jaundice, oedema, malaise, drowsiness, loss of seizure control.<br>• If these symptoms are present, cease therapy immediately. |
| FBC | Periodically, before surgery and if spontaneous bruising or bleeding occurs | • May cause blood dyscrasias and bone marrow suppression including thrombocytopenia, anaemia, leucopenia and pancytopenia.<br>• Withdraw therapy if spontaneous bruising or bleeding occur. |
| Plasma valproate level | If poor compliance is suspected or side-effects are a problem. If other anti-epileptics are started or stopped | • Not routinely monitored as dosage is usually established by overall situation and seizure control.<br>• Therapeutic range for plasma valproic acid levels is 40–100 mg/L (278–694 micromol/L).<br>• Sample in the middle of a dosage period.<br>• Steady state is achieved after 3 to 5 days.<br>• Free valproic acid is usually around 6–15% of the total valproic acid plasma levels. |

(continued)

## Monitoring (continued)

| Measure | Frequency | Rationale |
|---------|-----------|-----------|
| Serum amylase levels | If pancreatitis is suspected | • Pancreatitis can occur at any point of therapy although the occurrence is low.<br>• If pancreatitis is diagnosed therapy should be withdrawn.<br>• Caution: pancreatic enzymes frequently become slightly raised asymptomatically. |
| Ammonia levels | If mental confusion develops and before initiation if urea cycle abnormality is suspected | • Moderate hyperammonaemia occurs frequently and is usually transient. There is no need to stop therapy if the patient is asymptomatic.<br>• It may occur without altered liver function tests.<br>• If accompanied with vomiting, ataxia and ↑confusion therapy should be stopped. |
| Pregnancy | If pregnancy suspected | • Sodium valproate may be teratogenic; pregnancy should be discussed with a specialist. |

## Additional information

| | |
|---|---|
| Common and serious undesirable effects | *Immediate:* Rash and other hypersensitivity reactions have been reported.<br>*Injection/infusion-related:* Too rapid administration: Nausea or dizziness that usually disappears spontaneously a few minutes after injection.<br>*Other:* ↑LFTs, hyperammonaemia, thrombocytopenia, transient hair loss. Rarely severe liver damage, pancreatitis (signs: nausea, vomiting, acute abdominal pain), drowsiness, encephalopathy, ↓Na, anaemia, leucopenia, pancytopenia, toxic epidermal necrolysis, Stevens–Johnson syndrome, erythema multiforme. |
| Pharmacokinetics | Half-life is usually 8–20 hours. May be shorter if the patient is receiving multiple antiepileptics. |
| Significant interactions | • The following may ↓valproate levels or effect:<br>antidepressants-SSRIs (↓convulsive threshold), antidepressants-tricyclic (↓convulsive threshold), antidepressants-tricyclic, related (↓convulsive threshold), antipsychotics (↓convulsive threshold), mefloquine, primidone, St John's wort (avoid combination).<br>• The following may ↑valproate levels or effect (or ↑side-effects):<br>cimetidine, olanzapine (↑risk of neutropenia).<br>• Valproate may ↑levels or effect (or ↑side-effects) of primidone. |
| Action in case of overdose | Symptoms of overdose are unlikely at levels up to 5–6 times the maximum therapeutic plasma levels. If symptoms do occur, stop administration and give supportive therapy as appropriate. |
| Counselling | None specific to parenteral dosing. |

| | |
|---|---|
| Risk rating: **AMBER** | Score = 3<br>Moderate-risk product: Risk-reduction strategies are recommended. |

This assessment is based on the full range of preparation and administration options described in the monograph. These may not all be applicable in some clinical situations.

## Bibliography

SPC Epilim intravenous (accessed 2 February 2010).
SPC Episenta solution for injection (sodium valproate) (accessed 2 February 2010).

# Starch, etherified

**See products listed in Table S3 below (other products may be available)**

- Etherified starch preparations are plasma volume expanders. Most 6% solutions produce an expansion in plasma volume slightly in excess of the volume infused; the 10% solutions and HyperHAES produce an expansion of plasma volume of about 1.5 times the infused volume.
- Duration of effect is dependent on the molecular weight of the starch used; products containing higher-molecular-weight starches are generally retained in the plasma for longer.
- The etherified starches are used in the initial short-term management of hypovolaemic shock caused by conditions such as burns, septicaemia, haemorrhage, acute trauma or surgery. They are not a substitute for whole blood or plasma and have no oxygen-carrying capacity; blood products should be given as soon as available if appropriate.

## Pre-treatment checks

- Do not give to patients likely to develop circulatory overload, e.g. congestive cardiac failure, renal failure and pulmonary oedema, patients with intracranial bleeds or those undergoing dialysis.
- Caution if at risk of liver disease and bleeding disorders.
- Dehydration should be corrected prior to or during treatment.
- In metabolic alkalosis and clinical situations where alkalisation should be avoided, saline-based solutions should be preferred over those containing alkalising agents.

*Biochemical tests (not all are necessary in an emergency situation)*

Electrolytes: Na
FBC
Renal function: U, Cr, CrCl (or eGFR)

## Dose

**Hypovolaemic shock by IV infusion:** the volume given and rate of infusion will depend on the condition of the patient. Prolonged infusion should be avoided where possible because of the risk of depletion of plasma proteins, electrolytes and coagulation factors.

- Hetastarch 6%: 500–1000 mL, usual daily maximum 1500 mL.
- Pentastarch 6%: up to 2500 mL daily.
- Pentastarch 10%: up to 1500 mL daily; maximum suggested rate 20 mL/kg/hour.
- Tetrastarch 6%: up to 50 mL/kg daily.
- Tetrastarch 10%: up to 30 mL/kg daily.

**Hypovolaemic shock by rapid IV infusion (HyperHAES):** 4 mL/kg (or 250 mL for a 60–70 kg patient) as a single dose over 2–5 minutes. Repeated infusions are not recommended. Follow immediately by the administration of appropriate isotonic replacement fluids, dosed according to the needs of the patient.

## Intravenous infusion (not HyperHAES)

*Preparation and administration*

1. The infusion is pre-prepared for use. It should be clear and colourless to pale yellow. Inspect visually for particulate matter or discoloration prior to administration and discard if present.
2. Give by IV infusion at the required rate. Some manufacturers recommend that owing to the risk of anaphylaxis, the first 10–20 mL should be given slowly and the patient observed closely.
3. Discard any unused portion. Do not reconnect partially used infusion containers.

## Intravenous infusion (HyperHAES only)

*Preparation and administration*

Administration via a central line is preferable but a peripheral line may be used.

1. The infusion is pre-prepared for use. It should be clear to slightly opalescent, colourless to slightly yellow. Inspect visually for particulate matter or discoloration prior to administration and discard if present.
2. Give the required dose by rapid IV infusion over 2–5 minutes; pressure may be applied to the container to hasten administration.
3. Discard any unused portion. Do not reconnect partially used infusion containers.
4. Follow immediately by the administration of appropriate isotonic replacement fluids.

| Technical information | |
|---|---|
| Incompatible with | No information |
| Compatible with | **Flush**: NaCl 0.9%<br>**Solutions**: Not relevant<br>**Y-site**: Not relevant |
| pH | See Table S3 below. |
| Electrolyte content | See Table S3 below. |
| Osmolarity (plasma osmolality = 280–300 mOsmol/L)[1] | HyperHAES ≅ 2464 mOsmol/L.<br>Administration via a central line is preferable but a peripheral line may be used. |
| Storage | Store below 25°C. Do not freeze.<br>(HyperHAES no special precautions for storage.) |

| Monitoring | | |
|---|---|---|
| **Measure** | **Frequency** | **Rationale** |
| U&Es, renal function and acid–base balance. | Prior to and during treatment | • All aspects of fluid and volume replacement need to be taken into account.<br>• Dehydration should be corrected prior to or during treatment and adequate amounts of fluid provided daily.<br>• Close monitoring is required at all times as the patient's condition is likely to be unstable. |

*(continued)*

## Monitoring (continued)

| Measure | Frequency | Rationale |
|---|---|---|
| FBC and coagulation screen | Prior to and during treatment | • Adequate haematocrit should be maintained and not allowed to fall below 25-30%, early signs of bleeding complications should be observed for.<br>• Dilutional effects upon coagulation should be avoided.<br>• Coagulation factor deficiencies should be corrected. |
| Urine output | | • Monitor for oliguria or renal failure. |
| Signs of anaphylaxis | During treatment | • Severe anaphylaxis has occurred. |
| CVP (and signs of circulatory overload) | | • Monitoring of CVP during the initial period of infusion will aid the detection of fluid overload. |
| Serum osmolality | | • Particularly with hypertonic solutions and in diabetic patients. |
| Haemorrhage | | • ↑Risk with aggressive fluid resuscitation and ↑perfusion pressures. |

## Additional information

| | |
|---|---|
| Common and serious undesirable effects | *Immediate:* Anaphylactoid and other hypersensitivity reactions have been reported.<br>*Common:* Pruritus with prolonged administration - may not occur until weeks after the last infusion and may persist for several months. ↑Serum amylase: dose dependent, lasts for 3-5 days after administration. Dilutional effects: may result in a dilution of blood components and ↓haematocrit.<br>*Hypertonic solutions:* ↑Na, ↑Cl. If given to patients without marked hypovolaemic shock: ↓BP, LVF, arrhythmias, pulmonary hypertension. |
| Elimination half-life | Hydroxyethyl starch: approximately 4 hours (HyperHAES).<br>Tetrastarch: approximately 12 hours (Volulyte/Voluven). |
| Significant drug interactions | • Etherified starches may ↑levels or effect (or ↑side-effects) of heparins (may extend bleeding time).<br>• Etherified starches may affect the following tests:<br>  ↑amylase levels for 3-5 days after administration (limits use in diagnosis of pancreatitis). |
| Overdose | *Symptoms to watch for:* Circulatory overload and electrolyte imbalance.<br>*Antidote:* Stop administration and give supportive therapy as appropriate. |

| Risk rating: **GREEN** | Score = 2<br>Lower-risk product: Risk-reduction strategies should be considered. |
|---|---|

This assessment is based on the full range of preparation and administration options described in the monograph. These may not all be applicable in some clinical situations.

**Table S3** Further technical information of some etherified starch-containing fluids

| | Hetastarch | Pentastarch | | | Tetrastarch | | | Hypertonic |
|---|---|---|---|---|---|---|---|---|
| **Brand:** | Generic | HAES-steril | Hemohes | Hemohes | Venofundin | Volulyte | Voluven | HyperHAES |
| **Percentage:** | 6% | 10% | 6% | 10% | 6% | 6% | 6% | 6% |
| **Volume:** | 500 mL | 500 mL | 500 mL | 500 mL | 500 mL | 500 mL | 500 mL | 250 mL |
| Na (mmol) | 75 | 75 | 75 | 75 | 75 | 68.5 | 75 | 300 |
| K (mmol) | – | – | – | – | – | 2 | – | – |
| Mg (mmol) | – | – | – | – | – | 0.75 | – | – |
| Cl (mmol) | 75 | 75 | 75 | 75 | 75 | 55 | 75 | 300 |
| Acetate (mmol) | – | – | – | – | – | 17 | – | – |
| pH | 3.5–7 | 3.5–6 | | | | 5.7–6.5 | 4–5.5 | 3.5–5 |
| Mol. wt (ave) | 450 000 | 200 000 | 200 000 | 200 000 | 130 000 | 130 000 | 130 000 | 200 000 |

## Reference

1. Longmore M *et al.*, eds. *Oxford Handbook of Clinical Medicine*, 6th edn. Oxford: Oxford University Press, 2004.

## Bibliography

SPC HAES-steril 10%. www.fresenius-kabi.com (accessed 31 March 2010).
SPC Volulyte 6%. www.fresenius-kabi.com (accessed 31 March 2010).
SPC HyperHAES. www.fresenius-kabi.com (accessed 31 March 2010).

# Streptokinase

**250 000-unit dry powder vials; 750 000-unit dry powder vials; 1.5 million-unit dry powder vials**

* Streptokinase is a plasminogen activator derived from beta-haemolytic streptococci. It has thrombolytic activity.
* It is licensed for the dissolution of clots in MI, acute massive PE, peripheral arterial thromboembolism, and central retinal venous or arterial thrombosis.
* It may also be used to clear cannulas and shunts, and may be given intrapleurally as adjunct in empyema (all unlicensed).

## Pre-treatment checks

Streptokinase is contraindicated in the following:

* Existing or recent internal haemorrhages, all forms of ↓blood coagulability, in particular spontaneous fibrinolysis and extensive clotting disorders.
* Recent cerebrovascular insults, intracranial or intraspinal surgery, recent head trauma.
* Intracranial neoplasm, known neoplasm with risk of haemorrhage.
* Arteriovenous malformation or aneurysm.
* Acute pancreatitis, severe liver or kidney damage.
* Uncontrollable ↑BP with systolic values >200 mmHg and/or diastolic values >100 mmHg or hypertensive retinal changes grades III/IV.
* Recent implantation of vessel prosthesis.
* Simultaneous treatment with oral anticoagulants (INR > 1.3).
* Endocarditis or pericarditis.
* Known haemorrhagic diathesis.
* Recent major operations (6th to 10th postoperative day, depending on the severity of surgical intervention), invasive operations, e.g. recent organ biopsy, long-term (traumatic) closed-chest cardiac massage.
* *Caution:* repeat dosing may not be effective >4 days after initial exposure, with ↑risk of hypersensitivity reactions after this time owing to the formation of anti-streptokinase antibodies. Use of an alternative non-antigenic thrombolytic is recommended for repeat thrombolysis after this time.

*Biochemical and other tests (not all are necessary in an emergency situation)*

Blood pressure
LFTs
Renal function: U, Cr, CrCl (or eGFR)

Thrombin time (TT), activated partial thromboplastin time (APTT), haematocrit and platelet count (before commencing thrombolytic therapy).

## Dose

Streptokinase is antigenic and allergic reactions are common. Consider prophylactic administration of parenteral corticosteroid when used systemically.

**Myocardial infarction (initiated within 12 hours of symptom onset):** 1.5 million units by IV infusion over 60 minutes.

**DVT, PE, acute arterial thromboembolism, central retinal venous/arterial thrombosis:** 250 000 units by IV infusion over 30 minutes, followed by a maintenance dose 100 000 units/hour by IV infusion for 12–72 hours according to condition and response (12 hours is usually adequate for retinal thrombus). This may be followed with heparin by IV infusion, oral anticoagulants or platelet deaggregants as appropriate.

For other regimens, see product literature.

**Cannula occlusion (unlicensed):** 250 000 units (see below for method).

NB: Urokinase is licensed for this indication (see the Urokinase monograph).

**Clearance of thoracic empyema and pleural effusion (unlicensed):** 250 000 units intrapleurally as a single dose or once or twice daily for 3–5 days.[1]

## Intravenous infusion

*Preparation and administration*

1. Check that you have selected the correct strength of vial.
2. Reconstitute the vial with 5 mL NaCl 0.9%, directing the solvent against the sides of the vial rather than directly into the drug powder to minimise frothing.
3. Roll and tilt the vial gently to dissolve the powder. Do not shake (to avoid foam formation).
4. The solution produced contains:
   300 000 units/mL (1.5 million-unit vial)
   150 000 units/mL (750 000-unit vial)
   50 000 units/mL (250 000-unit vial).
5. Withdraw the required dose and add to a suitable volume of NaCl 0.9% (usually 100 mL) or make up to a suitable volume in a syringe pump. Mix well.
6. The solution should be clear and colourless. Inspect visually for particulate matter or discoloration prior to administration and discard if present.
7. Give by IV infusion via a volumetric infusion device or syringe pump at a rate appropriate to the indication. Do not use a drop-counting infusion device because streptokinase affects drop size.

## Clearance of occluded intravenous cannulas (unlicensed)

*Preparation and administration*

1. Add 2 mL NaCl 0.9% to a 250 000-unit vial, directing the solvent against the sides of the vial rather than directly into the drug powder to minimise frothing.
2. Roll and tilt the vial gently to dissolve the powder. Do not shake (to avoid foam formation).
3. Infuse the 2 mL dose over 25–35 minutes directly into the cannula, clamp for 2 hours, then aspirate and flush with NaCl 0.9%.

## Intrapleural administration (unlicensed)

*Preparation and administration*

1. Add 5 mL NaCl 0.9% to a 250 000-unit vial, directing the solvent against the sides of the vial rather than directly into the drug powder to minimise frothing.
2. Roll and tilt the vial gently to dissolve the powder. Do not shake (to avoid foam formation).
3. Withdraw 250 000 units and make up to 50 mL with NaCl 0.9% in a 50-mL syringe.
4. Introduce into the intrapleural space via an intercostal tube.
5. Clamp and release after 2–4 hours.
6. The patient should be given a streptokinase exposure card.

## Technical information

| | |
|---|---|
| Incompatible with | Bivalirudin |
| Compatible with | **Flush**: NaCl 0.9%<br>**Solutions**: NaCl 0.9% (preferred), Gluc 5%, Hartmann's<br>**Y-site**: Dobutamine, dopamine, glyceryl trinitrate, lidocaine |
| pH | 6.8–7.5 |
| Sodium content | Negligible |
| Storage | Store below 25 °C in original packaging. Do not freeze. |
| Displacement value | Negligible |
| Stability after preparation | From a microbiological point of view, should be used immediately, however, prepared infusions may be stored at 2–8°C and infused (at room temperature) within 24 hours. |

## Monitoring

| Measure | Frequency | Rationale |
|---|---|---|
| *In treatment of myocardial infarction* | | |
| Blood pressure | Continuously | • ↓BP – raise the legs and slow or stop infusion temporarily. |
| Heart rate | | • ↓Pulse may result from reperfusion. |
| ECG | | • Arrhythmias may result from reperfusion. |
| *In treatment of venous and arterial thromboses* | | |
| Thrombin clotting time | 4 hours after initiation then periodically | • Maintain the thrombin clotting time at a 2- to 4-fold increase above baseline for therapeutic effect.<br>• If the TT or any other parameter of lysis, after 4 hours of therapy, is <1.5 times the baseline discontinue therapy as excessive resistance to streptokinase is present. |

## Additional information

| | |
|---|---|
| Common and serious undesirable effects | *Immediate:* Anaphylaxis and other hypersensitivity reactions (rash, flushing, itching, urticaria, angioedema, dyspnoea, bronchospasm, ↓BP). Corticosteroids may be given prophylactically to ↓likelihood.<br>*Infusion-related:*<br>• Too rapid administration: ↓BP, ↑ or ↓pulse.<br>• Local: Haemorrhage at injection site.<br>*Other:* Bleeding from any site, development of anti-streptokinase antibodies, coronary artery reperfusion events, e.g. rhythm disorders, nausea, diarrhoea, epigastric pain, vomiting, headache, back pain, muscle pain, chills, fever, asthenia, malaise, transient ↑serum transaminases and bilirubin. |

*(continued)*

## Additional information (*continued*)

| | |
|---|---|
| Pharmacokinetics | Streptokinase is very rapidly eliminated where anti-streptokinase antibodies are present in the blood.<br>The elimination half-life of streptokinase based on activator formation is about 80 minutes. |
| Significant interactions | • The following may ↑risk of haemorrhage with streptokinase:<br>anticoagulants, heparins, antiplatelet agents, e.g. aspirin, clopidogrel, dipyridamole. |
| Action in case of overdose | *Symptoms to watch for:* Severe bleeding.<br>*Antidote:* No specific antidote. Stop administration and give supportive therapy as appropriate including fresh frozen plasma, fresh blood and tranexamic acid if necessary. Prolonged overdose may ↑risk of thrombosis due to ↓plasminogen. |
| Counselling | Report bleeding events and symptoms of allergic/anaphylactic reaction.<br>Advise on avoidance of repeat dosing due to antibodies. |

Risk rating: **AMBER**  Score = 4
Moderate-risk product: Risk-reduction strategies are recommended.

This assessment is based on the full range of preparation and administration options described in the monograph. These may not all be applicable in some clinical situations.

### Reference

1. Davies RJO, Gleeson FV. Introduction to the methods used in the generation of the British Thoracic Society guidelines for the management of pleural disease. *Thorax* 2003; 58(Suppl. II): ii1–ii7.

### Bibliography

SPC Streptase 1,500 000 IU, CSL Behring UK Ltd (accessed 31 March 2010)
SPC Streptase 250 000 IU and 750 000 IU, CSL Behring UK Ltd (accessed 31 March 2010).

# Streptomycin

**1-g dry powder vials**

- Streptomycin sulfate is an aminoglycoside antibacterial.
- It may be used with other antimycobacterials in the initial phase of treatment of tuberculosis.
- It may also be effective in the treatment of plague, tularaemia and, with a tetracycline, in brucellosis.
- Doses are expressed in terms of the base:
  Streptomycin 1 g ≡ 1.25 g streptomycin sulfate.

## Pre-treatment checks

- Do not give in myasthenia gravis.
- Ensure good hydration status (dehydration ↑risk of toxicity).

*Biochemical and other tests*

| | |
|---|---|
| Baseline check of auditory (audiogram) and vestibular function | Electrolytes: serum K, Ca, Mg |
| | FBC |
| Bodyweight | Renal function: U, Cr, CrCl (or eGFR) |

In the USA, Romberg testing of neurological function is also recommended.[1]

## Dose

**Tuberculosis (>50 kg and <40 years):** 15 mg/kg daily by IM injection (maximum of 1 g daily).
**Tuberculosis (<50 kg or >40 years):** 10 mg/kg daily by IM injection (maximum 750 mg daily).
**Other infections**: seek specialist advice.
**Dose in renal impairment:** adjusted according to creatinine clearance:[2]

- CrCl >20–50 mL/minute: give every 24–72 hours; dose according to levels.
- CrCl 10–20 mL/minute: give every 24–72 hours; dose according to levels.
- CrCl <10 mL/minute: give every 72–96 hours; dose according to levels.

## Intramuscular injection

See Special handling below.

*Preparation and administration*

1. Determine the required dose then reconstitute each vial with WFI to produce a suitable concentration of streptomycin, i.e.:

| Volume of WFI added | 4.2 mL | 3.2 mL | 1.8 mL |
|---|---|---|---|
| Approximate concentration of streptomycin | 200 mg/mL | 250 mg/mL | 400 mg/mL |

2. Withdraw the required dose.
3. Give by deep IM injection into a large muscle mass, preferably the upper outer quadrant of the buttock or the mid-lateral thigh (in children use mid-lateral thigh). Do not inject into the lower or mid-third of the upper arm. Rotate injection sites for subsequent injections.

## Technical information

| | |
|---|---|
| Incompatible with | Not relevant |
| Compatible with | **Solutions**: WFI |
| pH | 4.5–7 |
| Sodium content | Nil |
| Storage | Store below 30°C in original packaging. |

*(continued)*

## Technical information (*continued*)

| | |
|---|---|
| Displacement value | Approximately 0.8 mL/1 g |
| Special handling | May cause severe dermatitis in sensitised persons. Anyone who handles streptomycin frequently should wear masks and rubber gloves. |
| Stability after preparation | From a microbiological point of view, should be used immediately; however, reconstituted vials are stable at room temperature for 24 hours. |

## Monitoring

| Measure | Frequency | Rationale |
|---|---|---|
| Vestibular and auditory function | Daily | • Check that there is no deterioration of balance or hearing – may indicate toxic levels.<br>• Ototoxicity is a potential effect of overexposure to streptomycin and is more common than vestibular disturbances.<br>• An audiogram and vestibular testing should be repeated if there are symptoms of eighth nerve toxicity. |
| Renal function and electrolytes | Weekly initially | • ↑CrCl (or eGFR) may indicate nephrotoxicity and a dose adjustment may be necessary.<br>• ↓Ca, ↓Mg, and ↓K have been reported – levels need checking periodically. Imbalances should be corrected as required. |
| Streptomycin plasma concentration | Every 4 weeks in normal renal function; more frequently if renal function is impaired | • A trough level is taken just before the dose and should be <5 mg/L (<1 mg/L in renal impairment or in those over 50 years).<br>• A peak level is taken 1 hour after the dose has been given and should be 15-40 mg/L.<br>• For meaningful interpretation of results the laboratory request form must state the time the previous dose was given and the time the blood sample was taken. |
| FBC | Periodically | • Eosinophilia occasionally occurs. |

## Additional information

| | |
|---|---|
| Common and serious undesirable effects | Paraesthesia in and around the mouth. Less commonly neurological symptoms (including peripheral neuropathies, optic neuritis and scotoma), hypersensitivity skin reactions, nephrotoxicity. |
| Pharmacokinetics | Elimination half-life is 2.5 hours in normal renal function, but may be up to 100 hours in severe renal impairment. |
| Significant interactions | • Streptomycin may ↑risk of nephrotoxicity with the following drugs: ciclosporin, platinum compounds, tacrolimus.<br>• Streptomycin may ↑levels or effect of the following drugs (or ↑side-effects): diuretics-loop (↑risk of ototoxicity), muscle relaxants-non depolarising, suxamethonium.<br>• Streptomycin may ↓levels or effect of the following drugs: neostigmine, pyridostigmine. |
| Overdose | Antidote. IV calcium salts have been used to reverse neuromuscular blockade. Haemodialysis can aid removal from the blood. |
| Counselling | The patient should report in loss of hearing or problems with their balance. |

Risk rating: **AMBER**

Score = 3
Moderate-risk product: Risk-reduction strategies are recommended.

This assessment is based on the full range of preparation and administration options described in the monograph. These may not all be applicable in some clinical situations.

## References

1. American Thoracic Society, CDC, and Infectious Diseases Society of America (2003). *Morbidity and Mortality* Weekly Report Vol. 52(RR-11) Treatment of Tuberculosis. www.cdc.gov/mmwr/PDF/rr/rr5211.pdf (accessed 16 February 2009).
2. Ashley C, Currie A, eds. *The Renal Drug Handbook*, 3rd edn. Oxford: Radcliffe Medical Press, 2009.

# Sumatriptan

**12 mg/mL solution in 0.5-mL prefilled syringe and auto-injector; 12 mg/mL solution in 0.5-mL cartridges**

* Sumatriptan succinate is a $5HT_1$ agonist that causes vasoconstriction of cranial arteries.
* It is used as monotherapy for acute migraine, with or without aura, and for cluster headaches.
* Overusage of sumatriptan can lead to an exacerbation of symptoms.

## Pre-treatment checks

* Do not give if previous CVA or TIA; peripheral vascular disease; moderate and severe ↑BP, in ischaemic heart disease, previous myocardial infarction, coronary vasospasm (including Prinzmetal's angina).
* If cardiovascular disease is present, consider giving the first dose under medical supervision (possibly with ECG monitoring after administration as asymptomatic cardiac ischaemia can occur).
* Caution if there is a history of seizures or sensitivity to sulfonamides.
* Not recommended in elderly patients (>65).

*Biochemical tests*

LFTs – avoid in severe impairment
Renal function–use with caution (renally excreted)

## Dose

**Migraine and cluster headache:** 6 mg by SC injection as soon as possible after onset of headache symptoms; if symptoms recur, the dose may be repeated after at least 1 hour (maximum 12 mg in 24 hours). If no response is seen to the initial dose, a second dose should not be used for the same attack.

## Subcutaneous injection

*Preparation*

1. Open the case; break the red seal over one of the cartridges and open lid.
2. Remove the auto-injector pen – if the white rod is sticking out from the end of the pen, replace the pen and push firmly then remove the pen from the case.
3. Push the pen into the cartridge pack and turn clockwise as far as it will turn (approximately half a turn).
4. Pull the pen with the cartridge attached from the case – it may be necessary to pull quite hard.
5. Do not return the pen to the case until the dose has been administered, to avoid needle damage.

*Administration*

1. Place the blue end of the pen over a clean area of skin that has sufficient SC tissue to accommodate the needle, i.e. 5–6 mm (usually the outer thigh). Avoid inadvertent IV administration (can cause vasospasm resulting in arrhythmias, ECG changes or MI).
2. Press the pen firmly so that the grey part of the pen moves over the blue part to cover it – the safety catch has now been released.
3. Press the blue button on top of the pen to release the drug – count to 10 (slowly) holding the pen very still and secure. Removing the pen too soon will result in the dose being wasted.
4. Remove the pen, avoiding touching the needle.
5. Push the pen back into the cartridge slot and unscrew the pen by turning it anticlockwise and remove the pen.
6. Close the blue lid over the used cartridge and return the pen to the carry-case slot.

## Technical information

| | |
|---|---|
| Incompatible with | Not relevant |
| Compatible with | Not relevant |
| pH | 4.2–5.3 |
| Sodium content | Negligible |
| Storage | Store below 30°C in original packaging. |

## Monitoring

| Measure | Frequency | Rationale |
|---|---|---|
| Signs of intense chest/throat pain or tightness | Throughout therapy | • Discontinue treatment if these occur. |
| Injection site | Periodically | • Sumatriptan can cause erythema at the injection site. |

## Additional information

| | |
|---|---|
| Common and serious undesirable effects | *Immediate:* Anaphylaxis and other hypersensitivity reactions have been reported<br>*Injection-related:* Local: pain, stinging, burning, swelling, erythema, bruising and bleeding.<br>*Other:* Dizziness, drowsiness, flushing, nausea, vomiting, sensory disturbances, transient ↑BP, tightness (in any part of the body including the chest and throat – usually transient but may be intense), ↑ or ↓pulse, Raynaud's syndrome, ↑LFTs. |
| Pharmacokinetics | Half-life is about 2 hours. A clinical response is usually seen within 10–15 minutes of injection. |
| Significant interactions | • ↑Risk of vasospasm when sumatriptan given with the following drugs: ergotamine, methysergide (avoid for 6 hours after sumatriptan, avoid sumatriptan for 24 hours after these drugs).<br>• ↑Risk of CNS toxicity when sumatriptan given with the following drugs: citalopram, escitalopram, fluoxetine, fluvoxamine, MAOIs (avoid sumatriptan for 2 weeks after MAOIs), moclobemide (avoid sumatriptan for 2 weeks after moclobemide), paroxetine, sertraline (avoid combination), St John's wort (↑risk of serotonergic effects, avoid combination). |
| Action in case of overdose | Monitor the patient for at least 10 hours. Give supportive therapy as appropriate. |
| Counselling | Do not use prophylactically.<br>A second dose should not be administered if your headache does not go away after the first dose. If, however, your headache goes away and then returns, a second dose may be administered at least 1 hour after the first dose.<br>Do not use more than two doses (12 mg) in 24 hours.<br>Use of the auto-injector device and safe needles disposal. Counsel the patient to use an injection site with adequate skin and SC thickness, as the needle will penetrate up to 6 mm, and to rotate injection site.<br>Sumatriptan can cause drowsiness do not drive if affected. |

| Risk rating: **GREEN** | Score = 0<br>Lower-risk product: Risk-reduction strategies should be considered. |
| --- | --- |

This assessment is based on the full range of preparation and administration options described in the monograph. These may not all be applicable in some clinical situations.

## Bibliography

SPC Imigran injection, Subject, GlaxoSmithKline UK (accessed 21 April 2008).

# Tacrolimus

**5 mg/mL solution in ampoules**

- Tacrolimus is a potent macrolide immunosuppressant derived from *Streptomyces tsukubaensis* with actions similar to ciclosporin.
- It is used to prevent or manage organ rejection in transplant patients, but it is also licensed in some countries for use in treatment resistant myasthenia gravis, rheumatoid arthritis and Crohn disease.

## Pre-treatment checks

Do not give if there is hypersensitivity to tacrolimus, macrolides or polyethoxylated castor oils, and in pregnancy and breast feeding.

*Biochemical and other tests*

Blood glucose

ECG

Electrolytes: serum K, Na, Mg, Ca, $PO_4$

FBC

LFTs (in severe hepatic impairment (Child–Pugh score of 10 or higher) lower doses may be required)

Neurological and visual status

Renal function: U, Cr

## Dose

> IV administration carries a risk of anaphylaxis and should be reserved for patients who cannot tolerate the oral route. Tacrolimus should be given IV for no more than 7 days.
> In transplant patients it is crucial to seek specialist advice on any route or dose adjustments.

**Prophylaxis of liver transplant rejection starting 12 hours after transplantation:** initially 10–50 micrograms/kg daily by continuous IV infusion over 24 hours for a maximum of 7 days. Adjust dose according to response and blood level monitoring. Change to oral therapy (via NG tube if necessary) as soon as the enteral route becomes available.

**Prophylaxis of kidney transplant rejection starting within 24 hours of transplantation:** initially 50–100 micrograms/kg daily by continuous IV infusion over 24 hours for a maximum of 7 days. Adjust dose according to response and blood level monitoring. Change to oral therapy (via NG tube if necessary) as soon as the enteral route becomes available.

**Prophylaxis of heart transplant rejection (with or without antibody induction) starting within 5 days of transplantation:** 10–20 micrograms/kg daily by continuous IV infusion over 24 hours for a maximum of 7 days. Adjust dose according to response and blood level monitoring. Change to oral therapy (via NG tube if necessary) as soon as the enteral route becomes available.

**Rejection therapy:** seek specialist advice.

**Dose in renal impairment:** no adjustment is required for patients with impaired renal function; however, tacrolimus is nephrotoxic so monitoring of renal function is required.

**Dose in hepatic impairment:** in severe liver impairment keep blood trough levels within the recommended range.

## Continuous intravenous infusion

*Preparation and administration*

Tacrolimus must never be given undiluted and must always be given by continuous infusion. PVC containers and giving sets should not be used.

1. Withdraw the required dose and add to a suitable volume of NaCl 0.9% or Gluc 5% to give a solution containing 4–100 micrograms/mL (the total volume of infusion over a 24-hour period should be in the range 20–500 mL). Mix well.
2. The solution should be clear and colourless. Inspect visually for particulate matter or discoloration prior to administration and discard if present.
3. Give by IV infusion over 24 hours. Observe continuously for at least the first 30 minutes following initiation of the infusion and at frequent intervals for possible allergic reactions.

## Technical information

| | |
|---|---|
| Incompatible with | PVC containers and giving sets should not be used.<br>Aciclovir, ganciclovir. |
| Compatible with | **Flush**: NaCl 0.9%<br>**Solutions**: NaCl 0.9%, Gluc 5%<br>**Y-site**: No information but likely to be unstable |
| pH | 6.33 when diluted to 10 micrograms/mL in NaCl 0.9%[1] |
| Sodium content | Nil |
| Excipients | Contains ethanol (may interact with metronidazole, possible religious objections).<br>Contains polyoxyl castor oils (have been associated with severe anaphylactic reactions). |
| Storage | Store below 25°C in original packaging. |
| Stability after preparation | Use prepared infusions immediately. |

## Monitoring

| Measure | Frequency | Rationale |
|---|---|---|
| Tacrolimus blood concentration | Twice weekly in early post-transplantation period, then periodically or clinically indicated, e.g. during episodes of diarrhoea | • Also monitor: after dose adjustment, changes in the immunosuppressive regimen, and following co-administration of substances that may alter the tacrolimus level.<br>• Desired levels in transplant recipients are:<br>5-20 nanograms/mL in liver transplant recipients in the early post-transplantation period;<br>10-20 nanograms/mL in kidney and heart transplant recipients in the early post-transplantation period;<br>5-15 nanograms/mL in liver, kidney and heart transplant recipients during maintenance therapy. |

*(continued)*

## Monitoring (continued)

| Measure | Frequency | Rationale |
|---|---|---|
| Blood pressure and pulse | Regularly | • ↑BP and ↑pulse commonly occur – treat as appropriate. |
| Neurological and visual status | | • Neurotoxicity is possible especially at high doses. |
| Fasting blood glucose | | • Causes hyperglycaemia in almost half of patients (peripheral insulin resistance may also occur).<br>• Insulin therapy may be required. |
| U&Es + creatinine | | • ↑K may occur and usually responds to a dose reduction, or by using a polystyrene sulfonate resin or fludrocortisone (useful as ↓Na may also occur).<br>• Avoid high potassium intake and drugs that may cause ↑K.<br>• ↓K may also occur.<br>• Dose adjustment may be necessary if urea or creatinine rise and a switch to another immunosuppressant may be considered if the patient is unresponsive to a lower dose. |
| LFTs | | • Hepatic enzyme abnormalities, cholestasis and jaundice commonly occur. |
| FBC | | • Can cause RBC, WBC and platelet anomalies. |
| ECG | If clinically warranted | • May prolong QT interval.<br>• Consider echocardiography if there are clinical manifestations of ventricular dysfunction (myocardial hypertrophy). |
| Coagulation screen | | • Haemorrhage and coagulation disorders have been reported. |
| Albumin | | • Highly protein-bound drug: changes in albumin will affect the concentration of the unbound drug. |
| Symptoms of infection | | • Immunosuppression predisposes patients to infection. |
| Magnesium, calcium, phosphate | | • Can cause ↓Mg, ↓$PO_4$, ↓Ca. |
| Lipid profile | Occasionally | • Can ↑cholesterol and triglycerides. |

## Additional information

| | |
|---|---|
| Common and serious undesirable effects | *Immediate:* Anaphylaxis has been reported.<br>*Infusion-related:* Local: pain and discomfort.<br>*Other:* Infections, IHD, ↑pulse, ↑ or ↓BP, anaemia, thrombocytopenia, blood dyscrasias, tremor, headache, seizures, impaired consciousness, peripheral neuropathy, dizziness, blurred vision, photophobia, tinnitus, dyspnoea, pleural effusion, cough, nasal congestion, diarrhoea, nausea, stomatitis, GI ulceration, constipation, renal impairment, pruritus, rash, alopecia, acne, ↑sweating, muscle cramps, ↑blood glucose, ↑ or ↓K, ↓Mg, ↓PO$_4$, ↓Ca, ↓Na, hyperlipidaemia, altered LFTs, insomnia, anxiety |
| Pharmacokinetics | Elimination half-life is 43 hours (healthy adult); 11.7 hours (liver transplant); 15.6 hours (kidney transplant). |
| Significant interactions | • The following may ↑tacrolimus levels or effect (or ↑side-effects): atazanavir, chloramphenicol (systemic), clarithromycin, diltiazem, efavirenz, erythromycin, fluconazole, grapefruit juice, itraconazole, ketoconazole, nelfinavir, nifedipine, posaconazole (↓tacrolimus dose), quinupristin with dalfopristin, ritonavir, saquinavir (↓tacrolimus dose), telithromycin, voriconazole.<br>• The following may ↓tacrolimus levels or effect: caspofungin, phenobarbital, rifampicin, St John's wort (avoid combination).<br>• Tacrolimus may ↑levels or effect of the following drugs (or ↑side-effects): ciclosporin (avoid combination; allow 24-hour wash out if switching), droperidol (↑risk arrhythmias).<br>• Tacrolimus may ↑risk of nephrotoxicity with the following: amikacin, amphotericin, gentamicin, ibuprofen, tobramycin.<br>• Tacrolimus may ↑risk of ↑K with the following: amiloride, eplerenone, potassium salts, spironolactone, triamterene.<br>• Injectable preparation contains ethanol: may interact with disulfiram and metronidazole. |
| Action in case of overdose | No known antidote; stop administration and give supportive therapy as appropriate. Tacrolimus is not dialysable. Haemofiltration or haemodiafiltration may be effective at reducing toxic concentrations. |
| Counselling | Limit exposure to sunlight and UV light by wearing protective clothing and use sunscreen with a high protection factor.<br>If contraception is needed non-hormonal methods should be used.<br>Contact doctor if frequent urination or ↑thirst or hunger develops. |

| | |
|---|---|
| Risk rating: **AMBER** | Score = 5<br>Moderate-risk product: Risk-reduction strategies are recommended. |

This assessment is based on the full range of preparation and administration options described in the monograph. These may not all be applicable in some clinical situations.

## Reference

1. Correspondence with Astellas Pharma Ltd, 24 February 2009.

## Bibliography

SPC Prograf 5 mg/mL concentrate for solution for infusion (accessed 3 April 2009).

# Talc, sterile

#### 4-g and 5-g powder (other sizes may be available); 4-g Steritalc PF Puffer

- Sterile talc is an unlicensed product.
- It may be used as a sclerosant for pleurodesis in the management of malignant pleural effusions.[1]

## Pre-treatment checks

- An intercostal tube is inserted and the pleural effusion is drained.
- Administration of an anxiolytic should be considered prior to commencing pleurodesis.
- Lidocaine (3 mg/kg up to a maximum of 250 mg) has been given intrapleurally just prior to sclerosant administration.[1]

*Biochemical and other tests*

Chest X-ray: to ensure complete lung expansion and to confirm the position of the tube.

## Dose

**Standard dose:** 2–5 g of sterile talc is made into slurry and administered into the pleural space (doses used have ranged from 1 to 10 g).

If using the Steritalc puffer, a dose of 4 g can be administered directly into the pleural cavity.

## Intrapleural – slurry

*Preparation and administration*

1. Mix the required dose of sterile talc with 30 mL WFI using a bladder syringe.
2. Instil via the intercostal tube.
3. Clamp the tube for 1 hour and consider patient rotation to allow dispersion of the talc.
4. Release the clamp and drain the fluid off.

## Intrapleural – insufflation (Steritalc PF Puffer)

*Preparation and administration[2]*

1. Fix the silicone connector (included) onto the internal nozzle of the puffer.
2. Screw the male Luer-Lok connector to its maximum on the cannula while firmly holding it.
3. Hold the cannula and the puffer together and press smoothly several times on the puffer to spray Steritalc homogeneously into the pleural space.

## Technical information

| | |
|---|---|
| Incompatible with | Not relevant |
| Compatible with | Not relevant |
| pH | Not relevant |
| Sodium content | Nil |
| Storage | No special precautions |
| Stability after preparation | Use prepared slurry immediately. |

## Monitoring

| Measure | Frequency | Rationale |
|---|---|---|
| Position of patient | Following administration | • The patient's position should be rotated during treatment. |
| Pulmonary function | Periodically | • For signs of clinical improvement. |
| Temperature | | • Fever may occur. |

## Additional information

| | |
|---|---|
| Common and serious undesirable effects | *Common:* Chest pain, mild fever.<br>*Rare:* Respiratory distress syndrome or acute pneumonitis leading to acute respiratory failure, cardiac arrest. |
| Pharmacokinetics | Not relevant |
| Significant interactions | Not relevant |
| Action in case of overdose | Not relevant |

| | |
|---|---|
| Risk rating: **AMBER** | Score = 3<br>Moderate-risk product: Risk-reduction strategies are recommended. |

This assessment is based on the full range of preparation and administration options described in the monograph. These may not all be applicable in some clinical situations.

## Reference

1. Antunes G *et al.* BTS Guidelines for the management of pleural effusions. *Thorax.* 2003; 58 (Suppl. 11): ii29–ii38.
2. Novatech (2010). Steritalc. http://www.novatech.fr/en/pleura-concept-pulmonology-products/steritalcr.html (accessed 28 September 2010).

# Teicoplanin

**200-mg and 400-mg dry powder vials with solvent (WFI)**

* Teicoplanin is a glycopeptide antibiotic (it is a mixture of several components).
* It may be used as an alternative to vancomycin where other drugs cannot be used in the treatment of serious Gram-positive infections. These include the treatment and prophylaxis of infective endocarditis; peritonitis associated with continuous ambulatory peritoneal dialysis and suspected infection in neutropenic or otherwise immunocompromised patients.

## Pre-treatment checks

Caution in hypersensitivity to vancomycin.

*Biochemical and other tests*

FBC
LFTs
Renal function: U, Cr, CrCl (or eGFR)

## Dose

**Severe infections (joint and bone infection, septicaemia, endocarditis):** 400 mg by IV injection or infusion every 12 hours for three doses followed by 400 mg daily either by IM or IV injection or IV infusion (for patients >85 kg dose at 6 mg/kg). In some situations (e.g. severe burns, endocarditis) doses up to 12 mg/kg by IV injection or infusion have been given.

**Moderate infections (skin and soft-tissue infection, urinary tract infection, lower respiratory tract infection):** 400 mg by IM or IV injection or IV infusion on the first day followed by 200 mg daily thereafter (for patients >85 kg, dose at 3 mg/kg).

**Surgical prophylaxis:** 400 mg by IV injection as a single dose at induction of anaesthesia. Check local policies.

**Dose in renal impairment:** dose according to indication up to the fourth day of treatment then reduce the dose according to creatinine clearance:[1]

* CrCl >20–50 mL/minute: dose as in normal renal function.
* CrCl 10–20 mL/minute: give the normal loading dose then 200–400 mg every 24–48 hours.
* CrCl <10 mL/minute: give the normal loading dose then 200–400 mg every 48–72 hours.

**Peritonitis in continuous ambulatory peritoneal dialysis:** if the patient is febrile, give a 400-mg loading dose by IV injection or infusion, then 20 mg/L per bag for the first week, 20 mg/L in alternate bags for the second week and 20 mg/L in the overnight dwell bag only for a third week.

## Intravenous injection

*Preparation and administration*

1. Slowly add the entire contents of the solvent provided to the vial of teicoplanin.
2. Roll gently until the powder is completely dissolved (if the solution becomes foamy, leave it to stand for 15 minutes to settle). After reconstitution a 200-mg vial contains 200 mg/3 mL and a 400-mg vial contains 400 mg/3 mL.
3. Withdraw the required dose.
4. The solution should be clear and colourless to pale yellow. Inspect visually for particulate matter or discoloration prior to administration and discard if present.
5. Give by IV injection over 3–5 minutes.

## Intermittent intravenous infusion

*Preparation and administration*

1. Slowly add the entire contents of the solvent provided to the vial of teicoplanin.
2. Roll gently until the powder is completely dissolved (if the solution becomes foamy, leave it to stand for 15 minutes to settle). After reconstitution a 200-mg vial contains 200 mg/3 mL and a 400-mg vial contains 400 mg/3 mL.
3. Withdraw the required dose and add to a suitable volume of compatible infusion fluid (usually 100 mL NaCl 0.9% or Gluc 5%).
4. The solution should be clear and colourless to pale yellow. Inspect visually for particulate matter or discoloration prior to administration and discard if present.
5. Give by IV infusion over 30 minutes.

## Intramuscular injection

*Preparation and administration*

1. Slowly add the entire contents of the solvent provided to the vial of teicoplanin.
2. Roll gently until the powder is completely dissolved (if the solution becomes foamy, leave it to stand for 15 minutes to settle). After reconstitution a 200-mg vial contains 200 mg/3 mL and a 400-mg vial contains 400 mg/3 mL.
3. Withdraw the required dose.
4. Give by deep IM injection into a large muscle.

## Continuous ambulatory peritoneal dialysis

*Preparation and administration*

As for IM injection and add the required dose to dialysis solution.

| Technical information | |
|---|---|
| Incompatible with | Ceftazidime, ciprofloxacin, gentamicin, tobramycin. |
| Compatible with | **Flush**: NaCl 0.9%<br>**Solutions**: NaCl 0.9%, Gluc 5%, Gluc-NaCl, Hartmann's. Also peritoneal dialysis solutions containing glucose 1.36% or 3.86%<br>**Y-site**: No information |
| pH | 7.5 |
| Sodium content | Negligible |
| Storage | Store below 25°C in original packaging. |

*(continued)*

## Technical information (*continued*)

| | |
|---|---|
| Displacement value | Not relevant. Each vial contains an overage, so that when reconstituted as directed above the final solution contains: 200 mg/3 mL (200-mg vial) or 400 mg/3 mL (400-mg vial). |
| Stability after preparation | From a microbiological point of view, should be used immediately; however:<br>• Reconstituted vials may be stored at 2–8°C for 24 hours.<br>• Prepared infusions may be stored at 2–8°C and infused (at room temperature) within 24 hours. |

## Monitoring

| Measure | Frequency | Rationale |
|---|---|---|
| Physical signs of infection | Daily | • Monitor patient response for signs of infection resolution. |
| Renal function | Regularly, e.g. 2-3 times a week | • Especially in prolonged treatment in patients with renal impairment or if other potentially nephrotoxic drugs are added.<br>• Changes in renal function may require a dose adjustment. |
| Auditory function tests | | • Especially in prolonged treatment, or if other potentially neurotoxic drugs are added. |
| Signs of super-infection | Throughout treatment | • May result in overgrowth of non-susceptible organisms (especially if treatment is prolonged). |
| FBC | Periodically | • Thrombocytopenia (especially at higher doses), leucopenia, neutropenia, eosinophilia have been reported. Rarely agranulocytosis. |
| LFTs | | • Disturbances in liver enzymes occasionally occur. |
| Teicoplanin serum concentrations | Not usually considered necessary, but occasionally used to optimise therapy | • Consider monitoring in severe sepsis or burns, deep-seated staphylococcal infection (including bone and joint infection), endocarditis, renal impairment, in elderly patients, and in IV drug abusers.<br>• In severe infections, pre-dose (trough) serum concentrations should be >10 mg/L (>15–20 mg/L in endocarditis) but <60 mg/L.<br>• A relationship between serum concentration and toxicity has not been established - peak concentrations (1 hour post 400 mg IV dose) are usually in the range 20–50 mg/L. |

## Additional information

| | |
|---|---|
| Common and serious undesirable effects | *Injection/infusion-related:*<br>• Too rapid administration: Erythema or flushing of the upper body have rarely been reported but did not recur when the infusion rate was slowed and/or concentration decreased.<br>• Local: Local pain, thrombophlebitis, injection-site abscess.<br>*Other:* Nausea, vomiting, diarrhoea, rash and pruritus. |

(continued)

| **Additional information** (*continued*) | |
|---|---|
| Pharmacokinetics | Elimination half-life is 30-190 hours or more. 60 hours has been suggested for dosage calculations. |
| Significant interactions | No significant interactions. |
| Action in case of overdose | *Antidote:* No known antidote and not removed by haemodialysis. Stop administration and give supportive therapy as appropriate. |

| Risk rating: **GREEN** | Score = 2 Lower-risk product: Risk-reduction strategies should be considered. |
|---|---|

This assessment is based on the full range of preparation and administration options described in the monograph. These may not all be applicable in some clinical situations.

### Reference

1. Ashley C, Currie A, eds. *The Renal Drug Handbook*, 3rd edn. Oxford: Radcliffe Medical Press, 2009.

### Bibliography

SPC Targocid 200 mg and 400 mg (accessed 3 April 2009).

# Temocillin

### 1-g dry powder vials

- Temocillin sodium is a semisynthetic penicillin, and is resistant to a wide range of beta-lactamases.
- It is used to treat infections caused by beta-lactamase-producing strains of Gram-negative aerobic bacteria (including those resistant to third-generation cephalosporins).
- In mixed infections where Gram-positive or anaerobic bacteria are also likely it may be given with other appropriate antibacterial agents.
- Doses are expressed in terms of the base:
  Temocillin 1 g ≅ 1.11 g temocillin sodium.

### Pre-treatment checks

Check for history of allergy/hypersensitivity to penicillins and use with caution if the patient is sensitive to other beta-lactam antibiotics.

*Biochemical and other tests*

Renal function: U, Cr, CrCl (or eGFR)

## Dose

**Standard dose:** 1–2 g by IM or IV injection or IV infusion every 12 hours.
**Uncomplicated urinary tract infections:** 1 g by IM or IV injection or IV infusion every 24 hours.
**Dose in renal impairment:**

* CrCl >30–50 mL/minute: dose as in normal renal function.
* CrCl 10–30 mL/minute: 1–2 g every 24 hours.
* CrCl <10 mL/minute: 1–2 g every 48 hours.

## Intravenous injection

*Preparation and administration*

If used in combination with an aminoglycoside (e.g. amikacin, gentamicin, tobramycin), preferably administer at a different site. If this is not possible then flush the line thoroughly with a compatible solution between drugs.

1. Add 20 mL WFI to vial and shake vigorously.
2. Withdraw the required dose.
3. The solution should be clear and colourless to pale yellow. Inspect visually for particulate matter or discoloration prior to administration and discard if present.
4. Give by IV injection over 3–4 minutes.

## Intermittent intravenous infusion

*Preparation and administration*

If used in combination with an aminoglycoside (e.g. amikacin, gentamicin, tobramycin), preferably administer at a different site. If this is not possible then flush the line thoroughly with a compatible solution between drugs.

1. Add 20 mL WFI to vial and shake vigorously.
2. Withdraw the required dose and add to a suitable volume of compatible infusion fluid (usually 100 mL NaCl 0.9%).
3. The solution should be clear and colourless to pale yellow. Inspect visually for particulate matter or discoloration prior to administration and discard if present.
4. Give by IV infusion over 30–40 minutes.

## Intramuscular injection (maximum dose 1 g)

*Preparation and administration*

1. Add 2 mL WFI to vial and shake vigorously.
2. Withdraw the required dose.
3. Give by IM injection. If pain occurs, 0.5–1% lidocaine may be used for reconstitution (see the Lidocaine monograph for cautions and monitoring).

## Technical information

| Incompatible with | Amikacin, gentamicin, tobramycin. |
|---|---|
| Compatible with | **Flush**: NaCl 0.9%<br>**Solutions**: NaCl 0.9%, Gluc 5%, Hartmann's, Ringer's<br>**Y-site**: No information |

*(continued)*

## Technical information (continued)

| | |
|---|---|
| pH | 6-8.5 |
| Sodium content | 4.35 mmol/g |
| Storage | Store below 20°C in original packaging. |
| Displacement value | 0.7 mL/g |
| Stability after preparation | Use reconstituted vials and prepared infusions immediately. |

## Monitoring

| Measure | Frequency | Rationale |
|---|---|---|
| U&Es | Periodically | • ↓K sometimes occurs. Caution in patients with low K reserves or taking drugs that may exacerbate ↓K.<br>• Dose adjustment may be necessary if renal function deteriorates. |
| LFTs | | • Small elevations sometimes occur. |
| Development of diarrhoea | Throughout treatment | • Development of severe, persistent diarrhoea may be suggestive of *Clostridium difficile*-associated diarrhoea and colitis (pseudomembranous colitis). Discontinue drug and treat. Do not use drugs that inhibit peristalsis. |
| Coagulation tests | If any bleeding occurs | • More common in renal impairment and if concomitant with beta-lactam antibiotics. Stop drug and take corrective action. |

## Additional information

| | |
|---|---|
| Common and serious undesirable effects | *Immediate:* Anaphylaxis and other hypersensitivity reactions have been reported.<br>*Injection/infusion-related:* Local: Pain at IM injection site.<br>*Other:* Diarrhoea, nausea, urticaria, rash (discontinue if rash develops). |
| Pharmacokinetics | Elimination half-life is 4-6 hours. |
| Significant interactions | No significant interactions. |
| Action in case of overdose | *Symptoms to watch for:* Large doses may be associated with seizures.<br>*Antidote:* No known antidote but haemodialysis may be effective. Stop administration and give supportive therapy as appropriate. |

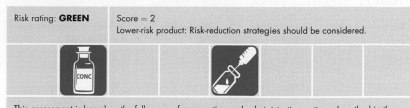

| Risk rating: **GREEN** | Score = 2<br>Lower-risk product: Risk-reduction strategies should be considered. |

This assessment is based on the full range of preparation and administration options described in the monograph. These may not all be applicable in some clinical situations.

## Bibliography

SPC Negaban 1 g, powder for solution for injection/infusion, published 1 September 2003.

# Tenecteplase

**8000 units (40 mg) dry powder vial with 8 mL WFI in pre-filled syringe**
**10 000 units (50 mg) dry powder vial with 10 mL WFI in pre-filled syringe**
* Tenecteplase is a fibrin-specific plasminogen activator. It has thrombolytic activity.
* It is licensed for the dissolution of clots in STEMI.
* Tenecteplase doses are expressed in units specific to tenecteplase, which are not directly comparable with units of other thrombolytic agents.

## Pre-treatment checks

* Contraindicated in recent haemorrhage, trauma, or surgery (including dental extraction), coagulation defects, bleeding diatheses, aortic dissection, aneurysm, coma, history of cerebrovascular disease especially recent events or with any residual disability, recent symptoms of possible peptic ulceration, heavy vaginal bleeding, severe ↑BP, active pulmonary disease with cavitation, acute pancreatitis, pericarditis, bacterial endocarditis, severe liver disease, and oesophageal varices.
* Use with caution if there is a risk of bleeding including that from venepuncture or invasive procedures.
* Caution in external chest compression, pregnancy, elderly patients, ↑BP, conditions in which thrombolysis might give rise to embolic complications such as enlarged left atrium with atrial fibrillation (risk of dissolution of clot and subsequent embolisation), and recent or concurrent use of drugs that ↑risk of bleeding.

*Biochemical and other tests (not all are necessary in an emergency situation)*

Blood pressure and pulse – do not give if systolic BP >160.
Bodyweight
LFTs

## Dose

**Acute myocardial infarction:** a single weight-based dose (Table T1) given by IV injection as soon as possible (within 6 hours) after the onset of symptoms.

**Table T1** Weight-based dosing of tenecteplase

| Bodyweight (kg) | Tenecteplase (units) | Tenecteplase (mg) | Volume of reconstituted solution (mL) |
|---|---|---|---|
| <60 | 6 000 | 30 | 6 |
| 60 to 69 | 7 000 | 35 | 7 |
| 70 to 79 | 8 000 | 40 | 8 |
| 80 to 89 | 9 000 | 45 | 9 |
| ≥90 | 10 000 | 50 | 10 |

**Dose in hepatic impairment:** do not give in severe disease.

## Intravenous injection

*Preparation and administration*

Tenecteplase is incompatible with Gluc solutions.

1. Select the correct vial size according to bodyweight: 8000 units for <80 kg, 10 000 units for 80 kg and over.
2. Screw the pre-filled syringe onto the vial adapter and penetrate the vial stopper in the middle with the spike of the vial adapter.
3. Add the WFI into the vial by pushing the syringe plunger down slowly to avoid foaming.
4. Reconstitute by swirling gently to give a solution containing 1000 units/mL.
5. Immediately prior to use invert the vial with the syringe still attached, so that the syringe is below the vial.
6. Transfer the appropriate volume of reconstituted solution into the syringe, based on the patient's weight (see Table T1).
7. Disconnect the syringe from the vial adapter.
8. The solution should be clear and colourless to pale yellow. Inspect visually for particulate matter or discoloration prior to administration and discard if present.
9. Give by IV injection over 10 seconds.

## Technical information

| Incompatible with | Tenecteplase is incompatible with Gluc solutions. |
|---|---|
| Compatible with | **Flush**: NaCl 0.9%<br>**Solutions**: NaCl 0.9%<br>**Y-site**: No information but unlikely to be stable |
| pH[1] | 7.0-7.6 |
| Sodium content | Nil |
| Excipients | Contains L-arginine (may cause hypersensitivity reactions). |

(continued)

## Technical information (continued)

| Storage | Store below 30°C in original packaging. |
|---|---|
| Displacement value | Negligible |
| Stability after preparation | From a microbiological point of view, should be used immediately; however, reconstituted solutions may be stored at 2–8°C and used within 24 hours. |

## Monitoring in treatment of myocardial infarction

| Measure | Frequency | Rationale |
|---|---|---|
| Heart rate | Continuously | • ↓Pulse may result from reperfusion. |
| ECG | | • Arrhythmias may result from reperfusion. |
| Blood pressure | | • ↓BP may occur. Raise the legs and slow or stop infusion temporarily. |

## Additional information

| Common and serious undesirable effects | *Immediate:* Anaphylaxis and other hypersensitivity reactions have been reported rarely.<br>*Injection/infusion-related:* Haemorrhage at injection site.<br>*Other:* Bleeding, ↓BP, ↑or ↓pulse, coronary artery reperfusion events, e.g. rhythm disorders, nausea, vomiting, headache, muscle pain, fever. |
|---|---|
| Pharmacokinetics | Biphasic elimination with terminal half-life of around 2 hours. |
| Significant interactions | • The following may ↑risk of haemorrhage with tenecteplase: anticoagulants, heparins, antiplatelet agents, e.g. aspirin, clopidogrel, dipyridamole, GP IIb/IIIa inhibitors. |
| Action in case of overdose | *Symptoms to watch for:* severe bleeding.<br>*Antidote:* No specific antidote. Stop administration and give supportive therapy as appropriate including fresh frozen plasma, fresh blood and tranexamic acid if necessary. |
| Counselling | Report bleeding events. |

| Risk rating: **GREEN** | Score = 2<br>Lower-risk product. Risk-reduction strategies should be considered. |
|---|---|

This assessment is based on the full range of preparation and administration options described in the monograph. These may not all be applicable in some clinical situations.

## Reference

1. Communication with Boehringer Ingelheim Ltd, 13 November 2009.

## Bibliography

SPC Metalyse (accessed 31 March 2010).

# Terbutaline sulfate

### 500 micrograms/mL solution in 1-mL ampoules

* Terbutaline sulfate is a direct-acting sympathomimetic with mainly beta-adrenergic activity and a selective action on beta$_2$-receptors.
* It can be given by various parenteral routes in the management of severe bronchospasm and by IV infusion to delay uncomplicated premature labour.

## Pre-treatment checks

* Avoid use in patients with underlying severe heart disease, e.g. ischaemic heart disease, arrhythmia or severe heart failure.
* Use with caution in thyrotoxicosis.
* In asthma, use should be combined with oxygen and corticosteroid therapy.
* Hypoglycaemic therapy in patients with diabetes may require review.

*Biochemical and other tests (not all are necessary in an emergency situation)*

| | |
|---|---|
| Blood glucose | Electrolytes: serum K |
| Blood pressure and pulse | Respiratory function: ABGs, pulse oximetry |

## Dose

**Severe bronchospasm:** 250–500 micrograms by SC or slow IV injection up to 4 times daily.
Alternatively, 90–300 micrograms/hour by IV infusion for 8–10 hours adjusted according to clinical response and heart rate.

**Premature labour:** Gluc 5% should be used to prepare the infusion to ↓risk of maternal pulmonary oedema.

Initially 5 micrograms/minute (300 micrograms/hour) by IV infusion increasing in steps of 2.5 micrograms/minute at 20-minute intervals until contractions have ceased.

More than 10 micrograms/minute is rarely required; 20 micrograms/minute should not be exceeded. Continue for 1 hour then gradually decrease every 20 minutes in steps of 2.5 micrograms/minute to the lowest dose that maintains suppression and continue at this dose for 12 hours. Continue with oral therapy or SC injections if required, bearing in mind ↑risk to the mother after 48 hours of treatment.

**Dose in renal impairment:** adjusted according to creatinine clearance:[1]

* CrCl >20–50 mL/minute: reduce the parenteral dose by 50%.
* CrCl 10–20 mL/minute: reduce the parenteral dose by 50%.
* CrCl <10 mL/minute: avoid the parenteral route.

## Continuous intravenous infusion via a syringe pump

*Preparation of a 100 micrograms/mL solution (other strengths may be used according to local policies)*

1. Withdraw 5 mg (10 mL) and make up to 50 mL in a syringe pump with Gluc 5%.
2. Cap the syringe and mix well to give a solution containing 100 micrograms/mL.
3. The solution should be clear and colourless. Inspect visually for particulate matter or discoloration prior to administration and discard if present.

*Administration*

Give by IV infusion at a rate appropriate to indication, and adjust according to clinical response and heart rate.

## Continuous intravenous infusion (large volume infusion)

*Preparation of a 5 micrograms/mL solution (other strengths may be used according to local policies)*

1. Remove 5 mL from a 500-mL bag of compatible infusion fluid and discard.
2. Withdraw 2.5 mg (5 mL) terbutaline injection and add to the prepared infusion bag. Mix well to give a solution containing 5 micrograms/mL.
3. The solution should be clear and colourless. Inspect visually for particulate matter or discoloration prior to administration and discard if present.

*Administration*

Give by IV infusion via a volumetric infusion device at a rate appropriate to indication, and adjust according to clinical response and heart rate.

## Subcutaneous injection

*Preparation and administration*

1. Withdraw the required dose.
2. Give by SC injection.

## Intravenous injection

*Preparation and administration*

1. Withdraw the required dose and dilute to 10 mL with NaCl 0.9%.
2. The solution should be clear and colourless. Inspect visually for particulate matter or discoloration prior to administration and discard if present.
3. Give by slow IV injection over 3–5 minutes.

| Technical information | |
|---|---|
| Incompatible with | No information |
| Compatible with | **Flush**: NaCl 0.9%<br>**Solutions**: Gluc 5% (preferred in premature labour), NaCl 0.9%<br>**Y-site**: Aminophylline, doxapram |
| pH | 3-5 |
| Sodium content | Negligible |
| Storage | Store below 25°C in original packaging. Protect from light.<br>Discoloured solutions must not be used. |
| Stability after preparation | From a microbiological point of view, should be used immediately; however, prepared infusions may be stored at 2-8°C and infused (at room temperature) within 24 hours. |

## Monitoring

| Measure | Frequency | Rationale |
|---|---|---|
| Respiratory function | Frequently during treatment | • For signs of clinical improvement. |
| Blood pressure and pulse | | • May cause ↑pulse, ↓BP and myocardial ischaemia. |
| Serum K | | • May cause ↓K. |
| Blood glucose | | • May ↑blood glucose levels. |

## Additional information

| | |
|---|---|
| Common and serious undesirable effects | *Immediate:* Hypersensitivity reactions have been reported.<br>*Other:* ↑Pulse, palpitations, ↓BP, ↓K (see also interactions), muscle spasm, fine tremor, anxiety, headache, hyperglycaemia (in diabetes). |
| Pharmacokinetics | Following SC injection, the mean terminal half-life is 5.7 hours. |
| Significant interactions | • Beta-blockers (including eye drops) may ↓terbutaline effect.<br>• Terbutaline may cause ↓K with the following drugs:<br>  acetazolamide, aminophylline, corticosteroids, diuretics, theophylline. |
| Action in case of overdose | The preferred antidote is a cardioselective beta-blocker, but use with caution in patients with a history of bronchospasm. Give supportive therapy as appropriate. |
| Counselling | Advise that shaking and a feeling of anxiety are common side-effects. Report palpitations or ↑heart rate. |

| Risk rating: **AMBER** | Score = 4<br>Moderate-risk product: Risk-reduction strategies are recommended. |
|---|---|

This assessment is based on the full range of preparation and administration options described in the monograph. These may not all be applicable in some clinical situations.

## Reference

1. Ashley C, Currie A, eds. *The Renal Drug Handbook*, 3rd edn. Oxford: Radcliffe Medical Press, 2009.

## Bibliography

SPC Bricanyl injection, 0.5 mg/mL, solution for injection or infusion (accessed 4 April 2010).

# Teriparatide

**250 micrograms/mL solution in 3-mL pre-filled multidose pen (28 doses)**

* Teriparatide is a recombinant fragment of human parathyroid hormone.
* It is used to treat osteoporosis in postmenopausal women, osteoporosis in men with ↑risk of fracture and osteoporosis associated with sustained systemic glucocorticoid therapy.

## Pre-treatment checks

* Avoid in pre-existing ↑Ca, severe renal impairment, metabolic bone diseases including hyperparathyroidism and Paget disease, skeletal malignancies or bone metastases or previous radiation therapy to the skeleton.
* Do not give if there is an unexplained ↑alkaline phosphatase.
* Caution in moderate renal impairment.
* Patients should have calcium and vitamin D supplements prescribed if dietary intake is inadequate.
* Women of child-bearing potential should take contraceptive precautions.
* The first injection should be given in an environment where the patient can sit or lie down if orthostatic ↓BP occurs.

*Biochemical and other tests*

Blood pressure
BMD

Electrolytes: serum Ca
Renal function: U, Cr, CrCl (or eGFR)

## Dose

**Standard dose:** 20 micrograms daily by SC injection for a maximum of 24 months. The course should not be repeated during the patient's lifetime.

**Dose in renal impairment**: no dose adjustment required in mild impairment; use with caution in moderate impairment; do not give in severe renal impairment.

**Dose in hepatic impairment**: no data available.

## Subcutaneous injection

*Preparation and administration*

1. The injection may be given immediately after removing the pen from the refrigerator. Insulin pen needles can be used with the device.
2. Give by SC injection into the thigh or abdominal wall in accordance with the Forsteo User Manual.
3. Return the pen to the refrigerator immediately after use.

| Technical information | |
|---|---|
| Incompatible with | Not relevant |
| Compatible with | Not relevant |
| pH | Not relevant |
| Sodium content | Negligible |
| Excipients | Contains metacresol (may cause hypersensitivity reactions). |

*(continued)*

## Technical information (continued)

| | |
|---|---|
| Storage | Store at 2-8°C at all times. Do not freeze.<br>*In use:* Once opened, the pen should be used for a maximum of 28 days and then discarded. Do not store the pen with the needle attached. |

## Monitoring

| Measure | Frequency | Rationale |
|---|---|---|
| Blood pressure | After initial administration and periodically | • May cause ↓BP, typically within 4 hours of administration. |
| Urinary calcium | Periodically | • In patients with suspected active urolithiasis or pre-existing hypercalciuria. |
| Serum uric acid | | • May ↑uric acid level.<br>• In trials this did not result in an increase in gout, arthralgia, or urolithiasis. |
| Biochemical markers of bone formation/resorption | If required | • E.g. serum total and intact osteocalcin, bone-specific Alk Phos to ensure that treatment is effective. |

## Additional information

| | |
|---|---|
| Common and serious undesirable effects | *Immediate:* Hypersensitivity reactions: acute dyspnoea, facial oedema, generalised urticaria, chest pain, oedema (mainly peripheral).<br>*Injection-related:* Injection-site reaction and erythema.<br>*Other:* Nausea and other GI disorders, pain in limb, headache, dizziness, palpitations, anaemia, sciatica, vertigo, dyspnoea, ↑sweating, muscle cramps, ↓BP, and depression. |
| Elimination half-life | About 1 hour. |
| Significant drug interactions | No significant interactions. |
| Overdose | *Symptoms to watch for:* Nausea, dizziness, headache, ↑Ca, orthostatic ↓BP.<br>*Antidote:* No known antidote; stop administration and give supportive therapy as appropriate. Monitor Ca. |

| | |
|---|---|
| Risk rating: **GREEN** | Score = 0<br>Lower-risk product: Risk-reduction strategies should be considered. |

| | | | | | | |
|---|---|---|---|---|---|---|
| | | | | | | |

This assessment is based on the full range of preparation and administration options described in the monograph. These may not all be applicable in some clinical situations.

## Bibliography

SPC Forsteo (accessed 14 September 2009).

# Terlipressin

**1-mg dry powder vial with 5 mL solvent**
**120 micrograms/mL (1 mg/8.5 mL) solution in 8.5-mL ampoules**

- Terlipressin acetate is an inactive pro-drug that is slowly converted in the body to lypressin. It has the pressor activity of vasopressin and some antidiuretic activity.
- It is indicated in the treatment of bleeding from oesophageal varices and reduces the relative risk of mortality by about one-third.
- It has also been used to treat hepatorenal syndrome and shock (both unlicensed).
- Doses are expressed in terms of terlipressin acetate.

## Pre-treatment checks

Caution in patients with hypertension, atherosclerosis, cardiac dysrhythmias or coronary insufficiency.

*Biochemical and other tests (not all are necessary in an emergency situation)*

Baseline plasma osmolality *or* baseline bodyweight (to enable monitoring of fluid balance)
Blood pressure
Electrolytes: serum Na, K

## Dose

**Acute variceal bleeding:** 2 mg by slow IV injection, followed by 1–2 mg every 4–6 hours until bleeding is controlled, up to a maximum of 72 hours.
**Hepatorenal syndrome (unlicensed):** 1 mg every 4–12 hours for 7–15 days appeared to improve renal function.
**Shock (unlicensed):** 1–2 mg by IV injection produced a progressive ↑mean arterial pressure over 10–20 minutes that was sustained for at least 5 hours, allowing reduction or cessation of noradrenaline therapy.

## Intravenous injection

*Preparation and administration*

1. *For dry powder vials:* reconstitute with the solvent supplied. Dissolve vial contents completely before withdrawing the dose.
2. Withdraw the required dose.
3. The solution should be clear and colourless. Inspect visually for particulate matter or discoloration prior to administration and discard if present.
4. Give by IV injection over 3–4 minutes.

## Technical information

| Incompatible with | No information |
|---|---|
| Compatible with | **Flush**: NaCl 0.9% <br> **Solutions**: NaCl 0.9% <br> **Y-site**: No information |
| pH | Not relevant |
| Sodium content | Negligible |

(continued)

## Technical information (continued)

| | |
|---|---|
| Storage | *Dry powder vials:* Store below 25°C in original packaging.<br>*Solution in ampoules:* Store at 2-8°C in original packaging. |
| Displacement value | Negligible |
| Stability after preparation | Use reconstituted vials immediately. |

## Monitoring

| Measure | Frequency | Rationale |
|---|---|---|
| Blood pressure | Frequently during treatment | • May ↑arterial BP. |
| Serum Na, K | | • May ↑urinary excretion of Na and K. |
| Fluid balance | | • Terlipressin has approximately 3% of the antidiuretic effect of vasopressin and could cause fluid retention and ↓Na.<br>• Review treatment if there is a gradual increase of the bodyweight, or serum sodium <130 mmol/L, or plasma osmolality <270 mOsmol/kg. |

## Additional information

| | |
|---|---|
| Common and serious undesirable effects | ↑Arterial BP, transient blanching, abdominal cramps, headache. |
| Pharmacokinetics | Lypressin reaches maximum plasma levels about 1-2 hours following IV administration and has a duration of activity of 4-6 hours. |
| Significant interactions | No significant interactions. |
| Action in case of overdose | *Symptoms to watch for:* ↑BP in patients with known hypertension. Manage symptomatically. Clonidine IV has been used. |

| | |
|---|---|
| Risk rating: **GREEN** | Score = 2<br>Lower-risk product: Risk-reduction strategies should be considered. |

This assessment is based on the full range of preparation and administration options described in the monograph. These may not all be applicable in some clinical situations.

## Bibliography

SPC Glypressin (accessed 3 July 2008).

# Testosterone and esters

**Sustanon 250 (mixed testosterone esters 250 mg) oily solution in 1-mL ampoules**
**Testosterone enantate 250 mg/mL oily solution in 1-mL ampoules**
**Testosterone propionate 50 mg/mL oily solution in 2-mL ampoules**
**Testosterone undecanoate 250 mg/mL oily solution in 4-mL ampoules**

- Testosterone is a hormone with anabolic and androgenic properties.
- The primary use of testosterone is as replacement therapy in male hypogonadal disorders.
- The plasma half-life of testosterone is only 10–100 minutes, therefore testosterone esters are usually formulated as oily solutions for IM use to give a longer duration of action.
- Some IM testosterone preparations are licensed for use in treatment of delayed puberty in boys and also of breast cancer in women.
- Doses below are expressed in terms of the specific ester or as millilitres of preparation.

## Pre-treatment checks

- Avoid in breast cancer in men, prostate cancer, past or present liver tumour, and ↑Ca.
- A detailed medical examination should be conducted prior to treatment to exclude the risk of pre-existing prostatic cancer.
- Caution in cancer patients at risk of ↑Ca.
- Caution in severe cardiac, hepatic or renal impairment or ischaemic heart disease: treatment with testosterone may cause complications characterised by oedema. Testosterone may also aggravate epilepsy and migraine.

*Biochemical and other tests*

| | |
|---|---|
| Blood pressure | Renal function: U, Cr, CrCl (or eGFR) |
| FBC | Serum electrolytes: serum Ca |
| LFTs | Serum testosterone level |
| Lipids | |

## Dose

**Androgen deficiency (adjust dose according to response):**
- *Sustanon 250:* usually 1 mL by IM injection every 3 weeks.
- *Testosterone propionate:* usually 50 mg by IM injection 2–3 times each week.

**Hypogonadism (adjust dose according to response):**
- *Testosterone enantate:* initially 250 mg by IM injection every 2–3 weeks. Usual maintenance dose 250 mg every 3–6 weeks.
- *Testosterone undecanoate:* 1 g by IM injection every 10–14 weeks. A second injection may be given after 6 weeks depending upon testosterone levels and clinical symptoms.

## Intramuscular injection

Contains arachis oil – should not be given in peanut allergy.

*Preparation and administration*

1. Withdraw the required dose.
2. Give very slowly by deep IM injection into the gluteal muscle.

## Technical information

| | |
|---|---|
| Incompatible with | Not relevant |
| Compatible with | Not relevant |
| pH | Not relevant - oily injection |
| Sodium content | Nil |
| Excipients | *Sustanon* brand only:<br>• Contains arachis oil (should not be used in peanut allergy).<br>• Contains benzyl alcohol. |
| Storage | Store below 25°C in original packaging. Do not refrigerate or freeze. |

## Monitoring

| Measure | Frequency | Rationale |
|---|---|---|
| Signs and symptoms of prostate (PSA) or breast cancer | Once or twice a year | • Review for prostate/breast cancer. |
| Testosterone levels | Periodically | • For signs of clinical improvement.<br>• Measure levels towards the end of an injection interval and use the same laboratory for measuring testosterone levels owing to variability in laboratory values.<br>• Normal adult ranges are male 300-1000 nanograms/dL, female 20-80 nanograms/dL and each diminishes with increasing age.<br>• Serum levels should be within the lower third of the normal range.<br>• Serum levels below normal range indicate the need for a shorter dosage interval.<br>• High serum levels may require an extension of the dosage interval. |
| Hb and Haematocrit | | • May increase both of these measures. |
| LFTs | | • Abnormal LFTs have been reported. |
| Lipids | | • May ↑triglycerides and cholesterol. |
| Blood pressure | | • May cause ↑BP. |
| Serum Na and Ca | | • May cause electrolyte disturbances including Na retention with oedema and ↑Ca. |
| Signs of osteoporosis | | • Especially in patients who have undergone oophorectomy (e.g. female-to-male transsexuals), as testosterone may not fully reverse the decline in bone density. |

## Additional information

| | |
|---|---|
| Common and serious undesirable effects | *Immediate:* Testosterone enantate and undecanoate - rarely coughing, dyspnoea and circulatory irregularities may occur. With testosterone enantate these symptoms may be reduced by injecting very slowly.<br>*Injection-related:* Local: Injection-site pain.<br>*Other:* Polycythaemia, weight gain, hot flush, acne, prostate abnormalities and prostate cancer. |
| Pharmacokinetics | Testosterone undecanoate elimination half-life is 50-130 days.<br>Testosterone enantate elimination half-life is 2-3 days.<br>Sustanon is a combination of different esters of testosterone with different durations of action. |
| Significant interactions | • Testosterone may ↑levels or effect of the following drugs (or ↑side-effects): coumarin anticoagulants (monitor INR), phenindione (monitor INR).<br>• Testosterone may affect the following tests: glucose tolerance, thyroid function. |
| Action in case of overdose | Stop treatment; once symptoms have disappeared consider resuming at a lower dose. |
| Counselling | Female patients should be asked to report any signs of virilisation such as acne, hirsutism and voice changes.<br>Male patients: if frequent or persistent erections occur, the dose should be reduced or the treatment discontinued to avoid injury to the penis. |

| | |
|---|---|
| Risk rating: **GREEN** | Score = 1<br>Lower-risk product: Risk-reduction strategies should be considered. |

This assessment is based on the full range of preparation and administration options described in the monograph. These may not all be applicable in some clinical situations.

## Bibliography

SPC Nebido (accessed 7 October 2009).
SPC Sustanon 250 (accessed 7 October 2009).
SPC Testosterone enanthate ampoules (Cambridge Laboratories) (accessed 7 October 2009).
SPC Virormone injection (accessed 7 October 2009).

# Tetracosactide (cosyntropin, tetracosactrin)

**250 micrograms/mL solution in 1-mL ampoules (Synacthen)**

**1mg/mL aqueous suspension (with zinc phosphate complex) in 1-mL ampoules (Synacthen Depot)**

* Tetracosactide is an analogue of corticotrophin (ACTH) and is used as a diagnostic test for the investigation of adrenocortical insufficiency.
* Tetracosactide is still licensed as an alternative to corticosteroids in conditions such as Crohn disease or rheumatoid arthritis; however, its value is limited by the variable and unpredictable therapeutic response and by the waning of its effect with time.

## Pre-treatment checks

* Do not give to patients who have allergic disorders, e.g. asthma.
* Treatment with corticosteroids in the hours prior to diagnostic testing may affect the test result.

*Biochemical and other tests*

In diagnostic testing, measure plasma cortisol concentration immediately before giving the dose.
In therapeutic use, measure Na and K.

## Dose

**Short or 30-minute test:** using the 250 micrograms/mL preparation, give 250 micrograms by IM or IV injection. Measure plasma cortisol concentration immediately before the dose, and exactly 30 minutes afterwards. Adrenocortical function is considered normal if the plasma cortisol concentration rises by 200 nanomol/L (70 micrograms/L) or more.

**5-hour test:** using the 1 mg/mL preparation give 1 mg by IM injection. Measure plasma cortisol concentrations immediately before the dose, and exactly 30 minutes and 1, 2, 3, 4 and 5 hours afterwards.
*Interpretation:* the 5-hour test is used where the 30-minute test is inconclusive or where it is necessary to determine the functional reserve of the adrenal cortex.

Adrenocortical function is considered normal if the plasma cortisol concentration increases 2-fold in the first hour, and continues to rise steadily. The values expected would be 600–1250 nanomol/L in the first hour, increasing slowly up to 1000–1800 nanomol/L by the fifth hour. Smaller rises in plasma cortisol may be attributable to Addison disease, secondary adrenocortical insufficiency due to a disorder of hypothalamo-pituitary function, or overdosage of corticosteroids.

**3-day test:** perform the 30-minute test just prior to giving the first day's dosing then, using the 1 mg/mL preparation, give 1 mg by IM injection each morning for 3 days. Repeat the 30-minute test on the fourth day.
*Interpretation:* the 3-day test is used to differentiate between primary and secondary adrenocortical insufficiency.

A marked improvement in the second assessment suggests secondary adrenocortical insufficiency.

## Intramuscular injection

*Preparation and administration*

1. If using the 1 mg/mL preparation, shake before use to re-suspend particles.
2. Withdraw the required dose.
3. Give by IM injection.

## Intravenous injection

*Preparation and administration*

1. Using the 250 micrograms/mL preparation, withdraw the required dose (1 mL).
2. The solution should be clear and colourless. Inspect visually for particulate matter or discoloration prior to administration.
3. Give by IV injection over 2 minutes.

## Technical information

| | |
|---|---|
| Incompatible with | Not relevant |
| Compatible with | Not relevant |
| pH | 3.8–4.5 |
| Sodium content | Negligible |
| Excipients | Synacthen Depot contains benzyl alcohol. |
| Storage | Store at 2–8°C in original packaging. |

## Monitoring

| Measure | Frequency | Rationale |
|---|---|---|
| Signs of hypersensitivity | For at least 1 hour after administration | • May provoke hypersensitivity reactions and anaphylactic shock.<br>• Most occur within 30 minutes of administration. |
| Electrolytes and fluid balance | Periodically during therapeutic use | • Fluid retention and electrolyte imbalance can occur during therapeutic use.<br>• A salt-reduced diet may be required (salt and water retention may occur).<br>• Potassium supplementation may be necessary. |
| Signs of psychological disturbances | | • These may be triggered or aggravated. |
| Signs of infection | | • Latent infections (e.g. amoebiasis, tuberculosis) may become activated. |
| Ophthalmological examination | | • Ocular effects, e.g. glaucoma, cataracts may occur. |
| Blood glucose and blood pressure | | • Dosage adjustments may be necessary in patients being treated for diabetes or ↑BP. |

## Additional information

| | |
|---|---|
| Common and serious undesirable effects | *Immediate:* Anaphylaxis and other hypersensitivity reactions (dizziness, nausea, urticaria, pruritus, flushing, dyspnoea, angioedema-particularly in asthmatics). <br> *Injection-related:* Local: Skin reactions. <br> *Other:* Unlikely with short-term diagnostic use; however, corticosteroid side-effects (as listed under hydrocortisone) would be expected if given long term. |
| Pharmacokinetics | IV tetracosactide exhibits triphasic pharmacokinetics. Most of a dose is excreted in the urine within 24 hours. The terminal half-life is about 3 hours. |
| Significant interactions | Treatment with corticosteroids in the hours prior to diagnostic testing can affect the test result. <br> Other interactions are unlikely with diagnostic use. For undesirable effects resulting from long-term corticosteroid use, refer to the BNF. |
| Action in case of overdose | Give supportive therapy as appropriate. |
| Counselling | Make patients aware of the risk of allergic reaction and advise them to report swelling in face or hands, swelling or tingling in the mouth or throat, tightness in chest, trouble breathing or itching. |

| | |
|---|---|
| Risk rating: **GREEN** | Score = 0 <br> Lower-risk product. Risk-reduction strategies should be considered. |

This assessment is based on the full range of preparation and administration options described in the monograph. These may not all be applicable in some clinical situations.

### Bibliography

SPCs Synacthen and Synacthen Depot (accessed 7 September 2008).

# Ticarcillin with clavulanic acid

### 1.6 g, 3.2-g dry powder vials

- Ticarcillin sodium is a carboxypenicillin. It is given in combination with the beta-lactamase inhibitor clavulanic acid to widen its spectrum of action.
- The combined preparation is used in the treatment of severe Gram-negative infections, especially those due to *Pseudomonas aeruginosa* including those in cystic fibrosis (respiratory tract infections), neutropenic sepsis, peritonitis, and septicaemia.

- Doses of ticarcillin are expressed in terms of the base:
- Ticarcillin 1 g ≡ 1.1 g ticarcillin sodium.
- Ticarcillin with clavulanic acid doses are expressed below as the combined mass (mg) of the two constituents:
  Ticarcillin with clavulanic acid 3.2 g ≡ ticarcillin 3 g with clavulanic acid 200 mg.

## Pre-treatment checks

Check for history of allergy/hypersensitivity to penicillins and use with caution if sensitive to other beta-lactam antibiotics.

*Biochemical and other tests*

FBC
LFTs
Renal function: U, Cr, CrCl (or eGFR)

## Dose

**Standard dose:** 3.2 g by IV infusion every 6–8 hours.
**Severe infections:** 3.2 g by IV infusion every 4 hours.
**Dose in renal impairment:** adjusted according to creatinine clearance:

- CrCl >30 mL/minute: 3.2 g every 8 hours.
- CrCl 10–30 mL/minute: 1.6 g every 8 hours.
- CrCl <10 mL/minute: 1.6 g every 12 hours.

## Intermittent intravenous infusion

*Preparation and administration*

If used in combination with an aminoglycoside (e.g. amikacin, gentamicin, tobramycin), preferably administer at a different site. If this is not possible then flush the line thoroughly with a compatible solution between drugs.

1. Reconstitute each 1.6-g vial with 5 mL WFI (use 10 mL for each 3.2-g vial) and shake well. Heat is generated as it dissolves.
2. Withdraw the required dose and add to a suitable volume of a compatible infusion fluid (usually 100 mL Gluc 5%). If using WFI dilute 1.6 g to 50 mL; 3.2 g to 100 mL.
3. The solution should be clear and a pale straw colour. Inspect visually for particulate matter or discoloration prior to administration and discard if present.
4. Give by IV infusion over 30–40 minutes.

## Technical information

| Incompatible with | Sodium bicarbonate. Amikacin, amphotericin, cisatracurium, drotrecogin alfa (activated), gentamicin, tobramycin, vancomycin. |
|---|---|
| Compatible with | **Flush**: NaCl 0.9%<br>**Solutions**: Gluc 5%, WFI<br>**Y-site**: No information |
| pH | 5.5–7.5 |
| Sodium content | 16 mmol/3.2 g |

*(continued)*

## Technical information (continued)

| | |
|---|---|
| Storage | Store below 25°C in original packaging. |
| Displacement value | 1.1 mL for 1.6 g; 2.2 mL for 3.2 g |
| Stability after preparation | Use reconstituted vials and prepared infusions immediately. |

## Monitoring

| Measure | Frequency | Rationale |
|---|---|---|
| Renal function and serum K | Periodically | • If renal function changes, a dose adjustment may be necessary.<br>• ↓K has been reported rarely in long-term treatment. |
| LFTs | | • Use with care in severe hepatic dysfunction. ↑AST and ↑ALT have been reported.<br>• Cholestatic jaundice occurs rarely but may be severe. May not present for several weeks after treatment. |
| Prothrombin time and FBC | | • Bleeding manifestations have occurred and are usually associated with renal impairment. Discontinue if bleeding occurs. Thrombocytopenia, leucopenia, eosinophilia and ↓Hb also observed rarely. |
| Signs of supra-infection or superinfection | Throughout treatment | • May result in the overgrowth of non-susceptible organisms - appropriate therapy should be commenced; treatment may need to be interrupted. |
| Development of diarrhoea | Throughout and up to 2 months after treatment | • Development of severe, persistent diarrhoea may be suggestive of *Clostridium difficile*-associated diarrhoea and colitis (pseudomembranous colitis). Discontinue drug and treat. Do not use drugs that inhibit peristalsis. |

## Additional information

| | |
|---|---|
| Common and serious undesirable effects | *Immediate:* Anaphylaxis and other hypersensitivity reactions have been reported.<br>*Infusion-related:* Local: Pain, burning, swelling, induration at the injection site and possible thrombophlebitis.<br>*Other:* Nausea, vomiting, diarrhoea, skin rashes. |
| Pharmacokinetics | Elimination half-life is about 1 hour for both components. |
| Significant interactions | No significant interactions. |
| Action in case of overdose | *Symptoms to watch for:* Large doses have been associated with seizures.<br>*Antidote:* No known antidote but haemodialysis may be effective.<br>Stop administration and give supportive therapy as appropriate. |

*(continued)*

| **Additional information** (*continued*) | |
|---|---|
| Counselling | Women taking the combined contraceptive pill should be should be advised to take additional precautions during and for 7 days after the course. |

| Risk rating: **AMBER** | Score = 3<br>Moderate-risk product: Risk-reduction strategies are recommended. |
|---|---|

This assessment is based on the full range of preparation and administration options described in the monograph. These may not all be applicable in some clinical situations.

## Bibliography

SPC Timentin 0.8 G, 1.6 G, 3.2 G (accessed 3 April 2009).

# Tigecycline

**50-mg dry powder vials**

- Tigecycline, a synthetic derivative of minocycline, is a glycylcycline antibacterial structurally similar to tetracyclines.
- It is active against a broad range of Gram-positive and Gram-negative bacteria, including tetracycline-resistant organisms and some anaerobic organisms.
- It is used for the treatment of complicated skin and soft-tissue infections or complicated intra-abdominal infections caused by susceptible organisms.

## Pre-treatment checks

- Do not use if the patient is hypersensitive to other tetracyclines or in pregnancy.
- Caution in cholestasis.

*Biochemical tests*

LFTs
Prothrombin time and activated partial thromboplastin time (APTT) – especially if the patient is taking anticoagulants.

## Dose

**Standard dose:** initially 100 mg, followed by 50 mg every 12 hours for 5–14 days (dependent on severity, site of infection and the patient's clinical response).
**Dose in hepatic impairment:** use with caution in severe hepatic impairment (Child–Pugh C), reduce to 25 mg every 12 hours after the 100-mg loading dose.

## Intermittent intravenous infusion

*Preparation and administration*

1. Reconstitute each 50-mg vial with 5.3 mL of NaCl 0.9 % or Gluc 5%. Gently swirl until contents dissolve to produce a solution containing 10 mg/mL.
2. Withdraw the required dose and add to a 100 mL Gluc 5% or NaCl 0.9%.
3. The solution should be clear and yellow to orange in colour. Inspect visually for particulate matter or discoloration prior to administration and discard if present.
4. Give by IV infusion over 30–60 minutes.

## Technical information

| | |
|---|---|
| Incompatible with | Amphotericin, diazepam, methylprednisolone sodium succinate, omeprazole, voriconazole. |
| Compatible with | **Flush**: NaCl 0.9%<br>**Solutions**: Gluc 5%, NaCl 0.9% (both with added KCl)<br>**Y-site**: Adrenaline (epinephrine), dobutamine, dopamine, fluconazole, metoclopramide, ranitidine |
| pH | 4.5-5.5 |
| Sodium content | Negligible |
| Storage | Store below 25°C in original packaging.<br>Vials are single use only – discard unused portion. |
| Displacement value | Not applicable. The vial contains a 6% overage and 5 mL of reconstituted solution contains 50 mg of tigecycline (10 mg/mL). |
| Stability after preparation | Use reconstituted vials and prepared infusions immediately. |

## Monitoring

| Measure | Frequency | Rationale |
|---|---|---|
| U&Es | Periodically | • ↑U commonly occurs. |
| LFTs | | • Dose adjustment may be necessary if hepatic function alters.<br>• ↑AST, ↑ALT and ↑bilirubin may sometimes occur after treatment. |
| Prothrombin time and APTT | Periodically especially if taking anticoagulants | • Both parameters may be prolonged and clearance of warfarin is additionally slowed by tigecycline (monitor INR more closely). |
| Signs of supra-infection or superinfection | Throughout treatment | • May result in the overgrowth of non-susceptible organisms – appropriate therapy should be commenced; treatment may need to be interrupted. |

*(continued)*

## Monitoring (continued)

| Measure | Frequency | Rationale |
|---------|-----------|-----------|
| Development of diarrhoea | Throughout and up to 2 months after treatment | • Development of severe, persistent diarrhoea may be suggestive of *Clostridium difficile*-associated diarrhoea and colitis (pseudomembranous colitis). Discontinue drug and treat. Do not use drugs that inhibit peristalsis. |

## Additional information

| | |
|---|---|
| Common and serious undesirable effects | *Immediate:* Anaphylaxis and other hypersensitivity reactions have been reported.<br>*Injection/infusion-related:* Local: Injection-site reaction, pain, oedema, phlebitis.<br>*Other:* Dizziness, nausea, vomiting, diarrhoea, abdominal pain, dyspepsia, anorexia, pruritus, rash, headache, acute pancreatitis. |
| Pharmacokinetics | Elimination half-life is 42.4 hours. |
| Significant interactions | No significant interactions. |
| Action in case of overdose | *Antidote:* No known antidote; haemodialysis is ineffective. Stop administration and give supportive therapy as appropriate. |
| Counselling | May be associated with permanent tooth discoloration if used during tooth development (therefore not recommended children under 8 years of age). |

| Risk rating: **GREEN** | Score = 2<br>Lower-risk product: Risk-reduction strategies should be considered. |
|---|---|

This assessment is based on the full range of preparation and administration options described in the monograph. These may not all be applicable in some clinical situations.

## Bibliography

SPC Tygacil 50 mg powder for solution for infusion (accessed 3 April 2009).

# Tinzaparin sodium

**10 000 units/mL pre-filled syringes: 2500 units/0.25 mL, 3500 units/0.35 mL, 4500 units/ 0.45 mL**
**10 000 units/mL solution in 2-mL multidose vials**
**20 000 units/mL pre-filled syringes: 10 000 units/0.5 mL, 14 000 units/0.7 mL, 18 000 units/0.9 mL**
**20 000 units/mL solution in 2-mL multidose vials**

* Tinzaparin is a low-molecular-weight heparin (LMWH).
* It is used in the treatment of venous thromboembolism (VTE) i.e. pulmonary embolism (PE) and deep vein thrombosis (DVT).
* It is used for prophylaxis of VTE in surgical patients and to prevent thrombus formation in the extracorporeal circulation during haemodialysis.
* Doses are expressed in terms of international anti-Factor Xa activity units:
Tinzaparin sodium 1 mg $\cong$ 70–120 units of anti-Factor Xa activity.

## Pre-treatment checks

* Avoid in acute bacterial endocarditis, major bleeding or high risk of uncontrolled haemorrhage including recent haemorrhagic stroke.
* Tinzaparin in treatment dosage is contraindicated in patients undergoing locoregional anaesthesia in elective surgical procedures.
* Placement or removal of a spinal/epidural catheter should be delayed for 10–12 hours after administration of prophylactic doses, whereas patients receiving treatment doses require a 24-hour delay. Subsequent dosing should be given no sooner than 4 hours after catheter removal.
* Caution with other drugs affecting haemostasis, such as aspirin or clopidogrel.
* Use with extreme caution in patients with a history of heparin-induced thrombocytopenia.

*Biochemical and other tests (not all are necessary in an emergency situation)*

Bodyweight (in certain indications)
Electrolytes: serum K
INR (in certain indications)

Platelet count
Renal function: U, Cr, CrCl (eGFR)

## Dose

*Prophylaxis*

**General surgery with low to moderate risk of VTE:** 3500 units by SC injection 2 hours before surgery and then once daily until the patient is mobile.
**General surgery or orthopaedic with high risk of VTE:** 4500 units by SC injection 12 hours before surgery followed by a once-daily dose until the patient is mobile, or 50 units/kg bodyweight by SC injection 2 hours before surgery followed by a once-daily dose until the patient is mobile.
**Prevention of extracorporeal thrombus formation during haemodialysis:** see product literature.

*Treatment*

**Treatment of VTE:** 175 units/kg bodyweight by SC injection once daily as indicated in Table T2 below (doses have been rounded to facilitate administration). Treat for at least 6 days and until INR > 2.

**Dose in renal impairment**: adjusted according to creatinine clearance:[1]
* CrCl >20–50 mL/minute: dose as in normal renal function.
* CrCl 10–20 mL/minute: dose as in normal renal function for prophylaxis only. For treatment doses either monitor anti-Factor Xa levels or use unfractionated heparin.
* CrCl <10 mL/minute: dose as in normal renal function for prophylaxis only. For treatment doses either monitor anti-Factor Xa levels or use unfractionated heparin.

**Dose in hepatic impairment:** the manufacturer advises avoid in severe hepatic impairment.

## Subcutaneous injection

*Preparation and administration*

1. Select the correct pre-filled syringe. Pre-filled syringes are ready for immediate use; do not expel the air bubble. If necessary expel excess tinzaparin to give the required dose.
2. If using multidose vials, withdraw the required dose using a needle suitable for SC administration.
3. The patient should be seated or lying down.
4. Pinch up a skin fold on the abdominal wall between the thumb and forefinger and hold throughout the injection.
5. Give by deep SC injection into the thick part of the skin fold at right angles to the skin. Do not rub the injection site after administration. Alternate doses between the right and left sides.

## Technical information

| | |
|---|---|
| Incompatible with | Not relevant |
| Compatible with | **Flush**: NaCl 0.9%<br>**Solutions**: NaCl 0.9%<br>**Y-site**: Not relevant |
| pH | Approximately 7 |
| Sodium content | Negligible |
| Excipients | Vials contain benzyl alcohol.<br>20 000 units/mL solution contains sulfites (may cause hypersensitivity reactions). |
| Storage | Store below 25°C.<br>*In use:* Vial contents should be used within 14 days of first use. |

## Monitoring

| Measure | Frequency | Rationale |
|---|---|---|
| Platelets | Alternate days from day 5 to day 21 | • Thrombocytopenia can occur in this period of therapy.<br>• A 50%↓ in platelets is indicative of heparin-induced thrombocytopenia and therapy should be switched to a non-heparin-derived agent. |
| Serum K | After 7 days | • Heparins inhibit the secretion of aldosterone and so may cause ↑K (especially in chronic kidney disease).<br>• K should be monitored in all patients with risk factors, particularly those receiving tinzaparin for >7 days. |

*(continued)*

## Monitoring (continued)

| Measure | Frequency | Rationale |
|---|---|---|
| Bleeding | Throughout treatment | • Low bodyweight: In women <45 kg and men <57 kg there is a higher risk of bleeding with prophylactic tinzaparin doses. |
| Anti-Xa activity | If indicated | • Not required routinely but may be considered in patients during haemodialysis (one hour after dosing should be within the range 0.4-0.5 IU/mL) or in those at ↑risk of bleeding or actively bleeding. |

## Additional information

| | |
|---|---|
| Common and serious undesirable effects | *Immediate:* Anaphylaxis has been reported rarely.<br>*Injection/infusion-related:* Pain, haematoma and mild local irritation may follow SC injection.<br>*Other:* Risk of bleeding with organic lesions, invasive procedures, asymptomatic thrombocytopenia during the first days of therapy, clinically significant ↑K in patients with diabetes or chronic renal failure. |
| Pharmacokinetics | Peak activity in blood is achieved 4-6 hours after SC injection. Detectable anti-Factor Xa activity persists for 24 hours. |
| Significant interactions | • The following may ↑risk of bleeding with tinzaparin:<br>  aspirin, diclofenac IV (avoid combination), ketorolac (avoid combination).<br>• Glyceryl trinitrate infusion may ↓tinzaparin levels or effect. |
| Action in case of overdose | *Symptoms to watch for:* Bleeding.<br>*Antidote:* Protamine sulfate may be used to ↓bleeding risk if clinically required. See the Protamine sulfate monograph. |
| Counselling | Report any bleeding or bruising.<br>Report injection site effects. |

| Risk rating: **GREEN** | Score = 1<br>Lower-risk product. Risk-reduction strategies should be considered. |
|---|---|

This assessment is based on the full range of preparation and administration options described in the monograph. These may not all be applicable in some clinical situations.

## Reference

1. Ashley C, Currie A, eds. *The Renal Drug Handbook*, 3rd edn. Oxford: Radcliffe Medical Press, 2009.

## Bibliography

SPC Innohep 10,000 IU/mL and Innohep Syringe 10,000 IU/mL, Leo Laboratories Ltd (accessed 24 November 2009).

SPC Innohep 20,000 IU/mL and Innohep Syringe 20,000 IU/mL, Leo Laboratories Ltd (accessed 24 November 2009).

**Table T2**  Tinzaparin treatment of VTE

| Preparation to use | Bodyweight | | Prescribed dose (anti-Factor Xa units) | Injection volume (mL) |
|---|---|---|---|---|
| | **kg** | **stones/ pounds** | | |
| 0.5-mL syringe | 40 | 6/4 | 7 000 | 0.35 |
| | 45 | 7/1 | 8 000 | 0.40 |
| | 50 | 7/12 | 9 000 | 0.45 |
| | 55 | 8/9 | 10 000 | 0.50 |
| 0.7-mL syringe | 60 | 9/6 | 11 000 | 0.55 |
| | 65 | 10/3 | 11 000 | 0.55 |
| | 70 | 11/0 | 12 000 | 0.60 |
| | 75 | 11/11 | 13 000 | 0.65 |
| | 80 | 12/8 | 14 000 | 0.70 |
| 0.9-mL syringe | 85 | 13/5 | 15 000 | 0.75 |
| | 90 | 14/2 | 16 000 | 0.80 |
| | 95 | 14/13 | 17 000 | 0.85 |
| | 100 | 15/10 | 18 000 | 0.90 |
| | 105 | 16/7 | 18 000 | 0.90 |
| Multidose vial | 110 | 17/4 | 19 000 | 0.95 |
| | 115 | 18/1 | 20 000 | 1.00 |
| | 120 | 18/12 | 21 000 | 1.05 |
| | 125 | 19/9 | 22 000 | 1.10 |
| | 130 | 20/6 | 23 000 | 1.15 |
| | 135 | 21/3 | 24 000 | 1.20 |
| | 140 | 22/0 | 25 000 | 1.25 |

# Tirofiban

**50 micrograms/mL solution in 250-mL infusion bags; 250 micrograms/mL solution in 50-mL vials**

* Tirofiban hydrochloride is an antiplatelet drug that reversibly inhibits binding of fibrinogen to the glycoprotein IIb/IIIa receptors of platelets.
* It is given with heparin and aspirin for the management of unstable angina, both in patients managed medically and in those undergoing PCI.
* Doses are expressed in terms of the base:
  Tirofiban 50 micrograms ≅ 55 micrograms tirofiban hydrochloride.

## Pre-treatment checks

* Avoid in abnormal bleeding within 30 days, stroke within 30 days or any history of haemorrhagic stroke, intracranial disease (aneurysm, neoplasm or arteriovenous malformation), severe ↑BP, haemorrhagic diathesis, ↑PT or INR, thrombocytopenia; and breast feeding.
* Caution in major surgery or severe trauma within 3 months (avoid if within 6 weeks); traumatic or protracted cardiopulmonary resuscitation, organ biopsy or lithotripsy within the previous 2 weeks; risk of bleeding including active peptic ulcer within 3 months; acute pericarditis, aortic dissection, haemorrhagic retinopathy, vasculitis, haematuria, faecal occult blood; severe heart failure, cardiogenic shock, anaemia; concomitant drugs that ↑risk of bleeding (including within 48 hours of thrombolytic administration).
* Discontinue if thrombolytic therapy, intra-aortic balloon pump or emergency cardiac surgery is necessary.
* Caution in hepatic and renal impairment, and in pregnancy.
* The number of vascular punctures and IM injections should be minimised during the treatment.
* IV access should be obtained only at compressible sites of the body.
* All vascular puncture sites should be documented and closely monitored (caution if there is puncture of non-compressible vessel within 24 hours).
* The use of urinary catheters, nasotracheal intubation and nasogastric tubes should be critically considered before commencing therapy.

*Biochemical and other tests (not all are necessary in an emergency situation)*

| | |
|---|---|
| APTT | FBC (including platelets, Hb and haematocrit) |
| Blood pressure | LFTs (avoid in severe impairment) |
| Bodyweight | Renal function: U, Cr, CrCl (or eGFR) |

## Dose

**Standard dose:** initially 0.4 microgram/kg/minute by IV infusion for 30 minutes, followed by a maintenance dose of 0.1 microgram/kg/minute by IV infusion. See Table T3 below. Infusion should ideally be started within 12 hours of the last anginal episode and continued for at least 48 hours.

**Concomitant therapy with unfractionated heparin:** 5000 units by IV injection at the start of tirofiban therapy, followed by 1000 units/hour by IV infusion, titrated to maintain APTT ratio at about 2.

* *Coronary angiography:* the infusion (and heparin) may be continued during the procedure and should be maintained for 12–24 hours after angioplasty or atherectomy.
* *If no coronary intervention procedure is planned:* discontinue infusion once the patient is clinically stable. Maximum duration of treatment should be no more than 108 hours.
* *If PTCA is required:* heparin should be stopped after PTCA, and the sheaths should be withdrawn once coagulation has returned to normal, i.e. when the ACT <180 seconds (usually 2–6 hours after discontinuation of heparin).

**Dose in renal impairment:** adjusted according to creatinine clearance:
* CrCl >30–50 mL/minute: dose as in normal renal function.
* CrCl 10–30 mL/minute: give 50% of the standard dose.
* CrCl <10 mL/minute: give 50% of the standard dose.

**Dose in hepatic impairment:** avoid in severe impairment.

## Continuous intravenous infusion using pre-prepared solution

*Preparation and administration*

NB: The loading infusion is given over 30 minutes and then the rate is reduced.

1. The 50 micrograms/mL strength in the infusion bag is pre-prepared for use.
2. The solution should be clear and colourless. Inspect visually for particulate matter or discoloration prior to administration and discard if present. Some opacity of the plastic is normal.
3. Remove the plastic protector from the outlet port at the bottom of the container and attach the giving set.
4. Give by IV infusion using a volumetric infusion device at the appropriate rate (see Table T3 below). Ensure that the initial loading infusion rate does not continue for longer than 30 minutes.

## Continuous intravenous infusion using concentrate

*Preparation and administration*

NB: The loading infusion is given over 30 minutes and then the rate is reduced.

1. Withdraw 50 mL from a 250-mL infusion bag of NaCl 0.9% or Gluc 5% and discard.
2. Using the 250 micrograms/mL strength, withdraw 50 mL tirofiban from the 50-mL vial and add to the prepared infusion bag.
3. Mix well to give a solution containing 50 micrograms/mL.
4. The solution should be clear and colourless. Inspect visually for particulate matter or discoloration prior to administration and discard if present.
5. Give by IV infusion using a volumetric infusion device at the appropriate rate (see Table T3 below). Ensure that the initial loading infusion rate does not continue for longer than 30 minutes.

## Technical information

| | |
|---|---|
| Incompatible with | Diazepam |
| Compatible with | **Flush:** NaCl 0.9%<br>**Solutions:** NaCl 0.9%, Gluc 5% (both with added KCl)<br>**Y-site:** Adrenaline (epinephrine), atropine sulfate, bivalirudin, dobutamine, dopamine, furosemide, glyceryl trinitrate, lidocaine, midazolam, morphine sulfate |
| pH | 5.5–6.5 |
| Sodium content | Concentrate: negligible<br>Infusion bag: 38 mmol/250 mL |
| Storage | Store below 25°C in original packaging. Protect from light. Do not freeze. |
| Stability after preparation | From a microbiological point of view, should be used immediately; however, prepared infusions may be stored at 2-8°C and infused (at room temperature) within 24 hours. |

## Monitoring

| Measure | Frequency | Rationale |
|---------|-----------|-----------|
| APTT | Regularly | • To check that heparin infusion is effective.<br>• Potentially life-threatening bleeding may occur, especially when heparin is administered with other products affecting haemostasis, such as glycoprotein IIb/IIIa receptor antagonists. |
| FBC and BP | 2-6 hours after start of treatment and then at least once daily | • Unexplained falls in haematocrit, Hb or BP may indicate haemorrhage.<br>• Treatment should be stopped if bleeding is observed or suspected.<br>• Consider testing stool for occult blood. |
| Platelet count | | • If the platelet count falls below 90 000/mm$^3$, further platelet counts should be carried out to rule out pseudo thrombocytopenia.<br>• If thrombocytopenia is confirmed, tirofiban and heparin should be discontinued. |
| Renal function | Periodically | • Changes in renal function may require an adjustment in infusion rate, but check APTT first.<br>• If CrCl < 60 mL/minute there is a greater chance of bleeding, so the patient should be closely monitored. |

## Additional information

| | |
|---|---|
| Common and serious undesirable effects | *Immediate:* Anaphylaxis has been reported rarely.<br>*Other:* Bleeding from any site, haemorrhage (haematoma) in the area of intravascular puncture sites, headache, nausea, fever. |
| Pharmacokinetics | Elimination half-life is about 2 hours. The antiplatelet effect persists for 4-8 hours. |
| Significant interactions | • The following may ↑risk of haemorrhage with tirofiban:<br>anticoagulants, heparins, antiplatelet agents, e.g. aspirin, clopidogrel, dipyridamole. |
| Action in case of overdose | *Symptoms to watch for:* severe bleeding.<br>*Antidote:* No specific antidote. Stop administration and give supportive therapy as appropriate including fresh frozen plasma or fresh blood if necessary. |

| Risk rating: **AMBER** | Score = 5<br>Moderate-risk product. Risk-reduction strategies are recommended. |
|---|---|

This assessment is based on the full range of preparation and administration options described in the monograph. These may not all be applicable in some clinical situations.

## Bibliography

SPC Aggrastat solution for infusion and concentrate for solution for infusion (accessed 30 March 2010).

**Table T3** Loading and maintenance infusion rates using a 50 micrograms/mL solution

| Patient weight (kg) | Patients with CrCl >30 mL/minute | | Renal impairment CrCl <30 mL/minute | |
|---|---|---|---|---|
| | 30-minute loading infusion (mL/hour) | Maintenance infusion (mL/hour) | 30-minute loading infusion (mL/hour) | Maintenance infusion (mL/hour) |
| 30-37 | 16 | 4 | 8 | 2 |
| 38-45 | 20 | 5 | 10 | 3 |
| 46-54 | 24 | 6 | 12 | 3 |
| 55-62 | 28 | 7 | 14 | 4 |
| 63-70 | 32 | 8 | 16 | 4 |
| 71-79 | 36 | 9 | 18 | 5 |
| 80-87 | 40 | 10 | 20 | 5 |
| 88-95 | 44 | 11 | 22 | 6 |
| 96-104 | 48 | 12 | 24 | 6 |
| 105-112 | 52 | 13 | 26 | 7 |
| 113-120 | 56 | 14 | 28 | 7 |
| 121-128 | 60 | 15 | 30 | 8 |
| 129-137 | 64 | 16 | 32 | 8 |
| 138-145 | 68 | 17 | 34 | 9 |
| 146-153 | 72 | 18 | 36 | 9 |

# Tobramycin

**40 mg/mL solution in 1-mL, 2-mL and 6-mL ampoules**

* Tobramycin sulfate is an aminoglycoside antibiotic.
* It has actions and uses similar to gentamicin and is used particularly in the treatment of pseudo-monal infections.
* Dose is calculated on the basis of renal function (as it is almost completely renally excreted) and bodyweight. However, tobramycin is not lipophilic so the dose should be based on ideal bodyweight (IBW) rather than actual body weight (ABW). Some authorities recommend using a 'dosing weight' calculated by adding IBW to 40% of the difference between ABW and IBW. Whichever method is employed, it is important to check these criteria to avoid overdosing, e.g. in short, obese individuals with impaired renal function.
* Doses are expressed in terms of the base:
  Tobramycin 40 mg ≡ 60 mg of tobramycin sulfate.

## Pre-treatment checks

* Do not give in myasthenia gravis.
* Ensure good hydration status (dehydration ↑risk of toxicity).

*Biochemical and other tests*

Baseline check of auditory and vestibular function

Bodyweight and possibly height if patient over-weight

Electrolytes: serum Na, K (Mg, Ca if long term)

FBC

Renal function: U, Cr, Cr Cl (or eGFR)

## Dose

To avoid excessive dosing, doses should be calculated on the basis of ideal bodyweight (IBW) in obese patients. (See Appendix 10.)

**Serious infections:** give every 8 hours by IM or IV injection or IV infusion to provide a total daily dose of 3 mg/kg/day.
**Life-threatening infections:** give every 6–8 hours by IM or IV injection or IV infusion to provide a total daily dose of 5 mg/kg/day. This should be reduced to 3 mg/kg/day as soon as clinically indicated.
**Cystic fibrosis:** give every 6–8 hours by IM or IV injection or IV infusion to provide a total daily dose of up to 8–10 mg/kg/day if required.
**Urinary tract infection:** 2–3 mg/kg daily by IM injection.
**Dose in renal impairment:** a loading dose of 1 mg/kg is given then doses are adjusted according to creatinine clearance and IBW. Either the dose interval can be adjusted (Table T4) or a reduced dose may be given every 8 hours (Table T5).

**Table T4**  Dose frequency adjustment of tobramycin in renal impairment

| Normal dose at prolonged interval: | IBW 50–60 kg: dose is 60 mg<br>IBW 60–80 kg: dose is 80 mg |
|---|---|
| **Creatinine clearance (mL/minute)** | **Dose frequency** |
| >70 | Every 8 hours |
| 40 to 69 | Every 12 hours |
| 20 to 39 | Every 18 hours |
| 10 to 19 | Every 24 hours |
| 5 to 9 | Every 36 hours |
| <4 | Every 48 hours (when dialysis not performed) |

**Table T5**  Dose adjustment of tobramycin in renal impairment

| Creatinine clearance (mL/minute) | Adjusted dose (mg) at 8 hourly intervals | |
|---|---|---|
| | **IBW 50–60 kg** | **IBW 60–80 kg** |
| >70 | 60 | 80 |
| 40 to 69 | 30-60 | 50-80 |
| 20 to 39 | 20-25 | 30-45 |
| 10 to 19 | 10-18 | 15-24 |
| 5 to 9 | 5-9 | 7-12 |
| <4 | 2.5-4.5 | 3.5-6 |

## Intramuscular injection

*Preparation and administration*

1. Withdraw the required dose.
2. Give by deep IM injection.

## Intermittent intravenous infusion

*Preparation and administration*

If used in combination with a penicillin or cephalosporin, preferably administer at a different site. If this is not possible then flush the line thoroughly with a compatible solution between drugs.

1. Withdraw the required dose and add to 50–100 mL of a NaCl 0.9% or Gluc 5%.
2. The solution should be clear and colourless. Inspect visually for particulate matter or discoloration prior to administration and discard if present.
3. Give by IV infusion over 20–60 minutes.

## Intravenous injection

*Preparation and administration*

If used in combination with a penicillin or cephalosporin, preferably administer at a different site. If this is not possible then flush the line thoroughly with a compatible solution between drugs.

1. Withdraw the required dose.
2. The solution should be clear and colourless. Inspect visually for particulate matter or discoloration prior to administration and discard if present.
3. Give by IV injection over 3–5 minutes. May be diluted to 10 mL with NaCl 0.9% or Gluc 5% to facilitate slow administration.

## Technical information

| | |
|---|---|
| Incompatible with | Administer at different sites and times from penicillins and cephalosporins. Amphotericin, drotrecogin alfa, heparin sodium, propofol. |
| Compatible with | **Flush**: NaCl 0.9%<br>**Solutions**: NaCl 0.9%, Gluc 5%, Gluc-NaCl, Hartmann's, Ringer's<br>**Y-site**: Aciclovir, calcium gluconate, ciprofloxacin, cisatracurium, clindamycin, fluconazole, foscarnet, furosemide, granisetron, labetalol, linezolid, magnesium sulfate, metronidazole, midazolam, ranitidine, remifentanil, tigecycline, verapamil |
| pH | 3.5-6.5 |
| Sodium content | Negligible |
| Excipients | Contains sulfites (may cause allergic reactions). |
| Storage | Store below 25°C in original packaging. |
| Stability after preparation | From a microbiological point of view, should be used immediately; however, prepared infusions may be stored at 2-8°C and infused (at room temperature) within 24 hours. |

## Monitoring

| Measure | Frequency | Rationale |
|---|---|---|
| Tobramycin serum concentration. For meaningful interpretation of results the laboratory request form must state the time the previous dose was given and the time the blood sample was taken | See right-hand column for details of first measurement, then twice weekly in normal renal function; more frequently if renal function is impaired | • The first measurements should be made around the third dose.<br>• A trough level is taken just before the dose and should be <2 mg/L.<br>• A peak level is taken 30 minutes after IV injection (60 minutes after IM injection) and should be ≤12 mg/L (the BNF suggests ≤10 mg/L). |
| U&Es | Twice weekly in normal renal function; more frequently if renal function is impaired | • Tobramycin is nephrotoxic (rarely this may develop after the drug has been discontinued).<br>• ↑Cr may indicated toxicity and require a reduction in dose.<br>• ↓Na and ↓K have been reported. |
| Vestibular and auditory function | Daily (if possible serial audiograms should be obtained in patients old enough to be tested) | • Ototoxicity is a potential effect of overexposure to tobramycin. Partial or total irreversible bilateral deafness may continue to develop after the drug has been discontinued.<br>• Check that there is no deterioration of balance or hearing - it there is this may be indicative of toxic levels. |
| FBC | Periodically | • WCC: for signs of the infection resolving.<br>• Blood dyscrasias reported rarely. |
| Urinalysis | | • To detect signs of renal damage: proteinuria, cells or casts. |
| LFTs | | • ↑AST, ↑ALT and ↑bilirubin have been reported. |
| Serum calcium and magnesium | Occasionally if prolonged therapy | • ↓Mg and ↓Ca have been reported. |
| Signs of supra-infection or superinfection | Throughout treatment | • May result in the overgrowth of non-susceptible organisms - appropriate therapy should be commenced; treatment may need to be interrupted. |

## Additional information

| | |
|---|---|
| Common and serious undesirable effects | *Injection/infusion-related:* Local: Pain at injection site.<br>*Other:* Dizziness, vertigo, tinnitus, roaring in the ears, hearing loss, fever, rash, itching, urticaria, nausea, vomiting, headache, lethargy, mental confusion, disorientation. |
| Pharmacokinetics | Elimination half-life is 2-3 hours (5-70 hours in renal impairment). |

(continued)

| **Additional information** (*continued*) | |
|---|---|
| Significant interactions | • Tobramycin may ↑risk of nephrotoxicity with the following drugs: ciclosporin, platinum compounds, tacrolimus.<br>• Tobramycin may ↑levels or effect of the following drugs (or ↑side-effects): diuretics-loop (↑risk of ototoxicity), muscle relaxants-non depolarising, suxamethonium.<br>• Tobramycin may ↓levels or effect of the following drugs: neostigmine, pyridostigmine. |
| Action in case of overdose | Haemodialysis or peritoneal dialysis will help remove tobramycin from the blood. IV calcium salts have been used to counter neuromuscular blockade. |

| Risk rating: **AMBER** | Score = 3<br>Moderate-risk product: Risk-reduction strategies are recommended. |
|---|---|

This assessment is based on the full range of preparation and administration options described in the monograph. These may not all be applicable in some clinical situations.

## Bibliography

SPC Tobramycin 40 mg/mL injection, Hospira UK Ltd (accessed 5 March 2010).

# Tramadol hydrochloride

**50 mg/mL solution in 2-mL ampoules**

* Tramadol hydrochloride is an opioid analgesic that also enhances serotonergic and adrenergic pathways, adding to its analgesic effect.
* It is used to treat and prevent moderate to severe pain. It has fewer opioid side-effects than other opioids and a lower potential for addiction.
* It is sometimes used as an alternative to pethidine for patient-controlled analgesia in morphine-intolerant patients.
* Tramadol may precipitate serotonin syndrome when used with other serotonergic drugs.

## Pre-treatment checks

* Do not use in uncontrolled epilepsy; acute porphyria.
* Caution in impaired consciousness and excessive bronchial secretions.
* Not suitable as a substitute in opioid-dependent patients.

*Biochemical and other tests*

LFTs
Renal function: U, Cr, CrCl (or eGFR)

## Dose

**Pain:** 50–100 mg by IM or IV injection every 4–6 hours.

**Postoperative pain:** 100 mg initially then 50 mg every 10–20 minutes when needed during the first hour (to maximum total 250 mg including initial dose), then 50–100 mg every 4–6 hours (to maximum 600 mg daily).

**Dose in renal impairment:** doses should be adjusted according to creatinine clearance:[1]

* CrCl 10–20 mL/minute: 50–100 mg every 8–12 hours.
* CrCl <10 mL/minute: 50 mg every 8–12 hours.

**Dose in severe hepatic impairment:** dose interval should be 12-hourly (or avoid tramadol).

### Intramuscular injection

*Preparation and administration*

1. Withdraw the required dose.
2. Give by deep IM injection.
3. Close monitoring of respiratory rate and consciousness is recommended for 30 minutes in patients receiving an initial dose, especially elderly patients or those of low bodyweight.

### Intravenous injection

*Preparation and administration*

1. Withdraw the required dose.
2. The solution should be clear and colourless. Inspect visually for particulate matter or discoloration prior to administration and discard if present.
3. Give by IV injection over at least 2–3 minutes (rapid IV administration ↑risk of adverse effects).
4. Close monitoring of respiratory rate and is consciousness recommended for 30 minutes in patients receiving an initial dose, especially elderly patients or those of low bodyweight.

### Patient-controlled analgesia[2]

Strength used may vary depending on local policies.

*Preparation and administration*

1. Make 500 mg (10 mL) tramadol up to 50 mL with NaCl 0.9% in a PCA syringe to give a solution containing 10 mg/mL.
2. The solution should be clear and colourless. Inspect visually for particulate matter or discoloration prior to administration and discard if present.
3. The usual setting for the PCA device is to deliver a 5-mg bolus with a 5-minute lock-out period. Lower doses are used in patients with renal failure.

### Continuous or intermittent intravenous infusion

*Preparation and administration*

1. Withdraw the required dose and add to a suitable volume of compatible infusion fluid (usually NaCl 0.9% or Gluc 5%).
2. The solution should be clear and colourless. Inspect visually for particulate matter or discoloration prior to administration and discard if present.
3. Give by continuous or intermittent IV infusion at a suitable rate via a volumetric infusion device.
4. Close monitoring of respiratory rate and consciousness is recommended for 30 minutes in patients receiving an initial dose, especially elderly patients or those of low bodyweight.

## Technical information

| | |
|---|---|
| Incompatible with | Aciclovir, clindamycin, heparin sodium. |
| Compatible with | **Flush**: NaCl 0.9%<br>**Solutions**: NaCl 0.9%, Gluc 5%, Gluc-NaCl, Hartmann's<br>**Y-site**: Dexamethasone sodium phosphate, metoclopramide, ondansetron, ranitidine |
| pH | 6-7 |
| Sodium content | Negligible |
| Storage | Store below 30°C in original packaging. |
| Stability after preparation | From a microbiological point of view, should be used immediately; however, prepared infusions may be stored at 2-8°C and infused (at room temperature) within 24 hours. |

## Monitoring

Close monitoring of respiratory rate and consciousness is recommended for 30 minutes in patients receiving an initial dose, especially elderly patients or those of low bodyweight.

| Measure | Frequency | Rationale |
|---|---|---|
| Pain | At regular intervals | • To ensure therapeutic response. |
| Blood pressure, heart rate and respiratory rate | | • ↓BP, ↓pulse, ↑pulse, palpitations and respiratory depression can occur, especially at higher doses.<br>• Rarely bronchospasm, dyspnoea or wheezing may occur. |
| Signs of serotonin syndrome | Throughout treatment | • Symptoms include: confusion, restlessness, fever, shivering, sweating, ataxia, exaggerated reflexes, muscle spasms and diarrhoea. |
| FBC | If prolonged use | • Tramadol can rarely cause blood disorders. |

## Additional information

| | |
|---|---|
| Common and serious undesirable effects | *Common:* Nausea and vomiting (particularly initially), constipation (to a lesser extent than other opioids), dry mouth, urticaria, pruritus, biliary spasm, ↑ or ↓pulse, hallucinations, euphoria, drowsiness, serotonin syndrome (see monitoring above).<br>*At higher doses:* ↓BP, sedation, respiratory depression, muscle rigidity. |
| Pharmacokinetics | Half-life is 5-6 hours (after IV administration) |
| Significant interactions | • The following may ↑tramadol levels or effect (or ↑side-effects): antidepressants-SSRI (↑risk of CNS toxicity), antidepressants-tricyclic (↑risk of CNS toxicity), antihistamines-sedating (↑sedation), MAOIs (avoid combination and for 2 weeks after stopping MAOI), moclobemide.<br>• Tramadol may ↑levels or effect of the following drugs (or ↑side-effects): acenocoumarol (monitor INR), sodium oxybate (avoid combination), warfarin (monitor INR). |

*(continued)*

| **Additional information** (*continued*) | |
|---|---|
| Action in case of overdose | *Symptoms to watch for:* ↑Sedation, respiratory depression.<br>*Antidote:* Naloxone (see the Naloxone monograph).<br>Stop administration and give supportive therapy as appropriate. |
| Counselling | May cause drowsiness, which may affect the ability to perform skilled tasks; if affected do not drive or operate machinery, avoid alcoholic drink (effects of alcohol enhanced).<br>Inform your doctor if you have epilepsy or a history of seizures.<br>Inform the patient of possible side-effects: see above.<br>Drink plenty of fluids to help avoid constipation. |

| Risk rating: **GREEN** | Score = 2<br>Moderate-risk product: Risk-reduction strategies are recommended. |
|---|---|

This assessment is based on IV or IM intermittent dosing (not PCA). This may not all be applicable in some clinical situations.

## References

1. Ashley C, Currie A, eds. *The Renal Drug Handbook*, 3rd edn. Oxford: Radcliffe Medical Press, 2009.
2. Walder B *et al.* Efficacy and safety of patient controlled opioid analgesia for acute postoperative pain. *Acta Anaesthesiol Scand* 2001; 45: 795–804.

## Bibliography

SPC Zydol (accessed 31 December 2009).

# Tranexamic acid

### 100 mg/mL solution in 5-mL ampoules

* Tranexamic acid is an antifibrinolytic agent that primarily acts by blocking the binding of plasminogen and plasmin to fibrin, inhibiting the breakdown of fibrin clots.
* It is used to prevent or treat bleeding associated with excessive fibrin breakdown, e.g. in prostatectomy, bladder surgery and dental surgery in patients with haemophilia; it is also used in the management of menorrhagia.
* It is used in haemorrhagic complications associated with thrombolytic therapy.
* It is also licensed for use in haemorrhage associated with DIC where activation of the fibrinolytic system predominates (see Pre-treatment checks below). It should not be used if activation of the coagulation system predominates.

## Pre-treatment checks

* Do not use if there is a history of thromboembolic disease.
* Caution in haematuria (clots formed in the renal system can lead to obstructive renal impairment).

- In DIC confirm predominant activation of the fibrinolytic system by checking haematological profile (prolonged prothrombin time; reduced euglobulin clot lysis time; reduced plasma fibrinogen, factor V, factor VIII, plasminogen and alpha-2 macroglobulin levels; normal plasma P and P complex levels; ↑plasma levels of fibrinogen degradation products; normal platelet count) assuming that the underlying disease state has not modified the elements of this profile.

*Biochemical and other tests (not all are necessary in an emergency situation*

Renal function: U, Cr, CrCl (or eGFR)

## Dose

**Local fibrinolysis**: 500 mg–1 g by IV injection three times daily. If IV treatment is likely to be required for more than 3 days, 25–50 mg/kg/day may be given by continuous IV infusion.
**Disseminated intravascular coagulation with predominant activation of fibrinolytic system:** 1 g by IV injection is usually sufficient to control bleeding, and maintain a reduced fibrinolytic level of activity for around 4 hours in normal renal function. Anticoagulation with heparin should be commenced to prevent further deposition of fibrin.
**Neutralisation of thrombolytic therapy**: 10 mg/kg bodyweight by slow IV injection.
**Dose in renal impairment**: adjusted according to creatinine clearance:[1]
- CrCl >20–50 mL/minute: 10 mg/kg every 12 hours.
- CrCl 10–20 mL/minute: 10 mg/kg every 12–24 hours.
- CrCl <10 mL/minute: 5 mg/kg every 12–24 hours.

## Intravenous injection (preferred method)

*Preparation and administration*

1. Withdraw the required dose.
2. The solution should be clear and colourless. Inspect visually for particulate matter or discoloration prior to administration and discard if present.
3. Give by IV injection at a rate of 1 mL/minute (100 mg/minute).

## Continuous intravenous infusion (longer duration of therapy)

*Preparation and administration*

1. Withdraw the required dose and add to a convenient volume of compatible infusion fluid. Mix well.
2. The solution should be clear and colourless. Inspect visually for particulate matter or discoloration prior to administration and discard if present.
3. Give by IV infusion at a dose of 25–50 mg/kg/day. Prepare a new infusion bag every 24 hours as required.

| Technical information | |
|---|---|
| Incompatible with | Benzylpenicillin |
| Compatible with | **Flush**: NaCl 0.9%<br>**Solutions**: NaCl 0.9%, Gluc 5%, Ringer's<br>**Y-site**: No information |
| pH | 6.5–8.0 |
| Sodium content | Nil |
| Storage | Store below 30°C in original packaging. |
| Stability after preparation | Use prepared infusions immediately and infuse within 24 hours. |

## Monitoring

| Measure | Frequency | Rationale |
|---------|-----------|-----------|
| Blood pressure | During injection or if symptomatic during infusion | • Rapid injection of tranexamic acid is known to cause ↓BP. |
| Renal function and LFTs | Periodically | • Monitor trends in renal function if impairment is suspected, as the dose may need to be reduced.<br>• Monitoring of LFTs is recommended for long-term therapy. |
| Occurrence/severity of bleeding | Throughout treatment | • Monitor the effectiveness of antifibrinolytic therapy. |
| Colour vision | | • Reported disturbances mainly on prolonged therapy.<br>• Discontinue immediately disturbance occurs.<br>• Recommendations regarding regular full eye examinations while on long term therapy are based on unsatisfactory evidence. |

## Additional information

| | |
|---|---|
| Common and serious undesirable effects | *Injection-related:* Too rapid administration: ↓BP, dizziness.<br>*Other:* Nausea, vomiting, diarrhoea, hypersensitivity-linked skin reactions, rarely thromboembolic events, disturbances in colour vision (usually following long-term therapy – discontinue). |
| Pharmacokinetics | Elimination half-life is 2 hours. |
| Significant interactions | No significant interactions known. |
| Action in case of overdose | Stop administration and give supportive therapy as appropriate. |

| Risk rating: **GREEN** | Score = 1<br>Lower-risk product: Risk-reduction strategies should be considered. |
|---|---|

This assessment is based on the full range of preparation and administration options described in the monograph. These may not all be applicable in some clinical situations.

## Reference

1. Ashley C, Currie A, eds. *The Renal Drug Handbook*, 3rd edn. Oxford: Radcliffe Medical Press, 2009.

## Bibliography

SPC Cyklokapron injection (accessed 14 May 2009).

# Triamcinolone

**40 mg/mL aqueous suspension in 1-ml vials; 1-mL and 2-mL pre-filled syringes**
**10 mg/mL aqueous suspension in 1-mL ampoules and 5-mL vials**

* Triamcinolone acetonide is a corticosteroid with mainly glucocorticoid activity.
* It is used in the treatment of conditions for which systemic corticosteroid therapy is indicated (except adrenal-deficiency states). Deep IM injections have a depot effect and may provide cover for several weeks.
* It may also be given by intra-articular, intrasynovial or intralesional injection for various inflammatory conditions.
* Doses for injection are expressed triamcinolone acetonide.

## Pre-treatment checks

* Avoid where systemic infection is present (unless specific therapy given).
* Avoid live virus vaccines in those receiving immunosuppressive doses.
* May activate or exacerbate amoebiasis or strongyloidiasis (exclude before initiating a corticosteroid in those at risk or with suggestive symptoms). Fungal or viral ocular infections may also be exacerbated.
* Caution in patients predisposed to psychiatric reactions, including those who have previously suffered corticosteroid-induced psychosis, or who have a personal or family history of psychiatric disorders.

*Intra-articular:*
* Do not inject into unstable joints.
* Do not give in the presence of active infection in or near joints.

## Dose

**Intramuscular:** initially 40 mg repeated at intervals according to patient response, maximum single dose 100 mg. Patients with hay fever may gain remission of symptoms lasting throughout the season after a single 40–100-mg dose.

**Intra-articular or intrasynovial or intradermal injection:** large joints: up to 40 mg; small joints: 2.5–10 mg; multiple joint involvement: up to a total of 80 mg; intradermal: 2–3 mg depending on the size of the lesion and using the 10 mg/mL strength. No more than 5 mg should be injected at any one site. If several sites are injected the total dose should not exceed 30 mg and multiple sites should be 1 cm or more apart. The injection may be repeated at 1- to 2-week intervals.

## Intramuscular injection

*Preparation and administration*

1. Shake vial well before withdrawing medication. If clumping occurs, do not use.
2. Withdraw the required dose.
3. Give by IM injection deep into the upper outer quadrant of the gluteal muscle (avoid the deltoid). Use alternate sides for subsequent injections.

## Other routes

*Preparation and administration*

1. Shake vial well before withdrawing the medication. If clumping occurs, do not use.
2. Withdraw the required dose.
3. Remove the IM needle that comes with the pre-filled syringe and replace with a needle appropriate to the planned route.
4. Inject into the affected area.
* In tenosynovitis care should be taken to inject into the tendon sheath rather than into the substance of the tendon. For short tendons the 10 mg/mL strength should be used.
* After intra-articular injections treatment failure is usually the result of not entering the joint space.

## Technical information

| | |
|---|---|
| Incompatible with | Not relevant |
| Compatible with | Not relevant |
| pH | Not relevant |
| Sodium content | Negligible |
| Excipients | Both preparations contain benzyl alcohol. |
| Storage | Store below 25°C in an upright position in original packaging. Do not freeze. |

## Monitoring (dependent on dose and site of injection)

| Measure | Frequency | Rationale |
|---|---|---|
| Serum Na, K, Ca | Throughout systemic treatment | • May cause fluid and electrolyte disturbances. |
| Withdrawal symptoms and signs | During withdrawal and after stopping systemic treatment | • During prolonged therapy with corticosteroids, adrenal atrophy develops and can persist for years after stopping. Abrupt withdrawal after a prolonged period can lead to acute adrenal insufficiency, ↓BP or death.<br>• The CSM has recommended that gradual withdrawal of systemic corticosteroids should be considered in patients whose disease is unlikely to relapse. In the UK full details can be found in the BNF. |
| Signs of infection | During systemic treatment | • Prolonged courses ↑susceptibility to infections and severity of infections. Serious infections may reach an advanced stage before being recognised. |
| Signs of chickenpox | | • Unless they have had chickenpox, patients receiving corticosteroids for purposes other than replacement should be regarded as being at risk of severe chickenpox.<br>• Confirmed chickenpox requires urgent treatment; corticosteroids should not be stopped and dosage may need to be increased. |
| Exposure to measles | | • Patients should be advised to take particular care to avoid exposure to measles and to seek immediate medical advice if exposure occurs.<br>• Prophylaxis with IM normal immunoglobulin may be needed. |
| Symptoms of septic arthritis | Following intra-articular injection | • A marked increase in pain accompanied by local swelling, further restriction of joint motion, fever, and malaise are suggestive of septic arthritis. |

## Additional information

| | |
|---|---|
| Common and serious undesirable effects | *Injection-related:*<br>• IM and intradermal: Severe local pain, sterile abscess, cutaneous and subcutaneous atrophy, hyper/hypopigmentation.<br>• Intra-articular: Transient pain, sterile abscess, hyper/hypopigmentation, Charcot-like arthropathy and occasional increase in joint discomfort.<br><br>*Short-term use:* Undesirable effects which may result from short-term use (minimise by using the lowest effective dose for the shortest time): ↑BP, Na and water retention, ↓K, ↓Ca, ↑blood glucose, peptic ulceration and perforation, psychiatric reactions, ↑susceptibility to infection, muscle weakness, tendon rupture, insomnia, ↑intracranial pressure, ↓seizure threshold, impaired healing.<br>*Long-term use:* In the UK for undesirable effects resulting from long-term corticosteroid use refer to the BNF. |
| Pharmacokinetics | Elimination half-life is 2-5 or more hours (biological half-life of 12-36 hours). |
| Significant interactions | • The following may ↓corticosteroid levels or effect:<br>barbiturates, carbamazepine, phenytoin, primidone, rifabutin, rifampicin.<br>• Corticosteroids may ↑levels or effect of the following drugs (or ↑side-effects): anticoagulants (monitor INR), methotrexate (↑risk of blood dyscrasias). If using amphotericin IV monitor fluid balance and K level closely.<br>• Corticosteroids may ↓levels or effect of vaccines (↓immunological response, ↑risk of infection with live vaccines). |
| Action in case of overdose | Give supportive therapy as appropriate. Following chronic overdose the possibility of adrenal suppression should be considered. |
| Counselling | Patients on long-term corticosteroid treatment should read and carry a Steroid Treatment Card.<br>Patients should be specifically warned to avoid overuse of joints in which symptomatic benefit has been obtained.<br>Severe joint destruction with necrosis of bone may occur if repeated intra-articular injections are given over a long period of time.<br>Repeated injection into inflamed tendons should be avoided as this has been shown to cause tendon rupture. |

| | |
|---|---|
| Risk rating: **GREEN** | Score = 2<br>Lower-risk product: Risk-reduction strategies should be considered. |

This assessment is based on the full range of preparation and administration options described in the monograph. These may not all be applicable in some clinical situations.

## Bibliography

SPC Kenalog intra-articular/intramuscular injection (accessed 14 May 2009).
SPC Adcortyl intra-articular/intradermal injection 10 mg/mL (accessed 14 May 2009).

# Triptorelin

**3-mg and 11.25-mg (Decapeptyl SR); 3.75-mg (Gonapeptyl Depot) dry powder preparations with solvent**

* Triptorelin acetate is an analogue of gonadorelin.
* It is used for the suppression of testosterone in the treatment of prostate cancer as an alternative to surgical castration.
* It is also licensed for use in the treatment of endometriosis, female infertility and uterine fibroids and in precocious puberty.
* Doses are expressed in terms of the base:
  Triptorelin 1 mg ≡ 1.05 mg triptorelin acetate.

## Pre-treatment checks

Caution in osteoporosis (or those at risk: i.e. chronic alcohol and/or tobacco use, strong family history of osteoporosis, or chronic use of drugs that can ↓BMD, e.g. anticonvulsants or corticosteroids).

*Biochemical and other tests*

Blood pressure
Pregnancy test (in endometriosis)

Testosterone level (in prostate cancer)
Consider BMD if treatment is to be prolonged

## Dose

**Prostate cancer:**
* *Decapeptyl SR:* 3 mg by IM injection every 4 weeks, or 11.25 mg by IM injection every 12 weeks.
* *Gonapeptyl Depot:* 3.75 mg by SC or IM injection every 4 weeks.
An anti-androgen agent may be given for 3 days before until 2–3 weeks after commencement of either therapy to ↓risk of disease flare, e.g. cyproterone acetate 100 mg three times daily.

**Endometriosis:** initiate treatment in the first 5 days of the menstrual cycle.
* *Decapeptyl SR:* 3 mg by IM injection every 4 weeks, or 11.25 mg by IM injection every 12 weeks for a maximum of 6 months.
* *Gonapeptyl Depot:* 3.75 mg by SC or IM injection every 4 weeks for a maximum of 6 months.

**Uterine fibroids:** initiate treatment in the first 5 days of the menstrual cycle.
* *Decapeptyl SR:* 3 mg by IM injection every 4 weeks for a minimum of 3 months and a maximum of 6 months.
* *Gonapeptyl Depot:* 3.75 mg by SC or IM injection every 4 weeks for a maximum of 6 months.

## Intramuscular injection (Decapeptyl SR)

*Preparation and administration*

1. Draw the solvent provided into the syringe using the pink needle and transfer into the powder vial. Do not remove the needle from the vial.
2. Shake the vial gently to produce a homogeneous mixture (make sure any clumps are dispersed) then draw the mixture back into the syringe without inverting the vial. The small amount of suspension left in the vial should be discarded as the vials contain an overage to allow the prescribed dose to be given.
3. Attach the green needle provided and give by IM injection into the gluteal muscle. Rotate injection sites for subsequent injections.

## Intramuscular or subcutaneous injection (Gonapeptyl Depot)

*Preparation and administration*

1. Remove the cap from the syringe containing the powder, keeping it upright to prevent spillage.
2. Without removing the connector from the packaging, screw the syringe containing the powder onto the connector and then remove it from the package.
3. Screw the syringe containing the solvent tightly onto the free end of the connector and empty the solvent into the syringe with the powder.
4. Shoot it back and forth between the two syringes (the first 2–3 times without pushing the injection rod all the way in). Repeat this about 10 times or until the suspension is homogeneous and milky.
5. If foam is produced, dissolve it or remove it from the syringe before giving the injection.
6. Attach the injection needle on to the syringe and give by SC injection (abdomen, buttock or thigh) or by deep IM injection. Rotate injection sites for subsequent injections.

## Technical information

| | |
|---|---|
| Incompatible with | Not relevant |
| Compatible with | Not relevant |
| pH | Not relevant |
| Sodium content | Nil (Decapeptyl SR). Negligible (Gonapeptyl Depot). |
| Storage | Decapeptyl SR: Store below 25°C in original packaging. Gonapeptyl depot: Store at 2-8°C in original packaging. |
| Stability after preparation | All presentations are intended for single use only, and should be given immediately after reconstitution. |

## Monitoring

| Measure | Frequency | Rationale |
|---|---|---|
| Prostate-specific antigen (PSA) and testosterone plasma levels | Periodically | • Monitored during treatment to assess efficacy.<br>• Testosterone levels should not exceed 1 nanogram/mL. |
| Blood pressure | | • ↓BP or ↑BP can occur (rarely) and may require medical intervention or withdrawal of treatment. |
| Plasma estradiol levels | If metrorrhagia occurs (other than in first month) | • If level is <50 picograms/mL possible associated organic lesions should be sought. |
| Bone mineral density | Consider if treatment is prolonged | • May lead to bone loss that enhances the risk of osteoporosis. |

## Additional information

| | |
|---|---|
| Common and serious undesirable effects | *Injection-related:* Transient pain, redness or local inflammation at the injection site.<br>*Other:* Hypersensitivity reactions; depressive mood; irritation; nausea; myalgia; arthralgia; tiredness; sleep disturbances; gynaecomastia; headache; perspiration.<br>*In men:* Hot flushes, ↓libido and impotence, ↑bone pain, worsening of genitourinary obstruction symptoms (haematuria, urinary disorders) and/or worsening of neurological signs of vertebral metastases (back pain, weakness or paraesthesia of the lower limbs). These often occur from the initial and transient increase in plasma testosterone and usually disappear in 1-2 weeks.<br>*In women:* Hot flushes, sweating, sleep disturbances, headache, mood changes, vaginal dryness, dyspareunia, ↓libido, symptoms of endometriosis (pelvic pain, dysmenorrhoea). These often occur from the initial and transient increase in plasma estradiol levels and usually disappear in 1-2 weeks. |
| Pharmacokinetics | Elimination half-life is 3-7.5 hours. |
| Significant interactions | No significant interactions. |
| Action in case of overdose | There is no specific antidote and treatment should be symptomatic. |
| Counselling | In women a non-hormonal method of contraception should be used throughout treatment and until resumption of menstruation or until another contraceptive method has been established (ovarian function resumes after withdrawal of treatment and ovulation occurs on average 58 days after the last injection, with menstrual bleeding resuming 7-12 weeks after the final injection).<br>Non-hormonal, barrier methods of contraception should be used during the entire treatment period. |

| Risk rating: **GREEN** | Score = 1<br>Lower-risk product: Risk-reduction strategies should be considered. |
|---|---|

This assessment is based on the full range of preparation and administration options described in the monograph. These may not all be applicable in some clinical situations.

## Bibliography

SPC Decapeptyl SR 11.25 mg (accessed 3 April 2009).
SPC Decapeptyl SR 3 mg (accessed 3 April 2009).
SPC Gonapeptyl Depot 3.75 mg (accessed 3 April 2009).

# Urokinase

**10 000-unit, 25 000-unit, 100 000-unit dry powder vials (other strengths are available on 'special order')**
* Urokinase is a plasminogen activator enzyme produced by the kidneys. It has thrombolytic activity.
* It is licensed for the dissolution of fibrin clots in intravascular cannulas, and also for the treatment of DVT, PE and peripheral vascular occlusion.

## Pre-treatment checks

* Caution when risk of haemorrhage is increased, e.g. surgery, cerebrovascular bleeding, severe ↑BP, peptic ulcer disease/risk of GI bleeding. Also in pregnancy and the immediate postpartum period, severe hepatic or renal insufficiency unless the patient is receiving renal replacement therapy.
* Caution in patients who have had recent repeated intravascular puncture.

*Biochemical and other tests (not all are necessary in an emergency situation)*

Bodyweight (in certain indications)
LFTs – do not give in severe disease

## Dose

**Cannula occlusion:** 5000–25 000 units (see below for method). Alternatively, for cannulas at risk of fibrin occlusion, an infusion of up to 250 000 units may be given through the cannula.
**DVT/PE loading dose:** 4400 units/kg by IV infusion over 10 minutes.
**DVT/PE maintenance:** 4400 units/kg/hour by IV infusion for 12–24 hours (12 hours for PE).
**PE via pulmonary artery:** 15 000 units/kg by injection into the pulmonary artery repeated up to three times in 24 hours. The dose is adjusted depending on the plasma fibrinogen concentration produced by the previous injection.
**Peripheral vascular occlusion:** see product literature for details.

## Clearance of occluded intravenous cannulas

*Preparation and administration*

1. Check that you have selected the correct strength of vial.
2. Determine the volume of NaCl 0.9% required to fill the lumen and use this to dissolve the vial contents (as little as 0.5 mL is sufficient).
3. Withdraw the required quantity of urokinase and mix with a further volume of NaCl 0.9% if necessary to make up to the required volume.
4. The solution should be clear and colourless. Inspect visually for particulate matter or discoloration prior to administration and discard if present.
5. Aspirate the cannula then instil the solution and cap for 20–60 minutes (up to 4 hours may be necessary in some cases).
6. Aspirate the cannula and repeat if necessary.

## Cannula infusion

*Preparation and administration*

Check that you have selected the correct strength of vial(s).
Urokinase is incompatible with Gluc solutions.

1. Reconstitute each vial with 2 mL NaCl 0.9% and shake gently to dissolve the powder.
2. Withdraw the required quantity of urokinase and add to a suitable volume of NaCl 0.9% to give a solution containing 1000–2500 units/mL.
3. The solution should be clear and colourless. Inspect visually for particulate matter or discoloration prior to administration and discard if present.
4. Infuse through the affected cannula over 90–180 minutes.

## Intravenous infusion (loading dose)

*Preparation and administration*

> Check that you have selected the correct strength of vial(s).
> Urokinase is incompatible with Gluc solutions.

1. Reconstitute each vial with 2 mL NaCl 0.9% and shake gently to dissolve the powder.
2. Withdraw the required dose and make up to a final volume of 15 mL with NaCl 0.9%.
3. The solution should be clear and colourless. Inspect visually for particulate matter or discoloration prior to administration and discard if present
4. Give by IV infusion over 10 minutes.

## Continuous intravenous infusion via a syringe pump

*Preparation and administration*

> Check that you have selected the correct strength of vial(s)
> Urokinase is incompatible with Gluc solutions.

1. Reconstitute each vial with 2 mL NaCl 0.9% and shake gently to dissolve the powder.
2. Withdraw the required dose and make up to a suitable volume with NaCl 0.9% in a syringe pump.
3. Cap the syringe and mix well.
4. The solution should be clear and colourless. Inspect visually for particulate matter or discoloration prior to administration and discard if present.
5. Give by IV infusion at a rate appropriate to the indication.

## Intra-arterial use

*Preparation*

As for IV use.

| Technical information | |
|---|---|
| Incompatible with | Urokinase is incompatible with Gluc solutions. |
| Compatible with | **Flush**: NaCl 0.9%<br>**Solutions**: NaCl 0.9%<br>**Y-site**: No information but likely to be unstable |
| pH | 6–7.5 |
| Sodium content | Negligible |
| Storage | Store below 25°C in original packaging. |

*(continued)*

## Technical information (*continued*)

| | |
|---|---|
| Displacement value | Negligible |
| Stability after preparation | Use reconstituted vials and prepared infusions immediately. |

## Monitoring

| Measure | Frequency | Rationale |
|---|---|---|
| Haemorrhage | Continuously | • Risk of bleeding. |
| Angiogram in peripheral arterial thromboembolism | 2-hourly | • Assessment of response to therapy. |

## Additional information

| | |
|---|---|
| Common and serious undesirable effects | *Immediate:* Allergic reactions including bronchospasm have been reported.<br>*Injection/infusion-related:* sensations of warmth, dull ache or pain may be felt in the vessel being treated.<br>*Other:* Bleeding, pyrexia and haematuria have rarely been reported. Embolic episodes following release of clot fragments, cholesterol embolism. |
| Pharmacokinetics | Elimination half-life is up to 20 minutes; increased in renal/hepatic impairment. |
| Significant interactions | • The following may ↑risk of haemorrhage with urokinase: anticoagulants, heparins, antiplatelet agents, e.g. aspirin, clopidogrel, dipyridamole. |
| Action in case of overdose | *Symptoms to watch for:* Severe bleeding.<br>*Antidote:* No specific antidote. Stop administration and give supportive therapy as appropriate including fresh frozen plasma, fresh blood and tranexamic acid if necessary. Avoid the use of dextrans. |
| Counselling | Report any bleeding.<br>Local sensations of warmth, dull ache or pain may be felt locally in the vessel being treated. |

| Risk rating: **RED** | Score = 7<br>High-risk product. Risk-reduction strategies are required to minimise these risks. |
|---|---|

This assessment is based on the full range of preparation and administration options described in the monograph. These may not all be applicable in some clinical situations.

## Bibliography

SPC Syner-KINASE 10,000 IU, 25,000 IU, 100,000 IU, 250,000 IU, 500,000 IU, 1,000,000 IU (accessed 2 April 2010).

# Vancomycin

**500-mg, 1-g dry powder vials**

- Vancomycin hydrochloride is a glycopeptide antibiotic.
- It is used IV in potentially life-threatening infections due to susceptible Gram-positive organisms including MRSA.
- Oral vancomycin is indicated for severe cases of antibiotic-associated pseudomembranous colitis (usually involving *Clostridium difficile*) and staphylococcal enterocolitis. The injection form may be given orally if necessary.
- Since it is not absorbed from the GI tract, vancomycin is not effective by the oral route for other types of infection.
- Vancomycin is **not** intended for IM administration.
- Doses are expressed in terms of the base:
  Vancomycin 1 g (1 000 000 IU) ≡ 1.03 g vancomycin hydrochloride.

## Pre-treatment checks

Caution in hypersensitivity to teicoplanin

*Biochemical and other tests*

Auditory function (especially if >60 years)
FBC
Renal function: U, Cr, CrCl (or eGFR)

## Dose

**Initial IV dose**: 1 g by IV infusion every 12 hours.
**Initial IV dose in elderly patients:** 500 mg every 12 hours, or 1 g every 24 hours.
**Antibiotic-associated pseudomembranous colitis (oral):** 125 mg orally every 6 hours (up to 2 g/day in severe cases) usually for 7–10 days.
**Dose in renal impairment**: initiate IV dose according to creatinine clearance then adjust according to serum vancomycin level (see *The Renal Drug Handbook* for further detail and other strategies):[1]
- CrCl >20–50 mL/minute: 500 mg–1 g every 12–24 hours.
- CrCl 10–20 mL/minute: 500 mg–1 g every 24–48 hours.
- CrCl <10 mL/minute: 500 mg–1g every 48–96 hours.
- Oral dose is as in normal renal function

## Intermittent intravenous infusion (preferred method)

*Preparation and administration*

1. Reconstitute each 500-mg vial with 10 mL WFI (use 20 mL for each 1-g vial) to give a solution containing 50 mg/mL.
2. Withdraw the required dose and add to a suitable volume of compatible infusion fluid. Each 500 mg must be added to a minimum of 100 mL.
3. The solution should be clear and colourless. Inspect visually for particulate matter or discoloration prior to administration and discard if present.
4. Give by IV infusion over a minimum of 60 minutes at a maximum rate of 10 mg/minute. To reduce the risk of 'red man' syndrome (see below) a 1-g dose is usually given over 2 hours.

**Fluid restriction:** the maximum concentration is 10 mg/mL, but ↑risk of infusion-related effects.

## Continuous intravenous infusion (use only if intermittent technique is not feasible)

*Preparation and administration*

1. Reconstitute each 500-mg vial with 10 mL WFI (use 20 mL for each 1-g vial) to give a solution containing 50 mg/mL.
2. Withdraw the total daily dose and add to a sufficiently large volume of compatible infusion fluid. Mix well.
3. The solution should be clear and colourless. Inspect visually for particulate matter or discoloration prior to administration and discard if present.
4. Give the total daily dose by IV infusion over 24 hours.

## Oral

*Preparation and administration*

1. Reconstitute each 500-mg vial with 10 mL WFI (use 20 mL for each 1-g vial) to give a solution containing 50 mg/mL.
2. Withdraw the required dose and dilute in 30 mL of water. May be mixed with common cordials immediately before administration to mask the taste.
3. Give to the patient to drink or administer via NG tube.

## Technical information

| | |
|---|---|
| Incompatible with | Aminophylline, amphotericin, ampicillin, aztreonam, cefotaxime, ceftazidime, ceftriaxone, cefuroxime, chloramphenicol sodium succinate, dexamethasone sodium phosphate, drotrecogin alfa (activated), foscarnet, heparin sodium, omeprazole, piperacillin with tazobactam, propofol, sodium bicarbonate, ticarcillin with clavulanate. |
| Compatible with | **Flush**: NaCl 0.9%<br>**Solutions**: NaCl 0.9%, Gluc 5%, Hartmann's (all including added KCl)<br>**Y-site**: Aciclovir, amikacin, atracurium, calcium gluconate, cisatracurium, clarithromycin, fluconazole, hydrocortisone sodium succinate, labetalol, levofloxacin, linezolid, magnesium sulfate, meropenem, midazolam, pantoprazole, ranitidine, remifentanil, tigecycline, vecuronium, verapamil |
| pH | 2.5–4.5 |
| Sodium content | Nil |
| Storage | Store below 25°C in original packaging. |
| Displacement value | Nil |
| Stability after preparation | From a microbiological point of view, should be used immediately, however:<br>• Reconstituted vials may be stored at 2–8°C for 24 hours.<br>• Prepared infusions may be stored at 2–8°C and infused (at room temperature) within 24 hours. |

## Monitoring

| Measure | Frequency | Rationale |
|---|---|---|
| Infusion-related reactions | Throughout infusion | • Stop the infusion if ↓BP or an erythematous rash develops.<br>• A longer infusion time or premedicating with an antihistamine may limit the reaction. |
| Temperature | Minimum daily | • For clinical signs of improvement. |
| Vancomycin serum concentration | Twice weekly in normal renal function; more frequently if renal function is impaired | • Trough level just before a dose should be 10–15 mg/L (15–20 mg/L for less sensitive strains of MRSA).<br>• Peak level 2 hours after a dose should be 30–40 mg/L.<br>• There is a trend to monitor trough levels only.<br>• For meaningful interpretation the laboratory request form must state the time of the previous dose and when the blood sample was taken. |
| Auditory and vestibular function | Daily and for several days after cessation of treatment | • Ototoxicity may occur on overexposure to vancomycin.<br>• Cease treatment if deterioration in hearing or onset of tinnitus occurs.<br>• Dizziness and vertigo have been reported occasionally. |
| Renal function | Twice weekly (more frequently in renal impairment) | • Vancomycin is nephrotoxic.<br>• ↑Cr may indicate toxicity: reduce the dose. |
| FBC | Periodically | • Reversible neutropenia occasionally occurs; rarely thrombocytopenia and eosinophilia.<br>• WCC: for signs of the infection resolving. |
| Signs of supra-infection or superinfection | Throughout treatment | • May result in the overgrowth of non-susceptible organisms - appropriate therapy should be commenced; treatment may need to be interrupted. |
| Development of diarrhoea | Throughout and up to 2 months after treatment | • Ironically, the development of severe, persistent diarrhoea during IV therapy may be suggestive of *Clostridium difficile*-associated diarrhoea and colitis (pseudomembranous colitis).<br>• Discontinue drug and treat (oral vancomycin is sometimes given concomitantly).<br>• Do not use drugs that inhibit peristalsis. |

## Additional information

| | |
|---|---|
| Common and serious undesirable effects | *Immediate:* Anaphylaxis and other hypersensitivity reactions have been reported.<br>*Injection/infusion-related:*<br>• Too rapid administration: Severe ↓BP, thrombophlebitis, flushing and a transient rash over the neck and shoulders ('red-man' or 'red-neck' syndrome).<br>• Local: Phlebitis, risk of tissue necrosis with extravasation.<br><br>*Other (after IV administration):* Nephrotoxicity, interstitial nephritis, ototoxicity, nausea, chills, fever, neutropenia (usually after 1 week or a cumulative dose of 25 g), rarely agranulocytosis and thrombocytopenia, exfoliative dermatitis, Stevens-Johnson syndrome, toxic epidermal necrolysis, vasculitis. |
| Pharmacokinetics | Elimination half-life is 4-6 hours in normal renal function (120-216 hours in haemodialysis). |
| Significant interactions | • Vancomycin may ↑levels or effect of the following drugs (or ↑side-effects):<br>ciclosporin (↑risk of nephrotoxicity), diuretics-loop (↑risk of ototoxicity), suxamethonium (↑effect). |
| Action in case of overdose | No known antidote, stop administration and give supportive therapy as appropriate. Monitor renal function. |
| Counselling | Warn the patient of its offensive taste when given orally. |

| | |
|---|---|
| Risk rating: **AMBER** | Score = 4<br>Moderate-risk product: Risk-reduction strategies are recommended. |

This assessment is based on the full range of preparation and administration options described in the monograph. These may not all be applicable in some clinical situations.

## Reference

1. Ashley C, Currie A, eds. *The Renal Drug Handbook*, 3rd edn. Oxford: Radcliffe Medical Press, 2009.

## Bibliography

SPC Vancocin powder for solution (accessed 3 April 2009).

SPC Vancomycin 500 mg & 1 g powder for solution for infusion, Wockhardt UK Ltd (accessed 3 April 2009).

SPC Vancomycin hydrochloride 500 mg and 1 g powder for concentrate for infusion, Hospira UK Ltd (accessed 3 April 2009).

# Vasopressin (antidiuretic hormone, ADH)

**20 argipressin pressor units/mL (400 micrograms/mL) solution in 1-mL ampoules**

* Vasopressin has a direct antidiuretic action on the kidney, increasing tubular reabsorption of water. It also constricts peripheral blood vessels and causes contraction of the smooth muscle of the intestine, gall bladder and urinary bladder.
* It may be used in the short-term treatment of pituitary (rather than nephrogenic) diabetes insipidus.
* It may be used to control variceal bleeding in portal hypertension prior to more definitive treatment. However, terlipressin and octreotide are now preferred treatments.
* Argipressin is a form of vasopressin obtained from most mammals including humans. Doses are usually expressed in terms of pressor units:
  Vasopressin 100 micrograms ≡ 5 argipressin pressor units.

## Pre-treatment checks

* Do not give in chronic nephritis with nitrogen retention.
* Caution in patients with hypertension and also in coronary artery disease (even small doses may precipitate anginal pain).
* If used in peripheral vascular disease the skin should be observed for signs of ischaemia.
* Caution in conditions which may be aggravated by fluid retention, e.g. epilepsy, migraine, asthma, heart failure.

*Biochemical and other tests*

Baseline plasma osmolality *or* baseline bodyweight (to enable monitoring of fluid balance)
Electrolytes: Serum Na, K

## Dose

**Diabetes insipidus:** 0.25–1 mL (5–20 units) by SC or IM injection every 4 hours. Tailor dose to allow a slight diuresis every 24 hours to avoid water intoxication.

**Variceal bleeding:** for the initial control of variceal bleeding give 1 mL (20 units) by IV infusion.

### Subcutaneous injection

*Preparation and administration*

1. Withdraw the required dose.
2. Give by SC injection.

### Intramuscular injection

*Preparation and administration*

1. Withdraw the required dose.
2. Give by IM injection.

### Intravenous infusion

*Preparation and administration*

1. Withdraw the required dose and add to 100 mL Gluc 5%.
2. The solution should be clear and colourless. Inspect visually for particulate matter or discoloration prior to administration and discard if present.
3. Give by IV infusion over 15 minutes. Monitor closely for signs of extravasation.

## Technical information

| | |
|---|---|
| Incompatible with | Furosemide, phenytoin sodium. |
| Compatible with | **Flush**: NaCl 0.9%<br>**Solutions**: Gluc 5%, NaCl 0.9%<br>**Y-site**: Adrenaline (epinephrine), ciprofloxacin, fluconazole, gentamicin, imipenem with cilastatin, linezolid, meropenem, metronidazole, noradrenaline (norepinephrine), pantoprazole, piperacillin with tazobactam, sodium bicarbonate, verapamil, voriconazole |
| pH | 2.5-4.5 |
| Sodium content | Nil |
| Storage | Store at 2-8°C. Do not freeze. |
| Stability after preparation | Use prepared infusions immediately. |

## Monitoring

| Measure | Frequency | Rationale |
|---|---|---|
| Signs of extravasation | During infusion | • Extravasation may cause tissue necrosis and gangrene. |
| Signs of hypersensitivity | During and immediately post injection | • Anaphylaxis has been observed shortly after injection. Urticaria and bronchoconstriction have also been observed. |
| Chest pain | During and post injection | • Anginal chest pain may occur in susceptible individuals.<br>• Treat with sublingual glyceryl trinitrate (but this may reverse some of the desired pressor properties of vasopressin therapy). |
| Peripheral ischaemia | | • May cause peripheral ischaemia in patients with peripheral vascular disease. Observe skin for signs of blanching, etc. |
| Fluid balance | Frequently during treatment | • Fluid overload may occur with repeated doses.<br>• Monitor fluid intake/output closely and check for fluid accumulation either by monitoring bodyweight or by determining plasma sodium or osmolality.<br>• Fluid intake must be reduced and vasopressin treatment interrupted if there is a gradual ↑bodyweight, or serum Na <130 mmol/L, or plasma osmolality <270 mOsmol/kg. |

## Additional information

| | |
|---|---|
| Common and serious undesirable effects | *Immediate:* Anaphylaxis and other hypersensitivity reactions have been reported.<br>*Injection/infusion-related:* Irritation at the injection site may occur.<br>*Other:* Tremor, sweating, vertigo, circumoral pallor, 'pounding' in the head, abdominal cramps, desire to defecate, passage of gas, nausea, vomiting, water intoxication. Peripheral vasoconstriction has rarely resulted in gangrene and thrombosis. |
| Pharmacokinetics | Vasopressin has a plasma half-life of about 10–20 minutes. Following SC or IM injection, the duration of antidiuretic activity is variable but usually 2–8 hours. |
| Significant interactions | No significant interactions. |
| Action in case of overdose | *Symptoms to watch for:* ↑Risk of water retention and/or ↓Na, i.e. water intoxication.<br>*Antidote:* No known antidote; restrict fluid intake and manage symptomatically. |

| Risk rating: **GREEN** | Score = 2<br>Lower-risk product: Risk-reduction strategies should be considered. |
|---|---|

This assessment is based on the full range of preparation and administration options described in the monograph. These may not all be applicable in some clinical situations.

## Bibliography

SPC Pitressin (received by e-mail 4 February 2009).

# Verapamil hydrochloride

### 2.5 mg/mL solution in 2-mL ampoules

- Verapamil hydrochloride is a calcium channel blocker and a class IV antiarrhythmic agent. It slows conduction through the AV node, thus reducing heart rate and cardiac output.
- It is indicated for the treatment of paroxysmal SVT and to ↓ventricular rate in atrial flutter/AF.

## Pre-treatment checks

- Do not give in cardiogenic shock, sinoatrial block, and uncompensated heart failure.

- Avoid in acute MI complicated by ↓pulse, marked ↓BP or LVF, in second- or third-degree AV block (except in patients with a functioning artificial ventricular pacemaker), and in sick sinus syndrome (except in patients with a functioning artificial ventricular pacemaker).
- Do not give in ↓pulse (<50 beats/minute) or ↓BP (<90 mmHg systolic).
- Avoid with concurrent or recent administration of an IV beta-blocker.
- Avoid if possible in patients with atrial flutter/AF in the presence of an accessory pathway (e.g. Wolff–Parkinson–White syndrome): may ↑conduction across the anomalous pathway, which may precipitate severe VT.
- Caution in first-degree AV block.

*Biochemical and other tests (not all are necessary in an emergency situation)*

Electrolytes: serum Na, K, Ca, Mg

## Dose

**Supraventricular arrhythmias**: 5–10 mg by slow IV injection.
**Paroxysmal tachyarrhythmias**: 5–10 mg by slow IV injection, followed by a further 5 mg after 5–10 minutes if required.

## Intravenous injection

*Preparation and administration*

1. Withdraw the required dose.
2. The solution should be clear and colourless. Inspect visually for particulate matter or discoloration prior to administration.
3. Give by slow IV injection over at least 2 minutes (3 minutes in elderly patients).

## Technical information

| Incompatible with | Sodium bicarbonate. Amphotericin, pantoprazole, propofol. |
|---|---|
| Compatible with | **Flush**: NaCl 0.9%<br>**Solutions**: NaCl 0.9%, Gluc 5%, (both with added KCl)<br>**Y-site**: Benzylpenicillin, bivalirudin, ciprofloxacin, clarithromycin, linezolid |
| pH | 4.5–6.5 |
| Sodium content | Negligible |
| Storage | Store below 25°C in original packaging. |

## Monitoring

| Measure | Frequency | Rationale |
|---|---|---|
| ECG | Continuously | • Response to therapy. |
| Blood pressure | | • May cause or exacerbate ↓BP. |
| Heart rate | | • May cause or exacerbate ↓pulse. |

## Additional information

| | |
|---|---|
| Common and serious undesirable effects | *Immediate:* Rarely bronchospasm with urticaria and pruritus.<br>*Other:* Seizures, transient asystole, ↓pulse, ↓BP, dizziness, headache. |
| Pharmacokinetics | Elimination half-life 2–5 hours. |
| Significant interactions | • The following may ↑verapamil levels or effect (or ↑side-effects): alpha-blockers (↑hypotensive effect), amiodarone (↑risk of ↓pulse, AV block), anaesthetics-general (↑hypotensive effect), beta-blockers (asystole, severe ↓BP, heart failure), clarithromycin, disopyramide (↑risk of asystole), erythromycin, everolimus, flecainide (↑risk of asystole), ritonavir, sirolimus.<br>• The following may ↓ verapamil levels or effect: barbiturates, primidone, rifampicin, St John's wort (avoid combination).<br>• Verapamil may ↑levels or effect of the following drugs (or ↑side-effects): carbamazepine, ciclosporin (monitor levels), digoxin (↑risk of AV block), everolimus, ivabradine (avoid combination), simvastatin (↑risk of myopathy), sirolimus, theophylline. |
| Action in case of overdose | *Symptoms to watch for:* Shock, ↓BP, ↓pulse, AV block, asystole.<br>*Antidote:* Stop administration and give supportive therapy as appropriate. This may include calcium gluconate, atropine and pacemaker therapy. |
| Counselling | Dizziness and other symptoms of ↓BP. |

| Risk rating: **GREEN** | Score = 1<br>Lower-risk product. Risk-reduction strategies should be considered. |
|---|---|

This assessment is based on the full range of preparation and administration options described in the monograph. These may not all be applicable in some clinical situations.

## Bibliography

SPC Securon IV (accessed 29 April 2009).

# Voriconazole

**200-mg dry powder vial**

• Voriconazole is a triazole antifungal and a synthetic derivative of fluconazole.
• It is used mainly in immunocompromised patients for the treatment of invasive aspergillosis, serious infections caused by *Scedosporium* spp., *Fusarium* spp., and invasive fluconazole-resistant *Candida* spp. (including *C. krusei*).

- Parenteral therapy should only be used where the oral route is unavailable; voriconazole has an oral bioavailability of 96%. The oral route is specifically preferred in ↓renal function because of potential toxicity resulting from one of the excipients of the IV form.

## Pre-treatment checks

- Do not give in acute porphyria.
- Use with caution in patients with potentially pro-arrhythmic conditions (cardiomyopathy, ↓pulse, symptomatic arrhythmias, history of QT interval prolongation, or concomitant use with other drugs that prolong QT interval), and in those at risk of pancreatitis.
- Check for specific drug interactions (many contraindications).

*Biochemical and other tests (not all are necessary in an emergency situation)*

| | |
|---|---|
| Bodyweight | FBC |
| Electrolytes: serum K, Mg, Ca (disturbances should be corrected prior to initiation of therapy) | LFTs |
| | Renal function: U, Cr, CrCl (or eGFR) |

## Dose

**Loading dose:** 6 mg/kg by IV infusion every 12 hours for 2 doses.

**Maintenance dose:** 4 mg/kg by IV infusion every 12 hours (reduced to 3 mg/kg every 12 hours if not tolerated). Voriconazole has a high oral bioavailability (96 %) so switch to oral administration as soon as possible.

**Dose in renal impairment:** dose as in normal renal function but if CrCl <50 mL/minute there is a risk of accumulation of the IV vehicle (sulfobutylether beta cyclodextrin sodium [SBECD]). The oral form should be used unless it is judged that the benefit outweighs the risk; Cr should be closely monitored.

**Dose in hepatic impairment:** in patients with a Child–Pugh Class A or B use the standard loading dose but half the maintenance dose. It has not been studied in patients with a Child–Pugh Class C.

## Intravenous infusion

*Preparation and administration*

1. Reconstitute each vial with 19 mL WFI. Discard the vial if the vacuum of the vial does not pull the diluent into the vial.
2. Shake until dissolved to give a solution containing 10 mg/mL.
3. Visually inspect and only use if clear and particle-free.
4. Withdraw the required dose and add to a suitable volume of compatible infusion fluid to give a solution containing 0.5–5 mg/mL.
5. The solution should be clear and colourless. Inspect visually for particulate matter or discoloration prior to administration and discard if present.
6. Give by IV infusion at a maximum rate of 3 mg/kg/hour over 1–2 hours.

| Technical information | |
|---|---|
| Incompatible with | TPN should be infused via a separate line.<br>Tigecycline. |
| Compatible with | **Flush**: NaCl 0.9%<br>**Solutions**: NaCl 0.9%, Gluc 5%, Gluc-NaCl, Hartmann's<br>**Y-site**: Vasopressin |
| pH | 5.5-7.5 |

*(continued)*

## Technical information (*continued*)

| | |
|---|---|
| Sodium content | 9.5 mmol/vial |
| Storage | Store below 25°C in original packaging. |
| Displacement value | 1 mL/200 mg |
| Stability after preparation | From a microbiological point of view, should be used immediately, however:<br>• Reconstituted vials may be stored at 2-8°C for 24 hours. Single use only - discard unused portion.<br>• Prepared infusions may be stored at 2-8°C and infused (at room temperature) within 24 hours. |

## Monitoring

| Measure | Frequency | Rationale |
|---|---|---|
| Infusion-related reactions | Throughout therapy | • Flushing and nausea are the most common   if severe consider stopping treatment. |
| Development of a rash | | • Although rare exfoliative cutaneous reactions may occur, e.g. Stevens-Johnson syndrome: monitor closely and discontinue if lesions progress.<br>• May cause photosensitivity reaction. |
| U&Es | Periodically | • ↓K should be corrected during therapy.<br>• Acute renal failure may occur.<br>• A reduction in creatinine clearance to <50 mL/minute may require a switch to the oral formulation. |
| Mg and Ca serum concentration | | • ↓Mg, ↓Ca should be corrected during therapy. |
| LFTs | | • Stop therapy if liver disease develops or worsens (serious hepatic reactions are uncommon). |
| Serum amylase or lipase | | • Patients with risk factors for acute pancreatitis should be monitored closely, e.g. recent chemotherapy, haematopoietic stem cell transplantation (HSCT). |
| FBC | | • Commonly causes pancytopenia, bone marrow depression, leucopenia, thrombocytopenia, purpura, anaemia. |
| Visual function | | • Visual acuity, visual field, and colour perception should be monitored if treatment lasts longer than 28 days. |

## Additional information

| | |
|---|---|
| Common and serious undesirable effects | ↑LFTs and ↑Cr, peripheral oedema, headache, dizziness, confusional state, tremor, agitation, paraesthesia, visual disturbance, papilloedema, optic nerve disorder, nystagmus, scleritis, blepharitis, acute respiratory distress syndrome, pulmonary oedema, respiratory distress, chest pain, abdominal pain, nausea, vomiting, diarrhoea, acute renal failure acute, haematuria, rash, exfoliative dermatitis, face oedema, photosensitivity reaction, maculopapular rash, macular rash, papular rash, cheilitis, pruritus, alopecia, erythema, back pain, hypoglycaemia, ↓K, gastroenteritis, influenza-like illness, ↓BP, thrombophlebitis, phlebitis, pyrexia, sinusitis, jaundice, cholestatic jaundice, depression, anxiety, hallucination. |
| Pharmacokinetics | Elimination half-life is 6 hours. |
| Significant interactions | <ul><li>Efavirenz may ↑voriconazole levels or effect (or ↑side-effects): Restrict doses of efavirenz to 300 mg/day and double the voriconazole dose. Monitor for any toxicity and/or lack of efficacy when given with efavirenz or nevirapine.</li><li>The following may ↓voriconazole levels or effect: carbamazepine, phenobarbital, rifampicin, high-dose ritonavir and St John's wort (avoid). Low-dose ritonavir should be avoided also unless risk/benefit justifies the use of voriconazole. Phenytoin should be avoided if possible - if it cannot, monitor phenytoin levels and increase maintenance dose of voriconazole to 5 mg/kg every 12 hours. Rifabutin should be avoided if possible - if it cannot, ↑maintenance dose of voriconazole to 5 mg/kg every 12 hours and monitor FBC and other ADRs of rifabutin more closely.</li><li>Voriconazole may ↑levels or effect of the following drugs (or ↑side-effects): Terfenadine, astemizole, cisapride, pimozide and quinidine ↑risk of QT interval prolongation (avoid). Causes very large increase in sirolimus levels and may increase levels of ergot alkaloids (avoid). Ciclosporin dose should be halved, tacrolimus dose decreased by a third and levels monitored with dose adjustment as necessary (process reversed on ceasing voriconazole). Monitor prothrombin time if given with warfarin or other oral anticoagulants. Monitor blood glucose closely if taking sulfonylureas - possible ↑levels causing hypoglycaemia. May ↑statin levels therefore ↓statin dose. Short-acting opioids, e.g. alfentanil, fentanyl, sufentanil and also methadone may require a dose reduction and closer monitoring of respiratory function. Halve the dose of omeprazole - levels of both drugs may be raised.</li></ul> |
| Action in case of overdose | There is no specific antidote: treatment should be symptomatic. Voriconazole and the IV vehicle (SBECD) may be haemodialysed. |
| Counselling | Avoid sunlight during the treatment. Visual perception may be altered/enhanced, blurred vision, colour vision change or photophobia occurs commonly - effects are transient and fully reversible (usually lasting about 1 hour). If in a position to do so the patient should not drive at night. Ensure effective contraception during treatment. |

| Risk rating: **RED** | Score = 6 |
| | High-risk product: Risk-reduction strategies are required to minimise these risks. |

This assessment is based on the full range of preparation and administration options described in the monograph. These may not all be applicable in some clinical situations.

## Bibliography

SPC VFEND 50 mg and 200 mg film-coated tablets, VFEND 200 mg powder for solution for infusion, VFEND 40 mg/ml powder for oral suspension (accessed 3 April 2009).

# Zidovudine (azidothymidine, AZT)

**10 mg/mL solution in 20-mL vials**

* Zidovudine is a nucleoside reverse transcriptase inhibitor (NRTI) with antiviral activity against HIV-1.
* It is used with other antiretrovirals in the management of HIV infection because viral resistance occurs rapidly if zidovudine is used alone.
* It may be used alone to prevent vertical transmission from mother to infant if combination antiretroviral therapy is not available.

## Pre-treatment checks

Do not use in acute porphyria or breast feeding.

*Biochemical and other tests*

Fasting serum lipids and blood glucose.
FBC (do not give if neutrophil count <7500 cells/mm³ (<0.75 × 10⁹/L) or haemoglobin <7.5 g/dL), vitamin B$_{12}$ level (↑risk of neutropenia if low).
LFTs.
Renal function: U, Cr, CrCl (or eGFR).

## Dose

**Management of HIV infection in patients temporarily unable to take zidovudine by mouth:** 1–2 mg/kg every 4 hours (approximating to 1.5–3 mg/kg every 4 hours by mouth) usually for not more than 2 weeks and as part of a multidrug treatment regimen.

**Prevention of maternal-fetal transmission:** pregnant women (over 14 weeks of gestation) should be given 500 mg/day orally (100 mg five times per day) until the beginning of labour. During labour and delivery 2 mg/kg should be given by IV infusion over 60 minutes followed by 1 mg/kg/hour by continuous IV infusion until the umbilical cord is clamped.

* In case of planned caesarean, the infusion should be started 4 hours before the operation.
* In the event of a false labour, the infusion should be stopped and oral dosing restarted.
* NB: newborn infants should be given 2 mg/kg bodyweight orally every 6 hours starting within 12 hours of birth and continuing until they are 6 weeks old.
* Infants unable to receive oral therapy should be given 1.5 mg/kg by IV infusion over 30 minutes every 6 hours.

**Dose in renal impairment:** adjusted according to creatinine clearance:

* CrCl 10–50 mL/minute: 1–2 mg/kg every 8 hours.
* CrCl <10 mL/minute: 0.5–1 mg/kg every 8 hours.

**Dose in hepatic impairment:** dose reduction may be necessary. If it is not possible to monitor plasma zidovudine levels, monitor for signs of intolerance e.g. anaemia, leucopenia, neutropenia and ↓dose and/or ↑interval between doses as appropriate.

## Intravenous infusion

*Preparation and administration*

1. Withdraw the required dose and add to a suitable volume of Gluc 5% to give a solution containing 2–4 mg/mL.
2. The solution should be clear and nearly colourless. Inspect visually for particulate matter or discoloration prior to administration and discard if present.
3. Give by IV Infusion over 60 minutes (see information above regarding the continuous infusion in prevention of maternal–fetal transmission). Discard the solution if it goes turbid during the infusion.

## Technical information

| | |
|---|---|
| Incompatible with | Meropenem |
| Compatible with | **Flush**: NaCl 0.9%<br>**Solutions**: Gluc 5% (with added KCl), NaCl 0.9%<br>**Y-site**: Aciclovir, amikacin, aztreonam, ceftazidime, ceftriaxone, cisatracurium, clindamycin, co-trimoxazole, dexamethasone, dobutamine, dopamine, erythromycin, fluconazole, gentamicin, granisetron, imipenem with cilastatin, linezolid, metoclopramide, ondansetron, oxytocin, pantoprazole, piperacillin with tazobactam, ranitidine, remifentanil, tobramycin, vancomycin |
| pH | 5.5 |
| Sodium content | Negligible |
| Storage | Store below 30°C in original packaging. |
| Stability after preparation | From a microbiological point of view, should be used immediately; however, prepared infusions may be stored at 2–8°C and infused (at room temperature) within 24 hours. |

## Monitoring

| Measure | Frequency | Rationale |
|---|---|---|
| FBC | At least weekly | • If Hb falls to between 7.5 g/dL and 9 g/dL; or neutrophil count falls to between 7500 cells/mm$^3$ (0.75 × 10$^9$/L) and 10 000 cells/mm$^3$ (1.0 × 10$^9$/L) the daily dosage may be reduced until there is evidence of marrow recovery. Alternatively, recovery may be enhanced by brief (2-4 weeks) interruption of therapy, with marrow recovery usually observed within 2 weeks after which time therapy at a reduced dosage may be recommenced.<br>• Other potential causes of anaemia or neutropenia should be excluded. |
| Renal function | | • Changes in renal function may require a dose adjustment. |
| LFTs | | • Changes in hepatic function may require a dose adjustment.<br>• Rapid ↑ALT and ↑AST may also be symptomatic of the patient developing lactic acidosis. |

(continued)

## Monitoring (continued)

| Measure | Frequency | Rationale |
|---------|-----------|-----------|
| Signs of lactic acidosis | Throughout treatment | • Discontinue if present.<br>• Symptoms include benign digestive symptoms (nausea, vomiting and abdominal pain), non-specific malaise, loss of appetite, weight loss, respiratory symptoms (rapid and/or deep breathing) or neurological symptoms (including motor weakness).<br>• More common in patients (particularly obese women) with hepatomegaly, hepatitis or other known risk factors for liver disease, hepatic steatosis (including certain medicinal products and alcohol), co-infection with hepatitis C and patients treated with alpha interferon and ribavirin. |
| Signs of immune reactivation syndrome | | • Inflammatory symptoms are more likely to occur in the first few weeks or months of initiation of therapy and should be evaluated with treatment instituted as appropriate.<br>• Complications that may occur include cytomegalovirus retinitis, mycobacterial infections, and *Pneumocystis carinii* pneumonia. |
| Viral load and CD4 cell count | | • To monitor efficacy of the combined treatment. |
| Fasting serum lipids and blood glucose | Periodically | • Treat as clinically appropriate. |

## Additional information

| | |
|---|---|
| Common and serious undesirable effects | *Infusion-related:* Local: May cause local reactions including pain and slight irritation.<br>*Other:* Anaemia, neutropenia, leucopenia, headache. Dizziness, nausea, vomiting, diarrhoea, abdominal pain. ↑liver enzymes and bilirubin, myalgia, malaise. |
| Pharmacokinetics | Elimination half-life is 0.5-3 hours. |
| Significant interactions | • The following may ↑zidovudine levels or effect (or ↑side-effects): fluconazole, ganciclovir (risk of profound myelosuppression, avoid combination if possible), probenecid, ribavirin (↑risk of anaemia, avoid combination), valproate (↑risk of haematological toxicity).<br>• The following may ↓zidovudine levels or effect: rifampicin (manufacturer advises avoid combination), tipranavir.<br>• Zidovudine may ↑levels or effect (or ↑side-effects) of phenytoin (monitor levels).<br>• Zidovudine may ↓levels or effect of the following drugs: phenytoin (monitor levels), stavudine (avoid combination). |
| Action in case of overdose | No specific antidote, management should be supportive as appropriate. |
| Counselling | Patients should be advised to seek medical advice if they experience joint aches and pain, joint stiffness or difficulty in movement - possible signs of osteonecrosis. |

| Risk rating: **AMBER** | Score = 3<br>Moderate-risk product: Risk-reduction strategies are recommended. |
|---|---|

This assessment is based on the full range of preparation and administration options described in the monograph. These may not all be applicable in some clinical situations.

## Bibliography

SPC Retrovir 10 mg/mL IV for infusion (accessed 3 April 2009).

---

# Zoledronic acid

**0.05 mg/mL solution in 100-mL vial (Aclasta); 0.8 mg/mL solution in 5-mL vial (Zometa)**

* Zoledronic acid is an aminobisphosphonate with properties similar to other bisphosphonates. It inhibits bone resorption, but appears to have less effect on bone mineralisation.
* Aclasta is a ready-to-use solution for infusion licensed for use in osteoporosis (postmenopausal women and men) and in Paget's disease.
* Zometa is a concentrate for use in advanced malignancy associated with bone involvement and ↑Ca.
* Doses are expressed in terms of the anhydrous form:
  Zoledronic anhydrous 1 mg = 1.066 mg zoledronic acid monohydrate.

## Pre-treatment checks

* Do not give to patients already receiving other bisphosphonates.
* Osteonecrosis of the jaw can occur: consider dental examination and preventive dentistry prior to *planned* treatment in patients with risk factors (e.g. cancer, chemotherapy, radiotherapy, corticosteroids, poor oral hygiene). Avoid invasive dental procedures during treatment if possible.
* Give cautiously to patients who have had previous thyroid surgery (increased risk of ↓Ca).
* Contraindicated in pregnancy and breast feeding. Women of child-bearing potential should take contraceptive precautions during *planned* treatment.
* For all indications other than ↑Ca prescribe oral calcium and vitamin D supplements in those at risk of deficiency (e.g. through malabsorption, lack of exposure to sunlight or inadequate dietary intake) to minimise ↓Ca.
* Hydrate the patient adequately before, during and after infusions (up to 4 L may be given over 24 hours but overhydration should be avoided; risk of cardiac failure). Especially important in especially elderly patients and those receiving diuretic therapy.

*Biochemical and other tests*

Electrolytes: serum Na, K, Ca, PO$_4$, Mg
FBC
Renal function: U, Cr, CrCl (or eGFR) – check before every dose[1]

## Dose

**Osteoporosis** (Aclasta): 5 mg by IV infusion once a year. Do not give in severe renal impairment (CrCl or eGFR <35 mL/minute).

**Paget's disease** (Aclasta): 5 mg by IV infusion as a single dose. Do not give in severe renal impairment (CrCl or eGFR <35 mL/minute). Specific information on re-treatment is not available.

**Tumour-induced hypercalcaemia**, i.e. corrected serum Ca ≥3 mmol/L (Zometa): 4 mg by IV infusion as a single dose. Repeat if clinically necessary after a period of at least 7 days. Do not give in severe renal impairment (Cr ≥400 micromol/mL).

**Prevention of skeletal-related events in patients with advanced malignancies involving bone** (Zometa): 4 mg given by IV infusion every 3–4 weeks. Reduce the dose in renal impairment (see Table Z1). Withhold if renal function deteriorates (see Monitoring).

**Table Z1** Dose adjustment in renal impairment

| Baseline CrCl (mL/minute) | Zometa dose (mg) for prevention of skeletal-related events |
|---|---|
| <30 | Not recommended |
| 30-39 | 3 mg |
| 40-49 | 3.3 mg |
| 50-60 | 3.5 mg |
| >60 | 4 mg |

## Intermittent intravenous infusion (Aclasta)

*Preparation and administration*

1. The solution should be clear and colourless. Inspect visually for particulate matter or discoloration prior to administration.
2. Give by IV infusion directly from the bottle via a vented infusion line, over at least 15 minutes.

## Intermittent intravenous infusion (Zometa)

The patient must be adequately hydrated using NaCl 0.9% before dosing for ↑Ca.
Zoledronic acid is incompatible with Hartmann's and Ringer's (contain Ca).

*Preparation and administration*

1. Withdraw the required dose (see Table Z2) and add to 100 mL of NaCl 0.9% or Gluc 5%.
2. The solution should be clear and colourless. Inspect visually for particulate matter or discoloration prior to administration.
3. Give by IV infusion over at least 15 minutes.

**Table Z2**  Volume of Zometa concentrate required

| Prescribed dose of Zometa (mg) | Volume of Zometa concentrate solution (mL) |
|---|---|
| 4.0 mg | 5.0 mL |
| 3.5 mg | 4.4 mL |
| 3.3 mg | 4.1 mL |
| 3.0 mg | 3.8 mL |

## Technical information

| | |
|---|---|
| Incompatible with | Zoledronic acid is incompatible with Hartmann's and Ringer's (contain Ca). |
| Compatible with | **Flush**: NaCl 0.9%<br>**Solutions**: NaCl 0.9%, Gluc 5%<br>**Y-site**: No information |
| pH | No information |
| Sodium content | Negligible |
| Storage | Store below 25°C in original packaging. |
| Stability after preparation | From a microbiological point of view, should be used immediately; however, opened vials (Aclasta) and prepared infusions (Zometa) may be stored at 2-8°C and infused (at room temperature) within 24 hours. |

## Monitoring

| Measure | Frequency | Rationale |
|---|---|---|
| Blood pressure and pulse | During infusion | • ↑BP, ↓BP and ↓pulse have been reported. |
| Fluid balance | Frequently during repeated dosing | • Hydration ↑Ca diuresis.<br>• Hydration reduces decline in renal function and decreases formation of calcium renal calculi. |
| Renal function | Before every dose and at least every 3-5 days during first 10 days post treatment, then as clinically indicated | • Enables appropriate dosing.<br>• If renal function declines during therapy, withhold further treatment until renal function returns to within 10% of the baseline value.<br>• Especially important in patients with pre-existing renal dysfunction; those of advanced age; those using concomitant nephrotoxic drugs or diuretic therapy; or those who are dehydrated.[1] |
| Serum K, Na, Ca, PO$_4$, Mg | | • ↑K, ↓K, ↑Na have been reported.<br>• Serum Ca may determine whether further treatment is necessary or appropriate. If ↓Ca develops, treat symptomatically.<br>• PO$_4$ and Ca share common control systems. Disruption to Ca metabolism affects PO$_4$ levels.<br>• ↓Mg occurs commonly during treatment. |

(continued)

| Monitoring *(continued)* | | |
|---|---|---|
| **Measure** | **Frequency** | **Rationale** |
| FBC | Every 3 months | • Anaemia, thrombocytopenia, leucopenia and pancytopenia have been reported. |

## Additional information

| | |
|---|---|
| Common and serious undesirable effects | *Injection/infusion-related:* Local: Injection-site reactions have been observed (redness, swelling, pain).<br>*Other:* Renal dysfunction, asymptomatic and symptomatic ↓Ca (paraesthesia, tetany), pruritus, urticaria, exfoliative dermatitis, fever and influenza-like symptoms, malaise, rigors, fatigue and flushes (usually resolve spontaneously), arthralgia, myalgia, bone pain (may resolve on stopping treatment); eye disorders: uveitis, scleritis, conjunctivitis; jaw osteonecrosis (see above). |
| Pharmacokinetics | Excreted unchanged via the kidney and taken up by bone in a triphasic process. The elimination half-life is 146 hours. |
| Significant interactions | None. |
| Action in case of overdose | *Symptoms to watch for:* clinically significant ↓Ca (paraesthesia, tetany, ↓BP).<br>*Antidote:* Calcium gluconate infusion. Stop administration and give supportive therapy as appropriate. Monitor serum Ca, PO$_4$, Mg, K. |
| Counselling | Maintain fluid intake during the post-infusion hours.<br>Inform of symptoms of ↓Ca (paraesthesia, tetany, muscle cramps, confusion).<br>Report any ocular discomfort/loss of visual acuity or injection-site reactions.<br>Advise on importance of taking calcium and vitamin D supplements as prescribed where these are indicated.<br>Advise patients with risk factors for osteonecrosis of the jaw (see Pre-treatment checks) not to undergo invasive dental procedures during treatment. |

| Risk rating: **AMBER** | Score = 3<br>Moderate-risk product: Risk-reduction strategies are recommended. |
|---|---|

This assessment is based on the full range of preparation and administration options described in the monograph. These may not all be applicable in some clinical situations.

## Reference

1. MHRA (2010). Adverse effects on renal function with zoledronic acid. *Drug Safety Update: Volume 3, Issue 9, April 2010.* www.nelm.nhs.uk/en/NeLM-Area/Evidence/Patient-Safety (accessed 11 April 2010).

## Bibliography

SPC Aclasta (accessed 1 March 2009).
SPC Zometa (accessed 1 March 2009).

# Zuclopenthixol acetate

**50 mg/mL oily solution in 1-mL and 2-mL ampoules**

This preparation must not be confused with the depot preparation.

* Zuclopenthixol acetate is a thioxanthene antipsychotic with a wide range of actions.
* It is used in the short-term management of acute psychoses including mania and exacerbation of chronic psychoses.
* The NICE clinical guideline on violence recommends that use of zuclopenthixol acetate may be considered in the following circumstances:
  * Where the patient is expected to be disturbed/violent over an extended period of time.
  * Where the patient has a past history of a good response to zuclopenthixol acetate injection.
  * Where the patient has a past history of requiring repeated parenteral administration of anti-psychotics or benzodiazepines.
  * Where an advance directive has been made.

## Pre-treatment checks

* Do not give to patients in comatose states, including alcohol, barbiturate or opiate poisoning.
* Do not give to patients who have never received antipsychotic medication or patients who are struggling.
* Caution in epilepsy and hepatic, renal or cardiovascular disease.

*Biochemical and other tests (not all are necessary in an emergency situation)*

Review the patient's physical health including current physical observations and recent ECG.
Blood pressure

LFTs
Renal function: U, Cr, CrCl (or eGFR)

## Dose

**Short-term management of acute psychoses:** 50–150 mg (1–3 mL) repeated if necessary after 2–3 days. If required, an additional injection may be given 1–2 days after the first injection. The maximum cumulative dose is 400 mg per course of treatment. The duration of treatment should not exceed 2 weeks (maximum 4 injections).
**Dose in renal impairment:** the dose should be reduced by half.
**Dose in hepatic impairment:** the dose should be reduced by half.

## Intramuscular injection

*Preparation and administration*

1. Withdraw the required dose.
2. Give by deep IM injection into the upper outer buttock or lateral thigh. Aspirate before injection to avoid inadvertent intravascular injection.

## Technical information

| | |
|---|---|
| Incompatible with | Not relevant |
| Compatible with | Not relevant |

*(continued)*

## Technical information (*continued*)

| | |
|---|---|
| pH | Not applicable - oily injection |
| Sodium content | Nil |
| Storage | Store below 25°C in original packaging. |

## Monitoring

| Measure | Frequency | Rationale |
|---|---|---|
| Therapeutic improvement | Daily | • To ensure that treatment is effective. |
| EPSEs | Every 15 minutes for the first 2 hours; then every 8 hours for 72 hours | • Causes extrapyramidal symptoms, e.g. dystonias. |
| BP, temperature, pulse rate and character, respiratory rate, levels of sedation and hydration. | | • Risk of arrhythmias, neuroleptic malignant syndrome. |

## Additional information

| | |
|---|---|
| Common and serious undesirable effects | EPSEs.<br>Other reported side-effects include orthostatic dizziness, reduced salivation, ↑pulse, abnormalities of visual accommodation, paraesthesia and convulsions.<br>Rare cases of QT prolongation, ventricular arrhythmias - ventricular fibrillation, ventricular tachycardia, torsade de pointes and sudden unexplained death have been reported. |
| Pharmacokinetics | Peak concentration are achieved 36 hours after injection. Elimination half-life is 25–39 hours. |
| Significant interactions | • Zuclopenthixol may ↑risk of ventricular arrhythmias with the following drugs:<br>amiodarone (avoid combination), disopyramide (avoid combination), erythromycin (avoid combination), moxifloxacin (avoid combination), sotalol (avoid combination). |
| Action in case of overdose | Treatment is symptomatic and supportive. Adrenaline must **not** be used. |

| Risk rating: **GREEN** | Score = 2<br>Lower-risk product: Risk-reduction strategies should be considered. |
|---|---|

This assessment is based on the full range of preparation and administration options described in the monograph. These may not all be applicable in some clinical situations.

## Bibliography

SPC Clopixol Acuphase (accessed 17 January 2008).

Bazire S. *Psychotropic Drug Directory 2010*. Aberdeen: HealthComm UK Ltd, 2010.

NICE (2005) *Clinical Guideline 25: Violence: The short-term management of disturbed/violent behaviour in in-patient psychiatric settings and emergency departments*.http://guidance.nice.org.uk/CG25 (accessed 14 July 2010).

# Zuclopenthixol decanoate

**200 and 500 mg/mL oily solution in 1-mL ampoules**

This preparation is a depot preparation and must not be confused with the rapid-acting injection.

- Zuclopenthixol decanoate is a thioxanthene antipsychotic with a wide range of actions.
- As a long-acting depot injection it is used in the treatment of schizophrenia and other psychoses, particularly with aggression and agitation.

## Pre-treatment checks

- Avoid in patients in comatose states, including alcohol, barbiturate, or opiate poisoning.
- Concomitant treatment with other antipsychotics should be avoided.
- Caution in epilepsy, Parkinson's disease, liver disease, renal failure, cardiac disease, depression, myasthenia gravis, prostatic hypertrophy, narrow-angle glaucoma, hypothyroidism, hyperthyroidism, phaeochromocytoma, severe respiratory disease or if there are risk factors for stroke.

*Biochemical and other tests*

| | |
|---|---|
| Blood pressure | LFTs |
| Bodyweight | Renal function: U, Cr, CrCl (or eGFR) |
| ECG | TFTs |
| FBC | |

## Dose

**Treatment of schizophrenia and other psychoses:**

- Test dose: 100 mg to assess tolerability. Reduce dose to 25 mg or 50 mg if the patient is elderly.
- Maintenance dose: To commence at least 1 week after test dose. Usual dose range is 200–500 mg every 1–4 weeks. The maximum dose is 600 mg weekly.

## Intramuscular injection

*Preparation and administration*

1. Withdraw the required dose.
2. Give by deep IM injection into the upper outer buttock or lateral thigh. Volumes >2 mL should be distributed between two injection sites. Aspirate before injection to avoid inadvertent intravascular injection. Rotate injection sites for subsequent injections.

## Technical information

| Incompatible with | Not relevant |
|---|---|
| Compatible with | Not relevant |
| pH | Not applicable – oily injection |
| Sodium content | Nil |
| Storage | Store below 25°C in original packaging. |

## Monitoring

| Measure | Frequency | Rationale |
|---|---|---|
| Therapeutic improvement | Periodically | • To ensure that treatment is effective. |
| EPSEs | During dose adjustment and every 3 months | • Causes extrapyramidal symptoms, e.g. dystonias. |
| Renal function | At least annually | • As part of regular health check. |
| LFTs | | |
| BP | | |
| Glucose | | |
| Lipids (including cholesterol, HDL, LDL and triglycerides) | | |
| Weight and obesity | | • As part of regular health check.<br>• May cause weight gain.<br>• Obesity measured by waist:hip ratio or waist circumference. |
| ECG | Annually | • Can ↑QT interval. |
| Prolactin | See Rationale | • If symptoms of hyperprolactinaemia develop. |

## Additional information

| Common and serious undesirable effects | Drowsiness and sedation more common at start of treatment and at high doses. EPSEs.<br>Other reported side-effects include orthostatic dizziness, reduced salivation, weight gain, hyperprolactinaemia, ↑pulse, ↓BP, abnormalities of visual accommodation, urinary incontinence and frequency, paraesthesia and convulsions.<br>Rare cases of QT prolongation, ventricular arrhythmias – ventricular fibrillation, ventricular tachycardia, Torsade de Pointes and sudden unexplained death have been reported. Blood dyscrasias. |
|---|---|

(continued)

## Additional information (continued)

| | |
|---|---|
| Pharmacokinetics | Elimination half-life is 17–21 days (after multiple doses). |
| Significant interactions | • The following may ↑zuclopenthixol levels or effect (or ↑side-effects): clozapine (avoid combination - depot preparation cannot be withdrawn quickly if neutropenia occurs).<br>• Zuclopenthixol may ↑risk of ventricular arrhythmias with the following drugs: amiodarone (avoid combination), disopyramide (avoid combination), erythromycin (avoid combination), moxifloxacin (avoid combination), sotalol (avoid combination). |
| Action in case of overdose | Treat EPSE with anticholinergic antiparkinsonian drugs.<br>If agitation or convulsions occur, treat with benzodiazepines.<br>If the patient is in shock, treatment with metaraminol or noradrenaline may be appropriate.<br>Adrenaline must **not** be given (may further ↓BP). |
| Counselling | Advise patients not to drink alcohol, especially at the beginning of treatment. Zuclopenthixol decanoate may impair alertness so do not drive or operate machinery until their susceptibility is known. |

**Risk rating: GREEN**  Score = 2
Lower-risk product: Risk-reduction strategies should be considered.

This assessment is based on the full range of preparation and administration options described in the monograph. These may not all be applicable in some clinical situations.

## Bibliography

SPC Clopixol (accessed 17 January 2008).
Bazire S. *Psychotropic Drug Directory* 2010. Aberdeen: HealthComm UK Ltd, 2010.
NICE (2009). *Clinical Guideline 82: Core interventions in the treatment and management of schizophrenia in primary and secondary care (update)*. http://guidance.nice.org.uk/CG82 (accessed 1 October 2009).

# Appendix 1
# The basics of injectable therapy

## The basics

The use of parenteral therapy is part of daily practice in hospitals and increasingly so in primary care. Using the parenteral route to administer medicines requires all practitioners to work in partnership to ensure the safe, effective and economic use of parenteral therapy.

Safe systems of practice must be put in place to ensure aseptic techniques are adhered to throughout all parenteral procedures and to minimise drug-related errors. All practitioners involved with any aspect of parenteral drug therapy must adhere to the recommendations of their own professional bodies, and must also work within their own organisation's procedures regarding medicines management and patient care.

This book may be used as a reference source by all practitioners: doctors, nurses, midwives, pharmacists, operating department practitioners (ODPs with NVQ Level 3 qualification) and other suitably qualified personnel who have been trained and assessed as competent to administer drugs by the parenteral route.

## General information

The monographs in this book detail appropriate methods of administration for medicines that can be given via the parenteral route. They must be used in conjunction with any polices and/or procedures recommended by the practitioner's own governing body, e.g. in the UK the most recent edition of The Royal Marsden Hospital Manual of Clinical Nursing Procedures[1] or a local Medical Devices Policy. Cancer chemotherapy agents are not included in this guide as they should only be administered by formally trained and qualified nurses and doctors. Practitioners requiring additional information relating to the handling and administration of these medicines should contact their own Pharmacy department.

There may be times when a patient's clinical status justifies a change from the instructions in the monograph. In this situation the nurse or doctor should contact their Pharmacy Medicines Information department or call their resident or on-call pharmacist for further instructions on how to administer the relevant drug.

## Sodium content

The sodium content of each medicine is included in this guide. Some medicines, e.g. many antibiotics, are formulated with a considerable sodium content; for example, metronidazole contains 13.15 mmol/500-mg bag. This may be clinically significant and may need to taken into account when therapeutic choices are made. In the monographs the sodium content is listed if a dose contains $\geq 1$ mmol sodium.

## pH

An indication of the acidity or alkalinity of injection solutions has been included in the monographs (as measured by their pH) to help practitioners predict possible Y-site incompatibilities of medicines when no compatibility information exists.

Injections with greatly differing pH values should not be administered concurrently down the same line as this may result in either precipitation or inactivation of the medicines[2]; for example, the pH of phenytoin injection is 12 and the pH of haloperidol injection is 3, making them incompatible; if mixed they would combine chemically to form a precipitate.

The pH can also give the practitioner an indication of the irritancy of the drug. Medicines that are either highly acidic or alkaline may be harmful if extravasation into the surrounding tissue occurs, causing tissue damage.

Injections in oily or other unusual vehicles do not have a pH value. This is because pH is a measure of the acidity or alkalinity of an aqueous solution and by its very nature an oily injection is not an aqueous solution.

## Light-sensitive infusions

Some drugs undergo photolysis and photodegradation if exposed to natural daylight (ultraviolet radiation) and fluorescent light during administration. This can result in loss of therapeutic effect and the production of toxic products.

To reduce these reactions, the products must be protected from light not only during storage but also once diluted and ready for use. The infusion bag, the syringe and sometimes the giving set need to be protected from light by covering with an opaque material or aluminium foil.

Periodic visual inspection of the diluted solution for the occurrence of discoloration and/or precipitation is recommended during its infusion.

Drugs that must be protected from light have this detailed in their individual monograph.

## Displacement value

Injection products formulated as dry powders or lyophilised cakes must be reconstituted with a suitable diluent before administration. Sometimes the final volume of the injection is greater than the volume of liquid added to the powder. This volume difference is called the displacement value; for example:

- The displacement value of amoxicillin injection 250 mg is 0.2 mL.
- If 4.8 mL of diluent is added to a 250-mg vial, the resulting volume is 5 mL, i.e. 250 mg in 5 mL.
- If 5 mL of diluent is added, the resulting volume is 5.2 mL, i.e. 250 mg in 5.2 mL or 240.38 mg in 5 mL.

Drugs that have a significant displacement have this detailed in their individual monograph and this must be taken into account when reconstituting the drug if only part of the vial is to be used. If the total content of a vial is to be given, the displacement value need not be taken into account when reconstituting the drug because the entire contents of the vial are withdrawn for administration.

## Visual inspection of prepared product

All products prepared for intravenous use make reference to this requirement as part of the preparation procedure. Products to be given by other routes should also be inspected prior to administration. This is because it is possible for particulate matter to be present in the final product, often from the rubber bung of the vial shedding material when punctured by a needle.

The following technique describes a method for visually checking the product. Hold the syringe or infusion container up to a light source and, while looking straight through the solution, invert the product. Usually all that is seen are air bubbles swirling and moving in a general upwards direction, but observe for a few seconds for anything (particles) moving downwards and any untoward colour changes as described in the specific monograph.

## Blood and blood products and parenteral nutrition (PN)

In the UK the Department of Health states that the co-administration of blood or concentrated red blood cells with any other medicine or vehicle is hazardous. The same caution should also be applied to bags of parenteral nutrition. The reason for such caution is that large molecules may form in the bag that could cause anaphylaxis or seed an embolism. As the contents of these bags are opaque, visual clues to such reactions cannot be seen.

If additional fluid or electrolytes are needed then these must be run separately via a different line if possible. If the same line must be used, all practitioners **must** check with their pharmacist about compatibilities as certain electrolytes/hyperosmolar fluids may cause precipitation of the PN/blood in the line.

## Flushing intravenous lines and cannulas[1,2]

Flushing between the administration of different medicines must always be carried out to avoid any problems with incompatibilities. Flushing also ensures the total drug dose is presented for systemic effect and prolongs the viability of the cannula or line.

If two drugs being administered one after the other are known to be compatible, then flushing the line or cannula need only be done before and after administration of the medicines. Commonly 5–10 mL of NaCl 0.9% or Gluc 5% is used to flush the dead space of a cannula, whereas 20 mL is usually needed for an administration set. The practitioner must check each monograph before deciding which flush to use, to ensure that both drugs are compatible with the chosen flush.

Frequent flushing of unused lines is also necessary in order to maintain patency of the line or cannula. The National Patient Safety Agency has recently recommended the exclusive use of NaCl 0.9% injection as a flush for maintaining peripheral intravenous cannulas.[3]

Occasionally NaCl with heparin is required to ensure that certain lines are kept patent, but such use should be kept to a minimum. If the use of a heparin flush is appropriate then it must be administered against a valid prescription. Practitioners should check their individual organisation's policies in order to determine when the use of a heparin flush is appropriate.

## Central versus peripheral access

Before a medicine can be administered intravenously, a suitable intravenous catheter must be inserted into the patient. These can either be central intravenous catheters, peripheral intravenous catheters or peripherally inserted central intravenous catheters (PICC lines). Choice of line is often dictated by the clinical condition of the patient; for example, a critically ill patient is more likely to require central access than a patient who only requires a few days' intravenous therapy.

Unlike peripheral catheters, central lines are generally thought to last longer, are more consistently accessible regardless of the patient's condition and can accept more irritant solutions, e.g. hyperosmolar or vasoconstricting drugs. Central catheters also carry the advantage of allowing a rapid rate of infusion of a drug and can be used to monitor central venous pressures as well as aid the passing of pulmonary artery catheters. However, insertion of central intravenous catheters requires greater skill and the risks associated with them are greater.[4]

A peripheral catheter is appropriate if the patient is not receiving irritant solutions intravenously, if intravenous therapy is likely to be short term and if suitable vein(s) are available for cannulation.

Central and peripheral catheters are often referred to in the vernacular as central lines and peripheral lines. For more information see Appendix 7 Intravascular devices.

## Glucose or dextrose: which term to use?

The term glucose (abbreviated to Gluc in this book) is used throughout the monographs to define the injection and infusion fluid of that substance. The term dextrose is used by some authorities and on occasion this been known to lead to confusion.

Glucose is a three-dimensional molecule that exists in two symmetrical forms (mirror images of each other) and the *dextro-* and *laevo-* prefixes are used to categorise the forms that can rotate plane-polarised light clockwise (to the right) or anticlockwise (to the left) respectively.

The word dextrose is a contraction of *dextrorotatory glucose* or *d*-glucose, which is the biologically active form of glucose, as opposed to *laevorotatory glucose* or *l*-glucose (which is not biologically active).

The colloquial naming system can lead to further confusion when applied to the less frequently used injection fructose, which has been referred to as laevulose as it is the laevorotatory form of fructose. It is however structurally different from glucose and is not the laevorotatory form of glucose.

## Osmolarity

Osmolarity is stated in some monographs only for those drugs that have a high osmolarity. The significance of this is that at a solution of high osmolarity can cause serious harm to small blood vessels and these drugs would not normally be appropriate for peripheral administration. In general solutions of high osmolarity should be given centrally.

It is worth explaining what the term means and how it differs from the similar term osmolality. *Osmolarity* is a measure of solute concentration in terms of osmoles per litre of solution (Osmol/L), whereas *osmolality* is a measure of the number of osmoles of solute per kg of solvent (Osmol/kg). Calculated figures for both are very similar and the terms are used interchangeably in practice with little consequence.

An osmole (Osm or Osmol) is a unit of measure that describes the number of moles of a chemical compound that contribute to a solution's osmotic pressure, that is, the pressure that must be applied to a solution to prevent the inward flow of water across a semi-permeable membrane.

## References

1. Dougherty L, Lister S, eds. *The Royal Marsden Hospital Manual of Clinical Nursing Procedures*, 6th edn. Oxford: Blackwell, 2004.
2. Pharmacy Department, University College London Hospitals NHS Foundation Trust. *Injectable Medicines Administration Guide*, 2nd edn. Oxford: Blackwell, 2007.
3. National Patient Safety Agency. *Rapid Response Report – Risks with Intravenous Heparin Flush Solutions*. Issued 24 April 2008.
4. Giuffrida DJ et al. Central vs peripheral venous catheters in critically ill patients. *Chest*. 1986; 90: 806–809.

# Appendix 2
# Good management principles

It is unacceptable to prepare medicines for administration by others. The practitioner administering the drug must be involved in the preparation and checking process. The following are exemptions from this principle:

* Injections and infusions prepared by the Pharmacy department.
* Drugs prepared for/by anaesthetists (however, this practice is only acceptable when carried out on the instructions and in the presence of a doctor who witnesses and checks the preparation).

Parenteral drugs must not be prepared in advance of their immediate use (except when prepared by the Pharmacy).

Parenteral medicines should be prepared in a designated clean area.

Parenteral medicines do not routinely need to be double-checked by another practitioner; however, each practitioner should check their own organisation's policy on this matter before administering a medicine. It is good practice to request a double check on administration if:

* The infusion involves the addition or mixing of drugs, e.g. the reconstitution of a powder to make a solution for injection does not need to be double checked.
* A Controlled Drug is involved.
* A calculation is involved.

Local circumstances may make involvement of a second practitioner desirable in order to minimise the potential for error, e.g. on a neonatal unit.

Each practitioner is responsible for maintaining his or her own knowledge on all drugs. Information on such products can be found in the monographs of this book, in the package insert and/or via the Pharmacy department.

In the UK practitioners requiring further information on the advantages and disadvantages of using any parenteral route and the principles of preparation and administration of intravenous drugs should see the Drug Administration Section of the most recent edition of The Royal Marsden Hospital Manual of Clinical Nursing Procedures or similar texts.

## Minimising risk of infections

Practitioners should ensure that they:

* Always use an aseptic non-touch technique (ANTT) when administering parenteral medicines.
* Minimise unnecessary disturbance or movement of the line/cannula.
* Cover the intravenous site with a transparent occlusive dressing so that the point of insertion into the vein is clearly visible.
* Inspect the site daily for signs of redness, swelling, inflammation; etc.
* Re-site all lines/cannulas that are thought to be infected and take cultures (see individual organisation's policies on taking blood cultures).
* Avoid using 3-way taps, ports, etc. wherever possible as these do not provide an effective barrier against entry of microorganisms.
* Change the line/cannula and the giving set at the intervals recommended by their own organisation's policies.

Practitioners should contact their Infection Control department for more guidance on aseptic non-touch technique (ANTT) in their organisation. Further information is also available at http://www.antt.co.uk/.

## Accountability

Parenteral therapy is a common and important part of the care received by many patients. It also carries the risk of potentially dangerous complications. In order to protect patients and provide staff with the means to deliver safe and effective treatment, the practitioner should always follow guidance issued by their own organisation.

In the UK the NHS requires that all practitioners involved in the administration of parenteral medicines should achieve an appropriate level of competence according to the procedure being undertaken, the drug involved and the device being used.

As nurses/midwives administer the majority of parenteral therapy, NHS organisations require that they provide evidence of competence through successfully completing an approved Parenteral Therapy course/programme before undertaking assessment in the clinical area.

In order to provide comprehensive patient care all nurses/midwives are expected to achieve competency at the earliest opportunity following appointment and may be called on to demonstrate their competency at any time. Although nurses/midwives can decline to perform duties in which they do not feel competent, they are obliged to adapt to new methods and techniques of administering medications and must work at a level commensurate with the grading of their role. Parenteral therapy, in particular, is an area that is continually evolving and can be considered to be an integral part of the nurse's or midwife's role and thus every effort must be made to achieve competence in this area of practice.

All practitioners have a duty of care to their patients, who are entitled to receive safe and competent care. If a practitioner is asked to perform a duty which is outside their area of expertise they must obtain help and supervision from a competent practitioner until they and the Trust consider they have acquired the requisite knowledge and skills.

## Bibliography

Association of Operating Department Practitioners. *Code of Conduct*. Lewes: AODP, 2001.

Dougherty L, Lister S, eds. *The Royal Marsden Hospital Manual of Clinical Nursing Procedures*, 6th edn. Oxford: Blackwell, 2004.

Nursing and Midwifery Council. *Midwives Rules and Standards*. London: NMC, 2004.

Nursing and Midwifery Council. *Standards for Medicines Management*. London: NMC, 2008.

Nursing and Midwifery Council. *The Code: Standards for Conduct, Performance and Ethics for Nurses and Midwives*. London: NMC, 2007.

# Appendix 3
# Usual responsibilities of individual practitioners

## The prescriber[1]

- The prescribing of parenteral medicines or fluids is the responsibility of a doctor, or an independent or supplementary prescriber. The prescription must clearly state:
  - Approved name
  - Dose and frequency of the drug
  - Method of administration and by which route – central or peripheral, intramuscular, subcutaneous, etc.
  - Type and volume of fluid for dilution or infusion
  - Final concentration
  - Calculated infusion rate.
- The prescriber must restrict the use of the parenteral route to situations where there is no clinically effective alternative method for administration of the medicine.
- The prescriber must review the patient on a daily basis to keep parenteral therapy to the minimum effective duration.
- The prescriber must ensure that the vascular access device to be used, e.g. Venflon, is appropriate for the needs of the individual patient and the drug to be administered.

## The pharmacist[1,2]

The Pharmacist (or Pharmacy service) has the role of:
- Monitoring the safety of the drug use process and alerting prescribers and other health care professionals to potential problems.
- Checking the selection of drugs and regimens to ensure appropriate treatment.
- Endorsing the prescription chart (or other prescribing system) with relevant and necessary information on dilution and rates of administration, etc. in accordance with pharmacy procedures.
- Providing information to specific enquiries raised by health care professionals on all aspects of intravenous therapy, e.g. diluents, drug stability, adverse effects and compatibility, etc.
- Checking the lines and/or administration devices, e.g. syringe and infusion bag, are labelled correctly.

## The practitioner administering the parenteral drug[3]

For in-patients the practitioner preparing and administering the drug (not the second checker) must:
- Appropriately identify the patient by checking their name and hospital identification number on an identity band (or an alternative as defined within the organisation's patient identification policy) before administering the drug.

In all cases the practitioner preparing and administering the drug must:

- Check the patient is not allergic and/or sensitive either to the drug or any of the constituents of the injection by checking the allergy status of the patient.
- Be in possession of sufficient information to ensure competence in the safe administration of the drug (including information on unlicensed medicines, clinical trial medicines or licensed medicines that are not licensed for the particular indication, dose, age group or route of administration).
- Seek advice if unsure of any aspect of the administration of a drug by the intravenous route.
- Ensure that any vascular access device used is appropriate for the needs of the individual patient and the drug to be administered.
- Check when the cannula in use was sited before administering any drugs through it, and ensure all peripheral cannulas are re-sited every 72 hours or earlier if any signs of phlebitis are evident.
- Ensure that an assessment of the venous access site is undertaken prior to, during and after drug administration, and that this assessment is documented in accordance with their own organisation's policies.
- Ensure that the cannula or line is flushed using the appropriate flush before and after the administration of all parenteral drugs as indicated under Flushing intravenous lines and cannulas in Appendix 1.
- Be familiar with and competent to use any equipment required as part of the drug administration process.
- Ensure the lines and/or administration device are correctly labelled.
- Monitor all infusions throughout administration to ensure that the infusion is being administered at the correct rate, that the infusion pump or device is working as intended, and that the patient is responding to the infusion therapy as intended.
- Be aware of, and be able to monitor for both immediate and delayed side-effects including hypersensitivity reactions or signs of extravasation and be able to respond appropriately if they occur.
- Ensure that accurate documentation of drug administration is maintained, including fluid balance for intravenous infusions.

## References

1. *British National Formulary*, No. 59. London: British Medical Association/Pharmaceutical Press, 2010.
2. The Royal Pharmaceutical Society of Great Britain. *Medicines, Ethics and Practice*. London: RPSGB, 2009.
3. The Nursing and Midwifery Council. *Standards for Medicines Management*. London: NMC, 2008.

# Appendix 4
# Advantages and disadvantages
# of parenteral therapy

There are many advantages to using the parenteral route to administer medicines, but because of the potential risks to the patient the practitioner should always carefully consider all advantages and disadvantages before using the parenteral route.

Advantages include:

- Rapid effect, e.g. useful in an emergency (myocardial infarction, anaphylaxis, status epilepticus)
- Usefulness for drugs that are not absorbed orally, e.g. insulin, heparin, some antibiotics
- Constant therapeutic effect, e.g. inotropes, antipsychotics
- The possibility of precise dosing, e.g. for anaesthesia, analgesia
- Controllable rate of administration, e.g. morphine
- Co operation of the patient is not needed, e.g. if the patient is unconscious, uncooperative or uncontrollable
- Usefulness if the patient is 'nil by mouth', not absorbing or unable to tolerate oral medicines (however, the topical and rectal routes may also be appropriate).

Disadvantages include:

- Risk of infection
- Dangerous and/or fatal if given incorrectly, e.g. potassium
- The dose is not retrievable
- Specialised technique is required to administer medicines
- Training is required before the practitioner can administer medicines
- Can be painful for the patient, or at the very least inconvenient
- Difficulty in self administration, e.g. for home intravenous antibiotics, which may lead to increased length of hospital stay
- High cost
- Complications, e.g. extravasation, side-effects usually more immediate and severe
- Compatibility and stability issues.

## Bibliography

Pharmacy Department, University College London Hospitals NHS Foundation Trust. *Injectable Medicines Administration Guide*, 2nd edn. Oxford: Blackwell, 2007.

# Appendix 5
# Injection techniques and routes

## Intermittent intravenous infusions

This is the technique used to administer an injectable drug in an intravenous infusion over a period of time ranging from 20 minutes to several hours. Repeated doses (e.g. benzylpenicillin) or single doses (e.g. furosemide) are given in this way.

The infusion may be connected to the primary intravenous giving set or to a secondary administration set via a Y-connector. Administration can also be via an in-line burette, which would normally constitute a section of the primary giving set.

The volume of intravenous fluid used to dilute the drug ranges from 50 mL (the smallest intravenous fluid bag) up to 500 mL. In clinical practice most drugs are given in 100 mL and are set to infuse over 20–30 minutes.

Advantages include:
- A volumetric pump can be used to deliver the dose in a controlled way.
- Fewer manipulations are required in preparation compared to use of a syringe driver.
- It is cheaper than using a syringe driver.

Disadvantages include:
- Aseptic technique is required for preparation – unless prepared by a central intravenous additive service (CIVAS).
- Bags usually have limited stability once prepared, possibly resulting in waste unless carefully managed by CIVAS.
- Patient mobility is restricted (at least during the administration).
- There is potential for extravasation at infusion site.
- Administration of intravenous fluid is required to maintain cannula patency.
- More invasive and expensive than enteral administration.
- Multiple doses may result in fluid overload.

The usual diluent solutions are NaCl 0.9% and Gluc 5%, which are available in a variety of volumes. These concentrations are used because they are isotonic with blood and thus do not cause haemolysis of blood cells.

The drug to be given may be compatible with one or both of these, although solubility and stability times may differ. Infusion bags may contain about a 5% overage so the practitioner must take this into account if only using part of the bag.

Mixing drugs in infusion bags is not advised without compatibility data, which can be found in reference sources such as the latest edition of Trissel's *Handbook on Injectable Drugs*[1] or via a website such as MedicinesComplete (www.medicinescomplete.com).

## Direct intravenous injections

Some drug products may be administered directly into the venous circulation in a relatively small volume of fluid over less than 5 minutes. This technique is sometimes referred to as an 'IV push' or 'IV bolus'. The injection may be given:

- Via an injection port in an infusion line
- Via an indwelling cannula, e.g. Venflon
- From a syringe and needle directly into a vein.

A direct intravenous injection (as opposed to an intravenous infusion) is used when:

- Administration is urgent (e.g. tenecteplase).
- A high concentration of the drug is required (e.g. adenosine).
- Time is limited (in the anaesthetic room prior to a surgical operation).
- The patient is fluid-restricted.
- Patient or carer convenience dictates (e.g. domiciliary antibiotics).
- It is recommended by the manufacturer.

Unless specifically directed otherwise by the manufacturer, a direct intravenous injection is given over 2–3 minutes, observing the patient and the injection site for signs of adverse reaction.

The volume of injection is usually 5 mL or less, although larger volumes may be necessary if the drug has low solubility, is likely to be an irritant to the vein or requires relatively slow administration.

Bolus injections into indwelling cannulas should always be preceded and followed by at least 2–5 mL of a flushing solution.

Some drugs are too irritant or toxic to be administered as a concentrated injection; for example, erythromycin is too painful and irritant to the vein, while potassium chloride 15% injection is too toxic to the myocardium in high concentration (and also extremely irritant).

## Intramuscular injections

Intramuscular injections are administered into the muscle beneath the subcutaneous tissue, and are generally absorbed faster than subcutaneous injections. They are most commonly given into the thigh or the gluteal muscle, and occasionally into the deltoid muscle (which attaches the upper arm to the shoulder).

The volume given at any one site is usually limited to 5 mL for the thigh (or 4 mL if it is a depot injection because depots can be more irritant), and 2 mL for the deltoid muscle.[2] Larger volumes are not effectively absorbed and if given may lead to abscess formation. If more than 5 mL has to be given, then more than one injection site should be used. If a series of injections are to be administered, injection sites should be used in rotation and a record of these kept.

The two most common ways of giving an intramuscular injection are by:

- *Direct injection* straight into the muscle, with the needle held at a 90° angle to the skin. Upon removal, pressure should be applied to the injection site to prevent leakage.[3]
- *Z-track technique* wherein the skin above the muscle is displaced sideways, so that when the needle is withdrawn the skin can be simultaneously released. This has the effect of sealing the injection under the skin and preventing leakage into the subcutaneous tissue.[2] The Z-track technique is notably recommended for iron injections to minimise subcutaneous irritation and staining.

### Relative bioavailability

There may be bioavailability differences between intramuscular and intravenous administration of certain drugs, and the intramuscular route is usually associated with a delayed onset of action. It is therefore incorrect to assume that a drug dose is interchangeable between the intravenous and intramuscular routes.

It is also considered to be an unsafe prescribing practice to specify alternative routes for the same prescription entry on a prescription chart.

## Subcutaneous injections[4]

Subcutaneous injections are given by injecting a fluid or a solid pellet into the subcutis (the fatty layer of tissue just under the skin). Subcutaneous injections of fluid are used to administer vaccines and medications, e.g. insulin. A pellet may be injected to deliver long-lasting doses of medication, e.g. goserelin. The technique provides slow and constant absorption of a drug or fluid.

Appropriate sites for a subcutaneous injection include:

- The outer aspect of the upper arm
- The anterior aspect of the upper arm
- The abdomen below the costal margins to the iliac crests
- The anterior aspect of the thigh
- The ventrodorsal gluteal area
- The scapular area.

The site must not be bruised, tender, hard, swollen, inflamed or scarred as this may hinder absorption and cause discomfort and injury to the patient.

Irritant medications should not be administered subcutaneously as they may cause tissue necrosis or a sterile abscess.

*Administering a subcutaneous injection*

Generally 25- to 27-gauge needles are used of varying lengths depending on the drug to be administered. Pinch up a skin fold between the thumb and forefinger and hold throughout the injection.

The angle of insertion of the needle depends on the length of the needle used and on the size of tissue fold pinched at the chosen site; for example, if there is a 2.5 cm tissue fold or if a longer needle is used, insert at a 45-degree angle; if there is a 5 cm tissue fold or a shorter needle is used, insert at a 90-degree angle.

Without aspirating, the medication should be injected with a slow, steady pressure. Aspiration after insertion of the needle is not recommended as this may cause tissue damage, hematoma formation and bruising. The likelihood of injecting into a blood vessel is small.

The site should not be massaged after administration as this can damage the underlying tissue and cause the medication to be absorbed faster than intended.

## Intra-articular injections

Intra-articular injections are made into the synovial space of a joint. They are typically given to relieve pain or inflammation and restore function to a joint or joints as in rheumatoid arthritis.

Steroid injections are used, e.g. triamcinolone, methylprednisolone (with or without lidocaine), hydrocortisone or dexamethasone. The size of the dose given depends on the size of the joint to be injected.

Injections should not be carried out if there is any suspicion of infection in the joint or in the surrounding tissue, i.e. if there are open sores or ulcers on the skin.

Once the needle is inserted, a small amount of synovial fluid should be withdrawn (aspirated) into a syringe to confirm correct positioning. A separate syringe is then used to give the medication. The joint is gently massaged and moved to aid mixing of the medication and the synovial fluid, and to reduce the risk of a permanent depigmented 'steroid scar' developing.

In practice, if multiple joints are to be injected, it is not normal to inject more than five joints on the same day.

Other types of material used intra-articularly are sodium hyaluronate and Hylan G-F 20. These are used for the sustained relief of pain in osteoarthritis of the knee, and Hylan G-F 20 is also used for temporary replacement and supplementation of synovial fluid.

## Intraosseous injection[5]

In children under the age of 6 years, and especially under 1 year, the intraosseous route of administration is used when venous access is difficult, e.g. in a hypovolaemic child.

A specially designed needle is placed into the tibia through which fluids and drugs may be administered into the bone marrow. Any drug or fluid that can be administered intravenously may be given in this way but it must be administered under pressure.

## Other routes of injection

### Intrathecal

Intrathecal injection is an injection into the spinal canal (the intrathecal space surrounding the spinal cord). The blood–brain barrier acts as a barrier to the brain and some drugs are unable to cross it. By administering these drugs intrathecally they are administered straight into the brain and so bypass the blood–brain barrier altogether. This route allows high concentrations of drugs – cancer chemotherapy agents, antibiotics etc. – to be administered directly to their site of action in the brain and spinal cord. Drugs given intrathecally have to be made up in a CIVAS unit because they cannot contain any preservative or other potentially harmful inactive ingredients that are sometimes found in standard injectable drug preparations.

### Epidural

An epidural is a form of regional anaesthesia involving injection of drugs through a catheter placed into the epidural space. The injection can cause both a loss of sensation and a loss of pain by blocking the transmission of signals through nerves in or near the spinal cord.

### Intracardiac

Intracardiac injection is administered directly into the heart muscles or ventricles. This route may sometimes be used in a cardiovascular emergency.

### Intradermal

Intradermal injection is injection into the skin itself. This route is used for skin testing, e.g. allergens, tuberculin PPD for Mantoux tests and for some vaccines, e.g. BCG vaccine.

### Intraperitoneal

The intraperitoneal involves an infusion or injection into the peritoneal cavity.

### Intravitreal

This is an injection delivered directly into the eye, usually into the vitreous cavity. 'Intravitreal' literally means 'inside an eye'.

## References

1. Trissel L, ed. *Handbook on Injectable Drugs*, 14th edn. Bethesda, MD: American Society of Health-System Pharmacists, 2007.
2. *Lippincott's Nursing Procedures*, 3rd edn. London: Lippincott, Williams & Wilkins, 2000.
3. Hayes C. Injection technique; intramuscular – 2 (practical procedures for nurses). *Nurs Times.* 1998; 94: 44.
4. National Institutes of Health (2002). *Patient Information Publications. Giving a subcutaneous injection.* http://nih.gov (accessed 12 March 2008).
5. Northern Neonatal Network, ed. *Neonatal Formulary*, 5th edn. London: Wiley-Blackwell, 2007.

# Appendix 6
# Extravasation

Extravasation is a complication of intravenous injection therapy. It manifests as tissue damage or irritation caused by inadvertent placement or leakage of a drug into the area around the injected vein.

Although most awareness of this problem relates to cytotoxic agents, it is important to note that it is a possibility for all drugs that can be given intravenously, e.g. antibiotics, drugs that are highly alkaline or acidic and glucose infusions.

Drugs can be classified as vesicant (literally meaning 'to cause blisters or blistering') which cause direct damage to the vasculature, or as non-vesicant, which are further classified as irritant or non-irritant. Vesicants can cause extensive necrosis. Irritants can cause pain at the injection site and along the vein, with or without inflammation.

The following general rules can help to minimise the risk of extravasation:

- Administration should be restricted to individuals familiar with the drugs and techniques used.
- The drug should be reconstituted appropriately to avoid administration of damaging concentrations.
- The drug should be given by via the injection port of free-flowing drip.
- The site of administration should be selected to take into account visibility, vessel size, amount of movement and potential damage if extravasation occurs. The optimum location is usually the forearm, which has superficial veins with sufficient soft tissue to protect tendons and nerves.
- The limb should be elevated with maintenance of gentle pressure after the needle is withdrawn.

## Suggested administration procedure

1. Insert a 23-gauge butterfly needle into the vein; a Teflon catheter may be preferred for longer-duration infusions.
2. Lightly tape the tubing in place; do not obscure the injection site by taping.
3. Connect a NaCl 0.9% infusion to the butterfly needle. Allow about 5 mL of the solution to run through, then withdraw a small amount of blood to test the vein integrity and flow. Observe for extravasation and if this is obvious select another site. Avoid a distal point on the same vein.
4. Repeatedly ask the patient if he/she feels any pain or burning, and visually check the site. For an infusion, check every 2–3 minutes that it is still running.
5. Following the drug injection, reconnect the NaCl 0.9% infusion and run through at least 5 mL of the solution to flush the drug from the entire tubing and needle.

If more than one drug is prescribed, inject the vesicant agent first; if all drugs are vesicant, inject the one with the smallest volume first.

Separate each drug administration by a 3–5 mL NaCl 0.9% flush. The rationale behind the administration of the vesicant first is that the integrity of venous access decreases with time and therefore if vesicants are administered first, all agents can be administered.

## Extravasation treatment

If extravasation occurs, treatment is critical and specific antidotes may be required for some drugs. The general recommendations in the management of extravasation are:

1. Stop the infusion/injection immediately.
2. Remove the infusion bag/syringe. Do not flush. Do not remove the needle. Mark the area with an indelible pen.
3. Attempt to aspirate as much of the drug as possible with a clean syringe.
4. Apply a cool compress, which should be maintained for 1 hour.
5. Check for specific antidotes if applicable.
6. Apply hydrocortisone 1% (cream is easier to apply than ointment) topically to the affected area.

In the UK all extravasation injuries should be recorded and details sent to the green card reporting scheme run by the National Extravasation Service (www.extravasation.org.uk/home.html).

## Bibliography

Allwood M et al. The Cytotoxics Handbook, 4th edn. Oxford: Radcliffe.

Hadaway L. I/V infiltration: not just a peripheral problem. Nursing. 2002; 32: 36–42.

National Extravasation Information Service (2007). http://www.extravasation.org.uk (accessed 12 March 2008).

# Appendix 7
# Intravascular devices

Central lines are long, hollow tubes made from silicone rubber, also referred to as skin-tunnelled central venous catheters. Examples of some of the branded devices that are used include Hickman and Groshong.

The central line is inserted (tunnelled) under the skin of the chest into a vein. The tip of the tube rests in the superior vena cava just above the heart (Fig. A7.1). They are frequently used in the administration of drugs and parenteral nutrition when the peripheral or oral routes are inappropriate. They are also used when the intravenous drug/infusion characteristics such as concentration, pH or osmolarity require their use.

All central venous catheters must be flushed before and after each drug administration and at least on a weekly basis with NaCl 0.9%. In some instances, a heparin solution, e.g. Hepsal is left in the device line (this is sometimes referred to as a 'lock technique'). The volume required depends on the line used. The tunnel insertion site on the skin surface of the chest should be covered with a dressing and changed twice a day.

A peripherally inserted central catheter (PICC) line is a long, thin, flexible tube that is inserted into one of the large veins of the arm near the bend of the elbow. It is then fed through the vein until the tip sits in a large vein just above the heart in a position similar to the central line (Fig. A7.2).

## Disadvantages

A number of problems can occur with both of these types of line, infection and clots being the most common.

Infections are treated empirically with systemic antibiotics and sometimes using an antibiotic lock technique whereby the antibiotic, usually teicoplanin (although gentamicin has been used) is injected into the catheter and left in place. This can be useful when trying to preserve the line. Alternatively, the line may be removed and replaced after resolution of any central infection.

Urokinase (licensed) or streptokinase (unlicensed) may be used to dissolve clots. See the relevant drug monographs for details.

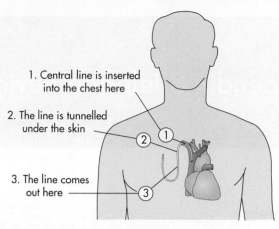

**Figure A7.1** Positioning of a central line.

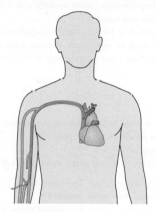

**Figure A7.2** Positioning of a PICC line.

## Bibliography

Anderson AJ et al. Thrombosis: the major Hickman catheter complication in patients with solid tumor. *Chest.* 1989; 95: 71–75.

Bard product information for Groshong and PICC lines. http://www.bardaccess.com/faq/q_a.html (accessed 10 March 2008).

Lokich JJ et al. Complications and management of implanted venous access catheters. *J Clin Oncol.* 1985; 3: 710–717 17.

Perry MC. *The Chemotherapy Source Book*, 4th ed. Philadelphia: Lippincott, Williams and Wilkins, 2007.

Raad II, Bodey GP. Infectious complications of indwelling vascular catheters. *Clin Infect Dis.* 1992; 15: 197–210.

Souhami RL et al. *Oxford Textbook of Oncology*, 2nd edn. Oxford: Oxford University Press, 2002.

Souhami RL, Tobias JS. *Cancer and Its Management*, 4th edn. Oxford: Blackwell Scientific, 2003.

# Appendix 8 Infusion devices

## General principles[1]

In the UK all pumps have been categorised as having either a high-, medium- or low-risk specification.

High-risk specification pumps infuse at higher accuracy rates, provide more consistent short- and long-term flow, incorporate comprehensive alarm features and deliver very low bolus doses on occlusion compared with medium- and low-risk pumps.

Practitioners should check with their Medical Devices department if they are unsure of the risk category of the pumps routinely used on their wards. It is the responsibility of the person administering the infusion to familiarise themselves with the type of infusion pump to be used and how to operate it safely.

## Using infusion pumps

An infusion pump must always be used in the following circumstances:
- To administer all infusions to patients under 16 years old.
- To administer parenteral nutrition.
- To administer certain other drugs (specified in the monographs of this book).

Before using an infusion pump always check the following:
- All previously used pump settings have been cancelled.
- The pump is clean – if not, ensure it is cleaned according to the manufacturer's instructions.
- The pump case and cable are intact – if not, return it to the Medical Devices department.
- If the pump displays a 'service due' message – return it to the Medical Devices department for an annual service.

An infusion pump should preferably be positioned at the same height as the infusion cannula insertion site. If positioned higher than 80 cm above the cannula insertion site the incidence of free flow and siphonage is increased, which may cause the pump to over-infuse.

Infusion pumps must be regularly checked throughout the administration of the infusion and the volume infused should be added to the patient's fluid balance chart.

All alterations to the settings of an infusion pump must be made by healthcare professionals who have been assessed as competent in using the device.

Infusion pumps must be cleaned by the practitioner disconnecting and removing the empty or unwanted infusion container after each patient.

All infusion pumps incorporate a backup battery. Infusion pumps should be kept plugged in to the mains when in use to ensure the backup battery is charged.

If an infusion pump is involved in an adverse incident the nurse in charge and the Medical Devices department must be informed immediately. The following actions must be taken:

- Close the roller clamp on the administration set.
- Assess the patient and summon assistance if needed.
- Disconnect the administration set from the patient but do not remove the administration set/ syringe from the pump.
- Record any alarms on the pump, contents of the infusion container and rate of administration of the infusion.
- Do not touch any of the keys on the pump except to switch it 'OFF'.
- Remove the pump from service and label it as defective.
- Complete an untoward incident form.

## Reference

1. Medicines and Healthcare products Regulatory Agency (2003). *Infusion systems and pumps. DB2003 (02) Infusion Systems.* http://mhra.gov.uk (accessed 8 June 2008).

# Appendix 9
# Syringe drivers

Syringe drivers are portable, battery-operated pumps delivering drugs at a predetermined rate by continuous subcutaneous infusion. The most common clinical use for the syringe driver is in palliative care when the oral route may not be available and other routes, e.g. rectal or sublingual, are not appropriate. Typical indications for their use are:[1]

- Dysphagia
- Unconsciousness
- Intractable nausea and vomiting
- Intestinal obstruction
- Malabsorption
- Intolerability of the oral route.

Common infusion sites used are the upper chest wall, the upper arm or thigh, the abdomen and occasionally the back. Excessively hairy areas should be shaved before use.

Sites to be avoided include oedematous areas (due to poor absorption), adjacency of bony prominences or joints, inflamed or infected sites, the upper abdomen if there is an enlarged liver, the upper chest wall if the patient is very cachexic, and previously irradiated skin (within the last 8 weeks).

There are two types of driver commonly in use. One delivers medication by the hour and the other delivers medication by the day (or 24-hour period).[2] Many hospitals have adopted the policy of using only one type of driver to avoid the confusion associated with two products which are calibrated differently. Practitioners should check with their Medical Devices department which type is used in their organisation.

Often several medicines are mixed together and administered via a syringe driver. Standard reference sources should be consulted to check for compatibility, e.g. *The Syringe Driver*[2] or the *Palliative Care Formulary*[3]. The *British National Formulary* also carries some limited information about compatibilities in the section 'Prescribing in palliative care'.

If it is not possible for a practitioner to verify whether a particular combination of drugs is compatible, options include:

- For a given indication, seeking alternate drugs for which compatibility has been validated
- Using a second driver at a different site
- Administering some drugs as subcutaneous injections, e.g. dexamethasone.

## Preparation of the syringe driver

1. Check that the driver is in full working order, and does not require a new battery.
2. Calculate the volume of drugs to be given (before dilution) and pick an appropriate size of syringe to hold the final volume.
3. Draw up the required drugs and diluent (usually WFI or NaCl 0.9%) into the syringe. Consideration should be given to the order in which the drugs are introduced into the

syringe because of possible incompatibilities during the preparation process.[2,3] This is particularly critical if dexamethasone is to be mixed with other drugs; in this case, as much diluent as possible should be added to the syringe before the addition of dexamethasone.[3]

4. If the giving line requires priming with fluid, draw up an extra 1 mL of diluent.

5. The syringe should be labelled with the patient's name, the time and date of preparation and the drugs and doses contained. The label should not totally obscure the fluid in the barrel as this requires subsequent measurement.

6. The infusion set can then be primed if necessary with the infusion fluid to expel all the air from the tubing. The length of fluid in the syringe is then measured against the scale on the driver. This length is dialled into the driver to set the rate of movement of the plunger over the next 24 hours.

7. If a new infusion set is being used it should be inserted into the site by grasping the skin firmly and pushing the butterfly needle into the subcutaneous tissue at a 45-degree angle. The skin is released and the butterfly is secured in position with a clear film dressing.

8. The start button can now be pressed, the transparent cover placed on the driver and the device placed in a safe, convenient place next to the patient. A fabric bag with a drawstring opening is often used to conceal the driver in a discreet fashion.

## Monitoring

The infusion site should be checked regularly, e.g. every 4 hours, and observed for viability, skin reactions or leakage. The driver should also be checked to ensure that it is functioning correctly and there is no sign of precipitation in the syringe.

Because of minor variations the accuracy of syringe driver infusion rates, the driver should be checked at least 1 hour before the anticipated finish of the infusion to check that a replacement is not required.

Drivers should be cleaned after each use with a disposable cloth dampened with a mild detergent. They should be calibrated annually.

### Troubleshooting

If the infusion has finished early this may indicate that:[1]
- The rate was incorrectly set.
- The scale length was measured incorrectly.
- The line was primed after the syringe was measured.

If the infusion finishes late this may indicate that:
- The rate was incorrectly set.
- The scale length was measured incorrectly.

If the infusion has stopped this may indicate that:
- The line is blocked.
- The battery is exhausted.
- There is precipitation.
- The infusion site has become inflamed.
- The syringe has not been correctly fitted to the driver.

## References

1. North Cumbria Palliative Care (2002). Protocol for the use of Graseby syringe drivers for subcutaneous use in palliative care. www.northcumbriahealth.nhs.uk/palliativecare/clinical/syringe/08.pdf (accessed 12 March 2008).

2. Dickman A et al. The Syringe Driver: Continuous Infusions in Palliative Care, 2nd edn. Oxford: Oxford University Press, 2005.

3. Twycross R et al. Palliative Care Formulary, 3rd edn. Oxford: Radcliffe Medical Press, 2007.

# Appendix 10
# Ideal bodyweight, dosing in patients with renal or hepatic impairment

## Ideal bodyweight (IBW)

For the dosing of some drugs and for calculation of creatinine, ideal bodyweight rather than actual bodyweight is used. This can be calculated as follows:[1]

For men :  IBW (kg) = 50 kg + 2.3 kg for each inch over 5 feet.
For women :  IBW (kg) = 49 kg + 1.7 kg for each inch over 5 feet.

If one wishes to obtain an approximately similar answer using only a metric measure of height, utilise the following equations:

For men :  IBW (kg) = 50 kg + 0.9 kg for each cm of height over 152 cm.
For women :  IBW (kg) = 49 kg + 0.7 kg for each cm of height over 152 cm.

## Dose adjustment in impaired renal function

If a drug is excreted from the body mainly by the kidneys then any reduction in renal function potentially means that the drug is not cleared at the same rate as would be expected in normal renal function. The drug might therefore accumulate in the body, potentially resulting in serious adverse effects. In order to prevent this, the dose should be adjusted or the drug avoided altogether if necessary. The monographs in this book give some guidance on this but specialist texts such as *The Renal Drug Handbook* should be consulted if necessary.[2] The degree of renal impairment is defined by the patient's creatinine clearance (CrCl), which is closely related to an individual's actual glomerular filtration rate (GFR). Some hospitals calculate an estimate of the glomerular filtration rate (eGFR) and it is acceptable in practice to use this figure as a substitute for creatinine clearance if available, except for patients at extremes of bodyweight or for drugs with a narrow therapeutic range.

In the absence of an eGFR value. the patient's creatinine clearance may be calculated using the Cockcroft and Gault equation.[3] For this the following patient-specific information is needed:

- Age
- Sex
- Serum creatinine level in micromol/L (should be relatively stable)
- Height – to calculate ideal bodyweight (IBW) if necessary.

$$\text{Creatinine clearance (mL/minute)} = \frac{F \times (140 - \text{age}) \times \text{weight (kg)}^*}{\text{Serum creatinine (micromol/L)}}$$

where $F = 1.23$ for a male; 1.04 for a female.

*If a patient is obese, use ideal bodyweight (IBW) because fatty tissue does not produce creatinine (for the purposes of the calculation, obesity is typically classified as actual bodyweight >120% of IBW).

## Dose adjustment in impaired liver function

Drugs metabolised or excreted by the liver may accumulate in the body if liver function is impaired. Doses should be adjusted or the drug avoided altogether if necessary. The monographs in this book give some guidance on this, but determining the degree of hepatic impairment is much more difficult than with renal function. Several methods exist but the most commonly used is the Child–Pugh classification,[4] which has been developed as a prognostic tool in chronic liver disease.

For the Child–Pugh classification, five clinical measures of liver disease are given scores of 1, 2 or 3 points in increasing severity as shown in Table A10.1. The scores for each parameter are added together and the degree of hepatic impairment is categorised as Child–Pugh class A to C as follows:

- 5–6 points Class A
- 7–9 points Class B
- 10–15 points Class C

**Table A10.1**  Scoring system for Child–Pugh classification of hepatic impairment

| Measure | Scores 1 point | Scores 2 points | Scores 3 points |
|---|---|---|---|
| Bilirubin - total (micromol/L or mg/dL) | <34[a] (<2) | 34-50[a] (2-3) | >50 (>3) |
| Serum albumin (g/L) | >35 | 28-35 | <28 |
| INR or prothrombin time (seconds) | <1.7 1 3 | 1 7-2.3 4-6 | >2.3 >6 |
| Ascites | None | Moderate or suppressed with medication | Refractory |
| Hepatic encephalopathy | None | Grade I-II (or suppressed with medication) | Grade III-IV (or refractory) |

[a] In primary sclerosing cholangitis and primary biliary cirrhosis, the bilirubin reference ranges are increased to <68 micromol/L (<4 mg/dL) for 1 point and 68-170 micromol/L for 2 points (4-10 mg/dL).

For the purposes of certain monographs this classification is all that may be needed. As a prognostic tool, however, the classification is used by clinicians to determine the survival chances of a patient.

## References

1. Halls.md (2003). *Health calculators and charts*. Edmonton, Alberta: Steven B. Halls Professional Corporation. www.halls.md/ideal-weight/devine.htm (accessed 18 August 2008).
2. Ashley C, Currie A, eds. *The Renal Drug Handbook*, 3rd edn. Oxford: Radcliffe Medical Press, 2009.
3. Cockcroft DW, Gault MH. Prediction of creatinine clearance from serum creatinine. *Nephron*. 1976; 16: 31–41.
4. Pugh RNH *et al*. Transection of the oesophagus for bleeding oesophageal varices. *Br J Surg*. 1973; 60: 649–549.

# Appendix 11
## Risk ratings

The risk ratings included in the *Injectable Drugs Guide* monographs are based on the NPSA tool for risk assessment of individual injectable medicine products prepared in clinical areas (see www.npsa.nhs. uk/health/alerts).

The risk scores are presented as a grid displaying pictorial icons for the individual risk category and the score is the summation of these categories. The eight risk categories are:

 **Therapeutic risk**: where there is a significant risk of patient harm if the injectable medicine is not used as intended. This risk is symbolised by skull and crossbones.

 **Use of a concentrate:** where further dilution after reconstitution is required before use, i.e. slow intravenous injection is not appropriate. This risk is symbolised by a bottle of a concentrated solution.

 **Complex calculation:** any calculation with more than one step required for preparation and/or administration, e.g. micrograms/kg/hour, dose unit conversion such as mg to mmol or % to mg. This risk is symbolised by a calculator.

 **Complex method:** where more than five non-touch manipulations are involved, or other steps including syringe-to-syringe transfer, preparation of a burette, the use of a filter. This risk is symbolised by a chain showing several links.

 **Reconstitution of powder in a vial:** where a dry powder has to be reconstituted with a liquid. This risk is symbolised by a liquid being injected into a vial of dry powder.

 **Use of a part vial or ampoule, or use of more than one vial or ampoule is required:** e.g. 5 mL is required from a 10-mL vial, or four 5-mL ampoules are required for a single dose. This risk is symbolised by showing more than one vial with the second vial only half used.

 **Use of a pump or syringe driver:** all pumps and syringe drivers require some element of calculation and therefore have potential for error; and the potential risk is considered less significant than the risks associated with **not** using a pump when indicated. This risk is symbolised by a syringe pump.

**Use of non-standard giving set/device required:** examples include light-protected products, low adsorption, use of an in-line filter or air inlet. This risk is symbolised by a square peg in a round hole to indicate something of a non-standard nature.

A **traffic light system** is used to denote broad risk banding together with a standard phrase to aid prioritisation for risk management in any given clinical area:

- **RED:** Six or more risk factors: high-risk product
  *Risk-reduction strategies are required to minimise these risks.*
- **AMBER:** Three to five risk factors: moderate-risk product
  *Risk-reduction strategies are recommended.*
- **GREEN:** Zero to two risk factors: lower-risk product
  *Risk-reduction strategies should be considered.*

NB: Although NPSA risk ratings only assess these eight categories, risk-reduction strategies could still be employed outside of these categories to further reduce risks in clinical areas; for example, staff training or standard operating procedures that could make even a zero rated product safer to use.

It is possible that the risk score may vary depending on the method of administration; for example, a direct intravenous injection may score lower than an infusion as there is no further dilution involved and therefore one less risk factor. In these scenarios the risk rating at the end of each monograph is always for the highest rated assessment unless otherwise stated.

It is vital that a local risk assessment accounts for method of administration in any given clinical area, so the risk score may be moderated to reflect local practice.

In all areas, appropriate competence is essential for healthcare professionals working with injectable medicines to give assurance of safety. Local policies and procedures must be adhered to but individuals should also include injectable therapy in their continuing professional development. The BMJ learning website provides such an opportunity with a free module on injectable medicines (accessible at http://learning.bmj.com/learning/search-result.html?moduleId=10009161) and this is strongly recommended.

# Index of cross-referenced terms